Clinical Neurology

A Modern Approach

Clinical Neurology
A Modern Approach

ANTHONY HOPKINS

Director, Research Unit,
Royal College of Physicians;
Consultant Neurologist,
St Bartholomew's Hospital
London

Oxford   New York   Tokyo
OXFORD UNIVERSITY PRESS
1993

Oxford University Press, Walton Street, Oxford OX2 6DP

Oxford New York Toronto
Delhi Bombay Calcutta Madras Karachi
Kuala Lumpur Singapore Hong Kong Tokyo
Nairobi Dar es Salaam Cape Town
Melbourne Auckland Madrid
and associated companies in
Berlin Ibadan

Oxford is a trade mark of Oxford University Press

Published in the United States
by Oxford University Press Inc., New York

A catalogue record for this book is available from the British Library

Library of Congress Cataloging in Publication Data
Hopkins, Anthony.
Clinical neurology : a modern approach / Anthony Hopkins.
Includes bibliographical references and index.
1. Neurology. I. Title.
*[DNLM: 1.Nervous System Diseases—diagnosis. 2. Nervous System
Diseases—therapy. WL 100 H793c]*
RC346.H66 1993 616.8—dc20 92-12789
ISBN 0–19–261474–6 (h/b)
ISBN 0-19-262262-5 (p/b)

Typeset by Cambridge Composing (UK) Ltd, Cambridge
Printed and bound in Great Britain by
Butler & Tanner Ltd, Frome and London

Preface

Every effort has been made to ensure that this single-author text on modern clinical neurology reflects the realities of clinical practice, and yet also reflects the great advances that have been made in our understanding of many neurological diseases in the past few years.

The aims and structure of this book are further outlined in Chapter 1, but in summary I have attempted to balance the insights gained from neurological and biological science with advice about the continuing support of those for whose disorders we can do little. Here I wish to acknowledge the help given to me over the years by Dr Jeffrey Gawler, Dr Charles Clarke, Dr Richard Greenwood and Dr Rodney Walker, my neurological colleagues at St Bartholomew's Hospital. I also thank Ms Joyce Bennett and Ms Barbara Durr, for their secretarial help with the manuscript. I am also grateful to the staff at Oxford University Press for their encouragement and careful attention to detail.

No attempt has been made to provide a reference for every statement made, as this interrupts easy reading, and I believe it unnecessary in a textbook. However, at the end of each chapter is a section with suggestions for further reading. Out of the enormous available neurological literature, preference has been given to recent review articles in generally available medical journals.

I am grateful to all those authors and publishers who have given me permission to reproduce figures and tables. Due acknowledgement is made where appropriate. I am particularly grateful to Dr Derek Kingsley, who has provided many of the magnetic resonance images (MRI) and computerized tomographic (CT) scans.

Although reference is made throughout the book to various aspects of the examination of the nervous system, technical aspects of clinical examination are better demonstrated on video. Readers can purchase two video recordings prepared by the author entitled 'Examination of the cranial nerves' and 'Examination of the motor and sensory systems'. Information about current prices and delivery can be obtained from:

Clinical Skills Unit
The Medical College of St Bartholomew's Hospital
Charterhouse Square
London EC1M 6BQ
Telephone: 071 982 6100
Fax: 071 983 6103

A.H.

London
September 1992

Dose schedules are being continually revised and new side effects recognized. Oxford University Press makes no representation, express or implied, that the drug dosages in this book are correct. For these reasons the reader is strongly urged to consult the drug company's printed instructions before administering any of the drugs recommended in this book.

Contents

Part I

An introduction to clinical neurology

1 Introduction

1.1 The aims of this book

Many medical students begin the neurological section of their training by fearing that this will be difficult, and many young physicians training in other branches of medicine are uneasy when confronted with a patient with neurological illness. Such anxieties appear to be based upon a misconception that an understanding of complex neuro-anatomy and neurophysiology is an essential prerequisite for the practice of clinical neurology. The first aim of this book is to demystify neurology and show that, as in other branches of medicine, a careful history and simple physical examination will allow an accurate diagnosis of the site of malfunction in most patients, without the need for vast stores of esoteric anatomical and physiological knowledge.

The separation of clinical neurology from the mainstream of general (internal) medicine is a historical and economic accident, brought about by the brilliant clinico-pathological correlations of neurological diseases described by the French school, led by Charcot, in the last quarter of the nineteenth century. At that time, neurology was the leading scientifically based medical speciality, a lead initially maintained in the UK by Wilson, Holmes, Head, Walshe, and Symonds, and in the USA by Adams, Denny-Brown, and Merritt. The intellectual prowess of these men seems to have made neurology something of a super-speciality, and for many years neurologists did not take an interest in the more common diseases such as stroke and dementia. The economic pressures of placing expensive radiological and clinical neurophysiological equipment on a limited number of sites led to the establishment of neurological and neurosurgical centres or special hospitals, thereby widening the separation of neurology from general medicine. In the great majority of hospitals in the UK, neurologists share the invidious distinction with dermatologists alone in not taking part in the acute-medical duty roster. Although many of the present generation of neurologists believe that such separation should continue, the second aim of this book is to show that clinical neurology is very much part of the mainstream of general medicine.

The third aim of this book is to bring into sharper focus the numeric and economic importance of certain neurological diseases. All textbooks of neurology must describe classical neurological illnesses such as syringomyelia and Wilson's disease. But readers must remember that in the whole of the USA (population 247 million) there will in one year be only about 600 new cases of syringomyelia, compared to 400 000 new patients with strokes, and a prevalence of 3.5 million people with varying degrees of dementia. This book attempts to give greater weight than most to the management of the more common neurological illnesses, without neglecting the major scientific advances that have increased our understanding of some of the less common neurological disorders.

A traditional jibe is that neurologists are only interested in diagnosis, and not in treatment, which is, in this view, largely ineffective anyway. No apologies are necessary for being interested in diagnosis. It is absolutely essential to 'get it right', or there is no proper basis for advice about prognosis and treatment. Accuracy of diagnosis is a need tempered only by what is kind and appropriate for any particular patient, and by the economic constraints of the medical system within which the neurologist is practising. However, that neurologists are not interested in treatment is—or should be—an unjustified slur. Specific pharmacological treatments are available for many neurological diseases, and there are drugs for the relief of less specific symptoms such as spasticity and pain.

However, neurologists know that one of their principal functions is to help their patients and their patients' families cope with situations that at first seem intolerable, and to come to terms with progressive disability. The fourth aim of this book, therefore, is to provide a core of useful practical knowledge about coping with physical or cognitive disabilities which any doctor can share with patients and their families.

A neurologist has to learn to advise about coping with symptoms such as headache and facial pain that are not accompanied by overt structural or biochemical neurological disease. Patients with such symptoms form the majority of those attending outpatient or office consultations, and yet the larger neurological textbooks are strangely silent about the management of such patients and the outcome of their symptoms. As a fifth aim, I hope to give some useful guidance here.

The sixth aim is to advise about the principles and appropriate use of technical neurological investigations. Older neurologists admit that the advent of computerized tomographic (CT) scanning, magnetic resonance imaging (MRI), and digital subtraction angiography have, to some extent, devalued their clinical skills so painstakingly acquired. Even those who do not acknowledge this willingly admit that imaging techniques now make many decisions simpler. A neurologist retains a prime role in deciding which symptoms warrant the expense of imaging techniques, in relating the symptoms and signs to any changes seen in the images, and, of course, in advising the correct future management, whatever the changes. He or she also soon learns that images may be normal in the face of obvious intracerebral disease, and abnormal images may be seen in the absence of relevant symptoms.

Finally, this book contains basic information about the principal neurological symptoms, syndromes, and diseases. In order to give a coherent structure to the whole, information about each disease is, wherever practical, presented in relation to the following:

(1) a brief definition;

(2) historical aspects;

(3) epidemiology
    (a) the incidence and prevalence;
    (b) causes and risk factors;

(4) pathophysiology;

(5) pathological findings;

(6) the patient's history;

(7) the findings on clinical examination;

(8) the differential diagnosis;

(9) the planning and results of appropriate investigations;

(10) pharmacological treatment and other management;

(11) the natural history and prognosis of the disease.

1.2   The structure of this book

This book is divided into four principal sections. Part I (Chapters 1–5) reviews the scope of neurological practice, the epidemiology of neurological diseases, neurological history-taking, and the principles of neurological diagnosis. There is no specific chapter on the techniques of neurological examination, but these are described, where appropriate, in Parts II and III. The author has prepared a series of video-recordings on which the techniques of examination are demonstrated.

Part II (Chapters 6–8) contains what I have termed 'the basic grammar of neurology'. An approach to common symptoms, such as dizziness or double vision, is described in Chapter 6. Chapter 7 describes the common neurological syndromes, such as an upper motor neuron lesion, found on examination, relating these to disordered integrative physiology. Chapter 8 describes the principal investigations currently employed in neurological practice, and indications for their use.

Part III (Chapters 9–25) describes the principal neurological disorders. Although headache is not usually considered to be a disease or disorder, as it is the most frequent presenting symptom in neurological practice the management of headache has been given a chapter in its own right.

Logical arrangement of diseases within the chapters of a medical textbook is notoriously difficult. For example, Charcot–Marie–Tooth disease could be included either in a chapter on genetic disorders, or in a chapter on peripheral neuropathy.

Vascular disease of the spinal cord could be included in the chapter on vascular disease or the chapter on spinal cord disease. I have made what I believe to be clinically relevant placements of such sections, and hope that careful cross-referencing and a good index will help the reader through any difficulty.

Part IV (Chapter 26) outlines an approach to coping with the physical disability that is associated with some chronic neurological illnesses.

2 The scope of neurology

What does a neurologist do? This is a question that many neurologists have faced at cocktail parties as, although most educated people have heard of neurologists, they have difficulty in knowing exactly what they do. The question is best answered from a historical perspective.

2.1   A brief history of neurology

Until the early part of the nineteenth century, sick people were cared for by surgeons, apothecaries, and physicians. Surgeons were the lineal descendants of barber surgeons but, until the advent of anaesthesia in 1843, surgery was largely confined to draining abscesses, amputations, and cutting for bladder stones. Apothecaries and physicians both practised supportive medicine, with different degrees of learning, and a gradually increasing pharmacopoeia. It was not until the middle part of the nineteenth century that the concept of diseases of different organ systems and the speciality of 'internal medicine' arose. In Europe, for example, Bright delineated many aspects of renal disease in 1827, Graves and Basedow aspects of thyroid disease in 1835 and 1840, and Laënnec hepatic cirrhosis in 1826.

Although an Englishman, Sir Charles Bell, wrote a substantial text, *The nervous system of the body*, in 1830, and Parkinson described the disease which bears his name in 1817, the origins of neurology are largely French. Romberg gave a good account of tabes dorsalis in 1840. In 1862 a physician named Charcot was appointed to the wards of the Salpêtrière, a large hospital in Paris, so called because it was a converted store for gunpowder (saltpetre). In the 1860s the Salpêtrière was an infirmary for those with chronic illness, including various forms of paralysis, and for dis-

eased prostitutes, many of whom, of course, had tertiary syphilis, including what we now know as neurosyphilis (see Section 17.4.1). By every contemporary account, Charcot was a superb clinician, and also an excellent morbid histologist. From the general mass of those with 'paralysis', he clearly defined a number of distinct entities. In the short years between 1865 and 1886 he described the clinical and histological features of what we now know as multiple sclerosis (see Chapter 14), motor neuron disease (see Chapter 20), and Charcot–Marie–Tooth neuropathy (see Section 19.3.8). He also made numerous original observations on many other neurological illnesses, particularly neurosyphilis, epilepsy, and the neuropathies and myopathies.

Charcot is generally acknowledged to have been responsible for initiating the speciality of neurology, although others in other countries also made important contributions, notably Weir Mitchell in the USA during the Civil War (upon the effects of peripheral nerve injuries) and Hughlings Jackson in the UK (upon epilepsy). A hospital devoted to the care of the 'Paralysed and Epileptic' was started in London in 1860. However, at the end of the nineteenth century and in the early part of the twentieth century few distinctions were made amongst the 'nervous' diseases that we would now regard as 'neurological' or 'psychiatric'. The very name for one syndrome of tertiary neurosyphilis—'general paresis of the insane'—is one indication of the difficulties then present.

Freud was a pupil of Charcot and was undoubtedly a skilled neurologist before his dissatisfaction with Charcot's teachings about hysteria—in particular, hysterical paralysis and hysterical seizures—led him to explore the effects of the unconscious mind upon human behaviour.

In Europe, and to a lesser extent in the USA,

this close link between neurology and psychiatry continued. Physicians styled themselves as 'neuro-psychiatrists'. Until the mid-1930s the principal journal in the USA for publication of neurological research was the *Journal of Nervous and Mental Disease*. Gradually, however, increasing experience in both neurological and psychiatric illness forced the realization that the training and practice in each speciality should follow different paths. None the less, an important part of consultant neurological practice continues to be the recognition of and appropriate management of 'minor' psychiatric illness, or distress presenting with physical symptoms that could be due to organic disease.

2.2   The role of a neurologist

A neurologist regards himself or herself as having special expertise in the management of the illnesses described in this book.

A neurologist must have special expertise in analysing symptoms, such as giddiness or pins and needles, for example, which might prove to be due to diseases within his or her sphere of interest, and in the clinical examination of patients with such neurological symptoms.

A neurologist must have expertise in planning the most cost-effective and comfortable investigations, if any, necessary to confirm or refute a diagnosis suggested by an analysis of the patient's history, and by his clinical examination (Chapter 5).

Some of a neurologist's patients will be acutely ill. Some will need urgent investigation in conjunction with a neurosurgeon. Many will be confused or in coma. A neurologist must have the necessary confidence and skills to cope with this branch of acute medicine.

A neurologist is often called upon by other specialist physicians to advise about neurological aspects of 'general' medical illnesses. Neurological complications of oncological disease, for example, are common, so a neurologist must have a broad knowledge of internal medicine.

Many of a neurologist's patients will not be acutely ill, presenting with symptoms, such as headache, which they fear have a basis in serious illness, but which turn out to be of no serious import. A neurologist must therefore have skills in reassuring patients, and in advising patients how to avoid or tolerate symptoms, such as giddiness, which may have a minor organic basis but for which pharmacological treatment is relatively ineffective.

Some patients with psychiatric illness present to a neurologist. Headaches, for example, are a common manifestation of a depressive illness (Section 9.3). Paralysis of a limb may occasionally be due to hysteria (Section 25.1.6). Severe depression in the elderly may mimic dementia (Section 11.3.2). Therefore a neurologist has to have a good knowledge of human behaviour and of psychological illness.

Some of a neurologist's patients will prove to have a serious and progressive illness, such as motor neuron disease (Section 20.1). Such an illness may present to the neurologist with symptoms that the patient himself had thought to be no more than a minor inconvenience, the solution to which should be found in a few weeks. Another skill a neurologist must possess, therefore, is the ability to help patients and their relatives come to terms with progressive illnesses which are unresponsive to pharmacological intervention.

A most important skill that a neurologist must possess is in the overall management of illnesses accompanied by increasing physical disability. An inability to help patients by pharmacological means must not mean that the neurologist may abandon the patient. Through liaison with members of other professions, such as social workers, physiotherapists, and occupational therapists, a neurologist should provide continuing support. He or she should advise competently about suitable accommodation for those with physical disability, about aids to mobility, aids to continuing work and to the fulfilment of normal domestic responsibilities, and about various systems for social support, including monetary allowances, that are available for disabled people in the community. These aspects are addressed in Chapter 26.

Further responsibilities of a neurologist are to advance the progress of his or her speciality by research, and by teaching others who may also advance his or her speciality by even better research or better clinical care. A neurologist also owes a responsibility to the vast majority of doctors in training who enter other types of medical practice. He or she should help them to recognize important neurological symptoms and illnesses, and to learn when they need the help of a neurologist.

2.3 Further reading

Aminoff, M. F. (1989). *Neurology and general medicine: the neurological aspects of medical disorders*. Churchill Livingstone, Edinburgh.

Hopkins, A. (1984). Different types of neurologist. *British Medical Journal* **288**, 1733–6.

Rose, F. C. and Bynum, W. I. (1981). *Historical aspects of the neurosciences*. Raven Press, New York.

3 Neurological epidemiology

3.1 Understanding the epidemiology of neurological disease

As in disorders of other tissues and organ systems, neurological diseases arise through an interaction of environmental factors and genetic predisposition.

A number of diseases are inherited through the actions of a single gene and, in the absence of the gene, the disease does not occur. Examples include the autosomal dominant transmission of Hunting-ton's disease (Section 13.6.2.4) and the sex-linked recessive transmission of Duchenne muscular dystrophy (Section 21.6.1.2). Sometimes in only a proportion of patients with a disease is clear-cut genetic transmission found. For example, about 10 per cent of cases of Alzheimer's disease (Section 11.5.1.4) are clearly familial, but the clinical features of this group are indistinguishable from sporadic cases.

In some diseases we postulate the interaction of environmental and genetic factors. For example, a patient who has had optic neuritis (Section 14.3.1) is far more likely to develop subsequent multiple sclerosis if he or she has both tissue haplotypes DR2 and DR3, and yet the familial incidence of the disease does not obey Mendelian laws.

In other diseases, polygenic transmission is responsible, at least in part. For example, the chances of stroke are related to the height of the blood pressure, which is believed to be polygeni-cally determined. However, other environmental risk factors, such as smoking, interact to vary the risk (see Fig. 10.4 on p. 138).

Isolated pockets of disease always raise the question of whether the disorder is localized through genetic transmission in a remote society without much outbreeding, or by some local dietary or other environmental factor. An example is the local very high incidence of motor neuron disease in some villages in Guam. The pendulum of neurological opinion has swung in recent years from a genetic to an environmental explanation of this cluster of cases (Section 20.1.3.2).

Other environmental factors are clear-cut. As examples, head injuries and brachial plexus injuries are commonly due to motor cycle accidents. Neuropathies occur in industrial workers exposed to certain solvents such as *n*-hexane, and in patients treated with some drugs such as vincristine. Meningitis is usually due to defined bacterial and viral causes.

Neurology shares with other clinical specialities a hard core of diseases in which the relative contribution of genetic and environmental factors is not known. We do not know what causes cerebral gliomas (Section 16.3.1). We do not know what causes Alzheimer's disease (Section 11.5.1.4), or Parkinson's disease (Section 13.1.4). However, increasing advances in biochemistry and immunology are at least elucidating the mechanisms of the diseases, even if the initiating steps remain unknown.

3.2 The burden of neurological symptoms and diseases in the community

As in disorders of other organ systems, systematic enquiry in the community reveals far more 'cases' of unrecognized neurological disease than ever emerge in outpatient clinics. For example, at one extreme, one study showed that 24 per cent of all respondents in an electoral roll survey had suffered a headache in the previous 14 days sufficient to require an analgesic, and yet other figures show that only about 2 in 100 of these will be referred in a year for a consultant opinion (see Fig. 9.1 on p. 114). Another study showed that for every patient with known Parkinson's disease in the community there were two more who had not sought medical advice. It is, of course, possible that in each of these examples neurological inter-

vention would make little difference to the outcome. However, every neurologist is only too well aware of late referrals of patients to whose management he could have made a useful contribution. Obvious examples include a progressive spastic paraplegia due to a spinal compressive lesion, or inadequately treated epilepsy or Parkinson's disease.

3.2.1 The incidence and prevalence of neurological diseases

The incidence and prevalence of neurological symptoms and diseases depends very much upon the methodology of case ascertainment, and upon the population studied. For some illnesses, such as acute bacterial meningitis, it is virtually certain that all patients will come under medical care in developed societies, and that the diagnosis will be

Table 3.1 Approximate annual incidence of some common neurological disorders per 100 000, per general practitioner, and per neurologist in England and Wales

Disease	per 100 000	per general practitioner	per neurologist
Herpes zoster	400	8	1100
Acute cerebrovascular disease	150	3	420
Epilepsy	50	1	140
Febrile convulsions	50	1	140
Dementia	50	1	140
Polyneuropathy	40	1	110
Transient ischaemic attacks	30	1	80
Bell's palsy	25	1	70
Parkinsonism	20	1 case every 2 years	55
Meningitis	15	1 case every 3 years	40
Subarachnoid haemorrhage	15	1 case every 3 years	40
Metastatic brain tumour	15	1 case every 3 years	40
Malignant primary brain tumour	5	1 case every 10 years	14
Trigeminal neuralgia	4	1 case every 12 years	11
Multiple sclerosis	3	1 case every 16 years	8
Motor neuron disease	2	1 case every 25 years	6
Infectious polyneuritis	2	1 case every 25 years	6
All muscular dystrophies	0.7	1 case every 70 years	2
Syringomyelia	0.4	1 case every 120 years	1
Huntington's disease	0.4	1 case every 120 years	1
Myasthenia gravis	0.2	1 case every 240 years	1 every 2 years
Wilson's disease	0.1	1 case every 480 years	1 every 4 years

Based upon Kurtzke (1984), 2068 registered patients per unrestricted general practitioner in England and Wales (*Annual Abstract of Statistics* 1988) and a census by the Association of British Neurologists (3.6 neurologists per million).

Table 3.2   Approximate prevalence of some neurological disorders

	per 100 000	per general practitioner in England and Wales	per neurologist in Engand and Wales
Epilepsy	650	13	1800
Cerebrovascular disease	600	12	1700
Dementia	250	5	700
Parkinson's disease	200	4	550
Multiple sclerosis	60	1–2	170
Syringomyelia	7	1 case per 7 doctors	20
Motor neuron disease	6	1 case per 8 doctors	16
Muscular dystrophy	6	1 case per 8 doctors	16
Primary brain tumour	5	1 case per 10 doctors	14

Sources as in Table 3.1

correct (even if only eventually). Theoretically, inspection of all hospital discharge records serving a confined community should provide an accurate indication of the incidence of this illness. However, all too often medical records are incomplete, incorrectly coded, or missing. None the less, a reasonable idea of the incidence of acute illness and prevalence of chronic illnesses sufficiently severe to require hospital care can be obtained by inspection of admission records, discharge records, autopsy records, and death certificates. The best available figures for the incidence and prevalence of some common neurological illnesses are shown in Tables 3.1 and 3.2. For those practising in the UK, these tables also show the number of patients with some common and uncommon neurological illness per family doctor (average list size 2068) and per neurologist (178 in England and Wales). Apart from providing a source for ready reference, another point of these tables is to stress the comparative rarity of some disorders, such as Huntington's disease, which are traditionally 'well known' because of their intrinsic biological interest.

3.2.2   *The neurological work of family doctors, neurologists, and specialist physicians*

Regardless of the burden of defined neurological disease in the community, perhaps the best guide to what family doctors and neurologists actually do, at least in the UK, is given in Fig. 3.1 and

Table 3.3. These data underline the need for both family doctors and neurologists to develop effective strategies in coping with rather ill-defined symptoms, such as headache and dizziness, as well as expertise in the management of more serious conditions. The vast majority of neurological symptoms are still coped with in general practice— for example, the Third National Morbidity Survey showed that only 3.5 per cent of patients with migraine and giddiness were referred to hospital for a further opinion, and only 20.4 per cent of those with cerebrovascular disease. These figures are not necessarily applicable to other European and other countries which do not have such a strong primary care system. In the USA, neurologists deal with many patients who in the UK would not be referred for a specialist opinion.

Information is available about the proportion of adults admitted to hospital with a primary neurological complaint. In a hospital in Northern Ireland serving a defined geographical area, patients with neurological symptoms and diseases accounted for 19 per cent of all admissions (mostly acute) over one year, and a further 2 per cent had an active neurological disorder which contributed to their admission. The special facilities of a neurological and neurosurgical centre were required for only 8 per cent of these neurological cases. That more than a fifth of all admissions had neurological features underlines the need for all physicians, whatever their speciality, to have an adequate understanding of neurological disease.

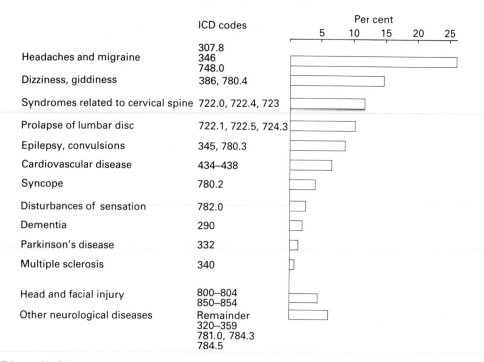

Fig. 3.1   Diagnosis of 411 consecutive new patients seen by 13 UK neurologists in one week (Hopkins 1989).

3.3   The organization of neurological practice

Neurologists are a relative luxury. They are found only in well-developed countries, as in Third World countries the burden of illnesses due to malnutrition and parasitic and bacterial infection consumes most of the available medical budget.

Although not every neurologist would admit it, neurosurgery has been the most important factor in determining the pattern of neurological practice.

Tumours of the nervous system have long been recognized, but their local effects upon different cerebral functions were first underlined by Broca in 1842, when he described a small tumour in the posterior part of the third frontal convolution, resulting in aphasia. Apart from the trepanation (making holes in the skull to let out evil spirits) practised in primitive societies, the first neurosurgical operation upon a cerebral tumour was not undertaken until 1878 by Horsley. Since then, access to a competent neurosurgeon has been a corner-stone of neurological practice.

There are at present in the UK approximately two neurosurgeons per million population. The epidemiology of disease in this population provides per neurosurgeon approximately 350 neurosurgical admissions and 200–250 neurosurgical operations per year. Although the ratio of neurosurgeons per million population is far higher in the USA (approximately 15 per million), it can reasonably be argued that, if the experience of major cranial surgery is less than about 200 operations a year, then specialist surgical skills are unlikely to be maintained or improved.

In order to allow an adequate duty roster, neurosurgeons have to practise in groups of at least three. Therefore the pattern, in the UK at least, has been the establishment of neurosurgical centres serving a population of 1–2 million. Apart from the duty roster needs of the surgeons involved, the establishment of such centres has also concentrated the very considerable capital costs associated with neurosurgical practice, nowadays principally the capital and revenue costs of imaging and theatres. A state-of-the-art CT scan-

Table 3.3 Patient consulting rates for various neurological syndromes and diseases of the nervous system—Morbidity Statistics from General Practice (1986)

Disorder	Diagnostic code (ICD9)	Patients consulting: rates per 1000 persons at risk	Referrals: per cent of patients consulting
Headache	784.0	13.2 ⎫	13.7
Tension headache†	307.8	4.1 ⎬ 25.5*	2.5
Migraine	346	8.2 ⎭	3.5
Dizziness, giddiness	780.4	10.0 ⎫ 14.9*	3.5
Vertiginous symptoms	386	4.9 ⎭	4.8
Syndromes related to the cervical spine	722.0, 722.4, 723	11.7	5.2
Prolapse or degeneration of lumbar disc, sciatica	722.1 pt, 722.5 pt, 724.3	10.1	11.7
Epilepsy	345	3.5	13.7
Convulsions	780.3	0.5	31.5
Faint, syncope	780.2	4.2	7.9
Cerebrovascular disease	430–434, 436–438 (not 437.2)	4.1 ⎫ 6.4*	20.4
Transient cerebral ischaemia	435	2.3 ⎭	11.1
Disturbance of sensation, paraesthesiae	782.0	2.6	11.1
Organic senile and pre-senile psychoses	290	2.1	16.7
Parkinson's disease	332	1.4	12.2
Multiple sclerosis	340	0.8	15.4
Involuntary movement	781.1	0.6	12.3
Disturbance of speech	748.3–784.5	0.8	27.9
Head injury without skull fracture	850–854	4.0	12.3
Fracture of skull and facial bones	800–804	0.7	25.8
Other diseases of the nervous system	Rem.320–359	4.8	18.1
(Facial palsy)		(0.3)	
(Primary cerebral tumour)		(0.1)	

Figures in brackets are derived from Second National Morbidity Survey when equivalent data are not available from the 1986 survey.
Figures marked with an asterisk indicate the sum of adjacent bracket figures for very similar conditions, about which it might reasonably be said that there was some doubt about the accuracy of coding.
† This code includes some cases of 'psychogenic backache and other pains of mental origin.'

ner (see Section 8.10.2) costs approximately £700 000 (1.25 million $US), and an MR scanner (see Section 8.10.3) approximately £1.4 million (2.5 million $US). Even before the advent of CT scanning in the early 1970s, X-ray machines capable of air encephalography, ventriculography, and angiography were exceedingly expensive.

The concentration of neurosurgical expertise and capital costs of imaging equipment has also concentrated into neurosurgical centres other associated specialities, such as neuroimaging, neuro-anaesthesia, neuropathology, radiotherapy, and,

Table 3.4   Neurologists per million population in England and Wales, and in the USA

	Number of neurologists	Population (million)	Neurologists per million population
England and Wales	178	49.8 (actual, 1987)	3.6
USA (1991)	7815 (adult) 1121 (child neurologists) (total 8936)	243.5 (projected, 1990)	36.6

Data from Kurtzke *et al.* (1991) and Association of British Neurologists.

not least, neurology. Neurologists also require close associations with these specialities, and also clinical neurophysiology and neuropsychology. The advantages of these associations were recognized in the UK during the first part of the twentieth century by the recruitment of specialists in these different fields to the National Hospital, Queen Square, the specialist neurological and neurosurgical hospital, and also by the experience of neurologists and neurosurgeons in different parts of the world during the Second World War.

3.3.1   *The numbers of neurologists*

The development of neurology and neurosurgery in the USA has been rather different, notably in the much greater numbers of neurologists per million population (Table 3.4). This reflects a number of different cultural factors, presumably not least the differences in income expectations and methods of payment of specialists on the two sides of the Atlantic. The broad perspective of British neurologists is that they cannot conceive that their American counterparts ever see any interesting clinical conditions, as the population each serves is so low. The broad perspective of American neurologists is that the small number of neurologists per million of the UK population means that the population is getting less than adequate care.

3.3.2   *The training of neurologists*

One approved training scheme (in the UK) suggests at least three years' general professional training in internal medicine, after graduation,

followed by training in neurology and related disciplines for a further four years. Experience should include exposure to neurosurgery, psychiatry, clinical neurophysiology, neuropathology, neuroradiology, neurophthalmology, clinical psychology, spinal injuries, and rehabilitation. Paediatric neurologists usually arise from the ranks of paediatricians, rather than neurologists, in training.

3.4   Further reading

Association of British Neurologists (1990). *Neurology services in the United Kingdom*. Association of British Neurologists, London.

Hopkins, A. (1984). Different types of neurologist. *British Medical Journal* **288**, 1733–6.

Hopkins, A. (1989). Lessons for neurologists from the United Kingdom Third National Morbidity Study. *Journal of Neurology, Neurosurgery and Psychiatry*, **52**, 430–73.

Hopkins, A., Menken, M., and De Friese, G. (1991). A record of patient encounters in neurological practice in the United Kingdom. *Journal of Neurology, Neurosurgery and Psychiatry*, **52**, 436–8.

Kurtzke, J. F. (1984). Neuroepidemiology. *Annals of Neurology* **16**, 265–77.

Kurtzke, J. F., Murphy F. M., and Smith, M. A. (1991) On the production of neurologists in the United States: an update. *Neurology* **41**, 1–9

Maurice Williams, R. (1987). Enough British neurosurgeons? *British Journal of Neurosurgery* **1**, 301–4.

Morrow, J. I. and Patterson, V. H. (1987). The neurological practice of a district general hospital. *Journal of Neurology, Neurosurgery and Psychiatry* **50**, 1397–401.

Royal College of General Practitioners, Office of Population Censuses and Surveys (1986). *Morbidity statistics from general practice 1981–1982*. HMSO, London.

4 The neurological history

Introductory texts of medicine give a broad overview of how to take a concise informative clinical history. This chapter records some aspects that are of particular relevance to neurology. Chapter 5 deals with the history of certain common neurological symptoms, and Chapters 9–25 deal with histories associated with specific diseases. There are, however, some general points that should be made in this introductory chapter.

4.1 The initial stages of the consultation

I begin by making an observation that is not strictly related to the history but arises even before the patient begins to recount his symptoms. General observation of the behaviour, dress, and movements of the patient as he or she first comes into the room may be extremely informative, and the physician would be most unwise to neglect the first few seconds of the encounter. These seconds may well focus his or her questions and subsequent examination. Patients do move differently when they are undressed and being formally examined from when they are dressed and acting 'socially', as in the early stages of a consultation. The first sight of a patient's bodily movements in the waiting room may be sufficient to raise the question of early Parkinson's disease (Section 13.1.6.2), for example, or the untidy dress of a patient whom

one knows to be a bank manager may raise the question of the social deterioration that is one of the features of dementia (Section 11.5.1.1).

4.2 The way in which patients describe their symptoms

Neurological symptoms are, with a few exceptions, outside normal experience. We have all felt one type of paraesthesia when we have hit our 'funny-bone'—the ulnar nerve behind the medial epicondyle of the humerus. We have, as children, mostly experienced rotational vertigo, induced by turning around rapidly on the spot and then stopping. However, neurological disease produces other types of sensory and vertiginous disturbances, strange feelings of heaviness or clumsiness of the limbs, and disorders of cognitive perception. Patients can only use the language of normal life to describe abnormal events for which there are no generally recognized words.

Patients often believe that a careful description of their tinnitus, vertigo, or disordered sensory perceptions, for example, will help us to analyse their illnesses. With rare exceptions, this is not so. It is sufficient to know that there is tinnitus, vertigo, or paraesthesiae, the events that precipitate these symptoms, and, in the case of paraesthesiae, their site. We cannot experience patients' perceptions, and the adjectives they use to describe them are often not helpful. None the less, what patients describe is important to them, and they will not have confidence in our judgement unless we pay close attention to what they say.

Unfortunately, patients may be not so precise as I have just indicated. Neurological disease often produces what can only be described as 'strange feelings in the head'. Vascular insufficiency, impaired cognitive function, even partial seizures (Section 12.4.1) may all be described in such uninformative terms as 'muzziness' or 'light-head-edness'. One physician colleague with polycyth-aemia told me that he always knew when he should have a further venesection as his head felt 'full', and his haematocrit showed that he was correct. It is, of course, necessary to question the patient closely in order to try to decide exactly what it is that he or she is describing, but there is a danger here—that of the effects of leading questions. It is all too easy, for example, to mislead a patient who has said no more than that he has 'muzzy spells' into what then appears to be a clear history of partial seizures arising from one temporal lobe, with feelings of unreality and *déjà vu* (Section 12.4.1).

Notwithstanding my strictures about the worth of patients' adjectival preferences when describing their symptoms, experience informs us that there are certain ways of recounting a story that are highly informative. In the English language, if a patient says a limb feels 'heavy', or a foot 'drags', it is very likely that he has a lesion affecting pyramidal pathways (Section 6.2.3). If one hand is said to be 'clumsy' there is very probably an organic lesion, although the disorder may be affecting pyramidal, cerebellar, extrapyramidal, or sensory pathways. Bizarre descriptions of abnormal sensory perceptions are often based upon organic disease. A disorder of afferent pathways in the posterior columns of the spinal cord may cause the patient to complain that his limbs feel 'swollen', or his hands 'encased in boxing gloves'. A patient with a spinothalamic tract lesion told me that it felt as though he had 'a cold, rough fish' inside his trouser leg. Periodic headaches that are described as of a 'bursting' quality always merit attention. Conversely, a description of 'continuous headaches, like an iron band around the head' or 'pins and needles all over the body' do immediately raise the question that the illness is not organically determined.

Some neurological symptoms are so diffuse that the patient writes them down on a piece of paper. It has for many years been suggested that this suggests a functional disorder (Section 25.1.6), but a follow-up study of such subjects has shown that this is not so, and organic disease is just as probable in those who make notes as in other subjects.

4.3   The effect of a disordered brain on the history; the frequent need for a relative's account

A patient suffering from cardiac disease is able to give an account of his or her symptoms which is in accord with his or her linguistic and educational abilities. Neurologists often have to deal with unconscious patients who can give no history at all. Apart from this extreme example, it must be remembered that, in the case of a patient with cerebral disease, the instrument that he or she will use to describe the symptoms may itself be disordered. One obvious example is aphasia (Section 6.1.1.1), in which language itself is impaired, compounding the patient's difficulties in describing what in itself is quite outside normal experience. On other occasions, confusion (Section 7.4), amnesia, or dementia (Chapter 11) will interfere with the patient's ability to give a history. In practice, inconsistencies and hesitations in the story usually make it readily apparent that further information must be sought from relatives, friends, or workmates.

A witness's account is also necessary in cases of transient disturbances of consciousness—'funny turns', 'fits', or 'blackouts'. Clearly, if consciousness has been disturbed, the patient can give no account of what went on during the blackout. A patient who has had a tonic–clonic (grand mal) seizure (Section 12.4), for example, cannot give a description of his stertorous breathing, cyanosis, convulsive limb movements, and post-ictal confusion, all of which will make the diagnosis clear. A relative's description of pallor during a 'turn', even if accompanied by some twitching, may make it clear that the causes of anoxic seizures (Section 12.7.1) should be considered.

4.3.1   *The possible importance of long past events*

Most physicians agree that it is best to begin one's questions by analysing the principal presenting complaint, and that a patient may well be irritated if a ponderous family and occupational history is taken before they are allowed to speak about why they have come. None the less, at some stage in the history it is important to ascertain what may be in the distant past. A previous history of blurring of the vision of one eye lasting a few days, for example, may immediately illuminate the nature of present symptoms of tingling and clumsiness in one limb, making a diagnosis of multiple sclerosis (Chapter 14) a real possibility.

In the case of some patients, and of all children with neurological symptoms, it is necessary to obtain a birth and developmental history, as failure to achieve milestones within the normal time limits often indicates neurological damage sustained in the perinatal period or early life.

A previous history of a seizure in childhood, or of a meningitic illness, or of a cranial injury may all suggest the aetiology of epilepsy in adult life.

Of course, a previous relevant medical history may not necessarily be a neurological one. Information about cardiac disease (for example, a past valvotomy or mitral stenosis) may be of great importance in understanding current symptoms.

It is essential to ascertain all drugs currently being taken by the patient. Many drugs cause confusional states in older people—notorious examples are benzhexol and orphenadrine used in the management of Parkinson's disease. Some drugs that were taken by the patient long ago may be responsible for current symptoms; for example, current involuntary movements may be due to past treatment with phenothiazines.

4.4   Timing of symptoms

4.4.1   *The onset of symptoms*

Most patients with symptoms of insidious onset are understandably vague about the date on which they first noted a problem. Other patients note the problem, and then assume that it began that day, even though there is evidence, such as wasting, that the problem is of much longer duration than

reported. Apart from ascertaining whether a problem was of abrupt or insidious onset, and the duration and chronology of different symptoms, the most important question is whether a symptom is improving, is static, or is worsening, as the answers will all influence decisions about investigation and management. For example, a hemiparesis of abrupt onset, with subsequent improvement, is likely to have a vascular origin. A steadily deteriorating hemiparesis of insidious onset is more likely to be due to a tumour.

4.4.2   *Episodic events*

The timing of episodic events in relation to other activities is important. For example, vertigo may only occur when the patient turns over in bed. Blackouts that occur only on assuming the erect posture are likely to be syncopal in nature. Seizures that always occur in front of the television set are likely to be of primary generalized type.

4.5   The family history

A number of neurological disorders are clearly mediated through genetic defects. Well-known examples include Duchenne muscular dystrophy (Section 21.6.1.2), Huntington's disease (Section 13.6.2.1), the spinocerebellar ataxias (Section 20.3), and some peripheral neuropathies (Section 19.3.8). Some disorders are recessively inherited through genes carried on autosomal or X-chromosomes, some are dominantly inherited. It follows that it may well be necessary to construct the fullest possible family pedigree when a disorder such as these is suspected. A firm diagnosis of, for example, Huntington's disease in an earlier generation will greatly influence thoughts about the present patient. It is often useful to question and examine members of the family other than the patient.

Less clearly defined, but none the less real, is the increased risk of the same disease in families of patients with hypertension and cerebrovascular disease (Section 10.1.4), epilepsy (Section 12.6.1), and multiple sclerosis (Section 14.1.3). Increased propensities to these diseases may be transmitted polygenically, or through the genes responsible for the tissue haplotypes which influence immunity. Although a family history of these disorders is not in itself diagnostic, it may well raise appropriate suspicions, and influence plans for investigation. For example, at the very least, a physician's knowledge that his patient's sister has multiple sclerosis will influence how he talks about his suspicions that his patient may have the same illness, and about the prognosis and management.

The family history is occasionally relevant in infective disorders of the nervous system. A child with chickenpox may precipitate herpes zoster in his grandparent. A clue to the cause of a meningitic illness may be given by the knowledge of a tuberculous relative in the household.

There is also an increased familial incidence of some cerebral tumours, but the excess risk is not great, except in the case of some Mendelian disorders such as neurofibromatosis 1 and 2 (Section 16.8.1).

4.6   The social history

The physician must always obtain a concise social history.

The patient's occupation may be of importance in the genesis of his or her neurological symptoms. For example, a bar-tender might have a peripheral neuropathy due to chronic alcoholism; a strawberry-picker might develop a common peroneal palsy due to the posture he or she needs to maintain for many hours each day. Neuropathies and encephalopathies due to environmental toxins are occasionally seen. Apart from this, a knowledge of the patient's occupation may well influ-

ence advice given. A youngster with chronic spinal muscular atrophy will need to be counselled about a suitable career. A bus-driver who has had a seizure will not be able to continue that occupation.

For those with chronic disabling neurological illnesses, the physician must know about his patient's housing. Are there stairs, and can the patient manage them? Can he or she cook a meal, or does the kitchen need to be modified? The physician must also enquire about the family background. Are there potential carers if his patient's condition deteriorates? What financial resources may be available?

4.7   Conclusion

It is, of course, often not necessary to obtain all information described in this chapter at the initial consultation, but by the end of his or her history-taking the physician should have a good grasp of the symptoms that the patient has experienced, of the disabilities that these symptoms have caused the patient, of relevant aspects of the patient's past personal and medical history, of the family history, and of the patient's station in life. As will be explained in the next chapter, the physician should also by this stage have developed a hypothesis about the likely anatomical site of the lesion causing the symptoms, so that he or she can focus the physical examination on aspects that will confirm or refute this hypothesis.

5 The principles of neurological diagnosis

This short chapter will, I hope, dispel some of the anxieties that seem to confront many medical students and young physicians when first confronted with patients with neurological disease. The details of neuroanatomy and neurophysiology seem to be vaguely remembered as being more detailed and more troublesome than those related to other clinical specialities. These recollections are a foundation for future unease in the setting of clinical neurology. Anatomists and physiologists do, of course, have to provide a basis for all human biology; they also, quite rightly, provide sufficient information and intellectual stimulus to attract students into a wide variety of careers, including research. However, complex details of the anatomy of the brain stem, for example, or of ion fluxes during synaptic transmission, are of little help when confronted with a patient with a weak hand or leg.

I certainly applaud excellence in cellular, mathematical, or biophysical research, and workers in these fields have made enormous advances in our understanding of the mechanisms of disease. One example is myasthenia gravis (Section 21.12.2), a disease in which much of the pathophysiology is now reasonably well understood, following contributions from physiologists, biophysicists, immunologists, and electron microscopists. The message for those engaged in clinical neurological diagnosis, however, is to 'keep it simple'. From experience in questioning senior medical students and those preparing for higher qualifications in medicine, I am often struck by the tortuous anatomical explanations they invoke to explain the clinical signs that they have, usually correctly, elicited. Table 5.1 summarizes a scheme to encourage clear thinking.

First, *listen to the history*. Points that should be elicited are covered in the previous chapter. All that needs to be remarked here is that, by the time you have finished the history, you should have *a clear hypothesis as to the probable anatomical site of the lesion responsible for the symptoms just recounted*. A 'full' clinical examination of every neurological patient is impossible through pressure of time. For example, it would be impractical to test carefully the sense of smell in every patient presenting with weakness and wasting of one hand. However, it would clearly be relevant to test smell in a patient who had noted progressive monocular failure of vision, as an olfactory groove meningioma could be compressing the optic nerve. Unless you approach the examination of your patient with some clearly defined hypothesis, or hypotheses, as to the site of the lesion, your examination will be diffuse, rushed, and unfocused.

The purpose of your clinical examination, therefore, will be to confirm or refute your initial hypothesis. For example, the history may have been of increased difficulty in walking due to stiffness and dragging of the right leg. You may, reasonably enough, have hypothesized a lesion affecting pyramidal pathways in the left hemisphere, and your examination does indeed confirm pyramidal signs (Section 6.2.3) in the right leg. However, in the course of your examination you note that there are no pyramidal signs in the right upper limb, which casts doubt upon your hypothesis, as it would be somewhat unusual for the leg alone to be affected in a hemisphere lesion. The observation of a *left* extensor plantar response (see Section 6.2.3.6) means that your original hypothesis is not correct, as there is clear evidence now of a disturbance of pyramidal pathways bilaterally, even if the patient had only noted problems with the right leg. The hypothesis has to be recast. A possible anatomical site causing pyramidal signs in *both* lower limbs, but leaving the upper limbs unaffected, would be the dorsal spinal cord (see Section 6.9). Again, supporting evidence for this new hypothesis should be sought by attention to relevant points in the examination. In this example, the finding of a sensory 'level'—a spinal segmental level below (caudal to) which sensation is impaired—would be convincing evidence of the rectitude of this recast hypothesis.

So far, then, we have listened to the clinical

story, hypothesized about the likely anatomical site of the lesion, and examined our patient with a view to confirming or refuting our hypothesis(es). One temptation to be resisted is to account for a multiplicity of signs by lesions at a multiplicity of anatomical sites. Multiple lesions certainly occur—in multiple sclerosis (Section 14.3), for example, or in diffuse vascular disease (Section 10.1.11.3 and 4), or with multiple secondary malignant deposits—but it is a necessary intellectual discipline to *think first how combinations of physical signs can be accounted for by a lesion at* one *site*, so that incorrect diagnoses are avoided and appropriate investigation and management can be planned.

Having tied down the patient's clinical story and abnormal neurological signs to a lesion at one site, the examiner should think as follows: '*From my knowledge of the natural history of diseases, and of pathology, what is the pathological nature of the lesion that is most probable at this particular anatomical site, with this particular history?*' For example, the physician may correctly localize a lesion to the left hemisphere, resulting in a right hemiparesis. The hemiparesis could be caused by a vascular lesion, or by a tumour. Vascular lesions, such as infarcts, are many times more frequent than tumours. However, a vascular lesion is characterized by an abrupt onset, but a slowly progressive hemiparesis will strongly suggest that the responsible lesion is a tumour.

Having made a provisional pathological diagnosis of a lesion occurring at a particular anatomical site, the physician may decide that further investigation is inappropriate. For example, few neurologists would feel it necessary to investigate an abrupt hemiparesis occurring in an elderly person with known diffuse vascular disease, with a previous history of hypertension and myocardial infarction. Very often, however, it is necessary to *consolidate a provisional pathological diagnosis by an appropriate plan of investigation*. This might include some imaging procedure, such as CT scanning or MRI, or more general investigations such as a chest X-ray, or various blood tests, as it must never be forgotten that neurological symptoms may be a manifestation of a systemic illness.

As in other branches of medicine, it is only necessary to investigate to confirm a diagnosis beyond reasonable doubt, or to establish modifiable risk factors that may influence prognosis, such as an elevated serum cholesterol in the case of vascular disease.

The final steps in our master plan are also identical to other branches of medicine—*to inform the patient of our conclusions* and *to give our advice about future management and prognosis*. An example of how one might inform the patient is given in Section 14.12 in relation to multiple sclerosis.

Table 5.1 A plan for neurological diagnosis

1. Listen to the history.
2. Form a hypothesis of the probable anatomical site of the lesion in the nervous system that could give rise to the symptoms described by the patient.
3. Examine the patient with this hypothesis in mind. The hypothesis will be supported, or perhaps refuted by the presence of inappropriate signs. A different anatomical hypothesis may be necessary.
4. Having established the anatomical site of the lesion, consider what is the most likely pathological process to occur at that particular anatomical site with that particular history.
5. Consider whether investigation is necessary to support the pathological diagnosis.
6. Plan management.
7. Inform the patient of your views and your plan.

If the steps outlined above, and summarized in Table 5.1, are followed, a student or young physician will approach a patient's problem in exactly the same way as the most experienced neurologist. A coherent plan of this sort will give confident competence, which will grow further on a secure base of understanding.

Part II

The basic grammar of neurology

6 Common neurological syndromes

Virtually any disorder of the special senses, communication, cognitive function, memory, mobility, or autonomic control can occur in neurological practice, and pain also is a feature of some neurological states. However, some symptoms are so common that they warrant discussion in their own right. Foremost amongst them is headache, the most common neurological symptom in family and specialist practice (see Table 3.3), and sufficiently important to be given its own chapter (Chapter 9). Another exceedingly common presenting symptom is what in English parlance is commonly known as 'a funny turn', analysis of which may suggest a fit, a faint, a transient ischaemic attack, or other event listed in Table 12.5.

In this chapter, I consider some other common

neurological symptoms and constellations of signs that crop up so often in neurological practice that it is justifiable to think in terms of a basic grammar of neurology. Familiarity with these basic syndromes will, I believe, eliminate most of the nervousness with which many young physicians approach a patient suffering from a neurological disorder. This approach is commonplace in other specialities. Throughout his clinical practice, a doctor will encounter groups of physical signs that frequently occur together, as they have a common basis in some physiological abnormality. In cardiology, for example, the syndrome of right ventricular failure is manifest by engorgement of the neck veins and gravitational oedema. On clinical examination the initial 'diagnosis' of right-sided heart failure is usually made mentally before proceeding to ascertain what the anatomical and pathological cause of that failure may be. Many students seem happy to accept this concept in cardiology and in respiratory medicine, but for some reason feel that neurology requires an entirely different and arcane approach. I hope that this chapter will dispel some of these misconceptions.

6.1 Disorders of higher cognitive function and behaviour

Abstract thought, language, reasoning, calculation, recognition of objects in space, and social behaviour are all functions of the cerebral cortex. The cortical mantle is vastly developed in humans in comparison with lower primates. Different areas of cortex have developed different functional specializations. Phrenologists recognized this, but were misguided in believing, first, that the extent of cortical development varied markedly between individuals and, secondly, that such variations could be detected in alterations of the shape of the skull. They also discounted the influence of social pressures in determining the response of humans to their environment.

A global impairment of cortical function is manifest as a dementia, which is fully reviewed in Chapter 11. This section is concerned with localized cortical lesions and the effects they produce. An outline of the principal syndromes is shown in Table 6.1, and these are now further elaborated.

Table 6.1 Cortical lesions and the syndromes they produce

Dominant hemisphere
  fronto-temporal
    Broca's aphasia
  temporo-parietal
    Wernicke's aphasia
  parietal
    Gerstmann's syndrome
  temporo-parieto-occipital
    acquired dyslexia
    dysgraphia
    auditory agnosia, word deafness
Non-dominant hemisphere
  parietal
    constructional apraxia
    spatial disorientation
    contralateral neglect
Bilateral frontal lesions
  social disinhibition
  impaired drive
  utilization behaviour
Bilateral temporal lesions
  amnesic syndrome
Bilateral occipital lesions
  occipital blindness
Diffuse cortical lesions
  dementia

6.1.1 Disorders of language

It is important to distinguish between language and speech. Language is written marks or sounds by which an understood symbolic meaning is communicated within a cultural group. The human voice is capable of only a limited number of phonemes (the name given to the shortest unit of sound, e.g. 'poo'). It is the culturally determined combination of phonemes that gives language its meaning. Hence a phoneme 'poo' will have a different cultural meaning in Chinese and English. The written symbols also have a different form. A disturbance of oral language is known as aphasia or dysphasia. A disturbance of written language is known as dysgraphia, and a disturbance of the ability to read written language is called an acquired dyslexia.

Speech, or articulation, is taken to refer to the

motor actions involved in the oral production of sounds that carry the symbolic meaning of language. Disorders of articulation are referred to as dysarthria (see Section 6.5.2).

The passage of expired air across the vibrating vocal cords is a necessary part of the production of meaningful sounds. A disturbance of this function is referred to as dysphonia (see Section 6.5.1).

6.1.1.1   *Aphasia*

Aphasia is now used more or less synonymously with dysphasia, although strictly speaking aphasia may be taken to imply a more complete loss of oral language.

Language is organized almost entirely in the dominant cerebral hemisphere; in those of European stock, the left hemisphere is dominant in about 95 per cent of subjects. Even in those whose left hand is preferred for skilled use (about 12–15 per cent of subjects), language is usually found to lie in the left hemisphere. The localization of language is confirmed, as may be necessary prior to temporal lobe surgery for epilepsy (Section 12.9.1), by the intracarotid injection of a small dose of amylobarbitone. If a carefully calculated dose of this drug is injected into the internal carotid artery supplying the hemisphere in which language is located, there will be a temporary arrest of language without impairment of consciousness. This is known as the Wada test.

Observations of aphasic patients illuminate but do not explain how language is organized in the dominant hemisphere. Phonemic confusions are common ('poor' for 'door', and 'flutter' for 'butter', for example), but the presence of confusions for semantically related words (table for chair) leaves it unclear as to whether language is organized on a phonemic or semantic basis. Furthermore, the ability to retrieve a word is determined by the run of pre-existing words—the contextual basis. Grammatical constructions may also be impaired in aphasia, indicating that linguistic rules can also be damaged by disease.

In 1861 Broca described a disturbance of language due to a tumour at the posterior end of the third frontal convolution. A lesion in this area produces an aphasia in which word production is so sparse that the term 'expressive aphasia' has often been used. Wernicke, in 1873, described a lesion of the angular gyrus which resulted in an aphasia in which comprehension was predominantly impaired—a 'receptive aphasia'. A closer analysis of the content of aphasic language, correlated with the responsible anatomical lesion identified with the newer imaging techniques, has led to a better understanding and newer classification.

First, it must be understood that the area of the brain in which language is organized extends over much of the posterior frontal, temporal, and lower parietal regions of the dominant hemisphere. A lesion anywhere in this area will give rise to some difficulty in word-finding (naming objects), so-called *nominal dysphasia*. The presence of nominal dysphasia is thus a useful screening test for a dominant hemisphere lesion. The ease with which a word is retrieved in pathological states has been shown to be related to its frequency of use in everyday life. This explains why 'yes', 'no', 'hallo', and 'goodbye' are often retained in severely affected patients. It follows that when testing patients with minimal nominal dysphasia, slightly unusual objects should be used, for example a screw, an eraser, or a magnetic compass. It is characteristic of nominal dysphasia that a patient will use a circumlocution—for a magnetic compass, 'the thing you find your way around with'.

Leaving aside nominal dysphasia, which is of no localizing value except to the dominant hemisphere, certain characteristic language disorders have been correlated with lesions of different parts of the dominant hemisphere. The following classification is based largely on the work of Geschwind and Benson, working at Boston.

Non-fluent aphasia (anterior aphasia, Broca's aphasia)

The lesion in this case is in the posterior part of the left third (inferior) frontal convolution, inferior motor cortex, and adjacent insula. Spontaneous language production is slow, with very few words per minute, and much effort is expended on initiation. Those words that are retrieved are often substantives (nouns), and therefore communication is often rich in meaning, even though few words are used, and these are often repeated (perseveration). Few or no conjunctions are used, and verb tenses are often incorrect. The normal prosody (rhythm) of speech is lost, and the low output is without much variation in pitch, literally monotonous. Comprehension of the language of others is good, but multiple commands may reveal some weakness. The proximity of Broca's area to the lower part of the pre-Rolandic motor strip means that an anterior aphasia is often associated with a contralateral facial palsy and a pyramidal deficit of the right hand (Section 6.2.3.4). There may also be a dissociation between the *idea* of non-verbal facial movements (e.g. mimicking kissing, or blowing a whistle) and their production—that is to say, associated with an anterior aphasia there may be an *apraxia of facial movements*. An apraxia is the inability to perform a movement or a task, the nature of which is understood, in the absence of paralysis (Section 6.1.2.2). This apraxia may also extend to the facial movements necessary for speech production, resulting in a defect in articulation, sometimes called a *cortical dysarthria* (although dysarthria otherwise invariably involves lower phylogenetic levels of the nervous system, (Section 6.5.2).

Patients with non-fluent aphasia are distressed, as considerable insight into the difficulty remains.

Fluent aphasia (posterior aphasia, Wernicke's aphasia)

In this type of aphasia, due to a lesion involving the posterior superior temporal gyrus, speech is fluent, but contains few substantives. Prosody and variations in pitch are normal, and grammatical constructions appear superficially to be normal. However, semantic and phonemic confusions are common, and these may be so prominent that muddled phonemes are strung together to make unknown meaningless words (neologisms). Comprehension is impaired. A similar defect is *auditory agnosia*, a loss of recognition of non-verbal sounds, for example the meaning of church bells. Writing and reading are also often impaired, but sometimes these functions remain intact, when one speaks of a pure word deafness.

Insight into the language difficulties may be markedly less than with anterior aphasias.

Conduction aphasia

Conduction aphasia is characterized by fluent speech with semantic confusions, nominal dysphasia, relatively well-preserved comprehension, but poor ability to repeat heard words. Although poor repetition used to be thought to be characteristic of lesions of the arcuate connecting bundles between the anterior and posterior parts of the

language areas, it is now known to occur with a variety of posteriorly placed lesions as well.

6.1.1.2 *Acquired dyslexia (alexia) and dysgraphia (agraphia)*

A lesion in the region of the dominant angular gyrus will result in an inability to comprehend written symbols. Acquired dyslexia is to be distinguished from the specific learning disability known as dyslexia, for which various explanations are advanced (Section 25.3.3). Acquired dyslexia is often associated with a posterior aphasia. Pure alexia without dysgraphia occurs in lesions of the left occipital lobe and splenium of the corpus callosum.

6.1.2 *Lesions of the parietal lobes*

Evidence of a lesion in either parietal lobe is commonly manifest on examination as a defect of attention in the contralateral visual field. A single powerful visual stimulus such as a finger movement may be readily perceived, but when this is accompanied by a similar synchronous stimulus in the opposite visual field, the stimulus in the affected field is not attended to, but ignored.

The parietal lobes are concerned with the integration into a perception of the somatosensory messages derived from the surface of the body, notably the hands. If there is a lesion of the left parietal lobe, the patient may be unable to recognize by touch alone, with his eyes closed, the nature of a common object, such as a key, placed in his right hand, even though the sensory threshold tested with cotton wool is within normal limits. This is known as *astereognosis*. A related defect may also be recognized by an inability to recognize with the eyes closed a number drawn by the examiner on the hand or leg.

Lesions of either parietal lobe may give rise to pseudoathetosis—abnormal posturings of the outstretched hands, with the eyes closed, due to a perceptual failure of integration of digit and limb position.

6.1.2.1 *Non-dominant parietal lesions*

Neglect of the contralateral field and space in lesions of the non-dominant parietal lobe may extend to neglect and even denial of the subject's own limbs. An affected patient may feel that the limbs contralateral to a non-dominant parietal lesion are not his, but belong to someone else in the same bed. An inability to comprehend patterns and structures within space leads to a patient getting lost even in familiar surroundings. An inability to recognize faces, known as *prosopagnosia*, may extend even to the patient's spouse. An ability to use and understand three-dimensional space is readily tested by Koh's blocks, small painted cubes with which patterns have to be constructed. An inability to do this is known as a *constructional apraxia*. (Apraxia is defined on p. 26.) Alternatively, the patient may be asked to draw a house, or a bicycle, or a clock. Often the clock is poorly constructed, with neglect of the left side of the face, and numbers entered only on the right. Disordered comprehension of space may extend to the patient's clothes, so that he is unable to orientate a sweater and his body and use appropriate movements to put it on. This is known as *dressing apraxia*. It is of great interest that neglect of space extends to the patient's own imaginary space. For example, if asked to describe the scene in a town square that he or she knows well, he or she may neglect to describe any of the shops on his left-hand side.

6.1.2.2   *Dominant parietal lesions*

Visual inattention and constructional apraxia is seen in dominant parietal lobe lesions, but neglect of contralateral space is not so prominent as in lesions of the non-dominant lobe.

Characteristic of a dominant parietal lesion is Gerstmann's syndrome. Gerstmann, in 1940, described dyscalculia (an inability to calculate), right–left disorientation, and an inability to name fingers (index, middle, etc.). This last phenomenon is known as finger agnosia.

A lesion of the dominant parietal lobe may also be associated with ideomotor apraxia—a disorder of the execution of movement that cannot be accounted for by weakness, incoordination, impairment of sensation, impairment of comprehension, or of attention. For example, if a patient is asked to imitate the turning of a key in a lock, he first has to comprehend the command, and then through association fibres to the motor cortex, the appropriate movement of the right hand must be undertaken. One hypothesis is that spatiotemporal

representations of skilled motor acts are stored in the dominant parietal cortex.

6.1.3   *Lesions of the occipital lobes*

What is curious about bilateral lesions of the tips of the occipital lobes is the neglect or denial of the virtual blindness due to bilateral occipital infarction caused by, for example, basilar artery occlusion. This phenomenon is known as Anton's syndrome. It seems that the neglect of blindness is due to preservation of some unconscious visual function, nicknamed 'blind-sight', preserved in the lateral geniculate bodies. These are phylogenetically important visual relay stations in which neurons are arranged in topological relationship to retinal ganglion cells, and clearly have an integrative function in some amphibians.

In occipital blindness, the pupils react normally to light, as the anterior visual pathways are unaffected.

6.1.4   *Lesions of the temporal lobes*

Lesions of one or other temporal lobe often produce seizures (Section 12.6.1). A lesion of the dominant temporal lobe will produce aphasia if it extends posteriorly beyond the anterior 6 cm. Changes in mood and potency may also be associated with temporal lobe lesions.

A characteristic high quadrantic hemianopia, as shown in Fig. 6.1(2a), may occur in extensive temporal lobe lesions, due to involvement of Meyer's loop of the optic radiation.

Occasionally both temporal lobes are damaged. The classic way in which this occurred was during the development of surgery for epilepsy when the 'wrong' temporal lobe was excised, the remaining one also containing a structural lesion. The bilateral temporal lobe damage so caused was manifest as a gross defect of recent memory, so much so that some of the affected patients were unable to remember even their own names.

Bilateral diffuse temporal lobe injury is said by some to be responsible for explosive rages seen occasionally after head injury. This so-called *episodic dyscontrol syndrome* may be helped by carbamazepine, even though it is not believed that the outbursts have an epileptic basis. Bilateral temporal lobe lesions in primates produce excessive aggression and hypersexuality—the Kluver–

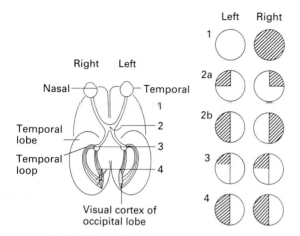

Fig. 6.1 Impairment of the visual field due to lesions at different sites (numbered) in the optic pathway. (The brain is seen from below.) The shaded areas indicate the areas in which vision is impaired or lost. At the chiasma (2), a lesion expanding upwards from the pituitary fossa will compress first the fibres that lie inferiorly in the chiasma, causing an upper quadrantic bitemporal hemianopia (2a). As the lesion increases in size the bitemporal hemianopia becomes complete (2b).

Bucy syndrome—but in humans the result is impairment of libido and potency.

6.1.5 Lesions of the frontal lobes

The frontal lobes are often contused in head injuries; they may be compressed by a meningioma growing slowly from the olfactory groove; they may be infarcted consequent to the rupture of an anterior communicating artery aneurysm. Survivors of such frontal insults are characterized by an impairment of normal social control. For example, inappropriate jokey remarks may be made to the attending neurosurgeon. After the acute stage, lack of social inhibitions may lead to urination or masturbation in public. Social drive and initiative is impaired, so that apathy is prominent. The patient may be irritable and disruptive of rehabilitation attempts. He or she may carry on doing one action when another is appropriate. This phenomenon is known as perseveration. Such patients may display what is known as 'utilization behaviour'. For example, the patient may see a

stethoscope, and inappropriately pick it up and attempt to listen to the doctor's heart.

These behaviours are readily recognizable on examination. The diagnosis is supported by groping and grasping reflexes. If the examiner's hand is placed on the back of the patient's hand, the patient may grope along the examiner's forearm. If the examiner's fingers are placed within the subject's palm, and the palm stroked from the lateral to medial aspect, the examiner's fingers may be firmly grasped. The patient finds it difficult to release the examiner's fingers even if so instructed.

The grasp reflex is a primitive reflex seen in the new-born, but subsequently inhibited by further myelination and frontal development. It may be 'released' in frontal lobe lesions. Other primitive reflexes that may be released in frontal lobe lesions are the sucking reflex and the palmo-mental reflex. The sucking reflex is elicited by stroking to one side of the mouth. The head turns towards the finger, and the lips make the movements of sucking. The palmo-mental reflex (Wartenburg's reflex) is a curious reflex, the biological significance of which is obscure. A gentle scratch across the thenar eminence of a patient with a frontal lesion results in dimpling of the chin as the ipsilateral mentalis muscle contracts.

Grasp, sucking, and palmo-mental reflexes, if present, all suggest frontal lobe dysfunction. In addition, the pout reflex and the jaw jerk may be increased. These are reflexes that are exaggerated whenever there is bilateral corticofugal impairment, for example in pseudobulbar palsy (Section 6.4.2), but they are also prominent in frontal lesions. The pout reflex is elicited by gently tapping centrally just above the upper lip. If the reflex is present, the lips form a pout, as if kissing. The jaw jerk is a monosynaptic reflex arising from masseteric muscle spindles. It is elicited by gently tapping the mandible when the patient's mouth is slightly open.

6.2 Syndromes of disordered motor function

6.2.1 The principles of normal motor control

This is extensively described in textbooks of physiology, but a brief review is necessary here on account of its central position in clinical neurology, where defects of strength and co-ordination are common presenting symptoms.

An example of a voluntary movement is stretching out the right hand to pick up a jug of water placed on a sloping surface. This movement is initiated as an 'act of will' in areas of the brain which are poorly defined, but which certainly largely involve the frontal lobes. An 'intention to move' can be recorded as a long-duration negative shift in the electroencephalogram, as long as 1000 ms before pyramidal cells in the motor cortex fire. This shift is known as the '*Bereitschaftspotential*' or readiness potential. Its initial stages appear to be due to firing of non-pyramidal neurons, the later stages to firing of pyramidal neurons. The interval between the onset of the first firing of pyramidal neurons and the first recorded electromyographic activity varies according to the type of movement willed. Once fired, however, some pyramidal cells have a powerful direct monosynaptic connection with, in this example, anterior horn cells in the cervical enlargement of the spinal cord. Before initiating this movement to pick up the jug, the brain has to integrate information from the visual cortex as to the distance and angle through which the hand must be moved in order to reach the jug. The brain has information from previous experience about the inertial mass of the limb, and therefore the number of motor units that will be required to generate the muscle tension necessary to launch the ballistic movement of the arm and forearm in the direction of the jug. Once launched, the ballistic movement cannot be aborted without a finite delay, so that if an unforeseen obstacle, such as someone else's hand reaching for the jug, travels across the path of the movement it is not possible to 'pull the punch', and each person's knuckles are hurt on contact.

A ballistic movement is not modified by feedback—there is insufficient time. Even if the jug is seen to slide away after the launch of the movement it will only be possible to grab it if it slides slowly, as visual information must be processed and passed to the motor cortex before any correction can be performed. This takes about 80 ms.

Although the movement just described is initiated by 'the will' and then by pyramidal cortical cells, the extrapyramidal system is also not idle. Stretching out an arm towards the jug will alter slightly the position of the centre of gravity of the body, so that reflex adjustments of posture must be made to prevent the body toppling. The extrapyramidal system can be regarded as controlling the posture on to which pyramidally mediated, purposive, skilled movements are grafted.

Cerebellar afferent and efferent pathways are concerned with stabilization of the arm extended towards the jug, particularly towards the end of the ballistic movement. Characteristic of abnormalities of cerebellar function are instability of the outstretched hand, and a tremor towards the end of a planned movement. Towards the end of a ballistic movement, receptors in muscle spindles provide information about the tension generated in the muscles employed in the movement. These afferents run up the spinocerebellar pathways and through the inferior cerebellar peduncle to the cerebellar cortex. Defects of these spindle afferents, as in the Miller Fisher syndrome (Section 19.3.9.2), produce an ataxia that is very similar to that of lesions of the cerebellum itself. After integration of information in the cerebellar cortex, efferent pathways run from the dentate nucleus to the red nucleus in the brain stem, and thence caudally as rubrospinal pathways to spinal cord segments, there again influencing motor control. Red nucleus afferents also pass to the lateral thalamus, and synapse there with neurons passing to the sensorimotor cortex, thereby allowing modification of motor output.

The pyramidal system is concerned with the dexterous movements necessary to control the position of the fingers around the handle of the jug, but sensory feedback is important, and a subject with a profound sensory loss in the relevant hand may well drop the jug as he picks it up, as he is unable to measure accurately the pressure with which he is holding on to the handle.

Another aspect of this scenario now comes into play. The subject has to decide how many motor units it is necessary to activate in order to generate sufficient tension to lift the jug. This will be based upon 'knowledge' of the same or similar jugs containing everyday fluids such as water. Suppose the jug unexpectedly contained mercury. The subject would soon perceive the jug as unexpectedly heavy, but even before this conscious perception, information from muscle spindles allows the recruitment of additional motor units in order that the planned action can be completed, with a latency of about 80 ms. This is considerably shorter than the fastest voluntary response of about 130 ms. (Those with very fast voluntary response times do very well in sprint races of 100 metres. Fast video-recordings show that the interval between the smoke from the starter's gun, and take-off from the blocks exceptionally may be as fast as 115 ms. The heavyweight boxer, Tyson, has been timed to throw six punches within 1 s.) The 80 ms latency described above occurs in pathways known as long-loop reflexes, passing through the cerebral cortex, but apparently not involving truly 'voluntary' control.

Clinical examination of the motor system analyses whether a defect is due to a lower motor neuron lesion, an upper motor neuron lesion, an extrapyramidal lesion, or a cerebellar lesion.

6.2.2   A lower motor neuron lesion

The lower motor neuron is the name given to the anterior horn cells in the spinal cord, and the axons which pass from them, through the ventral spinal roots. After mingling with afferent fibres running in the dorsal roots, the combined spinal nerves divide into anterior and posterior primary rami. The posterior primary rami largely supply paraspinal muscles and skin, and disorders of their function are seldom clinically apparent. The axons in the anterior primary rami become, in the thoracic region, the intercostal nerves. In other regions, they mingle with axons from other segments to form the cervical, lumbar, and sacral plexi, before entering one of the named peripheral

nerves, and finally branching pre-terminally to supply 10–400 muscle fibres. The anterior horn cell, axon, and its associated 10–400 muscle fibres are known collectively as a 'motor unit'.

An activated motor unit is the 'final common path', as Sherrington called it, of the integrative activity of the nervous system. Effective motor responses to an environmental stimulus or act of the will are mediated through these 'final common paths', whatever complex reflex or cognitive activity preceded them. As an example of a motor unit, an axon of an anterior horn cell neuron in the T1 segment leaves the spinal cord through the T1 ventral root, forms part of the lower trunk of the brachial plexus, passes through the anterior division and medial cord of the brachial plexus, enters the median nerve, and finally supplies about 150 muscle fibres in the abductor pollicis muscle in the thenar eminence. Analogous lower motor neurons are present in the brain stem, for example in the motor nuclei of the trigeminal and facial nerves.

Disorders of the lower motor neuron may arise at any point from anterior horn cell to neuromuscular junction. A simple example is a wound caused by falling into a window pane with the outstretched hand. The median nerve is commonly severed at the wrist in this sort of accident. Other lower motor neuron disorders can occur at the level of the anterior horn cell (for example, motor neuron disease, see Section 20.1), or as a metabolic disorder affecting motor axons (for example, an axonal neuropathy, see Section 19.2).

Whatever the cause of a lesion of a group of lower motor neurons, the clinical manifestations

Table 6.2   Lower and upper motor neuron lesions

	Lower	*Upper*
Wasting	present	absent
Fasciculation	present	absent
Tone	not increased	increased
Weakness	segmental, nerve, or distal pattern	pyramidal pattern with clumsiness
Tendon reflexes	decreased or absent	increased
Clonus	absent	present
Superficial reflexes (abdominal, cremasteric)	present	absent
Plantar reflex	plantarflexion of big toe ('flexor plantar response')	dorsiflexion of big toe ('extensor plantar response')

Not every change is found in mild or early lesions, but most or all signs are present in the fully developed syndrome.

are much the same. The distinctions between the signs of a lower and an upper motor neuron lesion are summarized in Table 6.2.

6.2.2.1   *Wasting*

A denervated muscle *wastes*, that is to say, its bulk is less. This is true at the microscopical level too, as the cross-sectional diameter of individual muscle fibres becomes less. There is usually no difficulty in distinguishing the generalized wasting, or cachexia, of malignant disease from the focal wasting affecting one limb as a result of, for example, a brachial plexus lesion. It is true that there is generalized wasting at the end stage of motor neuron disease (in which anterior horn cells are diffusely affected, see Section 20.1.2), but the natural history up to that point and the presence of fasciculation usually allows an accurate differential diagnosis. After nerve section, for example in the injury by a glass window pane postulated above, wasting takes 2–3 weeks to become clinically apparent.

Wasting occurs if there is loss of axonal continuity, and if there is disruption of the neuromuscular junction consequent upon Wallerian or axonal degeneration (see Section 19.2). The diameter of individual muscle fibres, and bulk of a muscle, is maintained by axonal contact.

The effects of nerve *compression* (as opposed to section) are described on p. 360. This may occur as the result of, for example, the overzealous use of a tourniquet. In nerve compression, there may be a transient block in conduction due to invagination of myelin and subsequent demyelination of the axon over a short segment. This is called *neuropraxia* (see Sections 19.2 and 19.4.2.3). Even though the axon is not conducting through the demyelinated segment, axonal continuity with individual muscle fibres is sufficient to prevent wasting. What 'trophic influences' maintain muscle fibre bulk in this case is not clear, but probably continued quantal release of acetylcholine and the generation of miniature end-plate potentials are important. Neuropraxia is the only type of lower motor neuron lesion that is not accompanied by wasting.

6.2.2.2   *Fasciculation*

A fasciculation is an involuntary, spontaneous contraction of a group of muscle fibres, making up part of a motor unit. Fasciculations are particularly common in disorders affecting the anterior horn cell, such as motor neuron disease (Section 20.1.4).

6.2.2.3   *No increase in tone*

Tone is defined on p. 33 as 'resistance to passive stretch'. Denervated muscles are floppy, or hypotonic, and can be stretched farther than is usual. If large groups of muscles are affected by lower motor neuron lesions, for example by a plexus lesion, the affected limb is said to be 'flail'. (A flail is a stout stick attached by means of a cord to a handle, and used in less-developed societies for threshing grain. The cord allows the stick to swing about freely.)

6.2.2.4   *Weakness*

Weakness is perhaps the most easily understood disorder of motor function, and occurs in upper motor neuron syndromes, too. However, the difference in *pattern* of weakness is crucial.

In lower motor neuron syndromes, the weakness 'makes sense' in terms of a lesion of one or more spinal segments or ventral roots, or spinal roots, or of part of a limb plexus, or of a peripheral nerve.

For some reason, the elucidation of the pattern of weakness strikes terror into the heart of many students and doctors unaccustomed to dealing with neurological patients. The schema shown in Table 6.3 is recommended. When examining a patient with a weak upper or lower limb, I recommend that those movements listed in the left-hand column are tested. If this schema is followed, then the integrity of each spinal segment and its ventral root is tested in sequence. Furthermore, the muscles selected are innervated by different nerves, so the integrity of each nerve can also be tested. If one of these listed muscles is found to be weak, then other muscles supplied by the same spinal segment can be tested to see if there is supportive evidence of a segmental or radicular lesion. If not, then other muscles supplied by the same peripheral nerve are next tested. In examining a patient with a weak hand, for example, the question should be mentally set—how can I best account for this weakness? Is it due to a first thoracic (T1) segment or root lesion? In both these cases, muscles in the hand innervated by T1 fibres

Table 6.3 Schema for the elucidation of patterns of weakness: movements, muscles, spinal segments, and peripheral nerves

Movement	Segment	Muscle	Nerve
Abduction of shoulder	C5	deltoid	axillary
Flexion of supinated forearm	C6	biceps	musculocutaneous
Flexion of mid-prone forearm	C6	brachioradialis	radial
Extension of forearm	C7	triceps	radial
Flexion of tip of thumb and index finger	C8	flexor digitorum profundus (2) and pollicis	median
Flexion of tip of ring and little fingers	C8	flexor digitorum profundus (4,5)	ulnar
Abduction of thumb (proximal phalanx)	T1	abductor pollicis brevis	median
Abduction of fingers	T1	dorsal interossei	ulnar
Flexion of hip	L1	iliopsoas	n. to iliopsoas
Adduction of hip	L2	adductor magnus	obdurator
Extension of knee	L3	quadriceps	femoral
Dorsiflexion of foot	L4	tibialis anterior	n. to tibialis anterior
Dorsiflexion of big toe	L5	extensor hallucis longus	n. to extensor hallucis longus
Eversion of foot	S1	peroneal muscles	musculo-cutaneous branch of common peroneal
Plantar flexion of foot	S1	gastrocnemius, soleus	posterior tibial
Flexion of knee	S2	hamstrings	sciatic
Extension of hip	S3	gluteus maximus	inferior gluteal

running in both median and ulnar nerve will be affected, and there will therefore be weakness of abductor pollicis brevis (median nerve), and the interosseous muscles (ulnar nerve). If abduction of the thumb is of normal strength, and yet the interosseous muscles weak, then clearly this cannot be a lesion of the T1 segment or root, as it is most unlikely that a lesion at this level could differentially affect fibres destined to run in the two different nerves. Attention must be directed to other muscles supplied by the ulnar nerve to see if there is supportive evidence for an ulnar nerve lesion. In this example, from a knowledge of the level at which branches are given off to different muscles, an anatomical diagnosis could be made of the level at which the ulnar nerve is damaged.

6.2.2.5   Depressed or absent tendon reflexes

If a lower motor neuron is damaged, it will not be able to carry the efferent response that is normally elicited by a tendon tap. In lower motor neuron

lesions, therefore, the tendon reflexes are depressed or absent. An example is the absent ankle reflex often found in association with a disc protrusion between L5 and S1, compressing the S1 root. In this particular case, however, part of the depression of the tendon reflex is due to compression of afferent as well as efferent fibres.

6.2.2.6   Superficial reflexes are normal

The term 'superficial reflexes' is given to muscle responses evoked by cutaneous stimuli. Those in common clinical use include the abdominal and cremasteric reflexes, and the plantar response. The abdominal and cremasteric reflexes are normal in patients with lower motor neuron lesions, unless the efferent limb of the reflex is affected by involvement of the relevant spinal segments (T7–11 for the abdominal reflex, L2 for the cremasteric reflex). This is only rarely clinically relevant. The plantar response is flexor.

6.2.3 *The upper motor neuron syndrome*

Although efferent paths from a number of different cell systems converge upon the anterior horn cell of the lower motor neuron, the term 'upper motor neuron syndrome' is usually considered to be synonymous with a disorder of pyramidal function. If the pyramidal syndrome arises from a lesion in the internal capsule of the hemisphere, then a *hemiparesis* results. If the pyramidal syndrome results from, for example, compression of the lateral corticospinal tracts in the dorsal spinal cord, then a *spastic paraparesis* occurs.

6.2.3.1 *Absence of wasting or fasciculation*

As the lower motor neuron is intact, maintaining a normal neuromuscular junction, there is no wasting or fasciculation.

6.2.3.2 *Increase in tone*

There is resistance to passive stretch of muscles.

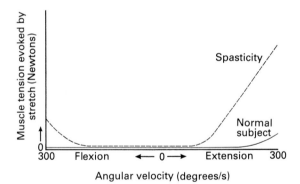

Fig. 6.2 The relationship between the angular velocity with which a muscle is stretched and the reflex muscle response. The ordinate shows, on an arbitrary scale, units of evoked muscle tension, the resistance felt by the examiner. Note that in a normal subject no stretch response is evoked on flexion however fast the rate of stretch. With very fast stretch a small response is evoked on extension. In subjects with spasticity, the threshold velocity at which a muscle response is evoked on extension is much reduced, and the slope of the curve relating muscle tension to stretch is much increased. The lesson is that, when testing for increased tone, a fairly vigorous stretch is required to be sure of eliciting the spastic response.

This is velocity dependent, as illustrated in Fig. 6.2. As there is a finite time before the myotatic reflex is elicited, the resistance is felt by the examiner as a sudden 'catch'. Increased tone is maximal in the pronators of the forearm, so the catch is felt during rapid supination. It is also prominent in biceps, so is felt during rapid extension of the elbow. In the lower limb, increased tone is most prominent in quadriceps, so is felt during brisk flexion of the knee.

A pyramidal lesion may also be accompanied by *clonus*. This is usually most easily elicited at the ankle, but may also be found at knee and wrist. At the ankle, a brisk passive dorsiflexion of the foot results in reflex plantar flexion. As long as pressure in the direction of dorsiflexion is maintained by the examiner's hand, rhythmic clonic reflex plantar flexion occurs. This is due to rhythmic facilitation of S1 anterior horn cells. It has been shown in animal experiments that this cyclical facilitation continues even when the tendon of tibialis anterior is severed, so it cannot depend upon alternating stretch of this muscle and the gastrocnemius.

A third way of demonstrating increased tone in the lower limb is to rotate the relaxed thigh and leg from side to side on the bed. If this is done fairly quickly in a normal subject, the foot flops from side to side at the ankle. There is a phase lag between the rotation of the tibia and the foot. If tone is increased, the phase lag is reduced as the resistance to passive stretch of the peroneal and tibial muscles splints the foot; the foot and leg appear to move in one block.

6.2.3.3 *Weakness*

The pattern of upper motor neuron weakness is characteristic. In the upper limb, the first muscles to be affected by an advancing pyramidal lesion are triceps and extensors of the fingers. The first affected muscles in the lower limb are the flexors of the hip, and dorsiflexors and evertors of the foot. The power of the extensors of the knee and plantar flexors of the foot is usually well preserved, even in advanced chronic pyramidal lesions. This is fortunate, as the preserved strength in these anti-gravity muscles allows a patient with an advanced pyramidal lesion due, for example, to multiple sclerosis, to stand, even if he cannot flex his thigh at the hip when lying on the bed.

6.2.3.4   *Clumsiness*

A patient with a pyramidal lesion, particularly of the cortex, loses fine dexterous movements of the thumb and fingers, even though power is preserved. Ablation of part of area 4 in a monkey results in it being unable to manipulate pelleted food out of a container, even though the strength in its finger flexors still allows it to hang by one hand from a bar in its cage. A similar loss of manual dexterity is often the first symptom of a pyramidal lesion. The examiner may overlook the evidence of a pyramidal lesion, as strength is normal, unless he asks the patient to oppose in rapid succession the tip of each finger to the thumb. Slowness and clumsiness of these movements is then readily apparent. Such clumsy movements are quite different from the ataxic incoordinate movements of a cerebellar syndrome (see Section 6.2.5).

6.2.3.5   *Increased tendon reflexes*

A lesion of descending pyramidal pathways removes a powerful inhibitory drive to anterior horn cells. Monosynaptic tendon reflexes, such as the knee and ankle jerks, are therefore exaggerated.

6.2.3.6   *Abnormal superficial reflexes*

The abdominal and cremasteric reflexes are absent in pyramidal lesions. The plantar response is extensor. An extensor plantar response is also known as a positive Babinski sign. It is most readily elicited from the lateral border of the foot, near the heel. As a pyramidal lesion advances, the zone from which the reflex can be elicited increases in area, to extend over the sole of the foot, then the dorsum of the foot and the front of the shin. Just as the afferent zone increases in area with the extent and severity of the pyramidal lesion, so does the efferent output. The threshold motor response is dorsiflexion of the big toe and fanning (abduction) of the other toes. In more advanced lesions, the reflex assumes more and more of the characteristics of the primitive flexor withdrawal response (which it is). It is unfortunate, in some ways, that dorsiflexion of the big toe is known as extension, thus concealing the primitive origins of this flexor withdrawal reflex. Just as a nociceptive stimulus

applied to the paw of a decerebrate cat results in flexor withdrawal of the limb from the stimulus, so a stimulus applied to the sole of the foot in a subject with a pyramidal lesion results firstly in dorsiflexion (extension) of the toe, then of the foot, then flexion of the knee and hip. In those with chronic spinal injuries, the reflex is often so easily elicited that the lightest touch of a bed sheet may precipitate a flexor withdrawal response—often called flexor spasms (see Section 18.1.4.4). A full bladder or a urinary tract infection in these circumstances lowers the threshold of the reflex so that flexor spasms are more troublesome.

The best instrument for eliciting the plantar response is a blunt wooden stick. No great force is necessary, nor indeed does the patient need to feel the stimulus—he certainly can't if he has a spinal transection, even though the response is very vigorous.

Extensor plantar responses are occasionally absent in those with clear-cut pyramidal lesions. The most frequent reason is such a degree of hallux rigidus that the big toe is virtually mechanically fixed. Another reason is if there is an associated disturbance of afferent or efferent peripheral pathways. For example, the peripheral neuropathy of vitamin B_{12} deficiency (Sections 19.3.4 and 23.2.5.3) may prevent an extensor plantar response, even though there is associated demyelination of the descending corticospinal tracts. Equally, loss of anterior horn cells in the L5 segment may prevent an extensor plantar response in motor neuron disease, even if there is associated degeneration of corticospinal tracts.

6.2.4   *The extrapyramidal syndrome*

The extrapyramidal system is the name given to the deep large nuclei in the hemispheres—the putamen and globus pallidus (together known as the striatum), the caudate nucleus, the subthalamic nucleus of Luys, the substantia nigra, and the red nucleus. Disorders of this central grey matter and their afferent and efferent connections result in movement disorders (see Chapter 13), which are quite distinct from the pyramidal syndrome just considered. Even though the extrapyramidal system is a group of neurons 'above' the lower motor neuron, if spoken or written without qualification, an upper motor neuron syndrome is usually taken to be synonymous with a pyramidal syndrome. Further discussion of the extrapyramidal syndrome will be found in Chapter 13.

6.2.5 *The cerebellar syndrome*

The functions of the cerebellum are best defined through the effects of disease or ablation as, in contrast to the pyramidal system, electrical stimulation of the human cerebellum at neurosurgical operations rarely produces any movement, and no sensation. On the other hand, the effects of ablation of one cerebellar hemisphere—perhaps for a localized tumour, or as the result of a local missile injury—are characteristic. They are listed in Table 6.4.

Table 6.4 Features of the cerebellar syndrome

Lesion of lateral lobe, including deep nuclei
   dysmetria, past-pointing
   action tremor (intention tremor)
   dysdiadochokinesis
   dysarthria
   rebound
   pendular reflexes
Lesion of vermis
   ataxia of stance and gait
If vestibular connections are involved:
   nystagmus

Some mechanisms underlying a typical voluntary act, reaching for a jug, were outlined on pp. 29–30. One function of the cerebellum is to turn off, or inhibit, a voluntary movement. After a unilateral cerebellar hemisphere lesion, the hand may shoot past the point of intended contact. This is sometimes called past-pointing, and is one manifestation of a more general disturbance in the self-measurement of voluntary movement—dysmetria. The outstretched arm of a subject with a unilateral cerebellar lesion is held reasonably steadily, that is to say, there is no postural tremor, but there is tremor on action. This action tremor is also called an intention tremor. The movements of a voluntary act are jerky and incoordinate, this unsteadiness being most pronounced towards the end of a movement. These abnormalities are easily tested by the well-known finger–nose and heel–knee–shin tests. In the former, the subject is asked to track

his index finger between his nose and the examiner's index finger. The test can be made more difficult by the examiner moving his finger from side to side. Tremor towards the end of each reaching movement and past-pointing can readily be demonstrated. In the heel–knee–shin test, the subject lies supine on the bed. He is asked to flex the thigh with extended knee, and then bring the heel gently down on the knee, and run it neatly down the front of the shin to the ankle. If abnormal, dysmetria is manifest by the heel crashing down heavily on or beside the knee, and then unsteadiness as the heel is moved down the shin, so that the heel falls off the bony anterior ridge of the tibia.

Another way of testing the influence of the cerebellum upon motor control is to ask the subject to pronate and to supinate alternately and rapidly the forearm. The movements will be chaotically organized in the affected arm. This is known as dysdiadochokinesis.

Action tremor affects speech as there is irregularity in phonation and in the orderly onset and termination of the movements of the muscles of articulation.

One test of the cerebellum's inhibitory function is for the examiner to ask the subject to flex strongly his or her forearm against the examiner's resistance. The examiner without warning then lets go. A normal subject is able to turn off the action of biceps within 80 ms, and brake the action of flexion. In a patient with an ipsilateral cerebellar lesion, the elbow may flex vigorously on release, and the hand hit the face.

6.3 Syndromes of impaired somatosensory perception

Many medical students and young doctors find sensory examination difficult, and wonder how there is possibly time to do a complete sensory examination in the course of a busy outpatient clinic or ward round. The explanation is that a careful sensory examination is necessary in only a few patients with neurological diseases. Perception of sensory stimuli is so sensitive that it is most unlikely that a subject with normal cognitive function will have sensory signs in the absence of sensory symptoms, and anyone with abnormal cognitive function will be unable to co-operate sufficiently accurately with a sensory examination for meaningful results to be obtained.

Another misconception is the use of the word 'subjective' to describe sensory impairment as in some way less convincing than 'objective' sensory loss. Any clinical examination of sensation—be it with cotton wool, pin, tuning fork, or thermal stimulation—depends upon the subject's co-operation. If he or she says that a pinprick feels less painful in one area of a limb compared to another, then that is a piece of evidence that has to be incorporated into the clinical picture.

6.3.1   *Modalities of sensation, and how to test them*

6.3.1.1   *Touch, pressure, and vibration*

The tactile sensations of touch, pressure, and vibration are initiated by deformation of Meissner's corpuscles, Merkel's discs, free nerve endings related or unrelated to hair follicles, Ruffini's endings, and Pacinian corpuscles. The rate of adaptation of firing of these various mechanoreceptors varies. All respond to some extent to all three stimuli; touch is no more than very light pressure, and vibration no more than rapidly varying pressure. Pacinian corpuscles adapt in a few milliseconds, and are therefore important in detecting vibration. They are served by large myelinated fibres of 12–15 μm diameter. Ruffini's endings are slowly adapting, and are therefore suitable for detecting maintained deep pressure. They are served by myelinated fibres of lesser diameter, 3–10 μm. Many degenerative and other illnesses of the nervous system, such as peripheral neuropathy, first affect fibres of largest diameter, so light touch and vibration are often impaired early in the course of the illness.

Light touch can be tested readily with the examiner's own fingertip, or with a piece of cotton wool fashioned into a fairly firm cone, which is used to prod the skin. If a wisp of cotton wool is drawn over the skin, the subject may perceive a sensation of tickle, mediated by unmyelinated nerve fibres, even if the threshold to light touch is considerably elevated. Vibration is easily tested with a common tuning fork vibrating at 128 Hz. A healthy young person should perceive vibration at the toes, but the ability to do so is lost in the sixties, and by age 70 about half the population cannot perceive vibra-

tion at the ankle, and many cannot perceive it at the knee.

For research purposes, the stimuli used in clinical practice are insufficiently reproducible, and abnormalities in any of these modalities can be more readily quantitated by electromechanical transducers. Thermal thresholds can be determined by a computer-controlled thermode.

The central processes of many axons subserving mechanoreceptors enter the spinal cord and pass upwards in the dorsal columns. As they ascend the spinal cord, the central processes from lumbar and sacral roots are displaced medially by those entering from the dorsal and cervical regions. The axons terminate on neurons in the gracile and cuneate nuclei. The axons of these second neurons decussate immediately in the medial lemniscus, and ascend in the brain stem, accompanied by equivalent fibres from the sensory nucleus of the trigeminal nerve, to the ventrobasal nuclear complex of the thalamus. These axons synapse with further sensory neurons which project through the posterior limb of the internal capsule to the parietal somatosensory cortex. Stimulation of the somatosensory cortex during the course of neurosurgical operations under local anaesthesia in humans has shown a topographic localization of axons projecting from the thalamus to the cortex, broadly similar to that portrayed in Fig. 12.3 for the pre-Rolandic motor cortex.

Another group of axons subserving mechanoreceptors enter the dorsal grey matter either in the segment in which they enter the spinal cord, or a few segments above. In the deeper laminae of the dorsal grey matter, they synapse with secondary axons which ascend just anterior to the dorsal horn as the spinocervical pathway. They synapse again in the high cervical grey matter, and then axons of the next order join the medial lemniscus to proceed to the thalamus, and, after a further synapse, to the parietal cortex.

Symptoms resulting from impaired function of nerve fibres subserving mechanoreceptors include tingling paraesthesiae, numbness, and a sensation of disturbed quality of tactile sensation, so that surfaces may be felt unexpectedly too smooth or too rough. Often the peripheral parts of the limb are described as feeling swollen. A patient with a plaque of demyelination in one cervical posterior column may say that the relevant hand feels as if it is 'enclosed in a boxing glove'. A woman who wakes at night with paraesthesiae due to compression of the median nerve in the carpal tunnel may say that her fingers feel like a 'bunch of bananas'.

6.3.1.2   *Discrimination between two points and stereognosis*

Lesions of central sensory axons in the internal capsule result in relatively less elevation of sensory threshold and less dense sensory impairment than those of axons in a peripheral nerve. However, discrimination between two points is greatly impaired in parietal lesions, even if the sensory threshold is not greatly elevated. On the fingertips, the points of a pair of blunted dividers will normally be felt when as close together as 2 mm. On other parts of the body, the threshold for normal discrimination between two points is substantially higher, up to 40 mm on the dorsum of the foot. In parietal lesions these distances are substantially increased, so that on the fingertips, for example, the dividers may have to be separated to more than 15 mm before they are felt to be separate stimuli. This failure to discriminate between points of light touch or pressure affects the ability to perceive the complex form of an object, such as a key. Failure to recognize common objects placed in the hand (with the eyes shut) is known as asterognosis (Section 6.1.2). The integrative action of the parietal sensory cortex can also be tested by the ability to recognize with the eyes shut a complex pattern, usually a single-digit number, drawn on the skin of the contralateral limb. This function is known as graphaesthesia.

6.3.1.3   *Sense of passive movement*

This is tested by the examiner taking a limb segment distal to a joint, initially usually the terminal phalanx of a finger or big toe, and flexing and extending it passively, with the subject's eyes closed. The subject is asked to indicate the direction of movement. It is a mistake for the examiner to move the digit under test too far and too briskly, as minor degrees of impairment of sense of passive movement will then be overlooked.

Although flexion and extension of a joint of a digit must pull on the associated tendons and muscle spindles, the sense of passive movement does not arise from these structures. An anaesthetic ring block at the base of the digit abolishes

the sense of passive movement, showing that the receptors responsible for detecting movement lie in the joint capsule, and not in the muscles. The principal receptors responsible are Ruffini's endings, but some Pacinian corpuscles also play a part. The central axons of the dorsal root ganglion cells subserving these receptors pass up the dorsal columns and spinocervical pathway, as do the axons of mechanoreceptors responsible for light touch, pressure, and vibration.

It is necessary to distinguish sense of passive movement from static position sense—that is to say, a consciousness of the orientation, with the eyes closed, of the limbs and body in space.

Parietal lesions are usually responsible for loss of static position sense, tested by asking the patient, with his eyes shut, to localize the position of one limb in space by pointing to or touching it with another, or by verbal description.

Profound sensory impairment due to multiple radicular lesions (e.g. in acute infective polyneuropathy) or lesions of the posterior columns may also interfere with static position sense, and give rise to illusions that the limbs are disposed in unreal ways. Subjects with such marked afferent impairment will possibly be moderately unsteady with their eyes open, but very much worse when the eyes are closed, as the stabilizing influence of visual fixation is removed. This is known as the Romberg test. In the upper limbs, such profound afferent impairment may result in pseudo-athetosis, vaguely wandering movements of the fingers of the outstretched hands, which is much more prominent when the eyes are closed.

6.3.1.4   *Painful sensations*

Perception of pain is usually tested clinically by pricking with a pin. Now that infection with human immunodeficiency virus is so prevalent in those with neurological disease, a fresh pin must be used for each patient, and the pin safely disposed of thereafter. The tradition of a neurologist carrying a pin in the lapel of his suit is dead.

A modest jab with a pin gives rise to a pricking sensation of pain. This is mediated by free nerve endings of small myelinated fibres of 2–4 μm diameter conducting at 12–24 m/s. A more substantial jab causes this sensation of initial prick, followed, after a slight delay, by a burning sensation of greater intensity. This delay is due to the fact that nerve endings responsible for this type of pain are the endings of unmyelinated nerve fibres conducting at only 0.5–2.0 m/s. Both small myelinated and unmyelinated pain fibres enter the spinal cord through the dorsal root, ascend or descend one or two segments in the tract of Lissauer in the dorsal horn, and then synapse in the dorsal horn with other neurons. The axons of these second neurons cross the mid-line of the spinal cord in the anterior commissure, and then ascend in the anterior and lateral spinothalamic pathways before terminating in the ventrobasal nuclear complex of the thalamus (pricking pathway) or reticular formation and intralaminar nuclei of the thalamus (burning pathway). Impairment of pain perception can arise as part of a peripheral neuropathy in which small myelinated or unmyelinated fibres are particularly affected (e.g. amyloid neuropathy, Section 19.3.8), or as a result of a dorsal ganglion neuronopathy affecting particularly the cell bodies of axons of small diameter, as may occur as a remote effect of carcinoma of the bronchus (Section 19.3.5). Pain fibres may also be affected as they cross the spinal cord by a syringomyelic cavity (Section 18.5.4.1) or by a tumour such as an ependymoma or astrocytoma within the spinal cord. If there is marked impairment of perception of pain, with reasonably preserved sensation of light touch and pressure, as may occur in syringomyelia, the sensory loss is said to be dissociated.

Impaired perception of pain is known as hypoalgesia, or analgesia if there is complete loss of pain sense in an area of the body. Rather surprisingly, many patients with marked hypoalgesia of, for example, one hand do not complain of anything other than a vague feeling of numbness. What usually brings the severity of the sensory impairment to medical attention is a blister or area of necrosis resulting from a burn sustained while cooking, or from a cigarette, that was unnoticed at the time.

Another syndrome of pain perception is hyperpathia, in which a stimulus that would be felt in a healthy person as no more than mildly unpleasant is perceived to have a burning quality of unusual intensity. This is found in patients with partial lesions of peripheral nerves (Section 19.4.2.2), as well as in patients with thalamic lesions (Section 10.1.5) and in those with incomplete spinal cord syndromes after injury.

For research purposes, pain can be more easily quantified by painful thermal stimuli. There are, of course, considerable difficulties in taking into account affective aspects of pain as perceived.

6.3.1.5   Thermal discrimination

Thermal discrimination is not often tested in day-to-day clinical practice as the pathways follow an identical route to the pain pathways. It is, however, sometimes useful to confirm an area in which there is a suspicion of hypoalgesia. The usual method of testing thermal sensation is to ask the subject to distinguish between two tubes containing what feels pleasantly warm and pleasantly cool to the examiner's own hand. For research purposes, rapidly adapting thermodes are used.

6.3.2   Findings on sensory examination in lesions of different parts of the nervous system

6.3.2.1   Sensory radicular lesions

Disturbance of sensation due to a radicular lesion commonly occurs as a result of a cervical or lumbar disc protrusion. Other causes include a neurofibroma on a spinal root, and herpes zoster (Section 17.12.7). It is through this last illness that the distribution of sensory fibres from each dorsal root to different parts of the skin was first ascertained, as the vesicles appear in the distribution of the sensory root. Figure 6.3 shows a map of the dermatomes—the name given to the areas of skin supplied by sensory fibres from any one spinal root. There is, however, considerable overlap between neighbouring dermatomes. The area of sensory impairment following a lesion of a single root is often smaller than the extent illustrated, and the margins of sensory impairment are often indistinct, as the nerve roots supplying adjacent dermatomes also supply receptors within the affected field.

6.3.2.2   Lesions of peripheral nerves

In contrast to dermatomal lesions, lesions of peripheral nerves result in areas of sensory impairment with a sharp border. For example, in the case of an ulnar nerve lesion, there is a sharp line down the centre of the ring finger demarcating the zone of impaired sensation medially from the lateral

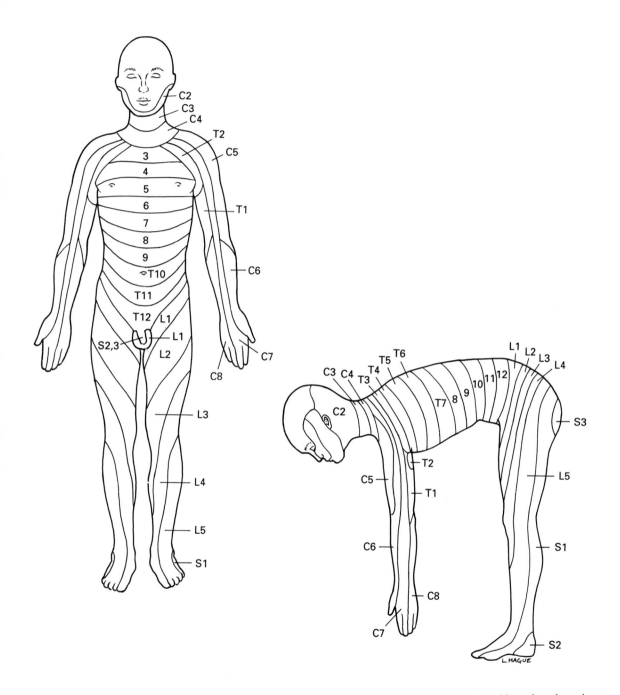

Fig. 6.3 Schematic representation of the cutaneous area supplied by each spinal nerve root. Note that there is considerable overlap between the root supply of adjacent segments. (Redrawn after Foerster 1933.)

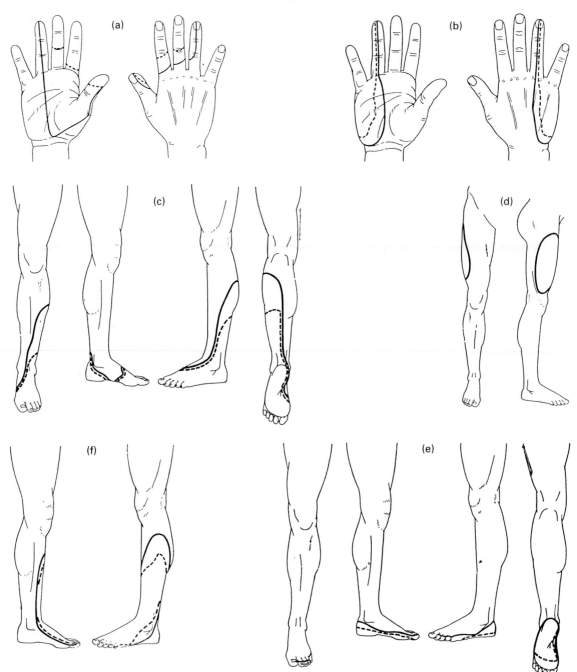

Fig. 6.4 The approximate areas within which sensory changes may be found in lesions of the following nerves: (a) median nerve; (b) ulnar nerve; (c) sciatic nerve; (d) lateral cutaneous nerve of the thigh; (e) posterior tibial nerve; (f) common peroneal nerve—high lesion; a lower lesion, below the origin of the anterior tibial nerve will cause disturbed sensation only in a V-shaped wedge running on the dorsum of the foot to the first and second toes. (Reproduced with permission from *Aids to the examination of the peripheral nervous system*. Baillière Tindall, London.)

area of normal sensation perceived through the median nerve. The areas of sensory impairment following lesions of the principal nerves in the limbs are illustrated in Fig. 6.4.

6.3.2.3 Lesions of the posterior columns

As explained on p. 36, the posterior columns carry the central axons of sensory nerve fibres from mechanoreceptors which serve the senses of light touch, pressure, vibration, and sense of passive movement. Impaired vibration sense and sense of passive movement are usually most easily detected.

6.3.2.4 Lesions of the spinothalamic pathways

Sensory changes due to lesions of the spinothalamic pathway are described in relation to the Brown-Séquard syndrome (Section 6.9.2), and to syringomyelia (Section 18.5.4.1).

6.3.2.5 Lesions of the parietal lobes

Characteristic of such lesions is the inability to discriminate between two points, and to recognize by touch an object placed in the hand—astereognosis (Section 6.1.2).

6.4 Brain-stem syndromes

The brain stem is a highly complex anatomical structure, carrying somatic afferent pathways from spinal cord to thalamus, and efferent pathways from the cerebral peduncles down into the spinal cord. The decussation of the somatic afferents (the medial lemnisci) takes place low in the medulla, as does the decussation of the corticofugal pathways in the medullary pyramids.

In addition to these long fibre pathways *en passage*, the brain stem is the site of origin of the IIIrd–VIIth and IXth–XIIth cranial motor nerves, and receives somatic, special sense, or visceral afferent input from the Vth, VIIth, VIIIth, IXth (very little), and Xth cranial nerve territories. The efferent output from the cranial motor nuclei is analogous to that of anterior horn cells in each spinal segment; the nuclear output is uncrossed (although many of the corticonuclear fibres from

the peduncles cross shortly before synapse with the cranial motor nuclear cells). Some of the somatic afferent input (e.g. fibres subserving light touch on the face) decussate. In addition to all this, the brain stem contains input and output pathways to and from the cerebellum, and association pathways between cranial nerve nuclei, for example the medial longitudinal bundle which yokes together the actions of the IIIrd, IVth, and VIth cranial nerve nuclei.

With all this to-ing and fro-ing, therefore, it is not surprising that brain-stem syndromes produce complex neurological symptoms and signs. As an example, Fig. 10.5 and accompanying text demonstrate the effect of a lateral medullary infarction. Figure 10.5 is a cross-section at one particular level of the brain stem. It is also helpful to think both in vertical terms, remembering the distribution of nuclei in the length of the brain stem, and in dorsoventral terms, remembering the dorsal (posterior) situation of the IIIrd and IVth cranial nerve nuclei (Fig. 6.5). Such an analysis will allow a rough approximation of the site of a lesion, as in

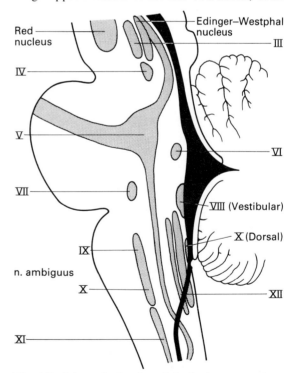

Fig. 6.5 Schematic drawing of the brain stem to show the distribution of brain-stem nuclei in the longitudinal and dorsoventral planes.

the example given in Fig. 10.5. However, it must be remembered that neither vascular lesions nor tumours respect neat anatomical boundaries.

There are, however, two more general 'brain-stem' syndromes—bulbar palsy and pseudobulbar palsy.

Table 6.5 (True) bulbar palsy

Loss of neurons; disorders within the brain stem
  motor neuron disease
  poliomyelitis
  infarction
  glioma
  syringobulbia
Disorders of lower cranial nerves outside the brain-stem
  infiltration by granuloma (e.g. sarcoid)
  infiltration by carcinoma (e.g. from nasopharynx, bronchus)
  Guillain–Barré syndrome
Disorders of myoneural junction
  myasthenia gravis

6.4.1 *Bulbar palsy*

This is the name given to the diffuse involvement of the lower motor cranial nerves (the IXth, Xth, and XIIth). Causes are given in Table 6.5. Whatever the cause, the clinical picture is one of difficulty in swallowing, often with nasal regurgitation due to palatal paralysis, or inhalation of liquids or food, dysarthria and often dysphagia. In advanced cases the tongue will be wasted. The muscles innervated by the VIIth cranial nerve, and eye movements, are, in general, not affected by diffuse disorders such as motor neuron disease. However, the VIth and VIIth nuclei and efferent pathways are commonly affected by pontomedullary infarctions.

Bulbar palsies due to extrinsic brain-stem lesions, such as carcinomatous meningitis, may have associated sensory signs in the trigeminal distribution, or in the tonsillar fossa, the somatic afferent zone for the glossopharyngeal (IXth) nerve.

6.4.2 *Pseudobulbar palsy*

This rather confusing term is used to describe bilateral lesions of upper motor neuron fibres as

they pass to the lower cranial nerve nuclei, as opposed to a (true) bulbar palsy in which lower motor neuron lesions occur. Pseudobulbar palsy may be due to the bilateral pyramidal degeneration of motor neuron disease (see Section 20.1) or the demyelination of these axons in multiple sclerosis (Section 14.3.2). It is also often caused by bilateral lacunar infarctions in the internal capsule. A patient recovering well from hemiparesis (due to the first lacunar infarction), without significant dysarthria, may develop sudden anarthria or dysarthria due to a small lacune in the opposite internal capsule. Release of brain-stem reflexes from higher cortical inhibiting centres results in a brisk jaw jerk and pout reflex, and emotional lability such that the patient may grimace and cry unduly easily when spoken to, or when watching a sentimental film. Conversely, he may laugh on inappropriate occasions.

Patients with pseudobulbar palsy may have few signs on neurological examination of the limbs, apart from generally brisk tendon reflexes and extensor plantar responses. However, the bilateral disturbance of outflow from each hemisphere is reflected in a defective pattern of organization of movement, most marked in walking, the gait being a hesitant shuffle, with short steps, the so-called *marche à petit pas*. Such patients often show a defect of organization of hand movements, and may be quite unable to copy the position adopted by the examiner's hands, even though there is no weakness. This is one type of apraxia (see p. 26).

The *marche à petit pas* bears a superficial (and only a superficial) resemblance to the gait of Parkinson's disease. On this account, the confusing notion of 'arteriosclerotic parkinsonism' used to be propounded. However, the natural history of diffuse lacunar arteriosclerosis resulting in pseudobulbar palsy and *marche à petit pas* is quite different from Parkinson's disease; the gait is not improved by L-dopa. These is no evidence that cerebral vasodilators, such as cyclandelate, have any beneficial action, although they are often prescribed.

6.4.3 *Other brain stem syndromes*

The syndromes arising from pontine infarction or haemorrhage and from lateral medullary infarction are considered in Section 10.1.5.

6.5 Dysphonia and dysarthria

It is important to distinguish between the mechanical functions of phonation and articulation, and disorders of language. Language may be defined as the cognitive processes involved in the communication and understanding of spoken and heard, written and read symbols which convey a shared meaning in a culture. Disorders of language are considered in Section 6.1.1.

6.5.1 *Dysphonia*

Dysphonia is the word used to describe a disorder of the ventilatory pump or vibrating vocal cords. The pump pushes the expired gases past the vibrating vocal cords, and so produces the sounds that are then further modified by the muscles of articulation to produce speech. The expired gases may be of low volume, and expired at low velocity, as may occur in a patient with myasthenia gravis or with acute infective polyneuropathy. Or one vibrating cord may be paralysed by a recurrent laryngeal palsy, so that the voice is hoarse. Or there may be a simple mechanical cause for dysphonia, such as a vocal cord polyp distorting the flow of expired air.

Some patients speak in a stage whisper, which is more readily recognized in life than described. This is usually a functional disorder (see Section 25.1.6), but in a few cases a similar voice may be produced by adductor spasm. This may occur in dystonic symptoms, or as part of a multisystem atrophy.

Patients with Parkinson's disease often shift their expired gases very slowly, so that their voice is quiet or soft. Other defects in extrapyramidal control of voice result in impaired variation in tone and prosody (rhythm) so that speech is monotonous.

6.5.2 *Dysarthria*

Just as the dexterous use of one hand may be disorganized by a variety of lesions at different levels, so may be the mechanisms of articulation.

Starting at the highest level of neuronal integration, a lesion in or adjacent to Broca's area (Section 6.1.1.1) may disturb the cortical pattern of lip and tongue movements so that speech is dysarthric (as well, in this case, as aphasic). A lesion of one internal capsule produces little in the way of dysarthria, apart possibly from that associated with any lip movements that are weak, as may be the muscles of the lower face in hemiplegia. However, lesions in both internal capsules—bilateral pyramidal lesions—result in a severe loss of cortical control of speech, which becomes slow and strained, a so-called 'spastic dysarthria'. This type of speech may be seen in patients with lacunar infarcts in each internal capsule, in those with the cortico-bulbo-spinal degeneration of motor neuron disease, and in those with diffuse white matter demyelination involving the same pathways, as in multiple sclerosis. A spastic dysarthria is usually accompanied by a brisk jaw jerk and pout reflex (Section 6.4.2). In extreme cases, speech may be entirely lost with the exception of vowel sounds, which are phonations such as 'aaah' or 'uugh' without articulation. This is called *anarthria*.

Lesions in the brain stem may result in a palatal palsy and nasal voice. If connections between brain stem and cerebellum are involved, then coordination of speech is impaired. Acute intoxication with alcohol or barbiturates produces a slurring and slowing of speech, and disorders of the brain stem and cerebellar connections have a similar, although exaggerated, effect. As equal or incorrect weights may be given to successive phonemes, the dysarthria may be said to be 'scanning' in character—typified by the patient with advanced multiple sclerosis.

Further down the motor pathways, lesions of the efferent nerves from the brain stem to the palate, larynx, and tongue will result in different types of dysarthria, as does myasthenia gravis by its effects on the neuromuscular junction. In lower brain stem lesions the dysarthric speech often has a nasal quality.

Impairment of afferent feedback from spindles in the tongue musculature may produce a dysarthria. This may happen as a result of bilateral damage to the lingual nerves during difficult extractions of the lower wisdom teeth.

Experience is necessary to analyse the different types of dysarthria, but certain 'tongue-twisters' may help. For example, the words 'thirty-seven, West Register Street, Edinburgh' may accent a slurring dysarthria of cerebellar type. A spastic dysarthria may be revealed by 'baby hippopotamus' or 'Daddy didn't do it', as both phrases require plosives and dental consonants which are poorly and slowly formed in those with bilateral pyramidal lesions.

6.6 Dizziness, giddiness, and vertigo

Many patients use the words dizziness or giddiness when they are attempting to convey some subjective experience in the head for which they know no better word. Other words used in the UK to describe symptoms which are probably similar include 'a muzzy feeling', 'light-headedness', and 'fullness'. More sophisticated patients with a greater vocabulary may use the words 'vertigo' to describe a similar unpleasant but non-specific sensation, which may indicate no more than an inner feeling of tension or anxiety. Indeed, 'dizzy spells' are a discriminant on the Goldberg short-scale for measuring anxiety (Table 25.1). Some patients may also use non-specific words such as 'dizziness' in order to convey organic symptoms such as impaired cognitive function, particularly due to non-dominant parietal lesions, which they understandably find difficult to explain. Other patients may describe a 'fullness' in the head in response to raised intracranial pressure, or some other organic disease.

Whatever the exact and individual sensations that patients are trying to convey by the use of these non-specific words, a physician is on much surer ground if his or her patient makes it clear that he or she experiences some sense of instability. True vertigo can best be defined as a *consciousness of disordered orientation in space*. Some authorities object to the use of the prefix 'true', rightly arguing that there is no such entity as 'false' vertigo. Be that as it may, it is often useful to make it clear when repeating a history that there is no doubt that the patient is describing a *consciousness of disordered orientation in space*, and not one of the vaguer symptoms of uncertain origin described in the preceding paragraph. All of us can experience rotational vertigo by spinning on the spot a few times and then stopping abruptly. However, some patients with true vertigo do not experience a sensation of movement, but to them the environment seems to tilt or slope. Unsteadiness accompanies true vertigo, as the patient makes inappropriate movements of his trunk, arms, and

legs in an attempt to orientate himself 'correctly' in the falsely perceived environment. However, although virtually all those who are vertiginous at the time of testing are ataxic, many ataxic patients are not vertiginous.

6.6.1 The orientation of the body in space

A number of sensory inputs keep us orientated in space. Probably the most important of these in everyday life is ocular fixation. Anyone who has had to wear a patch over one eye for a day or two after the intrusion of an ocular foreign body will feel fatigued and 'dizzy' by the end of the day. Diplopia also causes vertigo, as the false image disorients the body in space.

Additional important sensory information to describe the position of the body in space comes from the labyrinth. Angular accelerations of the head in any plane result in deflections of the cupola in one or more of the semicircular canals. The endolymph, due to its inertial mass, lags behind the turning walls of the canal. The semicircular canals are good detectors of change and of the rate of change in position of the head, but once the new position has been assumed for a few seconds, and the cupolae return to their original position, they can give no information about the static position of the head or body in space. This information is derived in part from the otolith organ, which detects vertical accelerations, including 'g'. Other sensory information is derived from joint receptors, and from pressure receptors on the surface of the body, particularly the feet. The role of input from the spindle receptors in the cervical muscles in spatial orientation in humans is not clear. Probably it is less important than in the cat and other quadrupeds. However, vertigo is a not uncommon symptom after a cervical whiplash injury.

Finally, our definition of vertigo, outlined a few paragraphs above, stresses the *consciousness* of the disorientation. Patients with Parkinson's disease may sit tilted 30° to one side, or tilt back dangerously while standing, and yet perceive no sense of misorientation of their trunk. Conversely, many of the tourists who stand on one of the west towers of Notre Dame feel intensely vertiginous, even though all receptors are working normally. They are aware of the low guard-rail and the crumbly nature of the stone on which they are standing.

Marked body sway may occur in these circumstances. It has been shown that this sway is immediately reduced by placing a cardboard cutout 'window' in front of them. A perception of 'safety' therefore may inhibit vertigo.

Other disorientations that technically fulfil our definition of vertigo include the peculiar and mildly unpleasant experience of walking up an escalator (moving staircase) that is not working. The differences in height of the first few steps, and the 'expectation' that such a staircase ought to move is presumably the cause of this generally acknowledged unusual perception. Fulfilled sensible expectations probably explain why vertigo is not generally experienced by passengers in an aeroplane as it takes off.

6.6.2 *Analysis of vertigo*

Hughlings Jackson, best known for his description of partial motor (Jacksonian) seizures (Section 12.4.1) remarked: 'I do not take the expression from a patient's mouth to always mean true giddiness . . . the investigator who simply asks leading questions . . . is not accumulating facts, but is organising confusion.' None the less, some organization of thought may help. A scheme of analysis is shown in Table 6.6.

Table 6.6 Analysis of vertigo

Duration of symptoms
Did some event precede the onset, e.g. a head injury?
Is the vertigo persistent or episodic?
If episodic,
  what is the frequency and duration of the attacks?
  what are the static or dynamic precipitating factors?
Are there associated symptoms
  suggesting a peripheral cause: tinnitus, deafness?
  suggesting a central cause: double vision?

Nausea, pallor, headache, and unsteadiness are of little help, occurring in vertigo due to both peripheral and central lesions.

Neurological disorders causing vertigo are usually due to pathological changes in the labyrinth or brain stem, or to abnormalities in the VIIIth nerve which connects them. Labyrinthine causes are usually referred to as peripheral, and brain-stem causes as central. Table 6.7 lists the common causes at each site. Before these are discussed

further, points to look for on the physical examination and the investigation of vertigo are described briefly.

On general physical examination, the presence of hypertension, cervical bruits, or peripheral arterial disease may suggest that the vertigo has a central, vascular origin. The external auditory canal and tympanic membrane should be inspected for signs of otological disease. Neurological examination should pay particular attention to hearing, stance, gait, and signs of incoordination of the limbs. Of particular importance is the examination of neighbours of cranial nerve VIII, notably the functions of V and VII. Much information is obtained from an analysis of eye movements, on account of the rich connections between vestibular and oculomotor nuclei. A gaze palsy or skew paresis (Section 6.8.4.1) will indicate that the vertigo has a central origin; deafness, a probable peripheral origin, although a plaque of demyelination at the VIIIth nerve entry zone can occasionally cause both deafness and vertigo.

6.6.2.1 *Nystagmus*

This is a convenient point to consider nystagmus, how it is caused, and the help that it may give in elucidating lesions of the labyrinth, the vestibular nuclei, and their connections.

Nystagmus is a rhythmical sequence of eye movements in opposite directions. The velocity of the movement in each direction is often different, hence one can speak of a fast phase and a slow phase. The fast component is nearly always in the direction of gaze. Nystagmus is usually not present when the eyes are in the neutral 'straight-ahead' position. It is elicited by asking the patient to follow a moving target, such as the examiner's finger. Care must be taken to remain within the binocular field, as otherwise monocular fixation may cause a few irregular jerky movements that may be mistaken for nystagmus.

A peripheral vestibular lesion affecting the horizontal semicircular canal results in unbalanced inputs to the vestibular nuclei on each side of the brain stem. A destructive peripheral lesion will allow the contralateral vestibular nucleus to dominate, with a tonic drive of the eyes towards the damaged side. The slow deviation towards the damaged side is interrupted by a quick saccadic return—the rapid beat of the nystagmus—away from the side of the lesion. An 'irritative' lesion of the labyrinth, such as may occur in Ménière's disease (Section 6.6.3.1), has an opposite effect, with rapid movement towards the side of the lesion.

Nystagmus induced by peripheral lesions is enhanced in the dark, or by some other manoeuvre which removes the power of the fixation reflex. Powerful magnifying glasses will do this, and also allow the examiner a magnified view of the eye which allows small movements to be more readily seen. In destructive vestibular lesions, closure of the eyes usually abolishes the nystagmus. In darkness, the velocity of the slow phase is induced, but the amplitude enhanced. Such examinations, of course, can only be undertaken by electrical recording of eye movements, a technique known as electronystagmography. The retinal dipole is readily picked up by surface electrodes mounted on the skin around the eye. Deviation of the globe causes shifts in the orientation of the retinal dipole relative to the electrodes. These are recorded on a machine similar to an electroencephalograph.

A nystagmus is described not only by the direction of its fast component, and by the direction of gaze by which it is induced, but also by its *degree*. A first-degree nystagmus to the left means that the nystagmus, with fast component to the left, is only present on left lateral gaze. If the fast phase to the left is present on central gaze, the nystagmus is one of second degree. If the fast phase to the left is present on looking to the right, then the nystagmus is of third degree. In practice, the vast majority of patients with nystagmus have a nystagmus of first degree.

Although a lesion of the vertical semicircular canal could, in theory, result in a vertical nystagmus, in practice all patients with a vertical or rotatory nystagmus can be assumed to have a central lesion. Occasionally, nystagmus will be present only on looking down. Such a 'down-beat nystagmus' is strongly suggestive of a lesion at the foramen magnum, such as an Arnold–Chiari malformation (Section 22.1.4).

6.6.2.2 Positional testing

Apart from observing nystagmus in different positions of gaze, the integrity of the labyrinthine and vestibulo-ocular pathways can be tested by the responses to sudden changes in position. This is

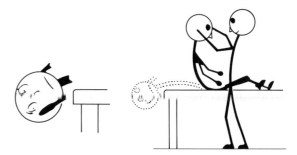

Fig. 6.6 Testing for positional nystagmus. (Reproduced by permission from the editor of *Brain*.)

illustrated in Fig. 6.6. If there is a peripheral labyrinthine lesion, there will be a short delay of a few seconds after tipping the head backwards, and then a horizontal or slightly oblique nystagmus occurs, with the fast component towards the downward ear. This is accompanied by intense vertigo. It is characteristic of peripheral lesions that the responses become less prominent, or 'fatigue', on repetition. A patient with a central (brain-stem) cause for vertigo will have immediate onset vertigo and nystagmus on positional testing, and this does not fatigue on repetition.

6.6.2.3 Caloric testing

Postional testing by rotation of the head obviously stimulates both labyrinths simultaneously. The advantage of caloric testing is that the function of each labyrinth can be individually tested. Water at 44 °C and 30 °C is irrigated through the external auditory canal. If the patient's head is at 30° to the horizontal, as it is if the backrest of the couch is elevated to this extent, then the horizontal canal becomes vertical. The conduction of heat into or away from the labyrinth induces thermal convection currents in the endolymph, and hence straining forces on the cupola.

Cold irrigation results in a slow tonic deviation towards the irrigated side, with a fast corrective component, that is the rapid phase of nystagmus, to the opposite side. As the nystagmus is always named after the direction of the fast component, the mnemonic *cows* may be useful (*c*old produces nystagmus to *o*pposite side, *w*arm to *s*ame side). With standardization of the duration of irrigation, the duration of the nystagmus can be used to assess the integrity of each labyrinth, and of the integrative functions of the vestibular pathways in the brain stem. The results are presented as shown in Fig. 6.7.

Canal paresis

A 'dead' labyrinth, e.g. due to advanced Ménière's disease, or a tumour on the vestibular component of the VIIIth nerve, will fail to transmit nerve impulses into the brain stem (Fig. 6.7, middle series).

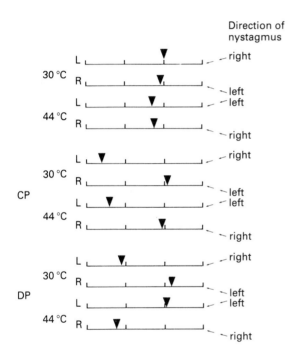

Fig. 6.7 Caloric responses. The continuous horizontal lines represent time, with minute intervals marked thereon. Irrigation of the external auditory canal with water at 30 °C and 44 °C induces nystagmus, the duration of which is marked by the solid arrowheads. Top series: normal responses; duration of nystagmus nearly 2 min for irrigation of each ear with both hot and cold water. Middle series: canal paresis (CP); the responses induced by irrigation of the left ear are substantially less than those induced from irrigation of the right ear. The abnormality must lie in the end-organ or VIII nerve. Bottom series: directional preponderance (DP); nystagmus induced to the left is greater than nystagmus induced to the right. This indicates a brain-stem lesion or distortion of the brain stem.

Directional preponderance

As Fig. 6.7 shows, the middle two traces of each series (cold right irrigation and warm left irrigation) record the duration of induced nystagmus to the left. In some brain-stem lesions, nystagmus to one side [in Fig. 6.7 (lower series) to the left] is much more prominent than to the other. This occurs in some brain-stem lesions, such as multiple sclerosis or a glioma.

6.6.3   *The causes of vertigo*

Tables 6.7, and 6.8 list some causes of vertigo. Some of these are now discussed.

Table 6.7   Causes of vertigo

Peripheral causes
    cranial trauma
    acute barotrauma (e.g. explosion)
    round or oval window rupture
    acute viral infections
    occlusion of the internal auditory artery
    Ménière's disease
    chronic bacterial otitis
Central causes
    toxic causes: alcohol and drugs
    vascular disease
    multiple sclerosis
    brain-stem tumours
    congenital lesions, e.g. Arnold–Chiari malformation
    acute vestibular neuronitis
    epilepsy
    hypoglycaemia

Tumours of the acoustic nerve seldom cause vertigo until they are big enough to distort the brain stem.

6.6.3.1   *Peripheral causes of vertigo*

Positional vertigo after cranial trauma is common. The cause is usually direct transmission of forces to the delicate labyrinth. However, in severe cases there may be some damage to the brain stem as well. Acute vertigo may also occur in association with an endolymphatic leak due to rupture of the round or oval window. This may occur spontaneously, or as the result of barotrauma, such as from an explosion.

A common cause of vertigo in family and

Table 6.8 Distinction of the various causes of vertigo

	Vertigo	Deafness	Tinnitus	Effect of changes in position	Results of caloric testing	Nystagmus on lateral gaze at rest
Benign positional vertigo	only on changing position	0	0	nystagmus ++ latency of a few seconds, fatigues on repetition	normal	0
Ménière's disease	episodic	+ → +++	++	nil in between episodes	canal paresis	0
Central lesions, e.g. infarct	+ worse on changing position	0 (unless VIII entry zone affected)	0	nystagmus +++, no latency, does not fatigue	directional preponderance	+ → +++
Cerebello-pontine angle tumour	late in course	early	±	not prominent	canal paresis and later directional preponderance	late in course
Cerebellar lesions	usually ataxia only	0	0	not prominent	may have directional preponderance	often nil

Cerebellar lesions result in nystagmus if the vestibular connections are involved, but not if the disorder is confined to the cerebellar cortex.

specialist practice is the entity known as *benign positional vertigo*. An otherwise healthy patient notices acute vertigo on changing position, often when turning over in bed. The occurrences of vertigo gradually diminish in frequency and in intensity over several weeks or months. The cause is believed to be otolith debris arising from a degenerate utricle. This collects upon the cupola of the posterior semicircular canal. In other subjects a similar syndrome appears to follow an acute viral infection. The diagnosis of an '*acute labyrinthitis*' is then made, even though pathological evidence is lacking. Those with chronic bacterial infections of the middle ear may have episodes of true acute labyrinthitis from time to time when their bacterial infection is more than usually active.

Acute vestibular neuronitis
This obscure condition results in vertigo similar to that experienced by those suffering from benign positional vertigo, from which it is separated only by the facts that occasionally small epidemics occur, suggesting a viral infection, and that, in contrast to benign positional vertigo, the caloric responses are abnormal.

Ménière's disease
Ménière's disease is characterized by recurrent episodes of vertigo, which may be prostrating, usually preceded by, or associated with, tinnitus (Section 6.7.1) or a sense of fullness in the ear. The disorder is due to increased endolymphatic pressure, but what causes this is totally unclear. After each episode, a little more hearing is lost, and eventually hearing may be totally lost. Treatment is often unsatisfactory, but there may be some benefit from betahistine. In severe cases it may be justifiable to destroy the labyrinth in order to prevent the recurrent attacks, and pre-empt the natural progression of the disease.

6.6.3.2 *Central causes of vertigo*

Table 6.7 lists some central causes of vertigo. Many older patients are labelled with a diagnosis of 'vertebro-basilar insufficiency' as the cause of episodic vertigo, but unless there is clear evidence of other transient brain-stem dysfunction, for example dysarthria or double vision, this is probably not justifiable. Older patients may well have

benign positional vertigo, as described above, and not arterial disease.

Other causes of vertigo
Occasional vertigo may be an initial symptom of a complex partial seizure (Section 12.4.1) or of hypoglycaemia. Alcohol and anticonvulsant drugs, particularly phenytoin and barbiturates, often produce vertigo if taken to excess.

6.7 Tinnitus and deafness

6.7.1 *Tinnitus*

Tinnitus is an unformed auditory hallucination of sound, usually of a whistling or pulsating nature. It is often combined with a sensorineural deafness, such as may occur with degeneration of the hair cells of the cochlea due to age, acoustic trauma, or Ménière's disease. Occasionally, tinnitus may arise through the auditory perception of a real bruit in the head, such as may be associated with a carotico-cavernous fistula. Tinnitus may intrude greatly into conscious awareness, and may be associated with depression. It is best treated with a masker, a device that produces noise across a broad range of frequencies—'white noise'. Many people find this less obtrusive than their own tinnitus. Pharmacological treatment of tinnitus is largely ineffective, although betahistine is widely used.

6.7.2 *Deafness*

Deafness due to middle-ear disease can be distinguished from that of sensorineural deafness, of greater interest to a neurologist, by tuning-fork tests. A 256 Hz tuning fork should be used, not the 128 Hz fork used for testing vibration sense (Section 6.3.1.1). In sensorineural deafness, hearing when the fork is placed adjacent to the external auditory meatus (air conduction) is better than when it is placed over the mastoid process (bone conduction), when the sound is conducted through the mastoid process to the ossicular chain. It is best to describe the result of the Rinne test, as this procedure is known, rather than just record 'Rinne positive' or 'negative', which causes confusion. It is essential to mask the contralateral ear, in which hearing may be so much better than in the ear under test that the tone is heard in the contralateral ear, concealing the extent and type of deafness. In practice, in any neurological case in which documentation of the type and extent of deafness is important, pure-tone audiometry is usually performed.

Some causes of sensorineural deafness are listed in Table 6.9.

Table 6.9   Causes of sensorineural deafness

End-organ	Advancing age
	Occupational acoustic trauma
	Ménière's disease
Nerve lesions	Acoustic neuroma
	Cranial trauma
	Inflammatory lesions
	neurosyphilis
	tuberculosis
	sarcoidosis
	Carcinomatous meningitis
Brain-stem lesions	Multiple sclerosis } damage to entry zone
	Lateral infarction } of cochlear nerve

6.8   Disorders of vision

Lesions of the visual pathways give rise to characteristic defects in acuity and in the visual fields. Disorders are best considered from the retina, proceeding backwards along the visual pathways, in conjunction with Fig. 6.1.

6.8.1   *Visual acuity*

Visual acuity is measured by a Snellen chart. The letters on the chart are constructed so that the height of the top letter at 60 m subtends the same angle at the retina as do the height of the letters on the 6 m line (usually the line next but one to the bottom) at 6 m. If a subject can read the 6 m line at 6 m, his acuity is said to be 6/6. If he can only manage the 60 m line at 6 m, his acuity is 6/60.

A neurologist, in general, is not interested in refractive errors, so visual acuity is always tested with the subject wearing his or her distance spectacles if appropriate. If these are not available, then any refractive error can be corrected by a pinhole, which functions as a perfect lens. However,

excellent illumination is necessary as the aperture is so small. Any residual failure of acuity after correction must have an ocular or neurological cause.

6.8.1.1   *Acuity and the visual field*

The concept illustrated in Fig. 6.8a, b is useful, first introduced by Traquair.

Imagine a South Pacific island (Fig. 6.8a, seen in cross-section in Fig. 6.8b). The ordinate scale at the left, instead of indicating height in metres, indicates increasing visual acuity. The abscissa

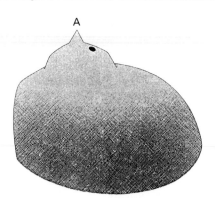

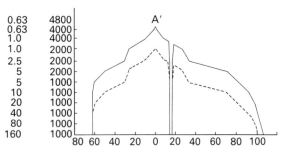

Fig. 6.8 Traquair's drawings of the field of vision; (a) regarded as an island and (b) seen in section. The horizontal abscissa ('sea-level') indicates the extent of the field in degrees; the ordinate, visual acuity for objects of different diameters (left hand column, mm) at different distances (right hand column, mm). For example, the apex of the hill (solid line) shows that an object 1.0 mm in diameter at 4000 mm can only be seen in the central 10° of vision. The deep chasm is the blind spot. A paracentral scotoma may be imagined as a deep crater near fixation. The dotted line indicates the alteration induced by a *uniform* depression of the visual field. (Redrawn from Traquair's *Clinical Perimetry* 1957.)

Hospital No. A. 45379

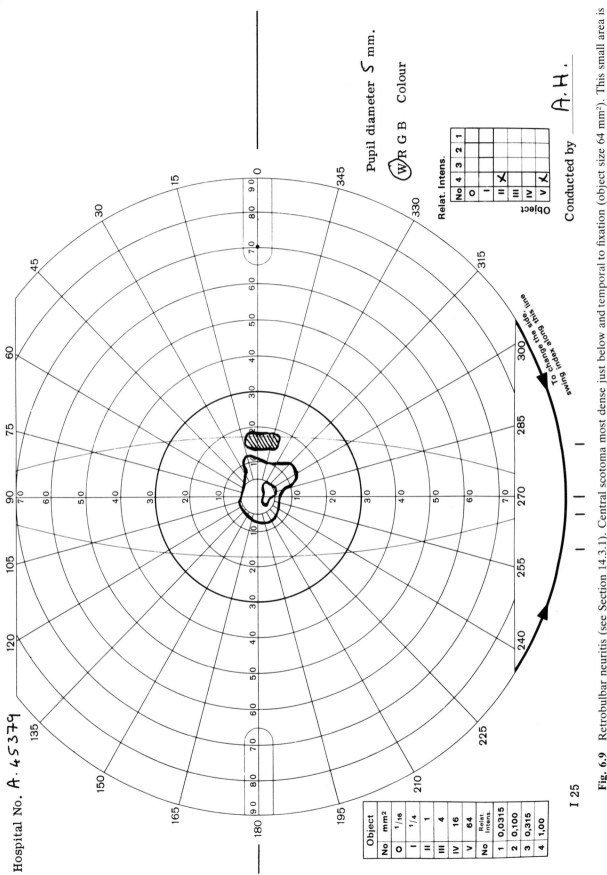

Pupil diameter 5 mm.

Ⓦ R G B   Colour

	No 4	3	2	1
O				
I				
II	✗			
III				
IV	✗			
V	✗			

Relat. Intens.

Object

Conducted by ___A. H.___

I 25

Object		
No	mm²	
O	1/16	
I	1/4	
II	1	
III	4	
IV	16	
V	64	

No	Relat. Intens.
1	0,0315
2	0,100
3	0,315
4	1,00

To change along this side:
swing index line

Fig. 6.9 Retrobulbar neuritis (see Section 14.3.1). Central scotoma most dense just below and temporal to fixation (object size 64 mm²). This small area is surrounded by the isoptre for the 1 mm² object. The blind spot is diagonally hatched.

represents not minutes of latitude or longitude as it would in a cross-section of a real island, but degrees away from fixation. The high peak on the island represents the excellent acuity at the macula. Acuity falls steeply at first over the central 10° adjacent to fixation, and then more slowly towards the 'sea level' of blindness outside the field of vision, about 70° away from fixation. The deep chasm on the temporal side of the island represents the blind spot—the part of the fundus occupied by the optic nerve, and devoid, therefore, of rods and cones.

The visual field, as usually plotted, translates the island into a contour map. A contour on a map joins up all points of equal height above sea-level. The analogous line on our map of visual acuity joins up all points of equal visual acuity. These lines are known as isoptres. The acuity at each point in the field is measured by a small object—a disc on a Bjerrum's screen, or a small circle of light on a Goldman scotometer. The relationship between the diameter of the disc (e.g. 2 mm) or circle of light, and the distance of the fovea from it (e.g. 2 m) is the tangent of the angle subtended by the disc. Isoptres join up all points at which the same visual angles can be distinguished.

Figure 6.9 illustrates the isoptre map of a patient with a large central scotoma due to multiple sclerosis.

6.8.2 Causes of monocular visual failure

Monocular impairment of acuity that cannot be improved by good illumination, refraction, or a pin-hole must be due to an impairment of that eye or its optic nerve. If not due to a cataract or other mechanical interruption of the transmission of light, or amblyopia (see below), the problem must lie in the retina or optic nerve anterior to the chiasma. Retinal lesions may be due to detachment or infarction. Infarction may be segmental (retinal branch artery occlusion) or total, due to central retinal artery occlusion. Central venous thrombosis also occurs, with venous retinal engorgement and infarction. These and some other causes of a monocular visual defect are listed in Table 6.10.

The special problem of amblyopia must be mentioned briefly. This has been greatly illuminated by the experimental work of Hubel and Wiesel. If a child is born with a major refractive error in one eye, retinal connections from the other eye make

Table 6.10 Causes of optic nerve lesions

Causes of lesions of one optic nerve
  Vascular lesions
    ischaemic optic neuropathy
    occlusion of central retinal artery or vein
    arteritis
      cranial arteritis
      syphilitic arteritis
  Trauma
    direct damage to nerve, commonly by fractures
  Tumour involving anterior cranial fossa, glioma,
    especially in neurofibromatosis
  Compression
    local compression by, for example, meningioma at
      sphenoid wing
  Retrobulbar neuritis

Causes of lesions of both optic nerves
  Papilloedema
    due to raised intracranial pressure
  Bilateral retrobulbar neuritis
  Toxic amblyopia—tobacco, alcohol, methanol
  Leber's optic atrophy
  Vitamin B_{12} deficiency

preferential connections in the lateral geniculate body and occipital cortex, as the brain matures during the first 2–4 years of life. Even if the refractive error is corrected after that age, it is too late for function to be restored. The retina and optic nerve of an amblyopic eye look perfectly normal on fundoscopy. It is the failure of physiological connections that results in an absence of useful function. Similar preferential connections are made if the child is born with a squint, and one eye then becomes amblyopic unless the squint is corrected sufficiently early.

6.8.3 Visual field defects due to lesions at different sites

Figure 6.1 illustrates some of the field defects that may be caused by lesions at different sites. The fibres from the nasal half of each retina, receiving images from the temporal fields of each eye, decussate in the chiasma. It follows that a lesion impinging on the decussation will produce a bitemporal hemianopia, beginning in the upper quadrants if the lesion is arising from below the chiasma (e.g. a large pituitary tumour), or in the lower quadrants if the lesion is arising from above (e.g. pressure from a dilated third ventricle in hydrocephalus).

Behind the chiasma, the optic tract and radiation contain uncrossed fibres from the temporal ipsilateral retina, and crossed fibres from the nasal contralateral retina. Inspection of Fig. 6.1 will show that a lesion of the right optic tract or radiation will therefore affect images received from the left nasal and right temporal retinae, both of which receive light rays from the left visual field. Lesions of the optic tract produce contralateral more-or-less homonymous scotomata, or, if larger, hemianopia. Lesions in the upper (parietal) part of the optic radiation produce a contralateral hemianopic loss, worse in the lower quadrants, whereas lesions in the temporal lobe, anteriorly affecting Meyer's loop of the radiation, produce a contralateral defect that begins in the upper quadrants. An occipital cortical lesion will produce a congruous crossed hemianopic deficit. If the lesion spares the tip of the occipital pole, the macular field may be spared.

6.8.4   *Double vision*

Double vision (diplopia) occurs if two images of a single object are perceived at two different points in space. It occurs if the ocular axes are not parallel, so that an object is not projected on to corresponding areas of the two retinae. Diplopia can be experienced by the reader if he looks at a distant object, at the same time displacing one eyeball medially by pushing with the index finger over the outer canthus, keeping the eye open.

Diplopia is an unpleasant experience. Most patients with a sudden diplopia will keep one eye shut if they cannot re-orient their head in order to keep single vision.

The position of the eyes is determined by the external ocular muscles. Their directions of action are shown in Fig. 6.10. The superior and inferior rectus muscles elevate and depress the abducted eye. The superior and inferior obliques depress and elevate the adducted eye.

From a knowledge of the direction of muscles shown in Fig. 6.10 and from the following rules, the affected muscle in a diplopia of recent onset can always be worked out.

The most peripheral image (the uppermost, the most lateral, the downmost) is always derived from the eye with the weak muscle. As a non-foveal retinal point is being stimulated in the eye with the weak muscle, the image from that eye appears less distinct.

The separation of images increases as the object is moved in the direction of action of the weak muscle. For example, in a left lateral rectus weakness there is *no* diplopia on looking to the right, nor straight ahead, but lateral displacement of images occurs on left lateral gaze, and the displacement increases as the object is moved farther and farther to the left.

In practice, many patients and examiners find the elucidation of a diplopia less than easy. Resourceful examiners will identify the images projected on to either retina by using spectacles with one lens red and the other lens green. It is then easy for the patient to explain the relative position of the red and green images.

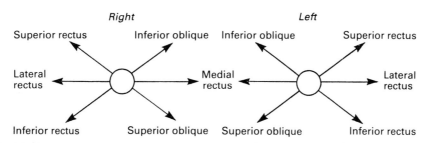

Fig. 6.10 The principal directions of actions of the external ocular muscles in each eye, drawn as the examiner faces the patient. For example, gaze upwards and to the right (dextroelevation) is undertaken by the right superior rectus and left inferior oblique muscles. There are also secondary actions of the muscles. The superior oblique and superior rectus muscles rotate (twist) the eyes inwards—intorsion. The inferior oblique and inferior rectus extort the eyes. In practice, torsion is only seen if there is an imbalance of action; for example, in the presence of a III nerve palsy, the superior oblique muscle will intort the eye on attempted adduction if the IV nerve is intact.

Table 6.11 Physical signs due to lesions of cranial nerves III, IV and VI

Cranial nerve	Muscles supplied	Physical signs
III	Superior rectus Medial rectus Inferior rectus Inferior oblique Levator palpebrae superioris Constrictor pupillae	Ptosis; dilated pupil; resting position of eye is down and out, due to unopposed actions of lateral rectus muscle; vertical separation of images, with tilt
IV	Superior oblique	Difficult to detect in isolation, but diplopia worse on looking down and away from affected side (towards tip of nose)
VI	Lateral rectus	Diplopia on lateral gaze to side of lesion

Diplopia may be due to local orbital lesions displacing the globe, to lesions of the muscles and neuromuscular junction (myasthenia gravis), to cranial nerve lesions, or to nuclear or internuclear lesions within the brain stem. The diplopia of myasthenia is virtually impossible to 'sort out', as the fatigue of neuromuscular transmission constantly alters the effectiveness of external ocular contraction. The signs caused by lesions of the IIIrd, IVth, and VIth cranial nerves are shown in Table 6.11. Once an ocular palsy has been present for more than a few weeks, then secondary changes occur, with contracture of the unopposed antagonist muscles. The resulting imbalance will need elucidation with a Hess test—a method of projecting the field of action of the imbalanced muscles.

6.8.4.1 Gaze palsy

A paralysis of conjugate movement of the two eyes in the same direction is known as a gaze palsy. For example, looking horizontally to the right requires the simultaneous and coordinated action of the right lateral rectus and the left medial rectus muscles, which must maintain a moving object of attention exactly on the fovea of each eye. Lateral gaze to the right can be induced by stimulation of the contralateral frontal lobe. A large frontal infarction therefore may result in a paralysis of this tonic direction of gaze, leaving the intact hemisphere to deviate the eyes towards the side of the lesion. There are also pontine gaze centres near each abducens nucleus, stimulation of which turns

the eyes to the side stimulated, and a lesion of which prevents the gaze of both eyes to that side.

Any lesion affecting the bundles of axons connecting the nuclei of the IIIrd, IVth, and VIth cranial nerves will result in a breakdown of conjugate gaze. The best-known example is a lesion, often demyelinating, that affects the medial longitudinal bundle, which connects the rostral IIIrd and IVth nuclei with the more caudal VIth nerve nucleus. When gaze is directed to the right, the left eye fails to adduct; when gaze is directed to the left, the right eye fails to adduct. There is also often nystagmus of greater amplitude in the abducting eye. As the lesion is in the bundle of axons connecting the nuclei of cranial nerves III, IV, and VI, this syndrome is often known as an *internuclear ophthalmoplegia*.

6.9   Spinal cord syndromes

The spinal cord may be compressed by what is known as an *extramedullary lesion* that takes up space in the spinal canal. Examples include extruded disc material and spondylotic bars (Section 18.2.3.1), or extramedullary tumours such as spinal meningiomas or metastases within vertebral bodies (see Table 18.1). Lesions within the spinal cord are known as intramedullary lesions. Examples include a plaque of demyelination (Section 14.1.4), or an astrocytoma (Section 18.5.3). Severe spinal trauma usually causes haemorrhage within and compression and distortion from out-side the spinal cord (Section 18.1.2).

Whatever the nature of the lesion, it is useful to think in segmental terms in order to define the anatomical site of the lesion. There will be inter-ruption of some sensory and motor functions below (caudal to) the level of the lesion. In the most obvious terms, a lesion of the dorsal spinal cord will affect the lower limbs, but leave the upper limbs unaffected. Usually a precise indication of the first involved segment preceding caudally can be defined by reference to Table 6.3, which indi-cates the principal spinal segment that supplies muscles that are easy to test. A common spinal injury, for example, is caused by diving into shal-low water (Section 18.1.1). The spinal cord is, in these circumstances, frequently damaged by hyperextension of the cervical spine, with injury to the C6/C7 segmental region. If C6 segment is intact, then the subject will retain abduction of the shoulder (deltoid muscle, C5), and flexion of the elbow (biceps muscle, C6). If C7 segment is severely damaged, he will have prominent weak-ness of extension of the elbow (triceps muscle, C7), and pyramidal signs (see Section 6.2.3) and sensory disturbance below. Sometimes a motor 'level' is more easily ascertained, sometimes a sensory level, this being the case particularly in thoracic spinal lesions, where testing the power of intercostal muscles is not practical. In early lesions, the level of the spinal segment involved may be given by the reflexes. For example, a lesion at C6 may depress the biceps and brachioradialis (supi-nator) reflexes, as these muscles are innervated by the C6 segment, but exaggerate the triceps reflex (C7), due to the partial interruption of the pyram-idal tracts as they pass through the damaged C6 segment.

Some features help distinguish extramedullary and intramedullary lesions.

6.9.1 *Extramedullary lesions*

Let us take as an example a meningioma growing at segmental level D10, on the left side of the spinal canal. As the meningioma takes up more and more room, the cord will first be pushed away, and then compressed. The patient will usually note dragging of the leg on the same side as the lesion, in this case the left, and pyramidal signs will first appear in this leg. Symptoms and pyramidal signs

will follow in the right leg as further distortion of the cord occurs. The arms, of course, will not be affected. Sensory impairment will then occur, affecting all modalities more-or-less equally, but it is unlikely that sensory loss will be severe until late in the progression of the expansion of the tumour. All areas of the skin below the level of the lesion are likely to be equally affected (compared to an intramedullary lesion, below).

Fibres controlling micturition lie just medial to the descending pyramidal tracts, and urgency of micturition is common. Impotence also occurs.

In the particular example described, the segmen-tal level of the lesion may be signalled also by a band of radicular pain in the tenth thoracic der-matome (Fig. 6.3). Remember that, as the spinal cord is considerably shorter than the vertebral spinal column, spinal cord segment D10 does not lie opposite vertebral body D10. Table 18.3 indi-cates the equivalent vertebral levels of different examples of spinal levels.

6.9.2 *Intramedullary lesions*

Examples of intramedullary lesions include pri-mary tumours, such as astrocytomas and ependy-momas (Section 18.5.3), syringomyelia (Section 18.5.4.1), vascular infarcts (Section 18.5.2), and, most frequently, a plaque of demyelination in association with multiple sclerosis (Section 14.3.3 and 18.5.1).

A centrally placed lesion, such as a syrinx or ependymoma, initially destroys the spinothalamic pathways subserving pain and temperature as they cross in front of the central canal to form the spinothalamic pathways. As the dorsal columns are usually spared, at least initially, sensory examina-tion shows a *dissociated sensory loss*, with impair-ment of painful and thermal sensations, and preservation of vibration sense and sense of passive movement. As the fibres from the sacral area are laminated on the periphery of the ascending spi-nothalamic tracts, centrifugal expansion of a cen-trally placed lesion affects these last, so there is 'sacral sparing' of impairment of pain and thermal sensation. This may help to distinguish an intra-medullary lesion from extramedullary compres-sion. Compression or destruction of the descending corticospinal pathways results in a spastic para-paresis below the level of the lesion, and bladder involvement is also common. Further clinico-pathological correlations of a centrally placed intra-medullary lesion, such as a syrinx, are described in Section 18.5.4.1.

A lesion placed laterally in the spinal cord, usually a plaque of demyelination, results in some of the features first described by Brown-Séquard in his experiments on hemisection of the cord. Consider a left-sided lesion. This will affect conduction in descending pyramidal fibres, causing weakness of the left leg, increased reflexes on the left, and a left extensor plantar response. There may also be impairment of the sense of passive movement and vibration sense on the left, due to involvement of the left posterior columns. However, as the spinothalamic tract on the left is taking upwards fibres that have crossed in front of the central canal from the right side of the body, there will be impairment of pain and thermal sensation from the *right* side of the body below the level of the lesion. So the patient may say in this instance 'My left foot drags, and my right leg feels cold and numb.'

Spinal cord syndromes are considered in further detail in Chapter 18.

6.10   The cauda equina syndrome

The spinal cord terminates at the lower borders of the body of L2. Any of the pathological processes described under extramedullary symptoms above can take up space within the lumbar spinal canal, but instead of resulting in compression of the spinal cord, below this level they result in compression of the cauda equina. For example, a large central disc protrusion at L4/L5 may result in compression not only of the L5 roots bilaterally, but also all sacral roots as they stream caudally. The patient will lose control of his sphincters, and be aware of numbness of the buttocks and the backs of his thighs. The distribution of weakness, which will of course be of lower motor neuron type, is dependent upon the level at which the cauda equina is compressed, but commonly the foot becomes flail, with paralysis of dorsiflexion of the foot (L4) and toes (L4, L5), and of eversion and plantarflexion (S1).

It is sometimes difficult to distinguish an acute lesion of the cauda equina from, for example, an acute plaque of demyelination in the conus medullaris, the lowermost part of the spinal cord. In both cases, there will be loss of sphincter control, and

weakness and sensory loss. In an *acute* conus lesion, all tendon reflexes in the legs may be lost, as they are in a high cauda equina syndrome. Depending, however, on the extent of a conus lesion, there may be signs suggestive of an intramedullary lesion, such as dissociated sensory loss (Section 18.5.4.1), or a Brown-Séquard lesion (Section 6.9.2), and the plantar responses may be extensor.

A patient who is numb to the waist (T8) and who has weakness of hip flexion (L1) clearly must have a lower cord lesion rather than a cauda equina lesion, as both motor and sensory levels are too high for the latter.

6.11   Urinary incontinence

Some degree of urinary incontinence is a common problem in the population. Surveys show that about one half of all women occasionally leak small quantities of urine when exercising physically (stress incontinence), and many older men are troubled by post-micturition dribbling associated with benign prostatic hypertrophy. About 2 per cent of the population are sufficiently troubled by some degree of incontinence to seek medical advice, most of them in the sixth and later decades.

Acute retention in men is a common symptom of benign prostatic hypertrophy, and in either sex this may occur as a result of the impaction of a urinary stone or blood clot in the bladder neck or proximal urethra.

A small proportion of all cases of retention or urinary incontinence will be found to have a neurological cause. A successful policy of restoring urinary control is a major determinant in rehabilitation and of long-term survival after spinal injuries.

6.11.1   *Physiology of control of the bladder musculature and urinary sphincter*

The smooth muscle of the lower urinary tract has, like all cells, a transmembrane potential. As the muscle is stretched, this transmembrane potential becomes smaller. To this extent, therefore, the muscle is its own stretch receptor, becoming more readily depolarized and ready to contract per unit of neurotransmitter release.

Afferent impulses recording the degree of bladder-wall tension are generated from tension receptors in series with the detrusor smooth muscle contractile fibres. They will, therefore, discharge in response both to passive dilatation of the bladder, and to detrusor contraction. The afferent fibres from these tension receptors pass in the pelvic nerves to the sacral segments 2–4 of the spinal cord. Somatic afferents also record exteroceptive sensations, such as pain. Efferent pathways from the lower sacral segments pass both in the parasympathetic pelvic nerves, and also in the pudendal nerves. The efferent parasympathetic nerves pass through the hypogastric plexus without synapsing, but then do synapse on post-ganglionic neurons in the bladder wall.

If we consider first the 'local' innervation, it is clear that control of bladder emptying could be self-sustaining. Gradual filling of the bladder from the ureters leads to progressive smooth muscle depolarization and hence readiness to contract. Afferent impulses from tension receptors in series in the bladder wall synapse in the cord with parasympathetic efferents, which in turn synapse with second-order neurons in the bladder wall, causing detrusor contraction and emptying of the bladder. There are, however, layers of complexity superimposed upon this local reflex.

First of all, detrusor contraction is unlikely to be sufficient to overcome the sphincter mechanism unless there is some way in which the sphincter mechanism can be 'turned off' as the detrusor muscle contracts. The internal urinary sphincter is constructed of striated muscle, innervated by axons in the pudendal nerve. These arise from a collection of anterior horn cells in sacral segments 2 and 3, known as Onuf's nucleus. In voluntary voiding of urine, the tonic discharge in Onuf's neurons is inhibited, allowing the internal sphincter to relax.

Secondly, it is known that the bladder neck receives a rich sympathetic innervation, arising from the thoracolumbar outflow and passing to the smooth muscle of the bladder neck in the presacral nerves and synapsing in the hypogastric plexus. It is not known how significant is the sympathetic control of the bladder neck in voluntary voiding, but it is certainly significant in ejaculation, preventing reflux of ejaculate into the bladder.

Thirdly, we are all aware that the desire to void urine can be inhibited for social reasons. One supraspinal mechanism is a loop passing between the superior frontal gyrus and the dorsal lateral tegmental nucleus of the pons. From this pontine nucleus descends a further pathway in the reticulospinal tracts to the sacral spinal cord.

6.11.1.1 Neurological abnormalities of bladder function

Injuries of the spinal cord
After a spinal cord injury, there will be a period of spinal 'shock' during which all bladder reflexes—just as tendon reflexes—are lost. Detrusor contractions then return after a period of a few weeks. In many patients, local reflexes as described above lead to the establishment of an 'automatic bladder', one that empties when it is filled by a sufficient volume. It is often possible to train this automatic bladder to empty at convenient times, either by increasing the intravesical pressure by manual pressure on the lower abdomen, or by providing further afferent input to the reflex by, for example, stroking the inner side of the thighs.

Disorders of the cauda equina
An acute central lumbar disc protrusion may result in acute retention of urine by disruption of detrusor afferent and efferent supply. A large atonic bladder with no detrusor contractions also occurs for similar reasons in many children with spina bifida and meningocele.

Disorders of the nerves in the pelvic floor
Electromyography of the urethral sphincter and adjacent pelvic muscle floor has shown evidence of chronic partial denervation and re-innervation (Section 8.7.1.2) in some women with retention of urine and/or incontinence. In some cases, damage to the nerves in the pelvic floor is clearly secondary to pelvic surgery. In others, it appears that the initial damage to the pelvic and pudendal nerves occurs at the time of childbirth, but then is exacerbated by repeated descent of the pelvic floor during straining at stool or during subsequent childbirth. The same explanation is probably responsible for some cases of ano-rectal incontinence in older women.

Disorders of somatic afferent supply
A large atonic bladder may occur in tabes dorsalis

and in diabetics with neuropathy, although in the latter case defects of autonomic function are also important.

Disorders of autonomic function

Patients with multiple system atrophy (Section 13.2) commonly have a large distended bladder with weak detrusor contractions. This is due probably in part to degenerative changes in the pontine nuclei and also basal ganglia, which have some function in control of bladder contractions and voiding. Patients with multiple system atrophy also have difficulty in voluntarily contracting the pelvic floor and striated sphincters in order to prevent leakage. These sphincters are innervated by Onuf's nucleus in sacral segments 2–3 (p. 57). Although in the anterior horn, and connected to striated muscle, Onuf's neurons must be significantly different from the vast majority of anterior spinal motor neurons. First of all, they are not affected by motor neuron disease (Section 20.1.2), although they are commonly affected in multiple system atrophies (Section 13.2). Secondly, they are unusual in maintaining a tonic discharge and contraction of the striated muscle fibre to which they are attached. It is of great interest that the only other muscle fibres known to be in a state of tonic contraction—the cricoarytenoid muscle, which is constantly active to maintain abduction of the vocal cords—is also affected in some cases of multiple system atrophy.

Frontal lobe disorders

Patients may lose social control of micturition, voiding inappropriately and without embarrassment, following damage to the medial frontal lobes, as may occur following, for example, a bleed from or a repair of an anterior communicating aneurysm. Social control of voiding is also gradually lost in Alzheimer's disease and other dementing illnesses.

6.11.1.2   *Urge-incontinence and its treatment*

The foregoing sections describe briefly the different anatomical and physiological causes of incontinence. In neurological practice, by far the commonest clinical type of incontinence is a desire to void very soon (urgency) followed by incontinence (urge-incontinence). This syndrome is particularly common in patients with multiple sclerosis and other spinal lesions. It is due to failure of synergic action between detrusor contractions and continuing tonic discharge of the internal sphincter so that a little urine escapes into the posterior urethra, thereby stimulating an urgent desire to micturate, and increasing intravesical pressure through increased detrusor contractions. The internal sphincter may then be inhibited, causing flow of more urine incontinently.

Urge-incontinence is best first treated by bladder training, that is to say an individualized schedule of voiding at certain hours, and not before the due hour, in order to maintain cortical control over spinal centres. It is also helpful to ensure easy access to the lavatory by suitable structural modifications and by adjustments to clothing. This may reduce some of the anxiety that is felt in relation to urgency and associated incontinence, an anxiety which may prove self-fulfilling. It is also right to ensure that urgency is not associated with urinary infection, commonplace in those with large residual volumes of urine after voiding.

However, many patients with, for example, multiple sclerosis or other spinal cord lesions require further help. Anticholinergic drugs such as propantheline hydrobromide (15 mg three times a day) successfully inhibit the detrusor contractions that occur at low bladder volumes and raise intravesical pressure. Another approach is to deafferent partly the bladder neck by the subtrigonal injection of phenol. For those with recurrent urinary infections resulting in urge-incontinence, long-term antibacterial treatment may well be useful, but resistant bacterial strains soon emerge. An alternative is to reduce bladder outflow obstruction by an α-adrenergic antagonist, such as phenoxybenzamine, or by transurethral resection of the bladder neck.

6.11.1.3   *Other measures for the management of incontinence*

For a few patients who are incontinent and whose spinal efferent pathway remains intact, it is worth considering the implantation of sacral nerve root stimulators. Their exact mechanism of action is not certain—it is probably more than simple maintenance of a tonic discharge to the striated sphincters. For carefully selected patients, sacral nerve root stimulation may prove dramatically successful.

Of more everyday use is the provision of appropriate aids for those whose incontinence is not controlled by some of the measures suggested above. For those who only leak a little urine, hydrophilic pads with a 'one way' backing worn in a pouch in a pair of knickers or trunks may be very useful. For men who leak larger amounts, the best solution is a penile sheath secured around the penis and draining to a leg-bag taped to the calf. Unfortunately there is as yet no satisfactory device for securing a collecting system externally to the vulva, and women with profuse incontinence may need to drain the bladder continuously through a catheter. For those with high residual volumes and overflow incontinence, intermittent self-catheterization is the better solution, if the neurological disorder allows sufficient manual dexterity, as rates of symptomatic infection are substantially lower than with continuous drainage. For some women ureteric diversion to a loop of ileum opening through an abdominal stoma may prove a successful solution, as the flat abdominal surface allows the successful watertight application of a standard ileostomy bag.

6.11.1.4 *Investigation of incontinence*

The vast majority of incontinent men and women are 'sorted out' by urologists and gynaecologists. For those with established neurological disease, joint investigation will include microscopical examination and culture of a mid-stream or catheter specimen, a cystometrogram, and often an intravenous urogram or video micturating cystogram. Cystometrography in normal subjects shows a slow rise in pressure as the bladder is filled. The first desire to void is felt at about 150 ml, and there is a marked sense of fullness by about 450 ml, with little further rise in pressure between these volumes. This is related to the law of Laplace, which links radius (R), pressure (P), and tension (T) in a hollow body $[P = (2T/R)]$. As the bladder becomes full in a normal subject, pressure rises sharply just before voiding. Disinhibited detrusor contractions, as may occur in spinal cord lesions, are revealed by irregular increases in pressure occurring at low infusion volumes. Atonic deafferented bladders receive large volumes of fluid with very little increase in pressure. Micturating video cystometrograms, combined with sphincter electromyography, allow the best possible analysis of possible dysynergies between bladder and sphincter contractions.

6.12 Impotence

Impairment of sexual function may arise from neurological disorders affecting the brain, spinal cord, and peripheral nerves. It is a frequent neurological symptom, though often not volunteered by reticent patients. Because patients, and indeed many doctors, are not used to talking about sexual activity, it is important to understand the vocabulary used.

Libido is sexual desire or, more briefly, lust. Potency is the ability to maintain an erection of sufficient rigidity that the vagina can be penetrated. Priapism is an erection that won't go away. Statues of Priaps, the Greek and Roman god of love, were often placed in gardens. Priapism may occur as a disinhibited erectile reflex in the early days after a spinal injury. It is also seen in patients with sickle-cell anaemia or leukaemia who have thrombosed veins draining erectile tissue. Emission is the emission of semen at the external urethral orifice. Ejaculation is emission accompanied by a brief series of rhythmic movements of the pelvic floor. Orgasm is the pleasurable feeling of sexual crisis that is largely, though by no means exclusively, referred to the genitals. Disjunctions of these various components can occur. For example, normal erections that are not necessarily libidinous occur on waking in the morning. Impotence with preserved libido may occur in cauda equina lesions. Preserved potency with impaired libido suggests dissatisfaction with the present sexual partner. Orgasm can occur without emission, and ejaculation without erection.

The blood flow through the cavernosal space in the flaccid penis is about 2 ml/min. During erection the penis can swell at a rate exceeding 100 ml/min. Both inflow and outflow channels for erection are neurally mediated. It used to be said that the obstruction to venous outflow was entirely mechanical in nature, as the intracavernosal pressure approaches the mean arterial pressure. However, if a balloon cuff is placed around an erect penis and inflated, so that further inflow cannot occur, the rate of shrinkage is faster if sexual stimulation is withdrawn than if it continues.

The nature of the neurotransmitters to the smooth muscles controlling arterial inflow and

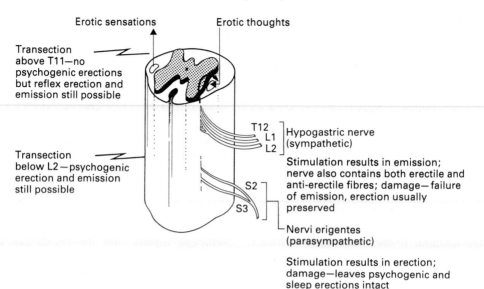

Erotic sensations   Erotic thoughts

Transection
above T11—no
psychogenic erections
but reflex erection and
emission still possible

T12
L1   Hypogastric nerve
L2   (sympathetic)

Stimulation results in emission;
nerve also contains both erectile and
anti-erectile fibres; damage—failure
of emission, erection usually
preserved

Transection
below L2—psychogenic
erection and emission
still possible

S2

S3

Nervi erigentes
(parasympathetic)

Stimulation results in erection;
damage—leaves psychogenic and
sleep erections intact

Fig. 6.11   Some of the pathways involved in sexual activity.

smooth muscles controlling arterial inflow and venous egress is uncertain. The intracavernosal injection of the α-adrenergic blockers, phenoxy-benzamine or thymoxamine, causes erections lasting for longer or shorter periods of time. However, it has also been noted that the intravenous infusion of a dopaminergic agent, such as bromocriptine, results in erection after a very short latency. Vasoactive peptide receptors have also been demonstrated.

Figure 6.11 shows some of the pathways involved in sexual activity. Stimulation of the upper part of the post-central gyrus in men results in a unilateral genital sensation, but without any erotic overtone. On the other hand, lesions on the medial surface of the hemisphere have been reported to result in sexually enjoyable sensations—sometimes unilateral, a phenomenon hard to imagine. Lesions in the temporal lobe may cause seizures with sexual imagery and, occasionally, result in a seizure in which the movements of intercourse occur. Much more commonly, however, lesions in the temporal lobe result in erectile impotence. Occasionally an impotent patient with complex partial seizures has potency restored by control of the seizures. Hypothalamic lesions may cause impotence, and frontal lobe lesions sexual disinhibition.

The information obtained from cordotomies car-ried out for the relief of pain suggests that pleasurable sexual sensations from the genitals are carried in the spinal cord in the lateral spinothalamic tract.

The genital apparatus in the male receives a dual nerve supply—from the thoracolumbar sympathetic outflow (T11–L2) and from the second and third sacral roots (parasympathetic).

From the thoracolumbar outflow, the hypogastric nerve is formed. This lies just to the left of the front of the aorta. Stimulation of this nerve results in contraction of the vas deferens, seminal vesicles, and bladder neck. It follows that lumbar sympathectomy, or damage to the nerve during dissection of the aortic glands or during an abdomino-perineal resection, will result in failure of emission—a 'dry orgasm'. Stimulation of the hypogastric nerve in the baboon results first in shrinkage of the penis, then erection, so this nerve contains both erectile and anti-erectile pathways. The anti-erectile pathway can be blocked by phentolamine, and it is presumably a similar block which causes erections in man after guanethidine—suggesting that there is usually tonic activity preventing erection.

The second and third sacral roots form the nervi erigentes, which lie on the pelvic floor. Stimulation of these causes erection that is resistant to adrenergic blockade and to atropine. Vasoactive peptide may be the relevant transmitter here. Reflex erections can occur on stimulating the relevant receptive field, which is confined to the genitalia and adjacent parts of the inner thigh. These reflex erections can be induced by a vibrator even when the mind is fully occupied by non-sexual thoughts—for example, by performing mental arithmetic under pressure.

Erotic libidinous thoughts, and erotic pleasure derived from non-genital stroking, pressure, and holding are, of course, the usual initiators of erection. A spinal transection above T11 will interrupt the descending pathways concerned in such psychogenic erections, but reflex erections through the sacral roots are still possible. Reflex emission is also sometimes possible, with adequate stimulation to the glans and frenum. Spinal transections below the thoracolumbar outflow allow psychogenic erections and emission, though without ejaculatory movements of the pelvic floor.

6.12.1   *Investigation and treatment of disorders of male sexual function*

Impaired libido without impaired potency is very common in those whose thoughts about work occupy their hours of relaxation—sometimes incorrectly called barrister's impotence. A brief holiday or change in sexual partner, if appropriate, may reassure the patient that all is well. Impaired libido is also very common after head injuries, and as a manifestation of depressive illness. It is common in other disabling neurological illnesses as a psychological reaction to a decline in self-esteem.

Impaired potency is very often of psychological origin. If morning erections or erections associated with dreaming occur (p. 431), then it is probable that all hormonal and neurological mechanisms are intact. If erections never occur, then investigation will be guided by other elements in the history, or by the findings on neurological examination. For example, the presence of back pain or generalized depression in tendon reflexes should make one think of possible spinal causes, or a neuropathy. If, after adequate investigation, it appears that full erection cannot be achieved, then consideration should be given to the use of a penile ring or splint, in the case of partial erections, or a silastic or inflatable implant.

Sometimes loss of libido and potency may be due to drugs. A number of drugs have been blamed, with varying degrees of probability. Among the most certain are oestrogens, cyproterone acetate, reserpine, and clonidine. Increased libido and resumed potency often follow the use of L-dopa or bromocriptine in the treatment of Parkinson's disease.

In partial lesions of the sympathetic outflow, emission may be aided by the use of a drug such as imipramine, which inhibits the uptake of noradrenaline. Those with partial lesions of the sympathetic, and some patients with spinal lesions, may wish to have children, and semen may be obtained for artificial insemination by either vibratory stimulation of the frenum or glans, or by the technique of electro-ejaculation. In this, electrodes mounted on a helper's gloved finger are inserted into the rectum, and the sympathetic nerve fibres stimulated on the lateral wall of the pelvis close to the obturator point.

Two other common disorders should be mentioned briefly, although they are not neurological. Retrograde ejaculation into the bladder is common after transurethral prostatectomy, which damages the sympathetic fibres, as they lie close to the bladder neck. Usually this occurs at a time of life when fertility is not overly important. Atheromatous disease of the iliac vessels may be responsible for erectile impotence.

6.12.2   *Sexual problems of the disabled*

Awareness of the sexual difficulties of the disabled has greatly increased in recent years. Counselling may help not only those with specifically disordered sexual function, as just discussed, but those who, by reasons of immobility or pain, are unable to imagine practical ways of sexual fulfilment. The charity SPOD (Sexual Problems of the Disabled) is available in the United Kingdom to advise couples about techniques they might use.

6.13   Further reading

General

Brazis, P. W., Masdeu, J. C., and Biller, J. (1990). *Localisation in clinical neurology*. Churchill Livingstone, Edinburgh.

Guarantors of *Brain* (1986). *Aids to the examination of the peripheral nervous system* (3rd edn). Baillère Tindall, London.

de Groot, J. and Chusid, J. G. (1991). *Correlative neuroanatomy*. Lange, New York.

Netter, F. (1985). The CIBA collection of medical illustrations, Vol. I. *Nervous system*. CIBA-Geigy, Basel.

Sudarsky, L. (1990). *Pathophysiology of the nervous system*. Little Brown, Boston.

Neuropsychology

McCarthy, R. A. and Warrington, E. K. (1991). *Cognitive neuropsychology*. Academic Press, London.

Motor control

Noth, J. (1991). Trends in the pathophysiology and pharmacotherapy of spasticity. *Journal of Neurology* **238**, 131–9.

Poizner, H., Mack, L., Verfaellie, M., Gonzalez Rothi L. J., and Heilman, K. M. Three dimensional computergraphic analysis of apraxia. *Brain* **113**, 85–101.

Rosenbaum, D. A. (1990). *Human motor control*. Academic Press, London.

Thilman, A. F., Fellows S. J., and Garms E. (1991). The mechanism of spastic muscle hypertonus. *Brain* **114**, 233–44.

Vertigo

Brandt, T. (1991). Man in motion. Historical and clinical aspects of vestibular function. Brain **114**, 2159–74

Sensorineural deafness

Douek, E. (1990) Sensorineural deafness. *British Medical Journal* **301**, 74–5.

Ludman, H. (1990). Ménière's disease. *British Medical Journal* **301**, 1232–3.

Vision

Walt, R. W. (1991). *Understanding vision*. Academic Press, London.

Micturition

Kirby, R. S. (1988). Studies of the neurogenic bladder. *Annals of the Royal College of Surgeons of England* **70**, 285–8.

7 Disorders of consciousness: coma and confusional states

In the previous chapter, I have described common symptoms and syndromes in which the history is an important contribution to accurate diagnosis. A neurologist often has to manage patients who are unconscious, and who can give no history, or who are confused, and whose history is therefore likely to be unreliable. In this chapter, I propose strategies for coping with these situations, which are often worrying even to those of considerable experience.

7.1 The unconscious patient

A doctor must learn to cope rapidly and effectively with the management of an unconscious patient. Before any diagnostic avenues are pursued, first thoughts must be directed towards the continuing safety of the patient—maintenance of or establishment of an airway, and of adequate ventilation and cardiac output. Continued cerebral perfusion by adequately oxygenated blood is, of course, the prime target of resuscitation, as irreversible neuronal changes occur within about 4 min of anoxia. Moreover, continued hypoxia, as may occur with a partly blocked airway or inadequate ventilation, in itself results in cerebral oedema. Hypoxia may therefore exacerbate the cerebral oedema associated with strokes and head injuries, although elective hyperventilation has not been shown to improve the outcome in either (Sections 10.1.7 and 15.5.2). In addition to ensuring a good airway, an unconscious patient must be positioned in such a way that any secretions or vomit drain out of the mouth and are not inhaled in the event of laryngeal reflexes being depressed. In practice, this means that the patient should be lain on his or her side, tilted over about 30° towards the prone position. In this position, gravity will help drain secretions from the mouth, and the tongue will fall forward, keeping the airways clear if no endotracheal tube is in place. This position can readily be maintained by appropriate positioning with pillows.

Also pre-eminent in ensuring an unconscious patient's continuing safety is to consider the possibility of insulin-induced hypoglycaemia and the possibility of intoxications requiring specific antidotes.

Careful attention must also be given in the unconscious patient to points of pressure at which pressure sores can rapidly develop. The sites at which sores are most frequent are over the greater trochanter, the ischial tuberosities, the sacrum, the heels, the spines of the shoulder blades, and the points of the elbows. The principles cited in Section 18.1.4.1 should be followed. Many physicians and nurses do not realize how rapidly tissue damage can occur, and although attention is usually carefully given to the protection of pressure points in bed, the care of pressure areas while patients are undergoing investigations, or being transported around the hospital, is often less good.

The eyelids often fail to close completely in deep unconsciousness, and the absence of normal blinking means that the cornea may develop an exposure keratitis. This can be prevented with hypromellose drops, and, if frank infection supervenes, with antibiotic eyedrops such as sulphacetamide or chloramphenicol.

Attention must also be directed to the bladder. Many patients, after severe infarctions, have retention of urine, and then overflow incontinence occurs from a grossly distended bladder. If the bladder is clearly palpable, then a urinary catheter should be inserted. Even if the bladder does not enlarge, continuous dribbling of urine into the bed enormously increases the chances of the development of pressure sores.

In order to prevent the development of pressure sores, and in order to prevent hypostatic changes in the lungs, the position of the patient must be changed from side to side at least every two hours. At least twice each day all limbs should be put through a full range of passive movements, in order to prevent fibrotic changes occurring in the joints, and the development of contractures. A fluid balance chart should be instituted, and adequate hydration ensured by either the intravenous or nasogastric route. If the patient remains unconscious for more than two days, attention must be given to calorie intake, most usually by naso-gastric tube.

7.1.1 Definitions and measurement of unconsciousness

Consciousness is best defined as a continuing awareness of self and of the environment. By this definition, most would agree that a dog or a cat are in their daily lives conscious, but we presume that somewhere back along the stages of ontological development there are primitive organisms which, although responding to the environment, are not conscious. Few would hold that an amoeba is conscious, even though its protoplasm responds

to changes in its local milieu. At what stage in evolution consciousness may be said to enter is a matter for ethical and philosophical discussion, exactly mirrored in discussions about the abortion of human fetuses. For example, some hold that a fetus 'becomes a human being' at 24 weeks after conception, others at conception itself. Others again fix on a different arbitrary interval. For no particular one of these can there be logical justification, although there may be moral views.

Although when asleep one is not aware of self, unless dreaming, or of the environment, sleep differs from unconsciousness in so far as from sleep one can be readily aroused. However, inappropriate drowsiness, from which the subject can be aroused, may be an early manifestation of organic cerebral disease. For psychiatrists and neurologists such 'clouding of consciousness' is often an important mark of distinction between organic and psychotic abnormal mental states.

The words 'stupor' and 'coma' are often seen as synonyms for 'lighter' and 'deeper' levels of consciousness, with 'comatose' presumably implying an intermediate state. Such indeterminate modifying words are best avoided in the management of the individual patient, and instead descriptions of consciousness should be based upon the internationally accepted Glasgow scale, which is described next.

7.1.1.1 The Glasgow scale

This is illustrated in Table 7.1. For each of the sections the best response is scored, with due reflection upon other factors of neurological significance. For example, it would be pointless to score the best verbal response of a patient who was drowsy after a stroke because of aphasia caused by the stroke. Likewise, the best motor response has to take into account the possibility of focal neurological damage causing hemiplegia, and the best alerting response to speech the possibility of analgesia and sedation. Leaving aside these points, which are difficulties more apparent than real in everyday clinical practice, the Glasgow coma scale has considerable inter-rater reliability, and is readily understood by nursing staff who are entrusted with the serial observations on which conclusions about improvement or deterioration are made. Figure 7.1 typifies the scores of a patient with an extradural haemorrhage (Section 15.5.1). The

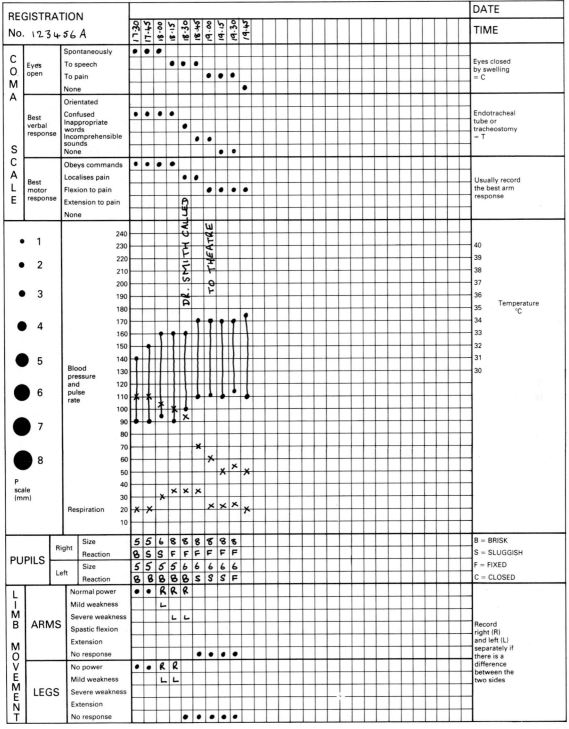

Fig. 7.1 Illustration of the use of neurological observations to detect deterioration associated with a right-sided extradural haematoma.

Table 7.1 Glasgow coma scale.
(The best response is scored)

Eye opening	
spontaneous	4
to speech	3
to pain	2
none	1
Best verbal response	
orientated	5
confused	4
inappropriate	3
incomprehensible	2
none	1
Best motor response	
obeys commands	6
localizes stimulus by appropriate movement	5
weak flexion	4
abnormal flexion	3
abnormal extension	2
none	1

changing scores allow rapid identification of a changing level of consciousness, even across nursing shifts, and prompt neurosurgical intervention.

All doctors are encouraged to use the Glasgow scale when communicating with each other and with nurses, giving the subscores in each section. In patients with diffuse cerebral damage, such as occurs in closed head injuries, the summated scores correlate strongly with outcome (see Fig. 15.3b).

7.1.2　An approach to the unconscious patient

I have already defined the first objective, to ensure the continuing safety of the airway, and of cardiopulmonary function (Section 7.1). After this, as always, the best possible history should be obtained. Clearly this cannot be sought from the patient himself, but the circumstances of the onset of the unconsciousness must be obtained from whatever source is available. Relatives or neighbours are often able to give an account of symptoms preceding unconsciousness, and of the patient's previous health, which may well be relevant. For example, if the patient is known to be diabetic, then the present episode of unconsciousness may well be due to hypoglycaemia or diabetic coma.

On other occasions, patients are brought to Accident and Emergency Departments, having collapsed and become unconscious in a public place, such as a railway station. The examining doctor must take the opportunity of speaking to the ambulance crew, as they may well have had an account of the circumstances, such as a convulsion, or a complaint of chest pain immediately preceding loss of consciousness.

Patients may be found unconscious, and then it is helpful to know when they were last seen to be well. Different classes of illness can then be considered. For example, an elderly woman unconscious and not seen for the three previous days may be unconscious due to meningitis. This could not be the case if she had been seen chatting in her doorway five minutes before.

It is often helpful to go through the patient's belongings. For example, a handbag may contain anticonvulsant drugs, an insulin syringe, or other drugs which indicate pre-existing and possibly relevant illnesses. More patients now carry bracelets or cards identifying illnesses that commonly lead to recurrent hospital care, and a search should be made for these.

A fair idea of the probable cause of the patient's unconsciousness may have been gained from the circumstances surrounding the onset but, if not, examination usually gives sufficient information on which a diagnosis can be based and management planned. The sequence next described will allow not only an adequate scaling of the level of coma, but also provide clues as to its probable cause. After recording temperature, pulse, and blood pressure, the degree to which the patient can be aroused is first assessed by calling or shouting his name, if known, or by using a painful stimulus. For this it is best to use sternal pressure, or by pressing strongly the side of a pen or pencil against a finger- or toe-nail. The patient may vocalize or, in order of increasing severity of coma, he may make a purposeful movement to avoid the stimulus, or flex all limbs, or extend all limbs. If limbs are withdrawn from a painful stimulus on one side but not on the other, then this indicates a probable hemiplegia.

At this point, it is right to search for evidence of external injury—not only the obvious, such as bullet wounds, but also the swelling of the scalp which indicates a recent cranial impact. It may be too early for discolouration of the skin to have occurred, but when there is bruising, the escaped blood collects in areas determined by fascial planes and local tissue resistance. For example, a 'black eye'—a periorbital haematoma—is common after impacts well above the eye. In fractures of the base of the skull, blood pigments drain to behind the ear (Battle's sign), even if the impact was to the vertex. A common combination is of a head injury associated with acute drunkenness. Care must be taken to avoid attributing a depressed level of consciousness to alcohol, thereby missing a head injury.

Neck stiffness should be next assessed as, if present, consideration should be given to the diagnosis of a subarachnoid haemorrhage (Section 10.6.2), meningitis (Section 17.1.2.2), or raised intracranial pressure.

Then look at the eyes. Very often they are in a neutral position, 'looking' straight ahead, in which case this provides little useful information. However, they may remain directed towards one side. This suggests a lesion of the frontal lobe towards which the eyes are directed, as the tonic deviating neuronal discharge from the contralateral frontal lobe is not balanced by that from the damaged one. On other occasions the eyes may be 'skewed', that is to say not conjugate. This may indicate a brain-stem lesion, or a combination of a tonic deviation and a cranial nerve palsy.

The efferent limbs of a number of brain-stem reflexes are related to the eyes, and it is necessary to consider them here. First and foremost are the pupillary responses to light. A patient in deep coma due, for example, to intoxication by barbiturates, will have bilaterally dilated pupils which do not respond to bright illumination with a torch. A patient who has a large hemisphere mass with depression of consciousness and herniation of the temporal lobe may have a third nerve palsy, with a fixed dilated pupil on the side of the lesion, which does not respond to light when either eye is illuminated (Section 15.5.1). A patient with a brain-stem haemorrhage, again interrupting the reflex arc, may have pupils in the mid-range of diameter, or pin-point pupils, neither being responsive to light.

Other brain-stem reflexes include two types of oculovestibular reflexes—commonly called the 'doll's eye' and 'caloric' reflexes. In the first, the labyrinth is stimulated by a sharp rotation of the head. If the reflex operates, the eyes will tend to deviate in the opposite direction in the orbits— that is to say, remain directed towards the point of original fixation. The caloric test depends upon the stimulation of the labyrinth by thermally induced currents (Section 6.6.2.3). The external auditory canal is first inspected to be free from wax, and then, in the case of the unconscious patient, is irrigated with 20 ml of iced water. If the reflex is operational, the eyes deviate towards the irrigated side. Other brain-stem reflexes include a gag response to the passing of an endotracheal tube or suction catheter.

In the limbs, a hemiplegia may be detected, as has already been remarked, by a failure to withdraw limbs in response to a painful stimulus on that side, or by an asymmetry of generalized flexor or extensor response to pain. Tone may be generally increased, or one side may feel much more 'floppy' than the other. The affected limbs of a hemiplegic unconscious patient will, if elevated, crash down upon the bed much more heavily on the plegic side than on the other side. The tendon reflexes may be helpful, as asymmetry clearly indicates a probable focal brain lesion. The plantar responses are often bilaterally extensor in deep coma, but again a unilateral response may well indicate a focal lesion.

7.1.3   *The causes of coma*

The preceding paragraphs have indicated one approach to the unconscious patient when there are no initial clues upon which the diagnosis of the cause of coma can be based. But, of course, in many instances, coma occurs on a background of known pre-existing metabolic or other disease. Table 7.2 lists some of the more common causes of coma. As in many lists and classifications, a cause could logically appear under more than one heading. For example, coma due to a subdural haematoma may reasonably be listed under the heading 'raised intracranial pressure' as well as under 'trauma'. None the less, the list provides a pragmatic basis for investigation and management.

7.1.3.1   *The investigation of the unconscious patient*

As already mentioned, the cause of coma in some

Table 7.2   The causes of coma

Trauma	encephalitis
head injury	malaria
diffuse cerebral injury	Epilepsy
extradural haemorrhage	after a seizure
subdural haemorrhage	status epilepticus
fat embolism	Metabolic
Toxicity	hypothermia
alcohol	hepatic failure
drugs, notably barbiturates, anticonvulsants,	renal failure
antidepressants, benzodiazepines	hypercapnia
Raised intracranial pressure	hyperglycaemia with ketosis
abscess	non-ketotic hyperglycaemia
tumour	hypoglycaemia
extradural or subdural haemorrhage	hypothyroidism
decompensated hydrocephalus	Anoxia
Cerebrovascular disease	after cardiac arrest
large infarcts	after near drowning
cerebral venous thrombosis	carbon monoxide poisoning
intracerebral haemorrhage	'End-stage' neurological disease
subarachnoid haemorrhage	e.g. sub-acute sclerosing panencephalitis;
hypertensive encephalopathy	Creutzfeldt–Jakob disease
Infections	Simulated unresponsiveness (psychogenic
meningitis	unresponsiveness)

patients is readily apparent from the preceding history, e.g. hepatic failure, or end-stage dementia. For those patients who present in the Accident and Emergency Department with an uncertain or an unknown history, examination will usually distinguish those patients with obvious focal neurological events, such as a large intracerebral haemorrhage, from those with more diffuse neurological dysfunction due to intoxication or infection. Initial metabolic investigations, which can be rapidly performed while the examination is proceeding, should include tests of blood sugar, bicarbonate, urea, sodium, and liver function. Blood should be saved for a subsequent drug screen. An electrocardiograph (ECG) may show evidence of a recent infarct, from which a period of possible cerebral hypoperfusion can be deduced. If the patient is febrile and/or the neck stiff, then meningitis or a subarachnoid haemorrhage may be suspected. A cranial CT scan should be done before lumbar puncture (see Section 10.6.3) unless facilities are not available and there is strong presumptive evidence of meningitis (see Section 17.1.2.3).

For some unconscious patients an electroencephalogram and CT scan are necessary prerequisites of a probable diagnosis, for example herpes simplex encephalitis (Section 17.12.3.3). On the other hand, for example, an elderly hypertensive man with two previous strokes and clinical evidence of a focal hemisphere lesion of sudden onset does not require further investigation of his presumed further stroke, unless unusual features are apparent.

Many patients presenting to Accident and Emergency Departments are subjects of drug intoxication. Examples that depress consciousness and ventilation include alcohol, phenobarbitone and other barbiturates, anticonvulsants such as phenytoin and carbamazepine, antidepressants such as amitriptyline, opiates, particularly when abused, neuroleptic drugs such as the phenothiazines, beta-blockers, and aspirin.

Before considering the causes of coma in general, it is necessary to explore the concept of brain death, originally described by the French physicians Mollaret and Goulon in 1959 as 'coma dépassé'.

7.2 Brain death

All doctors must be absolutely familiar with the concept of brain death. Confused statements distress relatives and contribute to the uncertainties that reduce the ready availability of organs for transplantation.

Some aspects of life continue after termination of an oxygenated circulation. The survival and further function of cadaveric transplanted kidneys is one example. At a cellular level, molecular reactions continue, at first ordered and then increasingly disordered, until decomposition. It may, at first thought, seem impossible to introduce an artificial discontinuity to mark the point of death in this continuous process of dissolution. The difficulty may, however, be resolved by remembering that there is a difference between the *meaning* of an abstract concept such as death, or time, and the *operations* used to determine it.

Our present concept of the meaning of death is the termination of an organism as an *integrated* functional unit, distinct from the death of some cells, such as a gangrenous toe, within a still living organism. The operational definition of death in former days depended upon observing absence of respiration, or an absent pulse. Before the advent of cardiopulmonary resuscitation, these observations, which could be applied by the man in the street, indicated that irreversible dissolution (decomposition) would surely follow. All that the development of artificial ventilation and other support in intensive therapy units has done is to shift, in the small proportion of the population who die there, the operational definition of death to brainstem death. We know that when brain-stem mechanisms fail, the disorders of integrative processes are so vast that irreversible dissolution begins, even though the heart continues to beat for a few days more. However skilled subsequent adjustment of intensive 'therapies' may be, circulatory arrest invariably follows. If ventilation and drugs to maintain the blood pressure are continued for some time after brain-stem death, frank autolysis may be visible to nurses, and always to the pathologist at autopsy.

Confusion often arises in press reports from the use of the words 'life-support machines'—artificial ventilators. When the patient is brain-stem dead, the machines are merely part of the mechanism for delivering oxygen to an organ that may be transplanted.

Many countries have now formalized the procedures necessary to diagnose brain-stem death. The first definite proposals were put forward by an *ad hoc* committee of the Harvard Medical School in 1968. In the UK, the Conference of Medical Royal Colleges and their Faculties formulated proposals in 1976, with an addendum in 1979. In 1981 the President's Commission for the Study of Ethical Problems in Medicine and Biochemical and Behavioural Research submitted a report on 'Defining death' to the President of the USA. The formulation is very similar to the UK formulation. This is conveniently laid out in the form of a protocol (Fig. 7.2).

The diagnosis of brain-stem death is a clinical one, and no special technically-based investigations, such as electroencephalography, are required.

7.2.1 *Pre-conditions for the diagnosis of brain-stem death*

First of all, certain 'pre-conditions' have to be satisfied. First, that the patient is apnoeic, and requires artificial ventilation, this requirement not being due to the effects of neuromuscular blockade. Secondly, that the patient is in coma, and that the cause is irremediable structural brain damage due to a disorder that can lead to brain death. The force of this pre-condition is to ensure that the diagnosis of brain-stem death is not even considered until a definite diagnosis of the cause of coma is made. The most common causes are severe cranial injury and subarachnoid haemorrhage, the diagnosis of which is without doubt. In such cases, it is the passage of time and total unresponsiveness to therapy that determine that the cause responsible for coma is irremediable. Apart from these obvious causes, potentially *reversible* causes of profound apnoeic coma that must be considered include drug intoxication, particularly with barbiturates, hypothermia, and metabolic and endocrine disturbances. The half-life of some barbiturate drugs is so long (50–140 hours in the case of phenobarbitone) that in practical terms the passage of time alone is not sufficient to exclude the possibility of intoxication. If cardiac arrest has been followed by coma, the diagnosis of brainstem death should not be considered until at least

Fig. 7.2 Protocol for the diagnosis of brain stem death

Criteria for the diagnosis of brain stem death

Patient's name _____ Ward _____

Date of birth _____ Hospital number _____

	Assessor A	Assessor B	Assessor A	Assessor B
Name				
Status				

If a patient in deep coma, requiring mechanical ventilation, is thought to be dead because of irreversible brain damage of known cause an assessment of brain stem function should be made according to the following guidelines. These follow the Department of Health and Social Security recommendations in *Cadaveric Organs for Transplantation: a Code of Practice, including the Diagnosis of Brain Death 1983.*

Assessments

Two assessments should be made by two doctors once the preconditions have been met. Diagnosis should not normally be considered until at least six hours after the onset of coma or, if anoxia or cardiac arrest was the cause of the coma (particularly in children), until 24 hours after the circulation has been restored, and then only if the preconditions have been satisfied.

(1) The assessments should be made by two medical practitioners who have skill and knowledge in the subject. One should be a consultant, the other a consultant or senior registrar, and they should assure themselves that the preconditions have been met before the examination.

(2) It is often convenient for the examination to be performed by one assessor and witnessed by the other.

(3) The respiratory disconnection test is usually performed by an anaesthetist and witnessed by one of the assessors.

What is the cause of the irremediable brain damage? _____

Why is it irremediable? _____

Start of coma: _____ Time: _____ Date: _____

Preconditions (All answers must be "No")

Time: _____
Date: _____

(1) Could primary hypothermia, drugs, or metabolic-endocrine abnormalities be contributing significantly to the apnoeic coma? (Where appropriate, check plasma and urine for drugs, plasma pH, glucose, sodium, and calcium.)

(2) Have any neuromuscular blocking drugs been administered during the preceding 12 hours?

(3) Is the rectal temperature below 35°C? (If so, warm the patient and reassess.)

Reproduced by permission from O'Brien (1990).

Examination

Do not proceed until the preconditions have been met.
The answer to all questions must be "No."

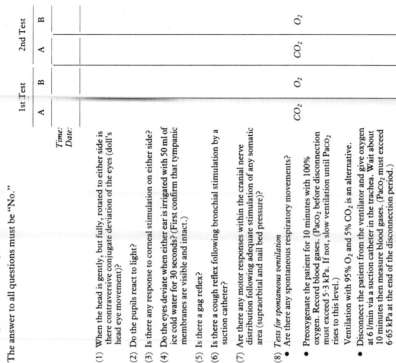

	1st Test		2nd Test	
	A	B	A	B
Time:				
Date:				

(1) When the head is gently, but fully, rotated to either side is there contraversive conjugate deviation of the eyes (doll's head eye movement)?

(2) Do the pupils react to light?

(3) Is there any response to corneal stimulation on either side?

(4) Do the eyes deviate when either ear is irrigated with 50 ml of ice cold water for 30 seconds? (First confirm that tympanic membranes are visible and intact.)

(5) Is there a gag reflex?

(6) Is there a cough reflex following bronchial stimulation by a suction catheter?

(7) Are there any motor responses within the cranial nerve distribution following adequate stimulation of any somatic area (supraorbital and nail bed pressure)?

(8) *Tests for spontaneous ventilation*
  • Are there any spontaneous respiratory movements?

  • Preoxygenate the patient for 10 minutes with 100% oxygen. Record blood gases. ($PaCO_2$ before disconnection must exceed 5·3 kPa. If not, slow ventilation until $PaCO_2$ rises to this level.)
    Ventilation with 95% O_2 and 5% CO_2 is an alternative.

  • Disconnect the patient from the ventilator and give oxygen at 6 l/min via a suction catheter in the trachea. Wait about 10 minutes then measure blood gases. ($PaCO_2$ must exceed 6·65 kPa at the end of the disconnection period.)

  • Is there any spontaneous respiratory movement?

| CO_2 | O_2 | CO_2 | O_2 |

Assessors' signatures:

24 hours after the time at which the circulation has been restored.

7.2.1.1   *Who should be responsible for diagnosing brain-stem death?*

It is right that the diagnosis of brain-stem death is made by doctors of sufficient experience. In the UK two are required. One should be the consultant in charge of the case and one other doctor. In the absence of a consultant, his deputy can undertake the tests with one other doctor, but he or she must have been registered for 5 years or more, and have had adequate previous experience in the care of such cases. If organs are to be removed for transplantation, the UK code of practice recommends two consultants or one consultant and a senior registrar, both of whom should have expertise in this field, but neither doctor should be a member of the transplant team. The two doctors may carry out the tests independently or together. Even if the tests confirm brain-stem death they should be repeated after an interval that is adequate for the reassurance of those directly concerned.

7.2.2   *Tests for brain-stem death*

The means by which total failure of the brain stem is assessed include:

1. No pupillary response to light; a bright focused torch is essential.

2. No corneal reflex.

3. No vestibulo-ocular reflex. Irrigation of the external auditory canal on each side with at least 20 ml of iced water must fail to induce any ocular movement. It is important to ensure that the canal is not blocked by wax or blood clot.

4. No motor responses within the cranial nerve distribution (e.g. no grimacing) in response to painful stimuli anywhere on the body.

5. No gag reflex or limb or chest movement in response to tracheo-bronchial stimulation induced by the passage of a catheter down the endotracheal tube or tracheostomy.

6. No ventilatory movements on disconnection from the ventilator for long enough to allow the $P_{a\,CO_2}$ to reach 6.65 kPa (50 mmHg). In practice, this is best achieved by pre-oxygenation by ventilation with 100 per cent oxygen for 10 min, and then by delivery of 100 per cent oxygen down an intratracheal catheter as the $P_{a\,CO_2}$ rises. Alternatively, patients may be ventilated with 95 per cent O_2, 5 per cent CO_2 for 5 min before disconnection, in order to generate an adequate $P_{a\,CO_2}$ drive to the respiratory centre in the event that it may still be functional. If there are no facilities for blood gas analysis, this pre-disconnection ventilation with 5 per cent CO_2 is essential. Apnoea should be observed for 10 min.

There are three further points to be considered. First of all, spinal cord reflexes may persist after brain-stem death. Consequently, limb movements and changes in heart rate and blood pressure may be seen in response to vigorous stimulation (e.g. in opening the abdomen to harvest kidneys for donation). Secondly, no high-technology test such as electroencephalography or measurements of cerebral blood flow are necessary to confirm the diagnosis of brain-stem death. Finally, it must be stressed again that the tests are not valid in the presence of sedative drugs, or of drugs that cause neuromuscular blockade.

7.3   Other states of altered consciousness

7.3.1   *The persistent vegetative state*

A patient who survives the initial stages of a severe cranial injury, or coma due to hypoxia such as may occur after profound hypotension or cardiac arrest, will, after a few weeks, open his eyes, and appear to 'look around' with roving conjugate eye movements. Spontaneous ventilatory control and movements of swallowing return. Periods during which the eyes open and close alternate over several hours, giving the impression of cycles of sleep and waking. The limbs are often very spastic, but their posture may change during the course of the day. However, it is apparent that the patient is not conscious in the sense of having any awareness of the environment, and all evidence equally points to there being no self-awareness. This state is known as the persistent, or chronic, vegetative state. The choice of the word 'vegetative', although unfortunate in its close similarity to the crude word 'vegetable', usefully conveys the fact that the body is driven only by its autonomic or vegetative reflex functions. The brain stem is functioning, but much of the cortex is dead. Autopsy studies of those who have survived months or years in this condition show varying degrees of cortical laminar necrosis, particularly prominent in the occipital and hippocampal regions. Although opening the eyes is a step in the road to recovery from any coma, it is unfortunate that many relatives interpret eye-opening in the persistent vegetative state as an indicator that there will be useful social recovery. They may fix their own gaze on the patient's eyes and feel that the patient is 'looking at them' or 'recognizing them'. Unfortunately, once 3–4 months have passed in the persistent vegetative state, such patients may, for all practical purposes, be considered to be permanently in this state.

7.3.1.1   Ethical considerations

There are considerable social and ethical problems about continuing to treat a patient in a persistent vegetative state. It takes some weeks for it to become clear that the patient is going to remain in a persistent vegetative state, rather than recover slowly from deep coma, so hydration and nutrition by nasogastric tube are, of course, being provided during this time. The consensus view is that it is right to continue hydration and nutrition in the persistent vegetative state, and skilled nursing to prevent pressure sores. It is usual to treat early infections with antibiotics, but as the months go by, and when there is no longer any doubt that the patient is in a persistent vegetative state, many physicians feel that it is inappropriate to use extraordinary methods of maintaining life, although what is extraordinary for one physician may be ordinary for another.

7.3.1.2   Prognosis

It is unusual for patients to survive for more than 5 years in a persistent vegetative state. About 1 per cent of younger people who have been in a persistent vegetative state for some months may regain some semblance of responsiveness to the environment, but even so remain grossly incapacitated.

7.3.2   *Akinetic mutism*

Akinetic mutism refers to a state of alert-appearing speechless immobility, without evidence of mental activity. In older descriptions, the term akinetic mutism was applied to many patients now regarded as being in a persistent vegetative state. The term 'akinetic mutism' is now reserved for those with focal neurological disturbances, some of which are at least potentially reversible. Examples include cysts in the region of the third ventricle, and lesions affecting the paramedian reticular system of the posterior diencephalon. A similar picture is produced also by large lesions in the basal and medial parts of both frontal lobes, as may be induced, for example, by rupture of an anterior communicating artery aneurysm. Advanced communicating hydrocephalus is another cause of akinetic mutism.

7.3.3   *Locked-in syndrome*

In this extraordinary syndrome, the patient is conscious, but may have great difficulty in communicating this. The usual cause is a large infarct in the anterior part of the pons. This results in total disconnection of the lower cranial nerves and all spinal anterior horn cells from the corticofugal outflow. The cortical pathways to cranial nerves III and IV, the nuclei of which lie in the dorsal mid-brain, are spared, so that the patient can make vertical eye movements. All other muscles are paralysed. It may take some time for nursing and medical staff to realize that the inert, immobile patient is conscious, but once they do it is often possible to help the patient communicate his wishes by a code based on vertical eye movements, for example up for 'yes' and down for 'no'. Few patients remain in such a state for more than a few weeks. Either a partial degree of recovery of motor function occurs, or the patient dies.

7.3.4   *Hypersomnia*

Prolonged periods of sleep from which the subject may be roused only with difficulty occur as a sequel of encephalitis lethargica (Section 13.1.4), and may occur during the phase of recovery from severe head injury. Hypersomnia of this type is usually distinguished from other disorders of excessive sleep, such as narcolepsy (Section 24.2.4) and daytime somnolence associated with obstructive sleep apnoea (Section 24.2.6).

The Kleine–Levin syndrome is a poorly understood disorder of episodic hypersomnia, associated with episodic excessive eating. The syndrome usually occurs in young men, and may be associated with changes in mood and psychotic features.

7.3.5   *Simulated unconsciousness*

Patients occasionally simulate unconsciousness, being totally unresponsive to shouting their name or to painful stimuli. These patients cause physicians and nurses great concern as the façade may be kept up for days. The preservation of normal brain-stem reflexes and preserved tendon reflexes in the face of apparent deep coma, and the tendency for the eyes to be screwed up on attempted fundoscopy of the less-sophisticated patients, are the best guide to the diagnosis. The electroencephalogram shows normal rhythms associated with wakefulness.

7.4   Organic confusional states

Many young doctors feel uneasy when first confronted by a confused patient. The physician's first ally, the patient, is incompetent to give a history or to help in his own relief. If confusion is admixed with agitation and even violence, then the task is even less easy.

The term 'organic confusional state' usually is taken to refer to episodes of acute or subacute onset. If confusion and agitation are prominent, the state may be called delirium. Patients with dementia are also confused due to organic brain disease, but their chronic state is best considered separately (Chapter 11). An organic confusional state may be defined as a transient organic mental syndrome characterized by a global disorder of cognition and attention, a reduced level of consciousness, and a disturbed cycle between sleep and wakefulness.

The first point is to distinguish an organic confusional state from the abnormal speech and behaviour that may be associated with an acute psychotic episode due to schizophrenia, mania, or depression. Patients with an organic state are characterized by clouding of consciousness, either drowsiness, or at the very least some obvious

difficulty in concentration and alertness. They are also disoriented in time and place and, as recent memory is impaired, they are unable to learn about their surroundings. For all these reasons the patients often appear perplexed or bewildered.

When consciousness is clouded, people and objects are misidentified, and illusions may cause agitation. Unconscious material that would normally appear only in dreams may surface into clouded consciousness, so that the patient may also be hallucinated. Delusions may also arise on the basis of the disordered perceptual experiences and disorientation. The paradigm for such states is the acute confusional state that accompanies alcohol withdrawal, delirium tremens (Section 23.4.2.1), in which the patient is drowsy, agitated, confused, and restless, and terrified by prominent visual hallucinations—in folklore, commonly pink elephants!

Table 7.3   Differences between organic confusional states and acute psychiatric states

Organic states	Psychiatric states
Clouding of consciousness	Alert
Disorientated	Orientated
Recent memory impaired	Recent memory retained
Lability of affect	No lability of affect
Usually no previous psychological history	May have previous psychological history
Often older age-group	Usually younger age-group
Evidence of organic disease (fever, etc.)	No evidence of organic disease
May have taken drugs known to cause confusion	No relevant drug history
	Positive evidence for schizophrenia, mania, or depression

Table 7.3 lists the differences between organic confusional and acute functional psychotic states. Table 7.4 lists the common causes of acute confusional states, on which appropriate clinical examination and investigation can be based.

Table 7.4 Causes of an acute or subacute organic confusional state

Infection	Tumours
generalized infections—bacteraemia associated with	cerebral metastases
renal infections can cause confusion with little fever	remote effects of carcinoma (limbic encephalitis)
in the elderly	Epilepsy
infections localized to the nervous system	complex partial or absence status
meningitis	post-ictal state
encephalitis	Metabolic causes
brain abscess	hypoxia
Intoxication	hypercapnia
alcohol (delirium tremens)	uraemia
drugs, e.g. orphenadrine, benzhexol, amitriptyline	hypoglycaemia
Drug withdrawal	hepatic coma
alcohol	hyponatraemia
heroin	hypercalcaemia
Trauma	hypothyroidism
recovery phase after acute head injury	porphyria
subdural haematoma	

7.4.1 *Immediate management of confusion*

A delirious patient should be nursed in a quiet well-lit room with minimal stimuli that could encourage misinterpretations and illusions. Constant reassurance by sympathetic nursing and medical staff is helpful.

The acutely agitated patient may need sedation for his/her own protection and for the protection of nursing staff. Haloperidol, 0.5–5 mg intramuscularly according to weight, age, and the extent of any underlying illness, is usually the most effective treatment. Some physicians prefer chlorpromazine, but this may cause prolonged sedation which makes further assessment difficult. The dose is 50–300 mg, again according to age, weight, and general health. Chlormethiazole is often used in the treatment of delirium tremens. This is most easily given as an intravenous infusion of 8 mg/ml (0.8 per cent). This is given at a rate of 4 ml (32 mg) per min until the patient feels drowsy, and then maintained at a rate of around 0.5–1.0 ml/min. An alternative is an infusion of diazepam.

7.5 Further reading

General

Plum, F. and Posner, J. B. (1980). *The diagnosis of stupor and coma*. F. A. Davis, Philadelphia.

Bates, D. (1991). Defining prognosis in medical coma. *Journal of Neurology, Neurosurgery and Psychiatry* **54**, 569–71.

Brain death

Health Departments of Great Britain and Northern Ireland (1983). *Cadaveric organs for transplantation. A code of practice including the diagnosis of brain death*. Health Departments, London.

O'Brien, M. D. (1990). Criteria for diagnosing brain stem death. *British Medical Journal* **301**, 108–9.

Pallis, C. (1983). *ABC of brain-stem death*. British Medical Journal Publications, London.

Pallis, C. (1990). Brain-stem death. In *Handbook of neurology*, (ed. P. J. Vinken, G. W. Bruyn, H. L. Klawans, R. Braakman), Vol. 13 (Revised series), pp. 441–69. Elsevier, Amsterdam.

Persistent vegetative state

Campbell, A. G. M. (1984). Persistent vegetative state. *British Medical Journal* **289**, 1022–3.

Organic confusional states

Francis, J., Martin, D., and Kapoor, W. N. (1990). A prospective study of delirium in hospitalised elderly. *Journal of the American Medical Association* **263**, 1097–101.

Lipowski, Z. J. (1989). Delirium in the elderly patient. *New England Journal of Medicine* **320**, 578–81.

8 Investigations commonly used in neurology

As already explained in Chapter 5, and illustrated in Table 5.1, the way forward to reaching a neurological diagnosis—a necessary prerequisite before advising on treatment—is to listen to the history, form a hypothesis as to the probable anatomical site in the nervous system that could give rise to those symptoms, and then support or refute that hypothesis on the basis of a careful physical examination. Some investigations in neurology, particularly imaging procedures (for example com-puterized tomographic (CT) scanning, magnetic resonance imaging (MRI), and myelography, can often confirm that a lesion does indeed lie at the presumed anatomical site. Characteristic changes in some images may also give a reliable lead as to the likely pathology; for example, an area of low attenuation in a CT scan surrounded by a ring of enhancing high density (see Section 8.10.2) may well prove to be a cerebral abscess or a malignant brain tumour. In other cases, the images may confirm the anatomical site, but leave the examiner very uncertain as to the probable pathology.

Faced with this situation, we still follow the principles outlined in Table 5.1. Having established the anatomical site, consider what is likely to be the most likely pathological process to occur at that particular site in a patient of that particular age with that particular history, and, if appropriate, plan further investigations accordingly. By appropriate, I mean in the most general way that the information likely to be gained from the investigation significantly outweighs the drawbacks of risk, discomfort, and anxiety. It must also be considered whether the information likely to be gained will influence significantly further management. For example, most would consider it inappropriate to image the changes in the brain arising after the third stroke in an 80-year-old man already in residential care.

Some investigations in neurology are concerned not so much with structural changes at anatomical sites, but with pathophysiological changes of importance. For example, electroencephalography (EEG) in a child with typical absences (Fig. 12.4) will confirm a diagnosis of primary generalized epilepsy (Section 12.5), a genetic disorder not accompanied by structural change at the macroscopic or microscopic level, but at the level of cellular metabolism.

Some investigations can help determine both abnormal physiology *and* abnormal location. For example, as Fig. 8.6 shows, nerve conduction studies can reveal slowing of conduction in the median nerve as it traverses a tight carpal tunnel.

8.1   Neurological investigation in relation to general medicine

In Chapter 1, I stress that neurology should be considered part of general medicine, and many of the investigations we necessarily perform reflect this. For example, tests of thyroid function may explain increasing ataxia in an elderly person (Section 20.3.3); examination of a blood film may show macrocytosis, and lead to the diagnosis of subacute combined degeneration of the cord (Section 23.24.2); a haematocrit is a relevant investigation in younger patients with stroke, as is an echocardiogram (Table 10.4). There are many other

possible examples. This chapter outlines briefly the background of the special investigations most commonly employed in neurology.

8.2   Examination of the cerebrospinal fluid

Cerebrospinal fluid (CSF) can be obtained by lumbar puncture or, much more rarely, by cisternal or ventricular puncture. As lumbar puncture (spinal tap) is often performed by doctors in training, the procedure is described briefly.

8.2.1   *Technique of lumbar puncture (spinal tap)*

There is no doubt that lumbar puncture is easier if the patient is relaxed and confident. Lumbar puncture enjoys a special and unreasonably feared reputation among the general public; many have heard of it as 'the lumbar punch'! A few minutes taken to explain the procedure and reassure the patient is time well spent. Only rarely is any premedication necessary, but very nervous adults could receive diazepam, 5–10 mg one hour before, and apprehensive children Vallergan, according to body weight.

The operator, too, must be confident and relaxed. The procedure is performed much less frequently than before, as the limited appropriate indications have become more clearly recognized (see Table 8.1). Relative unfamiliarity with the procedure may make the doctor, and any assisting nurse, tense. Indeed, in my experience, unless the lumbar puncture is undertaken in a neurological/neurosurgical unit, the nurse requires as much reassurance as the patient.

A lumbar puncture is most easily performed on an operating table, which firmly supports the lumbar spine, maintaining the spinous processes in a straight line. However, for practical reasons, most are undertaken with the patient in his or her own bed. Adequate support to the spine can be obtained if the patient lies on his or her side (the left side if the doctor is right handed) *right* on the edge of the bed, so much so that it looks as though the patient might fall off. The patient's shoulders and buttocks should be on the edge, and his or her head supported on pillows so that the cervical

Table 8.1   Appropriate indications for lumbar
               puncture

1. As a necessary preliminary to radiculography,
    myelography, or spinal anaesthesia
2. To prove or disprove the diagnosis of meningitis
    (see text; a scan may often be appropriate first)
       there may be an excess number of lymphocytes or
          granulocytes
       bacteria may be seen on Gram- or Ziehl–Neelsen
          stain
       micro-organisms in the CSF may grow on culture
       fungi may be seen
       bacterial or fungal antigens may be identified
       the CSF sugar may be unduly low
3. To search for abnormal proteins
       oligoclonal proteins in multiple sclerosis, in
          subacute sclerosing panencephalitis, etc.
       neurosyphilis
       acute infective polyneuropathy
4. To introduce intrathecal chemotherapeutic agents
       methotrexate, etc.

Only after CT scanning or MRI
5. To search for malignant cells
       in leukaemia
       in meningeal carcinomatosis
       in children with medulloblastoma
6. To search for red cells or haem pigments
       (xanthochromia) after subarachnoid haemorrhage
7. To measure pressure in the diagnosis and
       monitoring of benign intracranial hypertension

spine does not droop down. Two pillows should be
placed between the knees in order to prevent the
back rolling away from the operator. The hips and
knees should be strongly flexed towards the chin,
so that the spinous processes are separated, allowing greater access for the needle. However, strong
flexion usually pulls the buttocks away from the
edge of the bed, and further repositioning after
flexing is necessary. A towel or sheet of polythene
should be tucked between the body and mattress
to prevent soiling of the bed by topical skin disinfectant, spinal fluid, and, possibly, blood.

The operator must find a suitable stool, adjust
the height of the bed, make sure lighting is
adequate, and adjust the patient's garments to
provide some semblance of modesty, while allowing a broad area of the back to be displayed for

the operations. All this has to be undertaken
before the hands are scrubbed. As human immunodeficiency virus (HIV) infections in neurological practice are so common, gloves must be worn.

On returning to the patient, the skin of the back
and over the uppermost hip is widely cleaned with
whatever topical disinfectant is locally favoured.
The iliac crest is identified, and from this an
imaginary line drawn downwards will pass between
the spines of L3 and L4. After warning the patient,
a fine needle is inserted in the mid-line at this
point, between the spines of L3 and L4, and a
small volume of local anaesthetic, such as 1 per
cent lignocaine, introduced, sufficient to cause an
intradermal bleb. Local anaesthesia may also be
obtained, especially in children with their thinner
skin, by the topical application of lignocaine (pril-
ocaine cream) approximately one hour before the
procedure is carried out. If injected anaesthesia is
used, a limited quantity (<2 ml) intradermally and
immediately subcutaneously is adequate. More will
make identification of the landmark spinous processes difficult.

The needle used for local anaesthetic should be
left in place as a marker while the operator turns
to his or her tray to pick up the lumbar puncture
needle, which should never be thicker than 21
SWG, and finer in children. Thicker needles are
less whippy, but less kind to the patients, and more
likely to produce a post-puncture headache. The
needles are then exchanged, and the lumbar puncture needle pushed through the skin, subcutaneous
tissue and then the dense supraspinous ligament,
maintaining the needle parallel to the floor, at 90°
to the back, and pointing slightly towards the head
(by about 10°), rather than straight in as if towards
the umbilicus. Once the supraspinous ligament is
penetrated, the needle is relatively well splinted,
and the operator should pause to check the align-
ment in both axes. The needle is then slowly
advanced. As the probable depth from skin to dura
is approached, and this depends on the patient's
age and build, the stilette is withdrawn from the
needle every 2 mm or so, to see if CSF runs out.
Modern needles are so sharp that there is no
resistance felt when the dura is encountered. If the
needle meets the firm obstruction of bone, then it
has probably encountered the posterior surface of
an apophyseal joint. Either the patient has rotated
away from the examiner, or the needle has
deviated from its path parallel to the floor. Occa-

sionally the firm obstruction is due to the needle having been advanced too far, and hitting the anterior wall of the spinal canal. If the operator feels that the needle *ought* to be in the subarachnoid space, and yet no CSF runs, the needle should be rotated slightly as occasionally a nerve root may block the bevel.

Before beginning the procedure, the operator should have decided whether he or she really wishes to measure the opening pressure. To connect a manometer and tap is a fiddly business, and may dislodge the needle slightly. It is certainly *essential* to measure the pressure in some clinical situations, for example, the establishment of benign intracranial hypertension (Section 16.9), but in the vast majority of cases there is no point, the purpose of the examination being to collect fluid for microbiological, microscopical, or biochemical examinations. The pressure cannot be judged by the rate of flow through the needle, which is an exit pathway of high resistance.

Cerebrospinal fluid should be collected into three numbered tubes. If a small vessel has been penetrated on the way to the subarachnoid space, then red cells will enter the needle and appear in the first collection. The needle will then be flushed by CSF and, in the case of a mildly traumatic tap, no red cells will be present in the second and third bottles. For estimation of the CSF sugar, fluid should be collected into a fourth bottle containing sodium fluoride, as used for the collection of blood sugar. If it is thought that the CSF sugar is likely to be of considerable diagnostic importance, as in the case of tuberculous or carcinomatous meningitis, then blood for estimation of blood glucose should be obtained at the same time.

After collecting sufficient CSF—5 ml is enough for all tests, except when a search is being made for tubercle bacilli (Section 17.5.1.4)—the needle is then withdrawn, and a simple small Band-Aid dressing applied over the puncture site.

8.2.1.1   Headache after lumbar puncture

Some patients get a headache after lumbar puncture, probably because there is a continued slow leak of CSF from the subarachnoid space through the dural puncture into the extradural space. This is the principal reason for using a fine needle. Some hold that the bevel of the needle should lie in the sagittal plane, hoping that the dural fibres

be split parallel to their length. However, there is no evidence that this minor variation is of any significance.

What is clear from controlled studies is that the patient's expectation of the likelihood of headache is of crucial importance. If the nursing staff state, as they usually do, that bed rest on one pillow must be maintained for at least 12 h, or a headache will occur, then headaches commonly follow. If a robust attitude is adopted, that a lumbar puncture is no different in principal to a venepuncture, and no mention of headache is made, then headaches are rare. Indeed, in the USA, and increasingly in the UK, lumbar puncture for non-urgent reasons, for example in the case of multiple sclerosis, may be undertaken as an 'office procedure' or as a day case.

Occasionally, however, one is misguided in this cheerful expectant approach, and the poor patient does have a severe headache, which is exacerbated as soon as he or she tries to stand up. A period of bed rest followed by cautious mobilization then usually has to follow. In persistent cases, lasting for more than 5 days, 10 ml of the patient's own blood may be injected extradurally through a lumbar puncture needle at the same site. The resulting extradural clot may succeed in patching the transdural leak of CSF.

8.2.2   The risks of lumbar puncture

The most feared risk is of 'coning'. In the event of a large supratentorial, or even a small infratentorial mass lesion such as a tumour or abscess, the cerebellum and its tonsils may already be partly impacted into the foramen magnum. Withdrawal of cerebrospinal fluid from below increases the pressure gradient, and the cerebellar tonsils and inferior surface of the cerebellum are pushed firmly as a cone into the upper cervical canal, with resulting respiratory arrest.

Other complications of lumbar puncture include meningitis induced by the puncture (although this is excessively rare); puncture should be avoided if there is local skin sepsis. Another complication is persistent haemorrhage into the subarachnoid or extradural space. This may occur in those with haemophilia or on anticoagulants, and result in compression of the cauda equina.

8.2.3 *Appropriate indications for lumbar puncture*

Table 8.1 lists the appropriate indications for lumbar puncture. Note that firm advice is given as to those cases in which puncture should be preceded by CT scanning.

The relative places of CT scanning and lumbar puncture in the diagnosis of subarachnoid haemorrhage are now clear. Lumbar puncture may be hazardous in those with extensive bleeding and a high intracranial pressure. A cranial CT scan will usually reveal blood in the subarachnoid spaces in such patients, or the presence of a haematoma. However, about 20 per cent of those who have had a ruptured aneurysm, as proved subsequently by angiography, will not have visible blood on the CT scan, and of those about two-thirds will have blood in the CSF. In contrast to popular belief, it has been shown that in many cases in which blood is present, the supernatant after centrifuging does not show xanthochromia. The presence of red cells in the CSF without xanthochromia, if the history is suggestive, is some evidence therefore of subarachnoid haemorrhage, and the findings should not be lightly dismissed as a 'bloody tap'.

In the case of benign intracranial hypertension, usually presenting with headaches and papilloedema, CT scanning or MRI is clearly necessary, as a mass lesion such as a tumour is a far more likely initial diagnosis. Only after the scans have been rigorously reviewed should one proceed to lumbar puncture as a diagnostic procedure.

Finally, an acutely ill child or adult with headache and neck stiffness may well have meningitis. However, he may also have a cerebral abscess. Posterior fossa mass lesions can also cause severe occipital headache. Even if meningitis is strongly suspected on clinical grounds, it is wise to have a CT scan before proceeding to lumbar puncture. However, if a scanner is not readily available, and if meningitis seems very likely, the risks of delay in antibiotic treatment have to be balanced against the risks of coning.

8.2.4 *What tests should be done on the cerebrospinal fluid?*

From Table 8.1 the appropriate tests can be deduced for each clinical circumstance. For example in patients with suspected multiple scler-osis, the most important test is the presence of oligoclonal bands or myelin basic protein. In general, far more laboratory tests are performed on the CSF than is appropriate. One study reviewed 555 consecutive cases in which CSF had been sent to the laboratory. Among 334 cases (60 per cent) with a normal opening pressure, cell count, and protein, 1385 additional tests were done, but such tests were useful in only three patients, all with multiple sclerosis. In another phase of this study, among 148 consecutive cases of bacterial chronic infectious and malignant meningitis, the opening pressure, cell count, or protein were abnormal in all but three (two cases of childhood bacterial meningitis, one of cryptococcal meningitis with acquired immunodeficiency syndrome, AIDS).

A review of the findings on the analysis of CSF obtained during radiculography on nearly 400 orthopaedic patients showed that management was not influenced in a single patient. There are thus no reasons for sending the CSF to the laboratory in these circumstances.

8.3 Electroencephalography (EEG)

The electrical potentials generated by the more-or-less synchronized activity of large numbers of neurons can be detected by electrodes attached to the scalp, as first described by Berger in 1929. The potential at one electrode is either compared to a close neighbour (bipolar recording), or to an averaged reference electrode.

An occipital alpha rhythm can be recorded from most normal subjects over the back of the head. The alpha rhythm, typically of about 150 μV amplitude, and about 11 c/s in frequency (range 8–14 c/s) attenuates when the eyes are opened. It is usually of slightly higher amplitude over the non-dominant hemisphere. The alpha rhythm will be disrupted on one side by a large posterior cortical infarct, and may be attenuated if a subdural haematoma overlies the parieto-occipital cortex on one side. Apart from such abnormalities in the alpha rhythm, the clinical neurophysiologist will look out for abnormal rhythmic activity, such as slow 'delta' activity at less than 4 c/s which may be generated in the region of a tumour. It must be acknowledged, however, that most diagnoses of structural abnormality are made by CT scanning or MRI.

Electroencephalography is basically an investigation of cerebral *function*.

Rhythms intermediate in frequency between alpha and delta are termed 'theta' activity (4–7 c/s). Theta activity occurs normally in young people and during drowsiness, and abnormally (unhelpfully) in many conditions. Activity faster than 14 c/s is termed 'beta' activity. It is commonly recorded from normal subjects over the front of the head; if prominent and persistent, the consumption of drugs such as barbiturates should be suspected.

Apart from this more-or-less rhythmic activity, focal or generalized spikes, or spikes and slow waves, may be recorded (see Fig. 8.1). An example

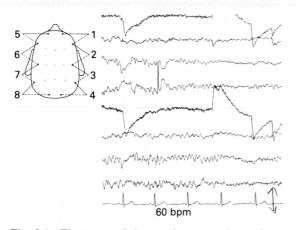

60 bpm

Fig. 8.1 Electroencephalogram between seizures in a patient with complex partial seizures. Note the sharp spike followed by a slow wave between the third and fourth channels over the right temporal lobe. There is phase reversal between electrodes T4–T6 and T6–02. The large deflections in the first and fifth channels represent eye movements.

of generalized epileptic activity recorded during a typical absence seizure (Section 12.4.2) is shown in Fig. 12.4. Abnormal spikes or spikes and slow waves may be seen inter-ictally over an epileptogenic focus in one temporal lobe. Other abnormalities include stereotyped complex waveforms. For example, generalized sharp waves every 0.5–1 s occur repetitively in Creutzfeldt–Jakob disease (Section 17.15.1), and high-voltage stereotyped delta wave complexes at longer intervals of 3–10 s in subacute sclerosing panencephalitis (Section 17.14.3.1). In other types of encephalitis, particu-

larly herpes simplex encephalitis (Section 17.12.3.3), or in association with a cerebral abscess (Section 17.2.1) or cerebral infarct, there may be periodic lateralized epileptic discharges, commonly known as PLEDS.

When the electroencephalogram (EEG) was introduced, it was hoped that it would have a major role in psychiatric practice, but these expectations have not been fulfilled. It is, however, occasionally useful in pointing to an organic cause for behavioural disorders in children, such as may occur in association with a lipidosis, and may help to distinguish between an agitated depression in middle age and early Alzheimer's disease.

The principal role of the EEG, however, is in the evaluation of patients with epilepsy. First of all, it must be remembered that about 50 per cent of those who have had an undoubted tonic–clonic seizure will have a normal EEG. It follows that a normal EEG does not prove or disprove a diagnosis of epilepsy. Conversely, more specific epileptic EEG features, such as spike–wave activity or focal spikes, are seldom found in subjects without a history of seizures. The probabilities of recording epileptic activity are increased by recording while the patient is drowsy, particularly after a period of deprivation of sleep, and during or shortly after hyperventilation. In some types of epilepsy, paroxysmal discharges may be induced by photic stimulation.

A major use of the EEG in epilepsy is to determine seizure type, as the choice of anticonvulsant medication for recurrent seizures depends on this (see Chapter 12). Continuing EEG abnormalities during anticonvulsant treatment, even if the seizures have been controlled, have been shown in some studies to be an unfavourable prognostic feature for the successful withdrawal of medication without further seizures recurring.

The EEG is also useful on occasions in the operating theatre and intensive care unit. For example, cerebral complications during cardiac bypass surgery can be monitored in the operating theatre. In the intensive care unit, changes in the EEG may be powerful predictors of good or bad outcome from coma.

8.3.1   *Other types of EEG recording*

If there is difficulty in deciding about the type of epileptic seizure, or in distinguishing true seizures from pseudoseizures, then it is often helpful to record the EEG long term on magnetic tape for several days, video-recording simultaneously the patient's activity on the same tape. If an event occurs, the physician and clinical neurophysiologist can review repeatedly patient movements and behaviour and the associated EEG activity on a split-screen monitor (Fig. 12.5).

Long-term monitoring may also be carried out by using a portable tape recorder, in a manner parallel to that used in Holter monitoring of cardiac rhythms. Up to eight channels of information can now be recorded. The method is useful in monitoring the frequency of epileptic activity in a patient's normal environment, and may sometimes be useful in distinguishing epileptic attacks from other causes of disturbed consciousness.

All the methods of recording so far described use electrodes attached to the scalp. These electrodes record from a comparatively limited volume of brain beneath them, as the amplitude of potential differences is rapidly attenuated by distance. It is occasionally helpful, therefore, to place electrodes nearer a site of suspected seizure discharge, either by placing an electrode in the nasopharynx, or as a fine wire inserted below the floor of the middle cranial fossa (sphenoidal electrode). When it is crucially important to determine the side and exact site of origin of a seizure discharge prior to attempts at surgical removal of a seizure focus (Section 12.9.1), then depth electrodes may be inserted into the brain, and recordings made for 2–3 weeks. Other techniques include a strip of electrodes fixed to plastic which can be inserted subdurally over the temporal lobe through one or more burr holes. Finally, at operation, tiny electrodes may be placed directly on the cortex around the suspected lesion. This is known as *electrocorticography*.

8.3.2 *The presentation of information derived from the EEG*

Rapid advances in electronics and computing mean that the potential changes recorded from the scalp or elsewhere can be readily manipulated. Some departments now record all their EEGs on tape or disc ('paperless EEG'), allowing subsequent hard-copy presentation only of interesting features. Mathematical processing of the information allows graphical presentation of results. Examples include

compressed spectral array, and brain mapping, the latter referring to computer-generated coloured images by which areas of difference can be highlighted. Fractal analysis is being assessed.

A simple and effective tool in the intensive care ward is the cerebral function monitor. Cerebral electrical activity is processed and recorded on slow-moving paper in such a way that a global view of cerebral function can be obtained. If coma is deepening, for example, this will be reflected in a downward slope of the trace; seizures will be reflected as sharp peaks in output on the monitor.

8.4 Evoked responses

A single flash will generate a change in occipital lobe potential that can readily be seen in the scalp EEG, although 'interfered with' by the alpha rhythm. As the response has a fixed latency after the flash, and the alpha rhythm can be considered as biological 'noise', the averaged response evoked by, say, 128 flashes can readily be extracted using computerized techniques of signal processing. In practice, a more stable visual evoked response (VER) is obtained if the subject looks at a chequer-board, the squares of which are made to alternate between black and white at a rate of about once a second.

An example of a normal VER is shown in Fig. 8.2a. The latency to the principal positive deflection is about 100 ms. In patients with optic nerve lesions, for example optic neuritis, the principal positive deflection is delayed, and of lesser amplitude. In the example shown in Fig. 8.2b, the positive deflection is no longer clearly visible after stimulation of the left retina.

Similar time-locked responses can be recorded from the scalp after a loud click, but the waveform is more complex; potentials in the so-called brainstem auditory evoked response (BSAER) can be identified as arising from the cochlea, cochlear nucleus, and auditory cortex. Other deflections have less certain origins. Somatosensory evoked responses can also be recorded from the parietal scalp if the skin of the contralateral hand is stimulated.

Any of these evoked responses may be deranged in any disease of the brain, and, in the case of somatosensory evoked responses, of the spinal cord as well. Their ease of recording with modern

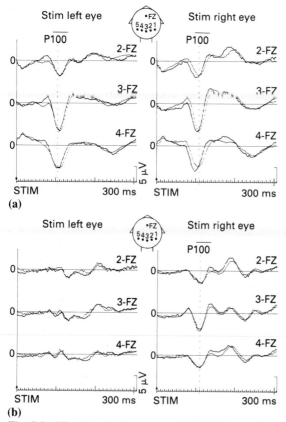

Fig. 8.2 Visual evoked responses (VERs) in retrobulbar neuritis. (a) Normal VERs from patient with an episode of sensory disturbance of acute onset in both lower limbs—suspected multiple sclerosis. The latency from the left eye is 104 ms and from the right eye 108 ms, both within normal limits. (b) One year later, after an episode of acute retrobulbar neuritis, the left VER is no longer detectable. (Reproduced by kind permission of Mr R. Pottinger.)

electronic techniques has made them appear more important in clinical practice than they really are. However, the presence of an abnormal cochlear potential in the BSAER is a useful guide to probable deafness in infants, in whom hearing cannot otherwise be tested. Abnormal evoked responses may also provide laboratory support for the diagnosis of multiple sclerosis when a subject has had only one clinical event at an anatomical site other than that being neurophysiologically tested (see Section 14.4.2). For example, in a subject with an acute resolving spinal cord lesion, the presence of

an abnormal VER will suggest that the basis of his illness is multiple sclerosis. Somatosensory evoked responses are also potential monitors of function during spinal cord surgery, or during operations to correct scoliosis.

8.5   Magneto-encephalography

The electrical activity of neurons produces minute changes in magnetic field which can now be detected by sensitive super-conducting quantum interference devices (SQUIDS). In contrast to electrical fields, which are variably impeded by grey and white matter, and considerably attenuated by the skull, magnetic fields are not greatly affected by the material through which they pass. It is therefore possible to deduce more accurately the site of origin of neuronal discharges by minute variations in the recorded magnetic field. EEG and magnetic recordings from a patient with epilepsy may show the same event (an EEG inter-ictal spike), with totally different wave forms, and with different temporal relationships on magneto-encephalography. This difference presumably reflects different physiological processes or signal generators. Magneto-encephalography is at present a research technique, which may prove to be of increasing value in epilepsy. The high capital cost of the necessarily sensitive detectors militates against the widespread introduction of magneto-encephalography at the present time.

8.6   Magnetic brain stimulation

The principle of this procedure is that a current passed through a flat circular copper coil (familiarly known as 'the magic halo') held over the scalp will induce a magnetic field in the centre of the coil, and this in turn will induce current flow sufficient to discharge Betz cells in the motor cortex. If the resulting muscle contractions are recorded electromyographically, it is possible to calculate a central motor conduction time between cortex and muscle (Fig. 8.3). It is of physiological interest that single motor units can be made to discharge by threshold scalp stimuli, and that these motor units are those that are first activated by voluntary contractions. Central motor conduction time is moderately prolonged in some patients with

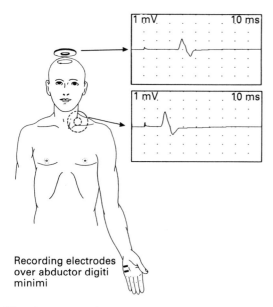

Recording electrodes
over abductor digiti
minimi

Fig. 8.3 Magnetic brain stimulation. The muscle response evoked from the left abductor digiti minimi after magnetic stimulation of the brain (top record) and brachial plexus (lower record). (Figure kindly provided by Dr J. A. Jarratt.)

multiple sclerosis and motor neuron disease. Similar estimates of central motor conduction time may be made by percutaneous electrical stimulation of the cortex, by means of a large capacitor discharged through an electrode over the scalp. This procedure is rather more uncomfortable than magnetic stimulation. As magnetic stimulation is also capable of stimulating peripheral nerves, and as magnetic stimulation is painless, it is possible that it will replace electrical stimulation in conventional nerve conduction studies (Section 8.8). Recently magnetic stimulation has been used in research on epilepsy. It is possible to activate seizure foci by external magnetic stimulation.

8.7 Electromyography

This is the technique whereby the electrical activity of muscle fibres is recorded. The changes in voltage are amplified and displayed on an oscilloscope, and also monitored through a loudspeaker, as the qualities of sound resulting from different abnormalities of muscle fibre electrical discharge activity are, in some cases, more readily recognized by the ear than by the eye.

8.7.1 *Normal and abnormal muscle activity*

Muscle activity can be recorded readily through surface electrodes placed on the skin, and indeed may prove a troublesome artefact when attempting to record the smaller potentials of the electro-encephalogram. However, because surface electrodes pick up changes in voltage from large volumes of tissue, they are really only of use when the overall pattern of activity of large groups of muscle fibres is required. Their principal use is to record the muscle response evoked by nerve stimulation in the measurement of motor conduction velocity (Section 8.8). There are, however, other applications. Studies of gait, for example, may use surface electrodes over a number of different muscles so that the timing of contraction during various phases of a step can be studied. Surface electrodes may also be of use when there is doubt about the presence of fasciculation (Section 6.2.2.2) in, for example, motor neuron disease (Section 20.1.4).

The electrical activity of individual muscle fibres and of motor units is studied by inserting a sterile concentric needle electrode percutaneously into the muscle belly. Such an electrode is a hollow steel needle through which runs a silver, steel, or platinum wire that is fully insulated except at its exposed tip. Here it remains separated from the cylindrical wall of the needle shaft. The needle tip and the needle shaft form two electrodes about 200 μm apart. Such an electrode therefore only 'sees' changes in voltage in its immediate vicinity, and by careful manipulation it is possible to detect the activity of a single fibrillating muscle fibre (Fig. 8.4). Other, rather larger, needles with a number of different recording channels and pick-up points at intervals down the needle shaft are used in specialized studies on neuromuscular transmission (Section 8.8.1).

8.7.1.1 *Normal muscle*

A normally innervated muscle at rest is electrically silent, unless the electrode happens, by chance, to be inserted into a region where there are many end-plates. Very small (10–30 μV), short duration (up to 1 ms) potentials occur at high frequency,

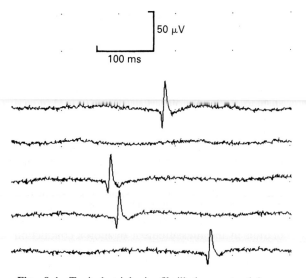

Fig. 8.4 Typical triphasic fibrillation potentials, as found on electromyography of denervated muscle.

making a steady 'sssshing' *end-plate noise* through the audio-amplifier. These are miniature end-plate potentials recorded extracellularly.

When a single anterior horn cell is activated, all the muscle fibres to which it is connected are also activated. The number of muscle fibres making up such a *motor unit* vary from 10 in the external ocular muscles to 400–500 in quadriceps. Owing to slight differences in conduction times down the branches of the pre-terminal axon, the muscle fibres do not contract synchronously. The *motor unit potential* therefore has a compound form, and lasts up to 12 ms.

During a weak voluntary contraction, individual motor unit potentials can be distinguished. Initially the same one fires at an increasing rate, but very soon it is joined by a second, which can be distinguished by its wave form. Increasing voluntary activity, however, soon results in a running together on the oscilloscope screen of motor unit potentials. They 'interfere' with each other, and the pattern of discharge is therefore called an '*interference pattern*'.

8.7.1.2   *Partial denervation*

Figure 20.2 illustrates what happens in a partly denervated muscle. It shows that anterior horn

cells A and C have incorporated, by axonal sprouting, the muscle fibres that originally belonged to anterior horn cell B. Electromyography in chronic partial denervation therefore reveals motor units that are of larger amplitude than normal (>5 mV). As conduction through the new axonal sprouts to distant muscle fibres takes longer than normal, the duration of the action potential is also increased, and reversals of polarity have a greater chance of occurrence. The hallmark of chronic partial denervation, therefore, is long-duration, high-voltage, polyphasic potentials which, because there are fewer motor units remaining, are seen firing in relative isolation in a reduced interference pattern.

When a muscle fibre is denervated, individual muscle fibres begin to contract spontaneously after an interval of about 17 days, and continue indefinitely thereafter until re-innervation occurs. The accompanying electrical activity is known as a fibrillation potential. Figure 8.4 shows a series of typical fibrillation potentials. These have an amplitude of up to 300 μV, and a duration of up to 5 ms, and a simple bi- or triphasic contour. They are not prevented by curare. It has been shown that the resting membrane potential of denervated muscle fibres tends to fluctuate rhythmically, and fibrillation potential is probably a spike generated when such fluctuations reach a critical level. Fibrillating muscle fibres cannot be seen through the skin, but may be visible under the mucosa of the tongue in, for example, motor neuron disease.

When a needle electrode is inserted into a normal muscle, there is a brief (<2 s) burst of activity due to mechanical stimulation of muscle fibres. This activity is prolonged in denervated muscle, which is unusually sensitive to mechanical deformation. A shower of fibrillation potentials or positive sharp waves may continue for several seconds after needle movement. These are biphasic potentials of about the same amplitude as fibrillation potentials, but of rather longer duration (up to 10 ms). Such a prolonged discharge is reported as *increased insertion activity*.

Fasciculation potentials have the same dimensions as motor unit potentials, but arise spontaneously in denervated muscle, discharging once every 3 or 4 seconds. They not uncommonly occur in normal calf muscles, but such benign fasciculations usually occur at a rather faster rate—at about once a second. A sufficient number of muscle fibres take part in a fasciculation to cause a twitch visible through the skin. Fasciculations are therefore important clinical evidence of denervation. They are particularly prominent in diseases of the anterior horn cells, such as motor neuron disease (Section 20.1.4). However, the origin of fasciculations is obscure. They do not necessarily represent spontaneous motor unit discharges, as it has been shown that the wave form of a fasciculation potential is usually different from that recorded from the identical site during weak voluntary contraction. It is probable that most are generated in the proximal branches of the pre-terminal axon.

8.7.1.3   *Myopathies*

Myopathic disorders are characterized by a reduction in the average number of fibres per motor unit. Motor unit potentials are therefore of smaller amplitude than normal, and are also of shorter duration, as the geographical limits of each motor unit shrink due to advancing primary muscle disease. The spikes generated by surviving fibres may be sufficiently separated so that they do not have the chance to summate and produce the more smoothly rounded contours of a normal motor unit potential. As each diseased motor unit exerts less tension than a healthy one, more units have to be recruited to produce the desired force. Myopathies, therefore, are characterized by a full interference pattern at low levels of voluntary effort, individual motor units being of small amplitude, short duration, and highly polyphasic. Through a loudspeaker, this pattern has a characteristic crackling noise.

8.7.1.4   *Other types of muscle fibre activity*

Myotonic discharges are seen in myotonic dystrophy (Section 21.7.1), and in other rare types of muscle disorder. Mechanical or electrical stimulation of a myotonic muscle results in a high-frequency discharge (up to 100 Hz) of action potentials, lasting 3–4 s. Characteristically, the frequency of the discharge falls towards its end. The signals so produced, when monitored through a loudspeaker, suggest a dive-bomber pulling out of its dive. The potentials making up a myotonic discharge are potentials derived from single fibres.
Pseudomyotonic discharges are complex, high-frequency polyphasic discharges that start and end abruptly. They are particularly frequent in polymyositis (Section 21.3).

Myokymia is the name given to quivering movements that may occur in fatigued periocular or calf muscles. Facial myokymia also occurs in tetanys, and in patients with the so-called stiff-man syndrome, a disorder of unknown cause (Section 21.12.4). In tetany, double or triple discharges of individual motor units can be seen.

If distant from the immediate periocular region, myokymia may be a manifestation of brain-stem multiple sclerosis or tumour. Electromyographically, myokymia is characterized by firing of single motor units for a few seconds, followed by a brief pause of a few seconds, before repetition. Alternate cycles in nearby motor units give rise to a worm-like wriggling under the skin.

Hemifacial spasm is a disorder characterized by brief spontaneous twitches occurring initially around the eye, and subsequently affecting the lower face. It is believed to be due to ephaptic transmission between adjacent nerve fibres of the facial nerve, at sites of compression just outside the brain stem. The usual source of compression is a redundant loop of artery, and decompression may result in complete cure. Electromyographically, hemifacial spasm is characterized by isolated bursts of repetitive high-frequency motor unit discharges.

Muscle cramps occurring in otherwise healthy people are due to repetitive high-frequency motor unit discharge. In rare circumstances cramping contractions can occur without motor unit discharge. An example is myophosphorylase deficiency (Section 21.8.1.1).

8.8   Nerve conduction studies

The principle of measurement of motor conduction velocity is illustrated in Fig. 8.5. Using the ulnar nerve as an example, surface recording electrodes are placed over abductor digiti minimi, and the nerve is stimulated supramaximally at wrist (stimulus 2) and above the elbow (stimulus 1), two points about 30 cm (0.3 m) apart. From the differences in latencies in the onset of the evoked muscle response (4.0 ms at the wrist, 10 ms at the elbow) the velocity of the fastest conducting fibres can be calculated: 0.3 m ÷ 0.006 s = 50 m/s. In this particular example, the latency on distal stimulation is of no great significance, but a characteristic feature

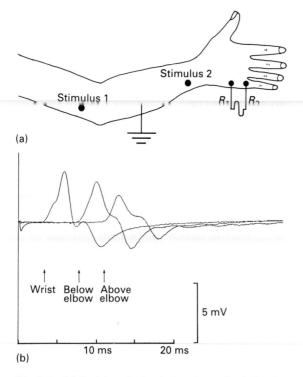

(a)

(b)

Fig. 8.5 (a) Position of stimulating electrodes (stimulus 1 and stimulus 2) and recording electrodes over abductor digiti minimi when recording motor conduction velocity. (b) Compression of the ulnar nerve at the elbow. The amplitude of the muscle action potential from abductor digiti minimi on stimulation of the ulnar nerve at the wrist is 4.0 mV; it is 3.0 mV below the elbow, and is much smaller again, and is dispersed, on stimulation above the elbow (2.1 mV). The maximal motor conduction velocity is 56 m/s from below elbow to wrist, but only 21 m/s across the elbow segment.

of the carpal tunnel syndrome is a prolonged distal latency (>5 ms) on stimulation of the median nerve at the wrist.

As measurements are made to the onset of the evoked muscle response, only the velocity of the fastest conducting motor fibre can be made. In disorders affecting anterior horn cells, therefore, such as motor neuron disease, motor conduction velocity remains near normal. It may be slightly reduced as there is a tendency for anterior horn cells with axons of largest diameter (and therefore fastest velocity) to be affected first. The amplitude of the evoked muscle response, although partly dependent upon electrode placement, will reflect the numbers of muscle fibres that remain innervated, so this declines as the disease progresses. Motor neuron disease (Section 20.1.5) and axonal neuropathies (Section 19.2) are therefore characterized by near normal motor conduction velocities, with reduced amplitude of evoked muscle response. However, in demyelinating (Schwann-cell) neuropathies (Section 19.2) conduction velocity is slowed, often to less than 25 m/s in the arms and to less than 20 m/s in the legs.

Useful information can also be obtained in compression neuropathies (Section 19.4.2.3). Figure 8.5b illustrates the findings in a chronic entrapment neuropathy at the elbow. Note the normal amplitude of the evoked muscle response when the ulnar nerve is stimulated at the wrist and the smaller dispersed amplitude when the stimulus is applied above the level of the block in conduction. Although it is not easy to measure small distances very accurately, it is clear that velocity through the compressed segment is also slowed compared to that below. Similar changes occur in the entrapment neuropathy of the common peroneal nerve at the knee.

Conduction in sensory fibres can also be measured. Figure 8.6 shows the usual arrangement whereby the purely sensory fibres in the digital nerves are stimulated by ring electrodes, and the evoked nerve action potential recorded at the wrist. The sural nerve in the leg can be studied in an analogous way. The amplitude of the sensory action potential is, broadly speaking, proportional to the number of surviving fibres, so it is diminished in axonal neuropathies. It is, however, also proportional to the degree of synchronization of the volley as it passes under the electrodes. Demyelinating neuropathies cause considerable slowing of conduction in some fibres, and the volley is desynchronized. In this type of neuropathy, therefore, sensory action potentials may also be reduced in amplitude or absent.

Other useful techniques include recording F waves and H reflexes. The F wave is a small muscle response occurring with a latency much longer than the directly evoked muscle response. It results from antidromic discharge of some anterior horn cells. F waves may occur with prolonged latencies or be lost at an early stage in radiculopathies and in acute infective polyneuropathy (Section 19.3.9). The H reflex is a monosynaptic response, obtained

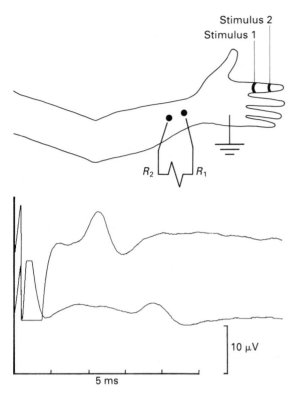

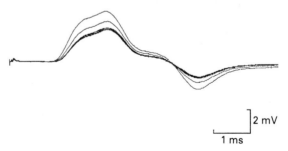

Fig. 8.6   (a) Position of stimulating electrodes (stimulus 1 and stimulus 2) and recording electrodes over median nerve when recording median sensory conduction velocity. For recording ulnar sensory action potentials, the fifth finger is stimulated, and the recording electrodes placed over the ulnar nerve. (b) Carpal tunnel syndrome. Top trace: normal ulnar sensory afferent volley recorded after stimulation of the fifth finger (amplitude 12 mV; latency 2.2 ms). Bottom trace: smaller and delayed sensory action potential recorded from the median nerve after stimulation of the index finger.

from weak stimulation of afferent fibres in the posterior tibial nerve. This evokes a reflex response from anterior horn cells supplying the gastrocnemius. This response will be delayed in cases in which peripheral nerve conduction is slowed. H reflexes may also be evoked from other muscles if the excitability of the motor neuron pool is increased, as is the case in upper motor neuron lesions.

   Conduction times with rough estimates of velocity can also be measured within the spinal cord. Surface electrodes can be placed over different spinal levels and, after peripheral nerve stimula-

tion, the ascending volleys in the posterior columns can be recorded and enhanced from background noise using computer averaging techniques. Descending central motor conduction time can be measured after cortical stimulation in humans, using transcranial electrical or magnetic stimulating techniques (Section 8.6).

8.8.1   *Studies of neuromuscular transmission*

Electrodiagnostic studies are an important tool in the analysis of the defects of neuromuscular transmissions that occur in myasthenia gravis (Section 21.12.2.4) and in the myasthenic syndromes (Section 21.12.3).

   These disorders are investigated electrophysiologically in the following way. Surface electrodes are placed over a convenient muscle, most frequently abductor digiti minimi, their position being adjusted so that occasional supramaximal stimuli to the ulnar nerve at the wrist evoke the largest possible response. The nerve is then stimulated at 3 Hz for 2 s. In normal subjects the amplitude of the fourth response should be at least 92 per cent of the amplitude of the first response. In myasthenia gravis the defect in neuromuscular transmission is exaggerated by repetitive stimulation, and the amplitude of the fourth response may be considerably less than that of the first (Fig. 8.7).

   Rather confusingly, at higher rates of stimula-

Fig. 8.7   Myasthenia gravis. Compound muscle action potential recorded from the abductor digiti minimi, the electrodes being placed as in Fig. 8.5a. The ulnar nerve was stimulated supramaximally at 3 Hz at the wrist. The first recorded response is the largest at 4.1 mV. The second is 3.2 mV, the third and fourth responses are superimposed and have an amplitude of only 2.4 mV, 59 per cent of the initial response. This decrement in amplitude of the evoked muscle response is typical of myasthenia gravis.

tion (30 Hz) there may be a brief period of facilitation of transmission, possibly due to release of stored quanta.

When a patient with the myasthenic syndrome is studied in the same way, the amplitude of the muscle response evoked at low frequencies of stimulation is smaller than normal. A brief period of voluntary contraction, or repetitive stimulation at 10 Hz, results in considerable facilitation so that the amplitude increases three- or four-fold.

Disorders of neuromuscular transmission are also studied by the use of the so-called single-fibre electrode, with more than one pick-up surface. The needle is inserted into a weakly contracting muscle. When an action potential is recorded, the voltage is used to trigger the oscilloscope sweep. Voltage changes derived from another fibre of the same motor unit are recorded through a second pick-up surface. There is a near-constant difference in latency between the two fibres in normal muscles, but if there is a defect in neuromuscular transmission, the interval will be variable. The second potential is seen to 'jitter' along the screen because of its variable time relationship to the first. Sometimes transmission to the second fibre fails completely. An example of 'jitter' is seen in Fig. 8.8.

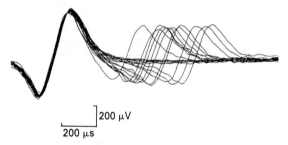

200 μV

200 μs

Fig. 8.8 Myasthenia gravis. The 'jitter' phenomenon (see text for details). In this example the difference in latency between the earliest and latest responses is about 400 μs.

8.9 Biopsy of brain, nerve, and muscle

One of the great difficulties that neurology has in relation to other clinical disciplines is that biopsy of central nervous system tissue is not nearly as practical as, for example, liver biopsy or intestinal biopsy. Although it is easy enough to make a burr hole, the passage of a cannula and removal of brain tissue carries a significant morbidity with a risk of hemiparesis or other disability. Brain biopsy is only rarely justifiable in the assessment of metabolic neurological disorders. It is often justifiable in an attempt to obtain histological confirmation of a malignant tumour that may prove to be radiosensitive, or bacteriological confirmation of an abscess.

Peripheral nervous system tissue can be biopsied rather more readily. The usual procedure is to resect a fascicle of a sural nerve. However, the procedure is painful if undertaken under local cutaneous anaesthesia, and many subjects are subsequently aware of unpleasant dysaesthesiae in the territory of the fascicle that has been removed. Although the procedure has enormously advanced our understanding of the range of structural abnormalities in peripheral nerves, it has to be admitted that sural biopsy in a patient with a peripheral neuropathy, the cause of which is difficult to elucidate, is often remarkably uninformative.

Biopsy of the rectal submucosa is an effective way of obtaining samples of neurons (lying in the plexi of Auerbach) that may help provide definitive evidence of one of the neurolipidoses (see Chapter 23).

Muscle biopsy is a standard procedure for investigating patients with possible metabolic myopathies, polymyositis, muscular dystrophies, or neurogenic atrophies (see Chapter 21). The muscle chosen should be clinically involved, but not so severely wasted that it is likely to be virtually replaced by fibrosis and fatty tissue. Common suitable sites are quadriceps or deltoid muscles. Needle biopsy has largely replaced open biopsy. The tissue obtained is commonly examined by histochemical and ultrastructural techniques. For example, in acid maltase deficiency (Section 21.8.1.2) both the deficiency of the enzyme and the excess accumulation of its substrate, glycogen, can be demonstrated.

8.10 Imaging procedures

8.10.1 *Plain X-rays*

8.10.1.1 *Chest X-ray*

One of many possible examples of reasons for needing a chest X-ray in neurological practice is the diagnosis of a bronchial carcinoma, which may be responsible for cerebral or spinal metastasis, or non-metastatic syndromes such as peripheral neuropathy (Section 19.3.5) or myasthenic syndrome (Section 21.12.3.1).

8.10.1.2   *Skull X-ray*

The role of the skull X-ray has diminished enormously since the advent of CT scanning and MRI. If there are already appropriate indications for CT scanning, the physician should ask himself whether plain films will of themselves contribute more, bearing in mind that a perfectly adequate lateral film is necessarily obtained as a 'scout' film in the initial stages of a CT scan. Sometimes a physician will use a skull X-ray as a relatively cheap investigation as a means of reassurance of a patient with a headache, whom he does not believe to be at significant risk of having a tumour; but, as explained in Section 9.11, there is no justification for this. Equally, skull X-rays cannot be used as a cheap 'screening' investigation in psychiatric practice. White and Barraclough showed that all their psychiatric patients who turned out to have abnormal CT scans had normal skull X-rays.

Table 8.2   Intracranial calcification

Normal calcification	Pathological calcification
Pineal body	Tumours
Falx cerebri	oligodendroglioma
Choroid plexus	craniopharyngioma
Petroclinoid ligaments	meningioma
Bridged sella	astrocytoma (rarely)
Carotid siphon	
	Other causes
	angiomatous malformations
	old haematomas
	tuberculoma
	toxoplasmosis
	cysticercosis
	tuberous sclerosis
	aneurysm (ring calcification in wall)
	hyperparathyroidism (in basal ganglia and dentate nucleus)

Skull X-rays may be needed after a head injury. The indications are discussed in Section 15.4.2 and listed in Table 15.3. Occasionally a skull X-ray taken in these circumstances may show an unexpected finding, such as abnormal calcification. Calcification may occur, for example, in oligodendrogliomas (Section 16.3.1.1), craniopharyngiomas (Section 16.6.5.1), or angiomatous malformations (Section 10.6.6). Other causes are listed in Table 8.2. Another chance finding is of an enlarged pituitary fossa, the management of which is discussed in Section 16.6.

8.10.1.3   *X-rays of the spine*

These are considered in Section 8.13.1.

8.10.2   *Computerized tomography (CT scanning)*

The original X-ray images produced by Röntgen depended upon the differential absorption by bones and soft tissues of X-ray photons as they passed through the imaged part of the body to fall upon a photographic plate. X-ray photons reduce a silver halide in an image reflecting the differential absorption. In computerized tomography (CT scanning), the conventional X-ray film is replaced by a series of photon detectors. The arrival or non-arrival of a photon is a yes/no piece of information, allowing the possibility of digital processing. In CT scanning of the brain, the patient lies horizontal, with his or her head within an orbiting focused X-ray beam housed in a gantry, which also houses a series of photon detectors located geometrically opposite the X-ray source. There is a central aperture in the gantry through which the patient, lying horizontally, is passed mechanically in a series of steps, usually at intervals of a few millimetres. The scanning system rotates around the patient during each scan cycle. Just as the silver halide molecules on Röntgen's plate acted as photon detectors, the receipt of the photon being marked by the reduction of the halide to metallic silver, so the photon detector signals the arrival of a photon.

Within the brain, any cube of tissue of, say, side 1 mm, is traversed a number of times as the beam rotates around the head. The relative value of the absorption of the volume of tissue is then solved through a computer processing a series of differential equations on the digital information. The software then constructs a digital map. A shade of grey between white and black is assigned to the digital value, and displayed as an image on a monitor screen and subsequent film for return to the neurologist or neurosurgeon. The image on the screen or film is made up of a matrix of individual squares known as pixels (picture elements). The third dimension, the slice thickness, adds the dimension of volume, the three-dimensional element being known as a voxel (volume element). The absorption values are assigned to a scale, known as the Hounsfield scale after the name of the British physicist who developed CT scanning. This linear scale assigns the value of 0 to water, −1000 to air, and +1000 to dense bone. High absorption (dense) structures are conventionally viewed as white. Air is therefore black, and soft tissue various shades of grey. The human eye can appreciate only a limited number of steps of greyness, so for this reason only a range of values can be distinguished simultaneously. The range of values for display appropriate to the tissue being examined can be set by controls on the imaging monitor. This range of density (absorption) values is known as the window width, the centre of the range being the window level. The smaller the range of absorption values represented by each grey scale step, the greater the contrast. When it is wished to display tissues with small differences in density, a narrow window width is therefore employed.

The long (vertical) axis of the patient passes through the axis of the gantry, so such scans are known as axial scans (hence the abbreviation sometimes used, CAT scan—computerized axial tomography—now usually further abbreviated to CT). However, the acquisition of digital information does allow the information to be processed in any plane of view required by the radiologist or surgeon. For example, the information acquired in a number of voxels round the pituitary fossa from a series of slices can be stacked vertically to provide a sagittal image. The resolution of such reconstructed images is dependent on slice thickness. Magnetic resonance imaging (MRI), creates sagittal images which are much superior in resolution to reconstructed CT images (see Fig. 8.19).

The digital information coming from the CT scanner can be used in other important ways,

notably to provide the possibility of sterotaxic biopsy. For example, in a patient with epilepsy who has an area of low density in one frontal lobe, the coordinates of the low density area on CT

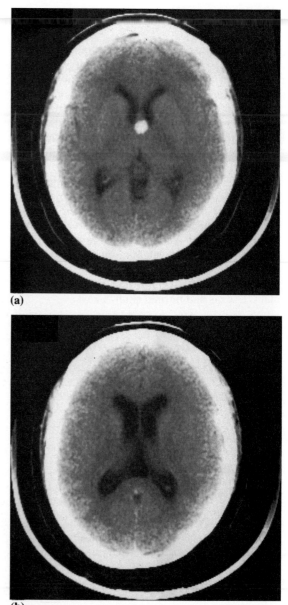

(a)

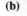

(b)

Fig. 8.9 Colloid cyst. (a) The spherical white lesion in the centre of the image is a colloid cyst. (b) A section 10 mm adjacent shows no cyst but prominent dilatation of the lateral and third ventricles.

scanning can be used to design an appropriate approach to the biopsy needle guided by a stereo-tactic frame. The information can be re-processed so that the surgeon can rotate and re-view the image, and consider the least damaging passage for the biopsy needle.

As noted above, the X-ray absorption of a voxel, the resulting number of Hounsfield units assigned, and the resulting level of greyness on the image depend upon the characteristics of the voxel—bone absorbing most X-ray photons largely because of the characteristics of the calcium atoms in it, and air and cerebrospinal fluid very few. The cerebrospinal fluid is thus clearly visualized in the ventricles as dark (low attenuation) cavities. They are clearly outlined in most of the scans used to illustrate this chapter, but are particularly promi-nent in Fig. 8.9. In this case the lateral ventricles are dilated as a result of a colloid cyst at the foramen of Monro. The cyst itself contains fluid which highly attenuates the passage of X-ray pho-tons, and is therefore imaged as a white circle (sphere in three dimensions).

Most tumours and other pathological tissues do not contrast so sharply with normal brain as the colloid cyst shown in Fig. 8.9. In order to enhance the distinction between different types of tissue, a contrast agent is commonly used. Most of these agents contain three atoms of iodine in each molecule. Enhancement results from the increased absorption (attenuation) of X-rays caused by the high atomic number of iodine. Circulating blood is imaged as the amount of iodine after intravenous injection significantly raises absorption (1 mg/ml of iodine raises the attenuation of blood by about 25 Hounsfield units). In the normal subject, there is slight overall enhancement of grey matter com-pared to white matter, as grey matter has a richer blood supply than the white. In the normal subject, an intact blood–brain barrier prevents the extra-vasation of the iodine-containing contrast medium through the tight capillary junctions. If there is a breakdown in the blood–brain barrier, as com-monly occurs in patients with cerebral tumours, then there is a considerable increase in the atten-uation of the tumour tissue as iodine leaks into it (Fig. 8.10). There is also often some enhancement in the early days of a cerebral infarct (Fig. 10.2c,d),

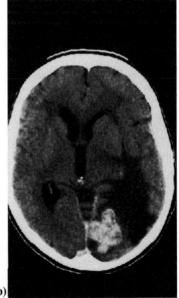

(a)   (b)

Fig. 8.10 CT scan: cerebral metastasis, probably from a bronchial carcinoma. (a) The left parieto-occipital region shows a large, irregular-shaped area of low attenuation. Posteriorly in the occipital lobe is an area of higher density. (b) After the injection of contrast, the area of high density enhances remarkably. These images also show a shift of the mid-line structures to the right, and some ventricular dilatation, particularly of the lateral ventricle opposite to the side of the lesion.

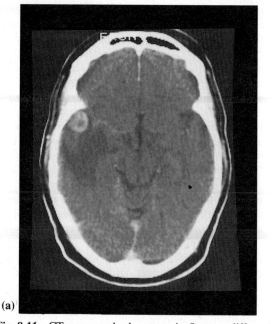 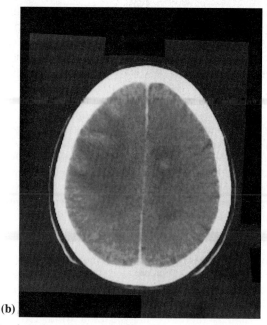

(a)   (b)

Fig. 8.11 CT scan: cerebral metastasis. Scans at different levels at the same examination. This patient had a bronchial carcinoma. Image (a) shows an anterior temporal enhancing lesion with adjacent oedema on the right. Image (b) is of an axial scan near the vertex. Notice the very extensive oedema on the right, and another enhancing, small, circular lesion close to the mid-line, again surrounded by oedema, on the left.

and pronounced enhancement in brain tissue surrounding an abscess.

An enhancing cerebral tumour is often surrounded by a zone of low-density brain due to cerebral oedema, the excess brain water showing as an area of low attenuation (Figs 8.10, 8.11). It is often difficult therefore, to estimate the true extent of tumours. After initial treatment of a patient with a brain tumour with dexamethasone alone (see Section 16.3.1.2), there may be a striking reduction in the volume not only of the surrounding brain oedema, but also in the volume of enhancing tissue, although there is no reason to believe that the extent of histologically abnormal glial cells has been altered by the dexamethasone. Multiple enhancing lesions are most likely to be due to cerebral metastases from tumours elsewhere in the body, most commonly from the bronchus, breast, or kidney (see Section 16.4). Similar appearances may result from multiple cerebral abscesses. Occasionally a glioma may be multicentric in origin.

Figures 8.10 and 8.11 show enhancing lesions

due to metastases, but many primary tumours also enhance after the injection of contrast. Figure 8.12 shows an enhancing malignant glioblastoma (Section 16.3.1). The bulk of this tumour is solid. In Fig. 8.13 another kind of primary tumour is illustrated—a largely cystic astrocytoma. After the injection of contrast medium, tumour tissue appears to be confined to a small nodule on the anterior wall of the cyst.

As haemoglobin contains a high-density iron atom at the centre of its molecule, blood has a high Hounsfield absorption number. An intracerebral bleed is therefore readily revealed by unenhanced CT scanning (Fig. 10.2a). Subarachnoid blood is also easily imaged after a rupture of a cerebral aneurysm. CT scanning should always precede examination of the cerebrospinal fluid in patients with suspected subarachnoid haemorrhage, for the reasons advanced in Section 10.6.3.

CT scanning is also useful in cranial trauma (Chapter 15). Figure 8.14 shows an extradural clot, with a high-density haemorrhage distorting the intracerebral contents (compare with Fig. 15.2c).

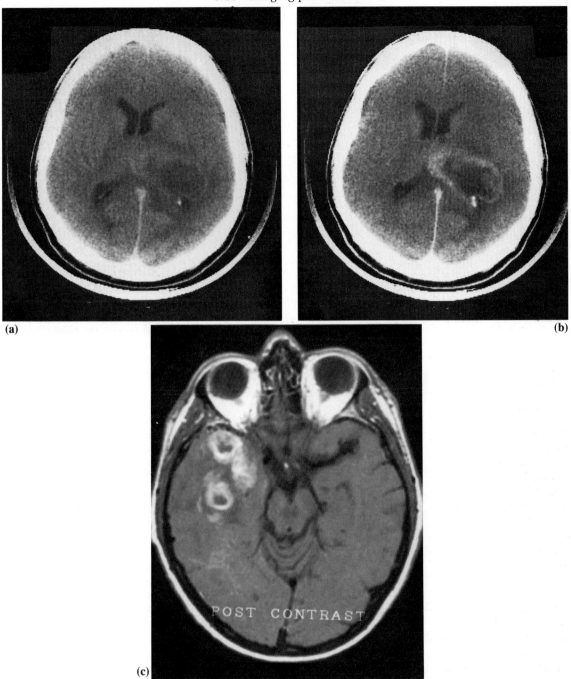

Fig. 8.12 Highly malignant glioblastoma (Section 16.3.1.1). Image (a) shows an area of low attenuation around the posterior horn of the lateral ventricle on the left. The high-density white spot in the middle is normal choroid plexus. After the injection of intravenous contrast medium (b), the periphery of the tumour enhances greatly. Note also the distortion of mid-line structures towards the right by the oedematous tumour on the left. (c) For comparison, MRI of another example of a malignant glioma seen in the right temporal lobe after injection of gadolinium DTPA. Six months before this patient had had a normal CT scan after a single seizure.

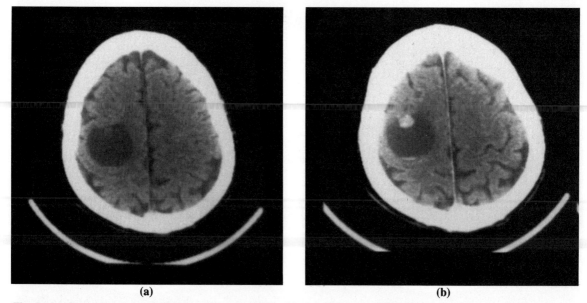

(a)   (b)

Fig. 8.13 Cystic astrocytoma (Section 16.3.1.1). Image (a) shows a large cystic lesion in the right hemisphere. In the anterior part an area of faintly greater density can be seen. In (b), after the injection of contrast, the tumour nodule enhances greatly.

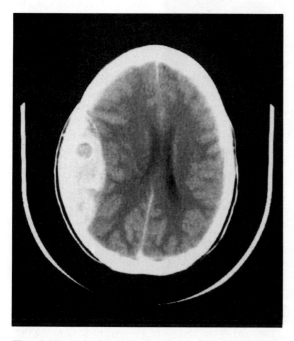

Fig. 8.14 Extradural haemorrhage (section 15.3.2). Note the large, lenticular-shaped area of high-density haemorrhage on the right, pushing the falx and lateral ventricles towards the opposite side. Compare with Fig. 15.2.

Unless such a clot is evacuated immediately, the patient is likely to die. Figure 8.15 shows a subdural haemorrhage. This figure has been chosen to show that as such a subacute clot gradually liquefies, the Hounsfield number falls, and at some stages of liquefaction the absorption coefficient may be similar to that of normal brain. So-called 'isodense' small subdural haematomas can therefore occasionally be overlooked unless consideration is given to the obliteration of the cortical sulci and a distortion of mid-line structures, as shown in Fig. 8.15c.

Figures 8.16 and 8.17 illustrate other structural abnormalities in the brain imaged by CT, due to differences in attenuation of the beam by tissues of different histological character. Figure 8.16 shows the scan of a child with tuberous sclerosis (Section 16.8.2). Patchy areas of low attenuation are due to dysplasia of white matter, common in this inherited disorder. Focal areas of dense hamartomatous glial proliferation are visible also as white dots in the subependymal region of the ventricles. Figure 8.17 shows multiple areas of high attenuation in a slowly growing tumour. These areas of high attenuation are flecks of calcium in an oligodendroglioma. This patient presented with seizures about 10 years before the scan was performed.

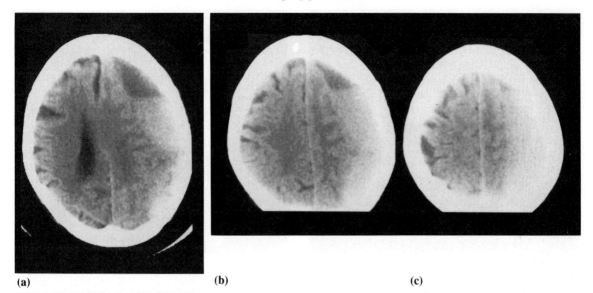

(a)   **(b)**   **(c)**

Fig. 8.15   Subdural haemorrhage (Section 15.6). (a) On the left there is a lenticular-shaped haemorrhage which must be several days old at least, as a horizontal fluid level can be seen, indicating some liquefaction of the cyst. Images (b) and (c) are at cuts progressively nearer the vertex. The uppermost cut (c) shows that the haemorrhage has a density similar to that of normal brain, which allows subdural haemorrhages occasionally to be overlooked at certain stages in their development. Note, however, that the sulci at the vertex cannot be clearly seen on this side, a clue to the underlying haemorrhage easily visible at more caudal sections. Compare with Fig. 15.2.

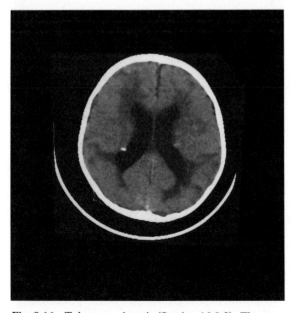

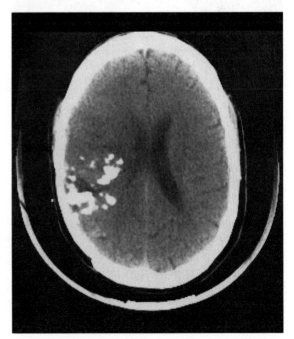

Fig. 8.16   Tuberous sclerosis (Section 16.8.2). The scan of this child shows much ventricular dilatation and numerous scattered areas of low attenuation, representing dysplasia of white matter. The high-attenuation, paraventricular white lesions are hamartomata.

Fig. 8.17   Oligodendroglioma (Section 16.3.1.1). The CT scan shows multiple areas of calcification in a slowly growing tumour.

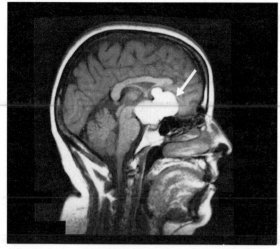

(a)

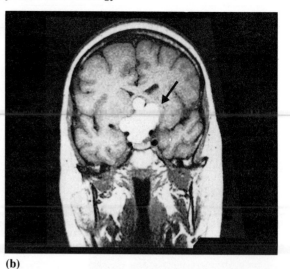

(b)

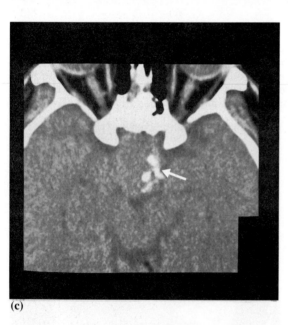

(c)

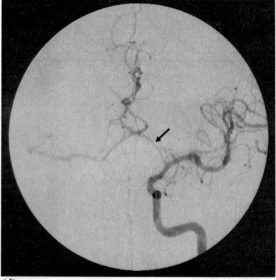

(d)

Fig. 8.18   (a) Craniopharyngioma (Section 16.6.5.1). MR sagittal image, showing a large region of high signal arising out of the pituitary fossa. (b) Coronal MRI of the same tumour. (c) Conventional CT image of the same tumour. Note that the attenuation of X-ray beam by the tumour is much less obvious than the area of high signal of the MRI. Flecks of calcium, indicated by an arrowhead, can be seen in the wall of the tumour. (d) Angiogram. Note the elevation by the tumour of the proximal part of the anterior cerebral arteries, indicated by an arrowhead on the left. The normal course of this artery is horizontal. Occasionally, suprasellar 'tumours' are large aneurysms arising from the proximal part of the internal carotid artery (see Fig. 8.25), so surgeons usually require angiography before proceeding to operation on suprasellar tumours.

8.10.3 *Magnetic resonance imaging (MRI)*

For historical reasons, computerized tomography (CT) tends to be referred to as CT scanning, and magnetic resonance imaging is abbreviated to MRI. The end products of the two are superficially similar in so far as both use a grey scale image to picture the physical state of each voxel, and both present that physical state as a two-dimensional image.

Nuclear magnetic resonance is the name given to the interaction between nuclei with an unequal number of protons or neutrons and radiofrequency pulses in a strong magnetic field. Hydrogen nuclei are single protons, and therefore unequal. As hydrogen both largely constitutes water and is abundant in hydrocarbons such as lipids, it is a very suitable proton for the purposes of MRI.

For MRI, the patient lies wholly within a magnetic tunnel. The axis of spin of protons in the brain is tilted and rotated by a strong and uniform external magnetic field, resulting in a motion known as precession. If a further pulsed magnetic field is applied briefly at right angles, the protons will be flipped out of the plane of the main external magnetic field through an angle dependent upon the duration of the additional external radiofrequency pulse. As the protons relax back towards their original positions, they emit a radiofrequency signal which can be analysed in digital form, allowing the construction of an image similar to that of CT scanning. The initial intensity of the emitted signal is proportional to the density of the protons in the tissues. The time that it takes for the protons to relax away from the vector induced by the resultant of the background homogeneous magnetic field and the short radiofrequency pulse can be measured. The relaxation time has two components. The T1 decay curve (spin lattice relaxation curve) depends upon the ability of protons to give up energy to their environment, and represents the rate at which the excited protons realign with the magnetic field. More compact tissues, and those with a lower water content, give up energy more quickly, and therefore have a shorter T1 decay surve and emit a high signal. Examples of high-signal tissues are fat and extravasated blood. Tumour and surrounding oedematous brain are less compact, have longer T1 decay curves, and give out a signal of lesser intensity.

The characteristic slope of the exponential T2 decay curve (the spin spin relaxation curve) is dependent upon the rate of spin of each proton differing from its neighbours due to the local magnetic effects from surrounding protons. The time taken for the protons to become out of phase is the T2 relaxation time.

The initial size of the emitted signal, and the characteristics of the T1 and T2 decay curves, determine the magnetic resonance parameters of the tissue under study, in turn determining the physical profile of the tissue. Different radiofrequency pulse signals produce signals weighted to proton density or different degrees of T1 or T2 relaxation times. A set of radiofrequency pulses, termed a sequence, is repeated a sufficient number of times over a period of minutes so that a sufficient sample can be analysed. Alteration of the variables within the sequences determines the relative dominance of proton density, T1 and T2 relaxation times, and the effect that each of these

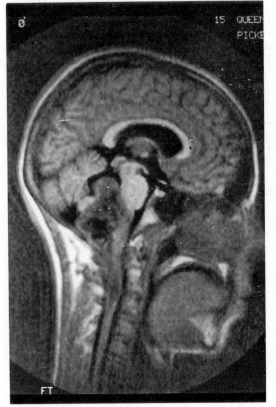

Fig. 8.19 MRI of a glioma in the region of the craniocervical junction.

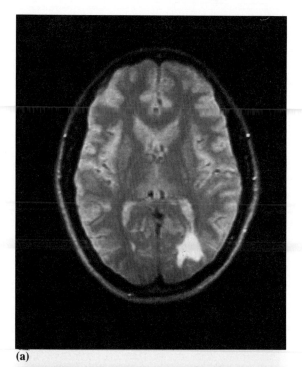

(a)

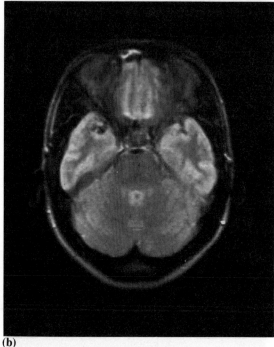

(b)

has upon the signal available for analysis. One common sequence is referred to as a spin echo sequence. The principal variables are the repeat time (the interval in milliseconds between each set of radiofrequency pulses at 90°) and the echo time (the time between the initial pulse and the beginning of the sampling period). A second commonly used sequence is known as inversion recovery, dependent upon varying the interval between the initial 180° and the 90° pulse, the T1 time.

The image produced by analysis of the emitted signals in MRI is affected also by flow of blood through the voxel. Fast flow rates, such as those seen in arterial blood, usually result in a low (black or void) signal, and high signal is seen if flow is slow. The signal void arising in large vessels can sometimes be of use by indicating displacement of these vessels by neighbouring masses.

Adjustment of MRI sequences results in images with good contrast and an excellent demonstration of anatomy (see Figs 8.18, 8.19). However, discrimination between different tissue types is sometimes rather poor, so that it is not always easy to see the boundary between a tumour and the surrounding oedema, and early stages after a cerebral infarction may also be rather unimpressive. A

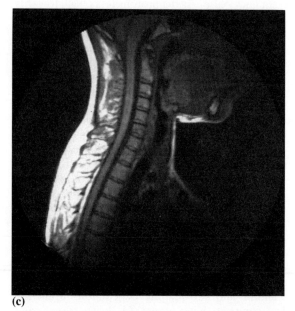

(c)

Fig. 8.20 Three MRIs from the same patient with multiple sclerosis. (a) Areas of high signal in the left occipital lobe, and around the posterior horns of the lateral ventricles; (b) a lesion in the right cerebellar hemisphere; (c) the sagittal image of the spinal cord shows multiple areas of high signal.

paramagnetic contrast agent such as gadolinium can be used. This is too toxic in its ionic form, but when chelated with diethylenetriaminepentaacetic acid (DTPA), it is less toxic and an effective contrast agent. It does not traverse the intact blood–brain barrier. The border between tumours and surrounding oedema can be well outlined, due to shortening of the T1 relaxation time.

A major clinical use of MRI is in the identification of areas of demyelination (Fig. 8.20). Plaques of demyelination appear as zones of long T2 relaxation times, both on inversion recovery and spin echo sequences. Plaques are particularly prominent in the periventricular white matter, the brain stem, the cerebellum, and the spinal cord (Fig. 8.20). There is, however, no necessary correlation between clinical events and the zones of demyelination and breakdown of the blood–brain barrier as imaged by MRI. (Section 14.11). The prognostic significance of an abnormal MRI in a patient with a unilateral retrobulbar neuritis is discussed in Section 14.11.

Areas of high signal of unidentified pathology are increasingly common after the age of 40. These also are often predominantly periventricular. These high signal areas probably represent areas of gliosis round tiny subclinical infarcts.

Acute cerebral infarctions tend to show poorly, at least initially, on MRI, unless they cause mass effect. In many patients, the breakdown in the blood–brain barrier can be demonstrated by the use of gadolinium, but the expense of this (about £75 per patient) must be taken into account.

8.10.4   *Comparison of CT scanning and MRI*

A major advantage of MRI is the absence of ionizing radiation. There is no evidence that magnetic fields in the strength used for MRI cause any significant biological damage. MR images can be acquired in any plane, and sagittal images are often particularly useful. Although sagittal images can be obtained by mathematical reconstruction of CT axially acquired information, the resolution is much less good. Both techniques have useful enhancing agents, but gadolinium DTPA is expensive, and the iodinated contrast agents used in CT scanning carry some risk of an allergic reaction. Patients find MRI more difficult to tolerate, as they have to lie in a much more confined space. It

is also difficult to look after acutely ill patients in an MR scanner, because of the difficulties of maintaining infusion lines and ventilation within the magnet tunnel. Patients with cardiac pacemakers cannot be imaged, as the magnetic field will interfere with the pacemaker signal. Patients who have had aneurysmal surgery, in which arterial clips containing ferrous material have been applied, cannot be imaged, as the clips may be displaced by the strong field.

MRI is the investigation of choice when imaging lesions in the region of the pituitary fossa. High-field, thin-section MRI using T1-weighted images is the investigation of choice. MRI in these circumstances is distinctly superior to demonstrating microadenomas of the pituitary region, and well demonstrates suprasellar extensions of pituitary lesions, or suprasellar tumours such as a cranio-pharyngioma (Fig. 8.18). Other MRI sequences can demonstrate the relationship of a large suprasellar tumour to the diaphragma sellae and surrounding vascular structures, such as the cavernous sinus or carotid artery, without the use of gadolinium. Suprasellar aneurysms (Fig. 8.26) can also be detected by MRI.

A particular disadvantage of CT is in relation to the posterior fossa, where the high absorption of bone in the petrous temporal region and posterior fossa immediately adjacent to normal brain or tumour impairs the resolution of the scan, as an individual voxel may contain both bone and brain, giving meaningless Hounsfield numbers. Small movements of the patient, transferring bone in and out of neighbouring voxels, also cause troublesome artefacts in this region. The lack of interference from bony structures on MRI very much facilitates the detection of lesions in close proximity to bone, such as cerebello-pontine angle tumours. It is also possible to obtain much better images of developmental abnormalities and tumours in the region of the cranio-cervical junction (Fig. 8.19).

MRI demonstrates high-signal lesions associated with multiple sclerosis very much better than CT scanning, which will only image large plaques, and then usually only if large volumes of contrast are used. As already noted, MRI is distinctly better for axial tumours, and tumours in the posterior fossa. For the management of gliomas or metastases in the hemispheres, the difference between the two techniques is not very important.

Fresh blood following a subarachnoid haemorrhage is often poorly imaged by MRI, but is readily visible in the cortical sulci, cisterns, or ventricles on CT.

MRI is also superior to CT for evaluation of the orbit and lesions arising in the region of the paranasal sinuses, for the same reasons as its superiority in the posterior fossa—the avoidance of bony artefact. MRI is also superior to conventional or CT myelography (see Section 8.13.2) for imaging the spinal cord. An example of a benign tumour (a meningioma) lying behind the high thoracic spinal cord is shown in Fig. 8.21. The nerve roots can also be well visualized in the lumbar dural sac, although not with the detail seen after the injection of contrast medium in radiculography. MRI does, however, show the roots outside the boundary of the theca, which radiculography cannot. MRI also successfully demonstrates the nucleus pulposus of the intervertebral disc, and vertebral bone marrow lesions such as metastases or myeloma.

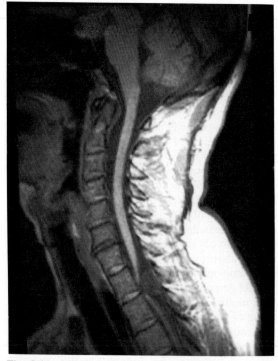

Fig. 8.21 MRI of tumour arising behind and outside the high thoracic spinal cord. Note the circular lesion pushing the cord forwards at the lower border of T_1. The tumour proved to be a spinal meningioma (Section 18.4.2.1).

Against the significant advantages for MRI listed above, it must be remembered that MRI is distinctly more expensive than CT scanning. The depreciation on capital, and running costs, are such that break-even costs are 1.5 to 4 times the cost of a CT installation. Although recent advances in speeding up the acquisition of an MR image by so-called low flip-angle techniques are likely to make MRI increasingly competitive, as will developments in MR angiography, a recent study of the cost-effectiveness of MRI was disappointing. Management changed after MRI in about a quarter of cases, and the confidence in an already considered diagnosis was increased in a further quarter. However, costs are added to by the use of MRI, largely because physicians still see it as an 'add-on' investigation rather than replacing other types of investigation such as CT scanning or evoked responses.

8.10.5 *Positron emission tomography*

Positron emission tomography (PET) uses positron-emitting radionucleides to map the physiology, biochemistry, and haemodynamics of the brain. A positron is of equal mass but opposite charge to an electron. It loses energy after travelling a few millimetres in tissue due to annihilation with an electron. When this occurs, mass is converted into energy in the form of two photons that are emitted at 180° to each other. The scanner detects these oppositely directed photons by a coincidence detection technique. Paired photon detectors around the transaxial cranial slice allow reconstruction of the image in a way analogous to the reconstruction of the CT image. The degree of attenuation of emitted photons can be assessed by a transmission scan performed with a ring containing a suitable positron-emitting isotope around the head. The transmission scan can then be used to correct each picture element of the emission scan for attenuation, which, with suitable calibration, allows absolute concentrations of isotope to be assessed in each local region.

It is necessary that a PET scanner is placed in close geographical proximity to a cyclotron, because the positron-emitting isotopes, such as ^{15}O, ^{11}C, and ^{18}F, are short lived. The present resolution of PET is in the order of relatively large volumes of brain (about 0.25 ml). One of the isotopes most commonly used is ^{18}fluoro-2-deoxy-

D-glucose. This is used to measure local cerebral glucose consumption. ^{15}Oxygen is used to show regional oxygen consumption. Studies using these isotopes in patients with cerebral infarction soon after the infarction have shown that there is a zone of brain tissue surrounding the infarct which strongly extracts oxygen, suggesting persistent mitochondrial function in an area of flow-limited reversible metabolic depression (Fig. 8.22). There

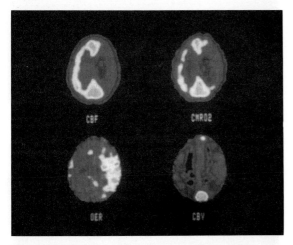

Fig. 8.22 Positron emission tomography (PET) scan using ^{15}O 8 hours after a left middle cerebral artery occlusion. CBF, reduced cerebral blood flow; CMRO$_2$ reduced oxygen utilization; OER, increased oxygen extraction ratio (i.e. oxygen consumption in relation to blood flow); CBV, cerebral blood volume. (Image kindly provided by Dr R. Frackowiack.)

has been, however, no evidence of the persistence of such a zone for more than a few hours. Other uses of PET have been in dementing illnesses. Regional reductions in blood flow are prominent in the superior parietal regions, later extending into the inferior parietal and temporal lobes in patients with Alzheimer's disease. In contrast, those with multi-infarct dementia can be shown on PET scanning to have multiple asymmetric regions of cortical and subcortical hypometabolism. PET scanning has also been used in patients with uncontrolled seizures who are being evaluated for the potential benefit of temporal lobe surgery. Interictal focal hypometabolism using ^{18}fluoro-2-deoxy-D-glucose has been shown to be a powerful indicator of the localization of the seizure focus, particu-

larly when subsequent resection shows that the epileptogenic lesion was due to mesial temporal sclerosis. PET has also been used on a research basis in patients with movement disorders. For example, those with progressive supranuclear palsy (Section 13.4) have areas of prominent frontal hypometabolism. Patients with Parkinson's disease, scanned after the administration of [^{18}F]L-dopa, show a lesser and delayed accumulation of dopa in the striatum than in normal subjects. The changes are particularly marked in those with the on–off syndrome (Section 13.1.8.4). The integrity of dopamine receptors can also be assessed by [^{11}C]methyl spiperone.

PET scanning, and the required close association with a cyclotron, requires a great investment of capital. However, it is clear that the technique allows a biochemical assessment of various brain disorders which, until the advent of this technique, had been largely impossible.

8.10.6 *Radio-isotope scanning*

Isotope scanning with a gamma camera without the use of tomographic software allows rapid imaging of the body skeleton for isotope that selectively accumulates in pathological areas. Examples are metastases from a carcinoma of the bronchus or prostate. However, isotopes such as ^{99m}technetium also accumulate at sites of Paget's disease of bone, and at areas of active joint involvement in, for example, ankylosing spondylitis.

Cranial radio-isotope imaging is of historical interest for its early use in the localization of intracranial tumours 30 years ago.

8.10.7 *Single-photon emission computed tomography (SPECT)*

Conventional CT scanning uses the absorption of transmitted X-rays through the brain to construct an image. Photon detectors and the appropriate software can be used in a similar way to construct an image from photons emitted from an isotope within the brain. Suitable isotopes include ^{99m}technetium hexamethylpropyleneamine oxime (HM-PAO) and ^{123}iodoamphetamine (IMP). SPECT has been used to show relative hyperperfusion after acute infarcts, hypoperfusion in those with epileptic foci in a temporal lobe, and increased tracer accumulation in disorders such as herpes simplex encephalitis. The development of further isotopes and improved gamma cameras and software are likely to improve the usefulness of this relatively simple investigation.

8.11 Angiography (arteriography)

Before the advent of CT scanning and MRI, cerebral angiography was an important diagnostic procedure in the evaluation of a patient with a suspected tumour, as distortion of vessels from their normal anatomical pathways could give useful information about the location of an avascular tumour. Pathological circulation in a vascular tumour, such as a glioblastoma or meningioma, further aided localization (Fig. 8.23). However, the role of angiography is now mainly limited to the demonstration of vascular anatomy prior to surgery, and, more particularly, to the demonstration of abnormalities of the circulation itself, such as atheroma, (particularly in the carotid arteries) an angiomatous malformation, or an aneurysm.

Contrast can be injected by both the arterial and intravenous routes. Ten years ago there was considerable interest in venous digital subtraction angiography. The faint contrast induced by dye reaching the arterial tree from a rapidly administered intravenous injection can be enhanced by computer software, which simultaneously subtracts surrounding soft tissue and bony image to leave a clear outline of the arterial lumen. However, the quality of the image obtained, even with large doses of contrast and the best software, is distinctly inferior to that obtained by a conventional intra-arterial injection, such as is used in coronary angiography. The rapid advent of MR angiography is likely to displace digital subtraction venous angiography as a useful tool. In MR angiography, the flow effects of the moving protons are analysed by time-of-flight or phase contrast software techniques to produce images, the quality of which is rapidly increasing. An example is illustrated in Fig. 8.24.

Digital subtraction angiography by intra-arterial injection, through a femoral or brachial catheter,

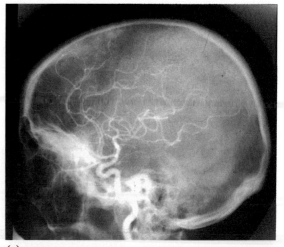

(a)

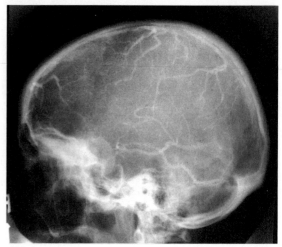

(b)

Fig. 8.23 Angiogram of a sphenoidal wing meningioma. (a) Both anterior cerebral arteries are filled, and pushed back from the sphenoidal wing and floor of the anterior cranial fossa. (b) Venous phase of the angiogram. The meningioma is outlined by the 'blush' of its circulation.

allows the use of more dilute contrast and shorter procedure times, but spatial resolution is less than with conventional direct photographic imaging. The relative restriction in size of the imaged field,

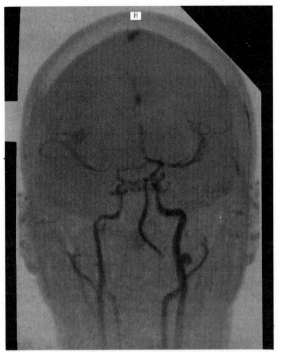

(a)

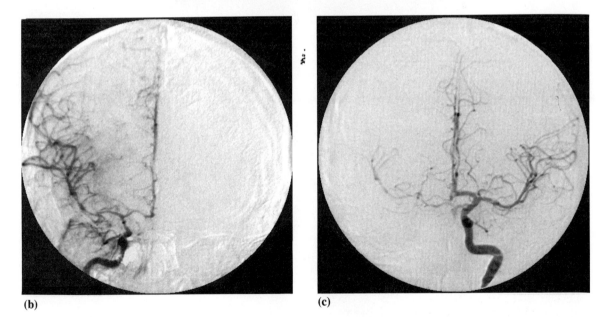

(b)   **(c)**

Fig. 8.24 Comparison of MR angiography and intra-arterial injection with contrast. Image (a) shows on MR angiography poor filling of the distal part of the right internal carotid artery, and anterior cerebral and proximal part of the middle cerebral artery, compared to better filling on the left. Images (b) and (c) show the confirmation of this asymmetry by intra-arterial injection of the right and left internal carotid arteries. It is likely that MR angiography will improve in resolution and will replace intra-arterial injections soon.

and the loss of bony detail due to the subtraction, may lead to some difficulty in orientation to those less expert in the field.

Whatever the methodology, angiography is the 'gold standard' for the demonstration of atheromatous lesions in the large extracranial vessls (Fig. 10.7), aneurysms (Figs 8.25, 8.26, and 10.7), and angiomatous malformations (Fig. 10.7b).

The standard ionic media (sodium, meglumine salts of iodinated acids) are reasonably innocuous agents, but severe allergic reactions occur in about 1 in 1000 injections, and result in death in about 1 in 50 000 injections. In recent years, some relatively expensive monomeric non-ionic iodinated compounds, with approximately half the osmolality of the corresponding ionic media, have become available. The difference in cost is considerable. It has been proposed that the less expensive ionic media can be used if the patient is protected with two doses of methylprednisolone, 30 mg orally approximately 12 hours and again 2 hours before the injection.

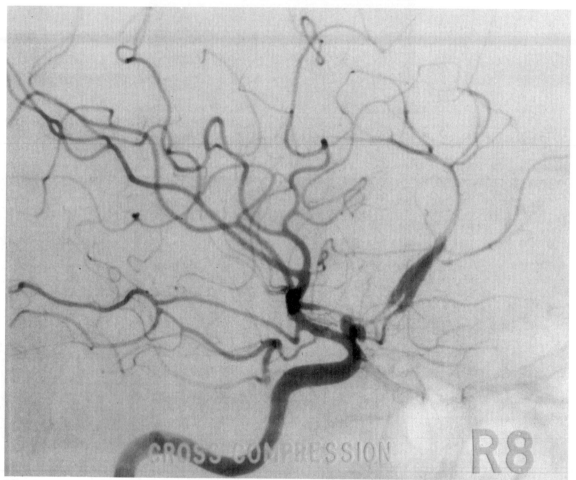

(a)

Fig. 8.25 Aneurysm on the anterior communicating artery. (a) A lateral image showing the aneurysm on the anterior communicating artery, with prominent spasm in the proximal segment of each anterior cerebral artery and dilatation of each distal of the spasm. (b) (Facing page) An oblique image of the same aneurysm.

8.11.1 *Interventional neuroradiology*

Although not strictly an investigation, this is a convenient place to consider endovascular techniques, such as embolization and occlusion, using detachable and non-detachable balloons to treat some highly vascular tumours. For example, highly vascular paragangliomas (see Section 16.3.4), such as glomus jugulare and carotid body tumours, are well treated by pre-operative partial embolization with polyvinyl alcohol foam particles. Dural arterio-venous malformations can also be treated by catheterization and embolization of the arterial supply with *N*-butyl cyanoacrylate. The tumours so far mentioned both have their blood supply from the external carotid system, so the risk of neurological complications resulting from embolization is comparatively low, although cranial nerve palsies may occur, as part of their course is supplied through the external carotid system.

A fistula between the internal carotid artery and the cavernous sinus may arise following a fracture of the skull base, or as a result of the rupture of a carotid aneurysm within the cavernous sinus. Such a fistula can be occluded by the placement of a small detachable balloon passed through the trans-

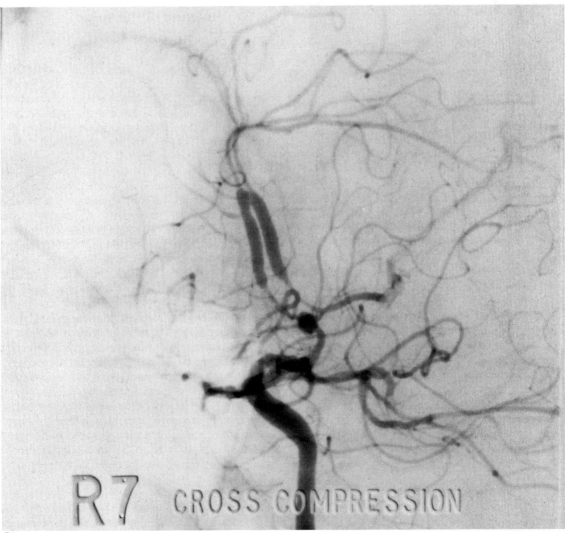

(b)

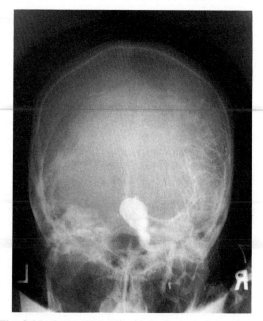

Fig. 8.26 Large supraclinoid aneurysm of the internal carotid artery. This patient presented with a bitemporal hemianopia, and was initially thought to have a pituitary tumour.

femoral route into the internal carotid artery, through the fistula and then into the cavernous sinus. Occasionally intracerebral aneurysms are occluded in the same way if the aneurysm does not have a neck which is safely accessible for neurosurgical clipping. A large aneurysm at the termination of the basilar artery is one example. The aneurysm may be occluded by placing a balloon within the aneurysm, or the vessel feeding it. In the latter case, if a trial occlusion lasting a few minutes produces no neurological deficit, it is considered safe to detach the balloon and leave it in place.

Balloon dilatation of extracranial atheromatous disease has not proved successful, largely due to the rigid character of most stenotic lesions. Some research centres are studying the use of tiny balloons in relieving spasm following subarachnoid haemorrhage of the type illustrated in Fig. 8.25.

8.12   Duplex sonography

Duplex sonography is a combination of real-time B-mode scanning and Doppler flow studies. It is a non-invasive test which is relatively sensitive at defining minor lesions at the carotid bifurcation. Duplex sonography is reliable at defining normal vessels, and may therefore avoid the need for angiography in many patients. The quality of the examination depends upon the skill and experience of the operator. The relatively cheap capital cost of the equipment means that in some cultures duplex sonography may be undertaken by those with comparatively little experience in the field, resulting in inappropriate surgical management of minor vascular lesions.

8.13   Imaging of the spine

8.13.1   *Plain X-rays*

For many years plain X-rays of the cervical and lumbar spine have been the mainstays of investigation of patients with cervico-brachial symptoms (see Section 18.2.2) and backache (see Sections 18.3 and 25.2.1). However, it has been shown that radiographic changes in the apophyseal joints, narrowing of the disc spaces, calcification in intervertebral discs, and osteophyte formation are almost equally common in middle-aged and older people with and without symptoms. It is very difficult to predict the severity of symptoms from the X-ray changes. The Quebec Task Force on spinal disorders has suggested that in the absence of any neurological deficit, plain X-rays are not indicated during the first week of an acute episode of back pain. X-rays are of dubious value in the next few weeks, but it is reasonable to do them if back pain persists beyond that length of time. Some other diagnostic tests, such as an erythrocyte sedimentation rate or the level of prostatic-specific antigen, may be of more value in suggesting a higher probability of underlying systemic disease than plain films in these circumstances.

Not only are X-rays of the lumbar spine comparatively uninformative, they also deliver a significant dose of radiation to the gonads. If X-rays of the lumbar spine are to be taken, much can be done to limit the number of views, as oblique views rarely add any significant information.

Plain films of the spine are, of course, the principal investigation used in the initial evaluation of those with spinal trauma. They also demonstrate

atlanto-axial subluxation as may occur in rheumatoid arthritis (Section 18.2.2) following inflammatory and degenerative changes in the transverse
ligament of the atlas (Fig. 8.27).

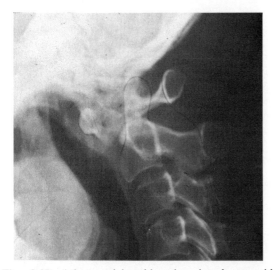

Fig. 8.27 Atlanto-axial subluxation in rheumatoid
arthritis. In this X-ray the head is flexed. The odontoid
peg (lightly outlined) has separated from the body of the
atlas, and its posterior surface is greatly reducing the
anterior–posterior diameter of the spinal canal.

8.13.2   *CT and MRI*

Excellent imaging of the vertebrae, the intervertebral discs, and the spinal canal is obtained either
by CT or MRI. However, the very excellence of
resolution of MRI results in comparatively low
specificity. Herniated discs can be seen in almost
10 per cent of asymptomatic young women, and
bulging discs in 45 per cent. It is therefore absolutely essential that the decision as to whether a
disc protrusion is responsible for clinical symptoms, and warrants surgical intervention, is based
very largely upon the history and findings on
examination, as outlined in Section 18.3.1.

Degeneration of the nucleus pulposus is imaged
on MR as a significant loss of MR signal relative to
neighbouring discs, and a reduction in disc height.
An annulus fibrosus bulging more than 2.5 mm is
usually associated with radial tears, which may
show as small streaks of relatively high signal on
MRI. However, MRI is not very good at dis-

tinguishing sequestrated fragments, which often
appear to remain in continuity with the disc.

8.13.3   *Myelography (radiculography)*

The original oil-based contrast medium for myelography ('Myodil') is now no longer used
because of the recognized risk of residual contrast
medium causing persistent arachnoiditis, with
fibrotic changes occurring in the arachnoid. These
tether the nerve roots in a mass of granulation
tissue, resulting in severe continued low-back pain
and radicular symptoms. A water-based contrast
medium such as iopamidol successfully outlines the
nerve root sheaths and allows conclusions about
the anatomy of the spinal cord, of nerve roots, and
of intramedullary and extramedullary tumours.
The use of such a contrast agent in cervical spondylosis is demonstrated in Fig. 8.28.

The routine examination of the spinal fluid
obtained at myelography (often also known as
radiculography) is not necessary (see Section
8.2.4).

Although iopamidol has not been shown to be
associated with arachnoiditis, like all other iodine-
containing contrast media, it may provoke an
anaphylactic reaction. Care also needs to be taken
in using the contrast medium with those patients
having functional impairment of the liver, kidneys,
or myocardium.

Iopamidol is epileptogenic in a small proportion
of subjects. For this reason, after myelography the
patient should be placed so that no contrast
medium enters the head. With the advent of MRI
there is now little reason to use contrast medium
in the posterior fossa. This was formerly undertaken in the evaluation of small tumours in the
cerebello-pontine   angle,   combined   with   CT
scanning.

8.13.4   *The relative value of different*
methods of imaging the spinal canal,
cord, and nerve roots

Even with MRI, it is not always easy to image the
extent of encroachment of extruded disc material
and osteophytes upon the spinal cord, with a view
to devising some measure of compression that
might allow guidance on the advisability of surgical
intervention. An anterior–posterior diameter of
less than 11 mm on a lateral view of the cervical

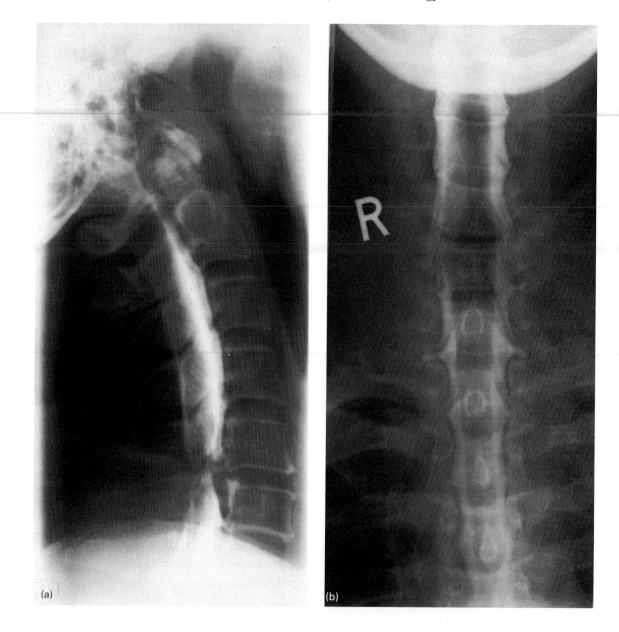

Fig. 8.28 Myelogram of cervical disc protrusion. Image (a) shows the narrowing of the disc space posteriorly between the fifth and sixth vertebrae, and deviation of the dura away from the posterior surface of the vertebrae, with consequent compression of the column of contrast. The AP image (b) shows widening of the grey shadow of the spinal cord at this point, and, on the right, an interruption of the contrast medium, imaged white, at the level of the C5/C6 discs. The AP image also shows that the root sheath at this level on the right does not fill out with contrast compared to the sheath at the same level on the left.

canal obtained at myelography, or a reduction in cross-sectional area to less than 30 mm² on CT scanning with contrast medium in the cervical/ canal, is associated with a poor outcome following decompression.

With regard to disorders of the spinal cord, the value of MRI is firmly established in the diagnosis of syringomyelia (Section 18.5.4.1), plaques of demyelination (Fig. 8.20), spinal tumours such as astrocytomas, and dysraphism. The diagnosis of a spinal angioma requires lumbar aortography, but MRI may define well the intramedullary extent of the angioma, and aid a decision about the advisability of surgery.

Limited observations about the nerve roots within the theca can be made on both CT and MRI, but it is not possible to predict reliably flattening or entrapment of intrathecal lumbar roots on CT, although displacement of fat from the intervertebral foramen at the clinically affected level may suggest this. MRI does have the advantage of showing the course of the nerve roots to a limited extent outside the lumbar canal, but for accurate observations of the anatomy within the theca, the addition of the injection of contrast medium into the subarachnoid space (myelography) is necessary.

8.14 Further reading

General

Matthews, P. M. and Arnold, D. L. (1991). *Diagnostic tests in neurology*. Churchill Livingstone, Edinburgh.

Lumbar puncture

Davson, H., Welch, K., Ingram, F. D., and Segal, M. (ed.) (1986). *The physiology and pathology of the cerebrospinal fluid*. Churchill Livingstone, Edinburgh.

Fitzgerald, R. and Davies, A. M. (1988). The value of routine CSF analysis during lumbar radiculography for low back pain. *Journal of Neurology, Neurosurgery and Psychiatry* **51**, 878–9.

Gibb, W. R. G. and Wen, P. (1984). Current practice of diagnostic lumbar puncture. *British Medical Journal* **289**. 530. (This article discusses headaches after lumbar puncture.)

Hayward, R. A., Shapiro, M. F., and Oye, R. K. (1987). Laboratory testing on cerebrospinal fluid: a reappraisal. *Lancet* **1**, 1–4.

MacDonald, A. and Mendelow, A. D. (1988). Xan-

thochromia revisited: a re-evaluation of lumbar puncture and CT scanning in the diagnosis of subarachnoid haemorrhage. *Journal of Neurology, Neurosurgery and Psychiatry* **51**, 342–4.

Electroencephalography

Daly, D. and Pedley, T. A. (ed.) (1990). *Current practice of clinical electroencephalography*. Raven Press, New York.

Nuwer, M. R. (1989). Uses and abuses of brain mapping. *Archives of Neurology* **46**, 1134–6.

Magneto-encephalography

Editorial (1990). Magneto-encephalography. *Lancet* **335**, 576–7.

Electromyography

Aminoff, M. J. (1987). *Electromyography in clinical practice*. Churchill Livingstone, Edinburgh.

Magnetic brain stimulation

Hess, C. W., Mills, K. R., Murray, N. M. F., and Schriefer, T. N. (1987). Magnetic brain stimulation: central motor conduction studies in multiple sclerosis. *Annals of Neurology* **22**, 744–52.

Imaging

Armstrong, P. and Keevil, S. F. (1991). Magnetic resonance imaging—I: Basic principles of image production. *British Medical Journal* **303**, 35–40.

Armstrong, P. and Keevil, S. F. (1991). Magnetic resonance imaging—2: Clinical uses. *British Medical Journal* **303**, 105–9.

Atlas, S. W. (ed.) (1991). *Magnetic resonance imaging of the brain and spine*. Rowen Press, New York.

Health and Public Policy Committee, American College of Physicians (1988). Magnetic resonance imaging of the brain and spine. *Annals of Internal Medicine* **108**, 474–6.

Kirkwood, J. R. (1990). *Essentials of neuroimaging*. Churchill Livingstone, Edinburgh.

Merran, S. (ed.) (1990). *CT and MRI radioanatomy*. Butterworth-Heinemann. London.

Szczepura, A. K., Fletcher, J. and Fitz-Patrick, J. D. (1991). Cost-effectiveness of magnetic resonance imaging in the neurosciences. *British Medical Journal* **303** 1435–9.

Steinberg, E. P., Sisk, J. E., and Locke, K. E. (1985).

X-ray, CT and magnetic resonance imagers. *New England Journal of Medicine* **313**, 859–64.

Teasdale, G. M., Hadley, D. M., Lawrence, A. *et al.* (1989). Comparison of magnetic resonance imaging and computed tomography in suspected lesions in the posterior fossa. *British Medical Journal* **299**, 345–55.

PET scanning

Brooks, D. J. (1991). PET: its clinical role in neurology. *Journal of Neurology, Neurosurgery and Psychiatry* **54**, 1–4.

The Therapeutics and Technology Assessment Sub-Committee of the American Academy of Neurology (1991). Assessment: positron emission tomography. *Neurology* **41**, 163–7.

Safety of angiography

Hirshfield, J. W. (1992). Low-asmolarity contrast agents—who needs them? *New England Journal of Medicine* **326**, 482–4.

Duplex scanning

Strandness, E. (1990). *Duplex scanning in vascular disorders*. Raven Press, New York.

Part III

The principal neurological disorders

9 Headache

Headache is one of the most common symptoms with which both general practitioners and neurologists are asked to deal. For many of the neurological illnesses described in this book, there is some professional consensus on the techniques of diagnosis and how the illness should be managed. A physician is very much more on his own when he comes to deal with headaches not associated with structural disease—the vast majority of headaches. Most standard textbooks gloss over the difficulties involved in helping ill-defined symptoms in patients who have, in some cases, difficulties in their situation in life, or psychological problems. This section attempts to provide a simple framework within which any physician should be able to make a contribution to the management of common headaches not associated with structural disease, and also to provide the description of those few specific headache syndromes that require more technical management.

9.1 Epidemiology

The vast majority of people who have headaches do not consult their family doctors, let alone a neurologist, about them. For example, one survey in 1971 sampled over 2000 people chosen at random from the electoral roll. Of these, no fewer than 24 per cent reported a headache in the 14 days prior to the doorstep interview. In about one-fifth of these, the subject graded his or her headache as severe. In another similar survey, nearly one-quarter of the population sampled had experienced, in the previous two weeks, a 'headache or migraine' sufficiently severe to lead the respondent to take an aspirin or other simple analgesic.

It is not surprising, therefore, that headache is one of the most frequent symptoms presented to a general practitioner. Table 9.1 shows information derived from the third National Morbidity Survey based on more than 200 000 consultations in gen-

Table 9.1 Patients consulting their family doctor per 1000 persons at risk in one year for tension headache (ICD 307.8), headache (ICD 784.0), and migraine (ICD 346) (Source: Office of Population Censuses and Surveys. Third National Morbidity Survey, 1986.)

| | Age (years) | | | | |
	15–	25–	45–	65–	75–
Men					
tension headache	2.6	3.6	3.2	1.5	0.9
headache	11.0	10.3	8.2	8.8	8.5
migraine	5.8	6.2	4.9	2.8	0.9
Women					
tension headache	6.8	8.8	6.6	3.6	2.1
headache	23.1	21.2	15.1	13.3	13.0
migraine	14.3	17.6	14.1	4.7	1.7

	Male	Female	Population
All ages			
tension headache	2.4	5.5	4.1
headache	9.4	16.7	13.2
migraine	4.7	11.3	8.2
total (if independent)			25.5

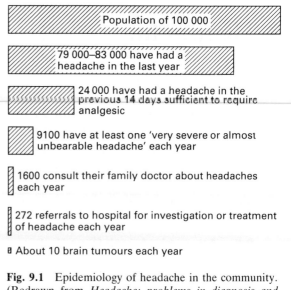

Population of 100 000

79 000–83 000 have had a headache in the last year

24 000 have had a headache in the previous 14 days sufficient to require analgesic

9100 have at least one 'very severe or almost unbearable headache' each year

1600 consult their family doctor about headaches each year

272 referrals to hospital for investigation or treatment of headache each year

About 10 brain tumours each year

Fig. 9.1 Epidemiology of headache in the community. (Redrawn from *Headache: problems in diagnosis and management*, W. B. Saunders, London, 1988.)

eral practice in the early 1980s. The overall figure for headache, tension headache, and migraine combined (these terms are further analysed in Section 9.3) was 25.5 per 1000. This can be placed in perspective alongside an annual consulting rate in the same study of 3.5 per 1000 for epilepsy, generally considered to be a common neurological problem. Table 9.1 also shows that women are far more likely to consult their family doctor about headache than men. More than 4 per cent of all women aged 25–45 will consult their general practitioner about headache or migraine in any one year, and that is excluding those in whom headache is a symptom secondary to, for example, a depressive illness.

Table 3.3 also shows that general practitioners do cope with the vast majority of patients with headache seen by them. Only about 3–14 per cent of patients with headache and migraine are referred on to hospital for a further opinion. None the less, studies based on the experience of a number of English neurologists show that consultations for headache make up about 15 per cent of all new outpatient referrals (Fig 3.1).

Figure 9.1 illustrates the statistics described above, and contains for completeness an illustration of the incidence of cerebral tumours, a diagnosis feared by many with continuing headaches. It is clear, therefore, that a physician has to develop strategies for sorting out those patients with headache who require investigation. This aspect is considered in Section 9.11.

It is clear from Fig. 9.1 that there is an enormous 'reservoir' of headache in the community, and, to use a well-known metaphor, neurologists only see the tip of the iceberg. If the number of neurologists were to be significantly increased, as it has been in the USA where the number of neurologists per head of population is something like 10 times the number prevailing in the UK (Table 3.4), then the ready availability of specialist help means that more of the tip is likely to float to the surface, and there will be an increased number of consultations for symptoms, such as headache, as the well-defined neurological diseases discussed elsewhere in this book are likely to remain broadly unchanged in prevalence for the foreseeable future. Equally, it could be seen that a small shift in the tolerance of subjects of their headaches, or in the referral patterns of general practitioners, could overwhelm outpatient clinics with requests for further opinions.

The main decision in our clinical approach to headache is whether the headache is a new event, or one of a recurrent series. As a general rule, it is more necessary to be alert to the possibility of an advancing neurological illness if the headache is a new event, arising in recent hours or days in a subject never much troubled previously by headache, than if the headache is one of a long-continued series.

9.2   Acute headaches of very recent onset

Table 9.2 lists some of the diagnostic possibilities to be considered if a headache occurs in an abrupt or subacute fashion. The headache of subarachnoid haemorrhage (see Section 10.6.2) is of such abrupt onset that the subject may think that he has actually been struck. Headache is usually severe, often generalized, though sometimes worse occipitally. With the benefit of hindsight, many substantial subarachnoid haemorrhages have been preceded by so-called sentinel headaches, which presumably represent either microscopic bleeds or stretching in the wall of the aneurysm from which the haemorrhage in many cases arises.

Similar severe occipital or generalized headaches, albeit of subacute onset, may occur in viral or bacterial meningitis. Meningeal irritation, whether it is due to blood in the subarachnoid space or infection, is associated with neck stiffness, or a positive Kernig's sign (see Section 17.1.2.2). Unpleasant generalized headaches often occur as part of a systemic infection, such as influenza, or in association with the bacteraemia that may accompany, for example, a renal infection. Such fevers may be associated also with neck stiffness or 'meningism' even if the infecting organism has not entered the spinal fluid. This is much more common in childhood than in adult life, and it is sometimes difficult to decide whether the spinal fluid should be examined in such circumstances. The general rule is that if in doubt a lumbar puncture should be undertaken.

Other causes of sudden 'first time' headache include infections of the paranasal sinuses, although in this case fever and local tenderness are usually prominent. Abrupt rises in intracranial pressure may follow a thrombosis in a major sinus, which may occur in the later stages of pregnancy or the puerperium (see Section 10.3).

Other headaches of acute onset, of which the cause is readily apparent, include headaches following a local injury to the head, and neurological investigations such as myelography. Finally, all the causes of chronic recurrent headaches listed in Table 9.3 must, of course, begin at some time, so it is necessary to consider whether the history is that of a first episode of, for example, cluster headaches (Section 9.6).

9.3   Chronic recurrent headache

The vast majority of headaches with which family doctors and neurologists have to deal are chronic recurrent headaches, and an approach to these is outlined in Table 9.4. Before going through the syndromes in Table 9.3, it is necessary to review current thinking about the specific headache diagnoses which are often made—tension headache and migraine. Until the 1980s, it was generally held that so-called tension headaches, that is to say the vast majority of headaches not due to structural disease and also not called migraine, had a basis in excessive muscular contraction. In support of this view there were observations that, under laboratory conditions, sustained voluntary contraction of scalp muscles could induce reported headaches.

Table 9.2   Acute headaches of very recent onset (hours or days), diagnostic possibilities

---

Vascular disease
  subarachnoid haemorrhage
  intracerebral haemorrhage
  acute athero-embolic infarction
  venous sinus thrombosis
Meningitis, cerebral abscess, encephalitis
Systemic infections, e.g. pyelonephritis with
  'meningism'
Extension of pain from local condition in:
  sinus, e.g. frontal or maxillary sinusitis
  eye, e.g. acute glaucoma, Tolosa–Hunt syndrome
  ear, e.g. otitis media
  tooth, e.g. erupting wisdom teeth

Additional causes include headaches following recent trauma, or neurological investigation such as myelography. Any first episode of the causes listed in Table 9.3 could figure here.

Table 9.3   Classification of chronic recurrent headaches

1. Common headache, including as variants/near
    synonyms: 'muscle contraction headache';
    'tension headache'; 'common migraine';
    'psychogenic headache'
    (a) with no obvious cause
    (b) as a response to an unsatisfactory life situation
    (c) as a manifestation of a definite depressive
        illness or anxiety state
    (d) as a specific anxiety in relation to the presence
        of cerebral tumour
    (e) subsequent to trauma
    (f) in association with cervical spondylosis or after
        whiplash injuries
    (g) induced or exacerbated by oral contraceptives
2. Headache with transient focal neurological
    symptoms, synonym: 'classical migraine'; if
    neurological deficit is more substantial,
    'hemiplegic', 'ophthalmoplegic', or 'basilar'
    migraine
3. Vascular headache
    (a) ischaemic vascular disease
    (b) carotid dissection
    (c) angiomas

    (d) cluster headache, synonym: 'migrainous
    neuralgia'
    (e) induced by sudden increases in blood pressure
        (i) with monoamine oxidase inhibitors
        (ii) in paraplegia
        (iii) with phaeochromocytoma
    (f) induced by general cranial vasodilatation
        (i) with CO_2 retention in chronic respiratory
            failure
        (ii) with amyl nitrite, etc.
    (g) cranial arteritis, synonym: 'temporal arteritis'
4. Headaches in association with raised intracranial
    pressure
    (a) primary or metastatic cerebral tumour
    (b) subdural haematoma
    (c) hydrocephalus
    (d) benign intracranial hypertension
    (e) cough headache
5. Lumbar puncture headache
6. Exertional and coital headache
7. Cranial neuralgias
8. Anatomical distortions or variations in the skull and
    facial bones

Table 9.4   Taking a history from a sufferer from chronic headaches

1. Background information
    age, sex, marital status
    occupation
    present social setting
    previous medical history
    family history of headaches
2. A typical headache attack
    Is there any warning before the headache begins?
    Whereabouts in the head is the headache?
    Does the pain radiate anywhere else?
    How severe is it?
    Of what character is the discomfort?
    Are nausea and vomiting associated with the
        attack?
    What does the patient do during the headache?
3. The time-course of the history
    When did the headaches begin?
    How frequent are they?
    How long do they last?
    Has the patient noticed any event that tends to
        bring on a headache?

    Do the headaches occur at any particular time of
        day, or on any particular day of the week?
    Do the headaches occur in bunches or clusters?
    For women, is there any relation to menstruation,
        oral contraception, or pregnancy?
4. Effect of the headaches
    How much do the headaches interfere with life?
    Has the patient missed work or even lost a job
        because of headaches?
5. Psychological factors
    Stressful recent life events
    Evidence of depression and anxiety, specifically
        anxiety about intracranial disease
6. Previous therapy and medical contacts
    What has the patient tried for headaches?
    How good is it?
    Has the patient previously consulted a doctor
        about these headaches?
    What did he or she do?

However, there are a number of studies that show that muscle contraction may be increased during episodes of classical migraine. Other studies have shown that no increased electromyographic activity occurs during many tension headaches and, even if there is some activity recorded, there is no correlation between electromyographic activity and clinical improvement.

Other ambiguities relate to the use of the word 'tension'. Many physicians have related chronic recurrent headaches to life stress or psychological 'tension', rather than to excessive muscular contraction. In fact, a review of the evidence does not suggest that psychological tension is often very important.

Clinical features that have been used to define 'migraine' include nausea or vomiting, and, for classical migraine, some sort of visual or other neurological phenomena. There is no doubt that in some headache syndromes focal neurological features occur, and visual phenomena, such as scintillating scotomata, are perceived in the visual field. However, many patients with severe headache complain of pain in the eyes, or photophobia, or blurred vision, which are symptoms certainly distinct from the visual phenomena mentioned above. Another distinguishing factor of so-called 'migraine' is that headaches in migraine are unilateral. Indeed, the word migraine is a corruption of 'hemi-crania'. However, many patients with the classical visual phenomena just mentioned may have generalized rather than unilateral headache.

Faced with these ambiguities, a number of researchers have instructed their computers to try to sort out a taxonomic classification of headaches. With the exception of so-called cluster headaches (see Section 9.6) such attempts at classification have failed. The present-day concept is that there is no clear-cut combination of symptoms of headache, or associated symptoms, that allows a separation into clearly distinct entities. A consensus has developed that patients with chronic recurrent headaches have at different times varying amounts of the features that have, in the past, been called migrainous (unilateral headaches of a throbbing type, associated with nausea) and at other times features of headaches that have, in the past, been called tension headaches or muscle-contraction headaches (pain at the back of the head, a headache described as like a band, or like a feeling of pressure on top of the head). Furthermore, from a

number of epidemiological studies it has emerged that the more severe the headache is graded by the patient, either in terms of severity of pain, or disruption of life, the more likelihood is there of other symptoms such as nausea or visual discomfort. This analysis at least fits in with the perspective of most patients, that there is a group of severe, nauseating, and often unilateral headaches which disrupt life, and which they, and many neurologists, until recently have called 'migraine'. Headaches with focal neurological symptoms (classical migraine, see Section 9.4.1) are clearly distinct, but variations in some classical attacks may well result in the patient experiencing some headaches without focal neurological events. Alternatively, common headaches are so common that a proportion of patients with classic migraine will have some common headaches by chance alone. It is for all these reasons that many neurologists find the classification of the International Headache Society, part of which is reproduced in Table 9.5, unsatisfactory. Although possibly a basis for future research, the classification is unrealistic for everyday use.

Table 9.5   Extract from the detailed classification of headache of the International Headache Society

2   Tension-type headache
  2.1   Episodic tension-type headache
    2.1.1   Episodic tension-type headache associated with disorder of pericranial muscles
    2.1.2   Episodic tension-type headache unassociated with disorder of pericranial muscles
  2.2   Chronic tension-type headache
    2.2.1   Chronic tension-type headache associated with disorder of pericranial muscles
    2.2.2   Chronic tension-type headache unassociated with disorder of pericranial muscles
  2.3   Headache of the tension-type not fulfilling above criteria

If, as the foregoing indicates, there is no real distinction between the vast majority of chronic recurrent headaches, it may be asked why it is necessary to take a history along the lines of the headings of Table 9.4. It is, of course, necessary still to take a full history in order to categorize those few headache syndromes that require specific management, such as cluster headaches (Section 9.6) and cranial arteritis (see Section 9.7). Another cogent reason for taking a careful history is that, despite the reality of the lack of distinction between most types of headache, patients at consultation expect matters to be gone into thoroughly. A number of studies have shown that outcome is related to the patient's perception that matters have been gone into properly at consultation.

Marital status, occupation, and present social setting are, in themselves, of no diagnostic importance, but do provide a framework within which attempts at treatment may be made. For example, if a patient attributes his or her headache to prolonged concentration at a visual display unit, then it is unlikely that therapy of any kind is likely to be effective unless this belief is recognized and the job modified in some way.

The previous medical history is often unimportant but, for example, if the patient had had a lump removed from one breast some years before, there may be some concern about the possibility of a cerebral metastasis. A family history of headaches is of uncertain value. Although there may be a genetic component to headache with focal neurological features, the occurrence of headaches in families may mean no more than illness behaviour in common—a learned way of coping with unfavourable life events, and of seeking support modelled upon the experience of other family members. The site and radiation of pain is not usually of much importance, though this certainly becomes so when considering the differential diagnosis of pain in the face (see Section 9.10). The patient's description of the character of the headache may be useful in so far as it has been shown that headaches described as 'crushing', 'spreading', 'stabbing', and other dramatic words are more likely to be associated with a psychiatric disorder. Equally, headaches that have been present 'all my life' or which have been continuous for many months are not likely to have an organic structural basis but may well prove to be a somatic manifestation of depression. Other features of the time-course of the history may be relevant, particularly in regard to clustering of the headaches in bouts

(see Section 9.6) and the time of day at which headache occurs. Headaches that are present on waking in the morning but which fade subsequently during the day do particularly suggest the possibility of raised intracranial pressure. However, many patients who turn out to have cerebral tumours have, on review of their history, rather unremarkable headaches.

Many patients report certain dietary or other factors that they think may precipitate or exacerbate a headache. Dietary factors include missing a meal, or certain dietary precipitants such as chocolate, cheese, red wine, or citrus fruits. Sometimes headaches are worse immediately before or at the time of menstruation. It is widely reported that oral contraceptives may bring on headaches in someone who has never previously suffered from them, or exacerbate the headaches of a long-term sufferer. Other recognized precipitants include sleeping in late at weekends, vigorous exercise, and, occasionally, sexual intercourse (see Section 9.5.1).

There are differences of opinion about the importance of psychological factors in the precipitation of headache. Controlled studies show no more unfavourable life events in those who have headaches than in the general population. However, patients with headache experience, or at least perceive that they experience, more everyday 'hassles', and seem to adopt less successful strategies in coping with them. It is interesting that it has been shown that patients who present to psychiatrists with an anxiety disorder have no more headaches than a control population. On the other hand, patients who present with depression are much more likely to have headaches.

There has been considerable discussion about the personality of patients with recurrent headaches. Patients with 'migraine' are said to be more intelligent than the general population, of a generally higher social class, and perfectionist in their actions. It is now realized that such reports are an artefact of the self-selection of patients to special migraine clinics. Surveys in the community suggest that sufferers from recurrent headaches do have a rather higher level of neuroticism than those without headache, and it does appear that such characteristic personality traits are not a result of the experience of headaches, but are present before the headaches start.

I should stress that there remain a substantial

number of patients who are not clinically depressed, and who seem to have entirely normal personalities, but who are specifically anxious about the possibility of serious neurological disease such as an intracranial tumour. It appears that such fears are often generated by hearing of an acquaintance with a tumour, or with a stroke, information about which turns the subject's headaches, previously thought to be trivial, into an object of specific anxiety. It is fortunate that simple reassurance of such patients is gratifyingly effective. It follows that such fears should always be explicitly explored, and firm and specific reassurance given, if that is possible, as it usually is.

There remain other patients for whom, as far as it can be judged, life at home and work is without any factors that are acknowledged by them to be stressful, nor do they hold any particular specific anxiety about serious disease. These puzzling patients are the most difficult to counsel. It is all too easy to seize upon some aspect of the patient's life, for example forthcoming examinations at school, or a difficult supervisor at work, and 'blame' the headaches on this factor, even though the patient may deny that the events cause sufficient stress to be responsible for the headaches, as the examiner chooses to believe. Whether it is that the stress is repressed and 'converted' to headache, or whether the subject is correct in being unconcerned about such factors in his private life is incapable of proof, but my impression is that many doctors too readily attribute the onset of common headaches to personal factors, even though these factors may not have changed for years. Such doctors find a way around this criticism by talking of a 'breakdown in coping mechanisms', again incapable of logical proof. The onset of many such headaches has to remain unexplained.

9.3.1   *Headache in children*

Just as in the case of adults, headaches not due to structural disease are very common in children and vastly predominate over those of serious import. The best epidemiological survey is based upon a review of more than 15 000 children born in one week in 1958 (the National Child Development Survey). By the age of 7, 5.3 per cent of children had had recurrent sick headaches; by the age of 11, 21.3 per cent, and by the age of 16, 49.7 per cent.

Many parents of children with headaches think first of a refractive error or squint as a likely cause. Reports of relief on refraction are non-critical, failing to take into account the tendency for most headaches in children to resolve. As long ago as 1881, a paediatrician reported 'Headaches in the young are for most part due to bad arrangements in the lives of children', a problem still applicable today. Children themselves, at least by the age of 16, commonly attribute their headaches to stress, but this may reflect no more than the prevailing view of their parents and doctors.

In one Danish study, 60 per cent of adults with headaches that were judged to be migrainous 20 years earlier had improved during adolescence, but headaches returned in about a third of these. It does seem, therefore, that a substantial proportion of children with headaches continue to have recurrent non-specific headaches in their adult life.

I have written at length about common or recurrent non-specific headaches as these are by far the most frequent of all headache syndromes. None the less, there are some specific neurological syndromes of headache which are considered next. The management of chronic recurrent headache, after exclusion of these, is considered in Section 9.11.

9.4   Headache with focal neurological symptoms

9.4.1   *Classical migraine*

There is a group of patients who have a neurological deficit prior to, or at the time of, their headache. The most frequent phenomena are visual—scintillating teichopsia (flashes of light in the visual field), scotomata, a perception that objects are too large (macropsia) or too small (micropsia). However, tingling in a part of a limb, usually a hand, or hemiparesis, or aphasia may all occur. For many years it has been believed that these neurological symptoms are the result of a spasm of intracerebral blood vessels, so that neurological dysfunction results from hypoxia. A number of arteriograms have, however, been taken during episodes of classical migraine, and the expected vasospasm has not been seen. Furthermore, although cerebral blood-flow studies using modern techniques, such as single-photon emission computerized tomography, do show hypoperfusion associated with attacks of classical migraine, this hypoperfusion develops independently of the territories of supply of the cerebral arteries. There is also a dissociation in time between reduced blood flow and the occurrence of focal neurological symptoms. One current hypothesis is that the neurological phenomena of classical migraine are due to a wave of cortical spreading depression, as first described by Leao more than 40 years ago. In experimental observations on animals, Leao observed that following a neuronal insult, such as pricking the cortex of a rat brain, all ongoing neuronal activity became completely extinguished for a period of a minute or so; this depression would propagate very slowly as a wave across a wide cortical region. This hypothesis certainly fits many of the observed features of classical migraine attacks, although the initial trigger of the wave of cortical-spreading depression is not known. Under this hypothesis, the cortical spreading depression is associated with a sharp reduction in cerebral blood flow which lasts for 2–6 h, although blood flow increases above resting levels in the phase of headache. The region of reduced blood flow in the initial stages gradually expands as the presumed cortical spreading depression moves anteriorly. Symptoms of aphasia or numbness, or the loss of use of one hand, appear when the cortical spreading depression arrives at the primary sensorimotor cortex. This hypothesis adequately explains the neurological dysfunction of migraine attacks, but is less successful at accounting for headache. The headache of migraine is probably due in part to dilatation of extracranial arteries. It may also be that cortical spreading depression alters activity in subcortical pain pathways in some way. Occasionally the neurological 'shut-down' may be so severe that a hemiplegia results. Cranial CT scanning at this stage may show hemispheric oedema. Very rarely, frank infarction ensues.

Another hypothesis brings together neural and vascular elements through a 'trigeminovascular reflex'. It is known that stimulation of the raphe nuclei and the locus coeruleus, which have a role in pain modulation, results in dilatation of extracranial arteries through axons running in the greater superficial petrosal nerve, and in the sphenopalatine and otic ganglia. Serotonin (5-hydroxytryptamine; 5-HT) constricts cerebral blood vessels. Free plasma serotonin drops markedly during an episode of classical migraine, and urinary excretion of its metabolite, 5-hydroxyindoleacetic acid, is increased. Some migraine headaches may be relieved by the infusion of serotonin during an attack, but only at the expense of unpleasant adverse effects. Sumatriptan, an agonist of one type of serotonin receptor (5-HT$_{1D}$) has also been shown to be effective (see Section 9.11). Ergotamine, an effective drug in the treatment of migraine, also has 5–HT$_1$-like actions. However, this model of migraine action is let down by the observation that the mean daily level of platelet serotonin in patients with chronic 'tension' headache is also lower than in normal controls.

Other observations made during acute episodes of classical migraine show elevated plasma levels of noradrenaline (possibly a secondary response to pain) and normal levels of vasoactive peptide, substance P, vasopressin, and β-endorphin.

9.4.2 Other variants of migraine

Hemiplegic migraine may run in families. Usually the first such episode requires fairly careful investigation to exclude an underlying lesion such as an angioma.

Another variant of headache with focal neurological symptoms is *basilar migraine*. In such patients, the neurological dysfunction seems to arise in the brain stem, and dysarthria, vertigo, nystagmus, and some degree of somnolence are all features. The patients are often younger than 20 years of age, and almost invariably younger than 50. There is often a history of other types of migraine with focal neurological features, and of a family history of similar disorders. The first such episode usually requires neurological investigation to exclude a posterior fossa tumour before the diagnosis can be made with any confidence.

A rather different syndrome is *ophthalmoplegic migraine*. In this, periocular and retro-ocular pain is accompanied by ptosis, and other features of a transient III nerve palsy, although the pupil is often spared. The differential diagnosis includes similar features arising from an expanding supraclinoid aneurysm, and arteriography will often be necessary. In ophthalmoplegic migraine, an arteriogram during the acute attack may show narrowing of the internal carotid lumen, which is taken to be evidence of oedema of the arterial wall.

Some authors consider *transient global amnesia* (see Section 10.1.10.1) to be a variant of migraine, but the evidence is at best circumstantial.

Migrainous neuralgia (cluster headache) seems to be quite distinct from other variants of migraine, and is considered in Section 9.6.

9.5   Headache and vascular disease

Many patients with headaches fear that a persisting headache may indicate an impending stroke. However, in any large series of patients with persistent headaches, strokes are not reported as a major outcome. From the opposite perspective, however, headache certainly occurs as a symptom of a stroke or transient ischaemic attack in about 25 per cent of all such patients. The incidence of headaches in lacunar infarcts (Section 10.1.2) is low.

Occasionally there may be a dissection of the wall of the common, or internal, or external carotid artery. In such cases, the pain is very severe, radiating from the neck up into the jaw, the eye, and the cheek. A Horner's syndrome commonly accompanies such dissections. (Section 19.7.2.4).

Other vascular headaches include headaches in association with intracerebral angiomas (Section 10.6.6). It is difficult to distinguish such headaches from attacks of classical migraine, but in those due to angiomas, the headache may precede a neurological deficit which is usually consistent in each attack. Occasionally a bruit may be heard.

9.5.1   *Other causes of vascular headache*

Sudden vascular headaches may arise in association with phaeochromocytomata, due to the sudden outpouring of circulating amines. A similar response may occur if certain foods containing monoamines are eaten in association with mono-amine-oxidase-inhibiting drugs, such as phenelzine. Such foods include cheese, broad beans, pickled herring, and Marmite, and red wine is also incriminated. Many nasal sprays or bronchodilators contain amines, and must also be avoided.

Paraplegic patients may suffer an acute pressor reaction to, for example, a full bladder, and this may result in a sudden vascular headache. Accel-erated hypertension, or acute hypertension in relation to acute nephritis, may be associated with headache, but there is no sound epidemiological evidence that headaches are more frequent in those with higher blood pressure in the general population.

Amyl nitrate, used for the relief of angina, or as an illicit drug, may induce headache through sudden vasodilatation. Nitrites are used in the preservation of meat and this may induce headaches in some susceptible people. Patients with chronic hypercarbic respiratory failure due to obstructive airways disease may be troubled by persistent headaches, and these have been attributed to the vasodilatation in relation to high $P_{a\,CO_2}$. However, vasodilatation does not invariably result in headache. For example, during a trial of extracranial–intracranial anastomotic bypass surgery for extracranial vascular disease (see Section 10.1.10.5), headache was not a common postoperative feature, even though postoperative arteriography showed considerable dilatation of the recipient vessels. It is probable that the speed of dilatation is important in the headaches reviewed above.

Some patients develop headaches during sexual intercourse at the moment of orgasm. This is unrelated to bodily passivity or otherwise at orgasm, and is probably due to a brief elevation of blood pressure at the time. In these cases, the headache may be so severe that a subarachnoid haemorrhage may be feared.

9.6   Cluster headache

As mentioned on p. 117, this variety of headache is one that seems to have a distinct pattern, and is justifiably distinguished from other headache syndromes. There are a number of synonyms for this condition (periodic migrainous neuralgia, ciliary neuralgia, Horton's syndrome). Some of the syndromes beloved by ear, nose, and throat surgeons, such as Sluder's neuralgia and Vidian neuralgia, are probably identical.

The word 'cluster' refers to the timing of the headache attacks, which is a characteristic feature. A cluster of attacks may last days or weeks, with remissions lasting months or years. The principal symptom is unilateral facial pain affecting principally the region of the eye, but spreading to the temple, the nose, the cheek, and the forehead. The build-up of pain is rapid, over 10 min or so, and at its peak the pain is extremely severe. The attacks seldom last for more than an hour. Lacrimation of the affected eye is a feature, and there may also be congestion of the conjunctiva, so the eye looks red during an attack.

The pain may wake the patient from sleep. The pain usually affects only one side, but occasionally the other side is independently affected. Simultaneous bilateral attacks do not occur.

Additional features include ipsilateral nasal stuffiness, and, if the nasal mucosa is inspected during an attack, it is seen to be congested in the same way as the conjunctiva. There may be a transient Horner's syndrome during an attack.

In contrast to all other types of headache, males are much more frequently affected than females. Most commonly, the onset is in the fourth and fifth decades.

All these features are clearly distinct from other types of migraine and headache in general. However, the cause of the syndrome is totally unknown, even though it is recognized that attacks may be precipitated by the injection of histamine or inhalation of nitroglycerine. The differential diagnosis usually presents no difficulty, although it is necessary to consider ophthalmoplegic migraine, or that the symptoms arise from a supraclinoid aneurysm, or from a lesion in the region of the trigeminal ganglion.

Treatment of cluster headaches is not easy. The pain is so abrupt in onset, and relatively so short-lived, that analgesia for the acute attack has little part to play. Most physicians use ergotamine tartrate in suppository form as a prophylaxis during the bouts. It is important not to exceed the safe weekly consumption of ergotamine (10 mg/week). In practice this means that a suppository is taken five nights a week, and withdrawn on two nights, so that it can be seen if the bout has spontaneously terminated. If ergotamine fails, lithium has proved to be an effective prophylactic in many patients. Just as in the treatment of mania, the serum levels of lithium must be monitored carefully. Other treatments include the inhalation of oxygen during the acute episode, and calcium antagonists, such as nifedipine, as prophylactic agents. Occasionally, surgical management is necessary, in which case a radiofrequency lesion of the trigeminal ganglion is probably the best method (see Section 9.10.1).

9.7 Cranial arteritis

Synonyms for this condition include temporal arteritis and giant-cell arteritis.

This is a rare disorder that commonly presents with headache, due to an acute inflammatory arteritis affecting branches of the carotid artery system. The disorder is rare under the age of 60. Over this age the annual incidence is approximately 10 per 100 000.

The cause of the illness is unknown. There is some association with polymyalgia rheumatica (Section 21.4), although it is much more common to find histological proof of the diagnosis of cranial arteritis on biopsy of a branch of a temporal artery than it is to find evidence of arteritis on muscle biopsy in cases of polymyalgia rheumatica. The most frequent presenting symptom is of unilateral persistent pain over the temple. The patient may notice a tender cord-like artery. Light pressure from wearing a hat or resting the head on a cushion or pillow may aggravate the pain. Although the temporal artery is the one most commonly involved, the occipital artery may also be affected and, less commonly, branches of the facial and maxillary arteries, when claudication of jaw muscles may occur during chewing. About half the patients with temporal arteritis have symptoms of polymyalgia, principally early morning pain and stiffness in proximal muscles. There are often systemic disturbances in such patients, with low-grade fever, weight loss, and general malaise.

Examination of patients with cranial arteritis may show that pulsations in the artery die out as the artery is tracked distally with the examining finger, and tender nodules may be felt.

The principal complication of cranial arteritis is visual loss produced by occlusive arteritis of the posterior ciliary arteries and/or the central retinal artery in its orbital and intraneural portion. Once visual loss has been present for more than a few hours, any improvement in vision is unlikely, however vigorous the treatment. However, some workers believe that it is worth infusing low molecular weight dextran, and giving high-dose intravenous steroids.

The risk of visual loss in something of the order of 10 per cent. Occasionally, the second eye is also affected. Therefore, it is certainly necessary not to overlook the diagnosis, and, as the condition is responsive to steroids, treat vigorously as soon as the diagnosis is confirmed. Associated features include an elevated sedimentation rate, although there are two difficulties about this. First of all, the sedimentation rate is commonly higher in older people in any event. Secondly, the sedimentation rate may be within normal limits in about 10 per cent of patients with cranial arteritis. The preferred course, therefore, is to confirm the diagnosis by biopsy of an affected artery. Unfortunately, there are difficulties here, too, as segments of the artery may be normal. It is certainly worth asking the surgeon to approach an area of the artery that is tender, or which seems to be enlarged in a nodular fashion. Bilateral biopsy may be necessary. The histological changes show an inflammatory arteritis with infiltration by giant cells, though with no clues as to the aetiology. There is also fragmentation and destruction of the internal elastic lamina, with extensive thickening of the intima and media. Arteries that normally contain little elastic tissue (such as the intracranial portion of the vertebral and carotid) are not commonly affected, suggesting that the disorder is due to some sort of immunological reaction against elastic tissue.

The arteritis may occasionally affect the small vessels along the course of the IIIrd, IVth, and VIth cranial nerves, resulting in external and internal ophthalmoplegia. The extracranial course of the internal carotid and vertebral arteries may also be affected, resulting occasionally in cerebral infarction, most commonly in the territory of the vertebrals, possibly because the calibre of these is less than that of the carotid system.

The effect on vision is so grave that while the diagnosis of cranial arteritis is suspected on clinical grounds, patients should be treated at once with prednisone, without waiting for histological confirmation. The only exception is the rare elderly patient with active peptic ulceration. However, most elderly patients tolerate long-term, high-dose steroid treatment poorly. A suitable compromise is to start the patient on 80 mg of prednisone each day, reducing the dose to 60 mg/day after 4 days, with further reductions by 10 mg at intervals of 4 days, and with regular estimations of the sedimentation rate, aiming to stabilize the patient on a minimum dose of corticosteroids that will keep the sedimentation rate below 35 mm in the first hour. It has to be acknowledged, however, that there are difficulties in those patients who have a normal sedimentation rate in the first place. It is also

difficult to decide how long to continue steroids, but it seems that the risk of ocular involvement after 6 months is small. At this stage it would be wise to attempt withdrawing steroids completely, in order to minimize the long-term adverse effects such as osteoporosis, vertebral collapse, and myopathy. If symptoms return, or the sedimentation rate becomes elevated again, then it is probably necessary to continue a maintenance dose of 10–15 mg/day indefinitely.

About half the patients with cranial arteritis will have aching and stiffness in cervical, posterior occipital, shoulder, and chest muscles that is worse on waking in the morning. This is polymyalgia rheumatica (Section 21.4).

9.8   Headaches due to changes in intracranial pressure

An anxiety experienced by all physicians is that they will falsely reassure a patient about a headache which eventually proves to be due to an intracranial tumour. As so many perfectly rational people with headaches fear that they might have a tumour (see p. 119), incorrect reassurance is doubly unfortunate, and may lead to litigation. As already written on page 118, the features of the headaches of many patients with proven intracranial tumours are no different from more banal headaches. There are, however, some features that should suggest the possibility of raised intracranial pressure and the need for further investigation. Headaches that are present on waking in the morning, or are initiated by change in posture, or by coughing or straining, should all be taken seriously. If the quality of headache is described as 'bursting', or in some other similar way, I would also be concerned. Clearly, a shorter history of weeks or months, rather than years, is a feature of most of the headaches caused by raised intracranial pressure. Apart from a tumour, a subdural haematoma, or decompensated hydrocephalus must also be considered.

Headaches that are initiated by coughing, or by other mechanisms that briefly raise the intrathoracic and therefore the intracranial pressure, do raise the question of a space-occupying lesion, particularly in the posterior fossa, or some sort of anomaly at the cranio-cervical junction. However, by no means all patients with cough headache have a structural cause, and the majority disappear spontaneously. It must also be remembered that any pre-existing headache, of the usual common and non-specific type, may also be exacerbated by coughing.

Headaches may also result from an intracranial pressure that is unduly low. For practical purposes, this really only arises as a consequence of lumbar puncture. Although the extent to which patients develop headache after lumbar puncture is dependent on their expectations (patients who are told that they may get a headache are more likely to get one than those to whom nothing is said), some patients undoubtedly develop headaches due to a transient dural fistula along the needle track. For this reason it is worth using a fine lumbar puncture needle (not larger than 21 gauge). Some hold that it is worth turning the bevel of the needle in a longitudinal direction at the moment of puncture so that the dural fibres are split rather than transected. Most such headaches are relieved by simple recumbency for a few hours, but if they continue to be troublesome for longer than this, it may be worth injecting 5 ml of the patient's own blood into the epidural space. This so-called 'dural patch' may seal off the dural fistula (Section 8.2.1.1). Other recommended treatments include brief overhydration by the use of antidiuretic hormone, but it is very rare indeed for such procedures to be needed.

9.9 Anatomical variations that may cause headache

Neurologists acknowledge that anomalies of the cranio-cervical junction may result in headaches through associated hydrocephalus, but they take a more jaundiced view of the attribution of headaches to other anatomical variations, such as styloid processes that are too long (Eagle's syndrome) or nasal septa that are not straight. On the whole, the reports of relief of headache following operation upon such minor abnormalities overlook the enormous placebo effect of an operation.

9.9.1 *Cervical spondylosis*

Headaches are commonly attributed also to disorders of the cervical spine, most commonly cervical

spondylosis. Experimental studies have shown that injections of hypertonic saline into the upper cervical muscles may cause an occipital headache radiating forwards. Furthermore, an occipital or generalized headache is a common feature after an acute whiplash injury, in which muscles and ligaments of the cervical spine are torn. It is not unreasonable, therefore, to believe that degenerative changes in the cervical spine may also cause chronic occipital headache radiating forwards. The difficulty is that the radiological features of cervical spondylosis are a virtually uniform finding in those over the age of 50. It is probable that many headaches attributed to dysfunction of the cervical spine are no different from the common or recurrent non-specific headaches reviewed in Section 9.3. The relief of such headaches by gentle cervical manipulation and massage may be no more than a non-specific relaxing effect, and such relief does not necessarily indicate that the original attribution of the headaches to cervical spondylosis was necessarily correct. There are equal reservations about the attribution of facial pain to disorders of the temporomandibular joint, reviewed in Section 9.10.3.

9.10 Facial pain

Most patients, and their doctors, make a distinction between pain in the cranial vault, which is called a headache, and pain in the face. Table 9.6 outlines the common syndromes of facial pain.

Table 9.6 Classification of pain felt predominantly in the lower part of the face

Extension of pain from local condition in
  sinus, e.g. maxillary sinusitis or neoplasm
  eye, e.g. acute glaucoma
  ear, e.g. otitis media
  tooth, e.g. root abscess
Cranial neuralgias
  trigeminal neuralgia
  glossopharyngeal neuralgia
Atypical facial pain

Pain due to dental or sinus disease is not considered further.

9.10.1 *Trigeminal neuralgia*

Trigeminal neuralgia is a common condition, with onset usually in the sixth or seventh decade of life. As it is an episodic disorder, it is more meaningful to consider the prevalence than the incidence. Calculations suggest that approximately 100 per 100 000 men and 200 per 100 000 women are affected. The right side of the face is more commonly affected than the left.

The character of the pain is the foundation of the diagnosis. First of all, for a diagnosis of trigeminal neuralgia to be made, the distribution of the pain has to be in the distribution of the trigeminal nerve. The mandibular and maxillary divisions are affected together in about 40 per cent of patients, the mandibular alone in about 20 per cent, and all three divisions in a further 15 per cent. It is rare for the ophthalmic division to be affected by itself.

The pain is described as sharp and stabbing, occurring in paroxysms of sudden onset, repeated at very short intervals. The pain may occur spontaneously, but is often precipitated by afferent stimuli in the field of the affected trigeminal nerve. Common stimuli include washing, shaving, eating, or talking. A light touch on the outside of the face in a 'trigger zone' may precipitate paroxysm. It is interesting that repeated triggering may temporarily 'exhaust' the nerve, so a paroxysm can then no longer be precipitated for 15 min or so. Patients may use this effect to induce a brief period in which they can eat in relative comfort.

The vast majority of patients with trigeminal neuralgia have no clearly defined cause on examination, although operative findings, reviewed below, indicate minor structural abnormalities in the region of the central branch of the nerve. Occasionally trigeminal neuralgia may arise during the course of multiple sclerosis, or as a presenting symptom of multiple sclerosis, and this diagnosis must certainly be considered if typical pain begins in someone under the age of 40. Other causes of symptomatic trigeminal neuralgia are rare, but an appropriately placed meningioma or acoustic neuroma may be responsible.

In recent years, operative findings have shown that a large number of people with 'idiopathic' trigeminal neuralgia have a redundant loop of artery or vein indenting the central portion of the trigeminal nerve. Gentle separation of these abnormal vessels from the root usually results in complete relief of symptoms. These observations, and the association of multiple sclerosis with trigeminal neuralgia, give some clues as to the aetiology. It is not sufficient to propose, as was originally suggested, that the neuralgia is produced by a short circuit between large-diameter tactile fibres and unmyelinated or small myelinated pain fibres, as peripheral damage to the nerve, for example by an injection into the ganglion or branches of the nerve distal to the ganglion, can abort the neuralgia. Probably, chronic irritation of the trigeminal sensory root produces a failure of segmental inhibition in the trigeminal nucleus, as well as ectopic spike production in the nerve. This combination leads to paroxysmal discharges of interneurons in the trigeminal nucleus in response to tactile stimulation.

These pathophysiological features are reminiscent of those of epilepsy (Section 12.3), and it is for these reasons that anticonvulsants were introduced in the management of trigeminal neuralgia. Carbamazepine is now the treatment of choice. Elderly patients should be started on not more than 100 mg/day, and the dose gradually increased until satisfactory relief has been achieved or until giddiness and drowsiness occurs. Just as in the management of epilepsy, carbamazepine has to be given three or four times a day, in view of the short half-life of the drug. If carbamazepine does not relieve symptoms, then phenytoin, baclofen, or the less commonly used anticonvulsant drugs may all be tried.

The medical treatment outlined above relieves pain satisfactorily in 70–80 per cent of all patients with trigeminal neuralgia. A surgical approach can be considered in the remaining 20 per cent, if the pain is sufficiently severe. The trigeminal ganglion can be destroyed by a radiofrequency lesion or the injection of glycerol into the extradural space around the ganglion. The radiofrequency probe, or injecting needle, is introduced through the anterior part of the face and passed through the foramen ovale under radiological control. In former days, when alcohol injection was used, experienced operators could pass the needle through the foramen ovale without radiological control, but the advent of effective medical treatment has meant that few now acquire this skill.

An alternative approach is a surgical exploration of the central portion of the trigeminal nerve, and the retraction and displacement of any redundant vessels found to be compressing the nerve. Critics of this operation, which has a low morbidity in skilled hands, suggest that the relief of symptoms is due to no more than minimal operative traumatization of the nerve, rather than to the relief of pressure. In any event, the medical and surgical approaches to trigeminal neuralgia are such that no elderly person should be allowed to put up with intolerable pain.

9.10.2 *Glossopharyngeal neuralgia*

Although not strictly a facial pain, it is convenient to consider glossopharyngeal neuralgia here. It is about 100 times less common than trigeminal neuralgia. The paroxysms of pain are identical to those of trigeminal neuralgia except in their distribution. Lancinating pain is experienced in the throat, tonsillar region, external auditory meatus, or tongue. Tactile triggers include swallowing, and talking and chewing. Many patients respond to carbamazepine. A neurosurgical approach has shown similar ectatic blood vessels as are described in trigeminal neuralgia, and a similar satisfactory response to operative decompression.

9.10.3 *Atypical facial pain*

There remains a group of patients with facial pain that is not 'typical' in the sense of being typical of trigeminal neuralgia. Such patients, almost invariably women, describe a dull, deep, aching pain in the cheek, often spreading to the lower jaw. It is certainly necessary to consider an invasive tumour of the maxillary sinus, but this is relatively easily excluded by simple sinus X-rays. The pain in the remaining patients was for many years attributed to dysfunction of the temporomandibular joint, so-called Costen's syndrome. The absence of clinical or radiological features pointing to true involvement of this joint was countered, by those in favour of this syndrome, by the argument that minor degrees of malocclusion could lead to aberrant muscular contraction on the two sides of the face, and unusual strains on the joint. There has never been adequate evidence for such a hypothesis. An interesting double-blind study showed that mock adjustment of occlusion, in which patients believed that their bite had been adjusted, was equally 'effective' in relieving facial pain as true occlusal adjustment.

It is now believed that many patients with facial pain are depressed, and, even if depression is not overt, the treatment of choice is tricyclic antidepressant drugs. Unfortunately, before such drugs are used, the patient has usually made many visits to dentists, ENT surgeons, and neurologists, and had a variety of analgesic preparations, dental extractions, and sinus wash-outs.

9.10.4 *Miscellaneous facial pain*

Other facial pains include facial post-herpetic neuralgia, the management of which is along the same lines as post-herpetic neuralgia in general (Section 17.12.7.3). Facial pain can also be a feature of cranial arteritis (Section 9.7). Cardiac ischaemic pain can radiate to the face and jaw, but its association with exertion usually makes this diagnosis apparent. Pain due to neoplasms of the head and neck, which have metastasized or spread by direct extension from the site of origin, is difficult to treat, largely due to the overlapping sensory representation of the various cranial and upper cervical nerves. All available operative procedures for the relief of such pain are major procedures. Multiple section of cranial nerves and cervical nerve roots, or stereotactic thalamotomy, may be considered occasionally.

Causes of periorbital pain other than cluster headaches include supraclinoid aneurysm, lesions in the middle fossa such as a meningioma, an acute diabetic cranial mononeuropathy (see Section 19.4.1.2), orbital tumours, and the Tolosa–Hunt syndrome. This is a disorder in which there is a granulomatous infiltration in the region of the superior orbital fissure. Orbital pain is accompanied by ophthalmoplegia, and sometimes by sensory loss in the ophthalmic division of the trigeminal nerve. The sedimentation rate is elevated. The condition responds to steroids. Recurrent attacks are not uncommon.

9.11 The management of the patient with chronic recurrent headache

The immediately foregoing sections have outlined the principal specific neurological syndromes associated with headache and pain in the face. It is now necessary to return to the management of the patient with common or recurrent non-specific headaches not due to structural disease.

The first point is this—after careful clinical examination that shows no evidence of structural disease, which patients with chronic recurrent headache should be investigated further? Some clinical pointers in relation to the character of the headache are given in Section 9.3. The difficulty is that, in developed countries at least, many patients with chronic headache now expect or specifically request a cranial CT scan. A number of studies have shown that CT scanning of patients without clinical pointers to structural disease is enormously expensive and virtually always unrewarding. Neurosurgeons, from their own perspective, can legitimately point to patients who have been incorrectly reassured, at an earlier stage of their management, that their headache were not due to significant intracranial problems. However, such exceptional cases should not be allowed to influence the considerate and economic practice of clinical medicine for the vast majority. Although there will always be patients who request a cranial CT scan for the investigation of their recurrent headaches, such difficulties should not be overestimated. It has been shown that both satisfaction with a neurological consultation and the relief of headaches are largely related to the patient's perspective that sufficient time has been given to an explanation of the symptoms and, in particular, what those symptoms mean to the patient in terms of his or her own life. Anxieties about specific disorders such as cranial tumours or an impending stroke should be specifically explored, and specific reassurance given.

Most patients who come to neurologists with their headaches have exhausted all the simple available over-the-counter analgesic preparations, and there is no evidence that stronger analgesics are appropriate in these circumstances. It is best to advise that the patient continue with whatever tablet has, so far, best suited him or her, and this, combined now with the reassurance of an adequate clinical examination, and the opportunity to ventilate anxieties, may well tide the patient over into a better time in which headaches are less troublesome.

In a proportion of patients, it may become clear that chronic headache is a manifestation of depres-

sion, and treatment with tricyclic antidepressant drugs may be rewarding.

As already noted in the earlier part of this chapter, there is little point in attempting to make a diagnosis of 'tension headache' or 'migraine'. My own practice in recent years has been to allow the patient to continue with a diagnosis of 'migraine' if that is the way in which the patient, or his or her other physicians, have seen his or her own headaches. For those patients with classical migraine, or periodic headaches with reasonable intervals of complete freedom between them, then some sort of prophylactic medication may be indicated. Most of the trials of prophylactic medication fail to acknowledge the tendency for patients to be recruited to trials at times when their headaches are severe and recurrent, a state from which change can only take place in one direction—towards improvement. It is difficult, therefore, to show a beneficial effect of any prophylactic medication, but probably propranolol and pizotifen are two reasonable drugs to employ. Propranolol should be used in dosages up to 320 mg/day. It is probable that other beta-blockers would be equally effective. There are, of course, unpleasant drawbacks to beta-blockers in high dosage—notably cold extremities, impairment of sleep, and impotence in males. Pizotifen is also probably an effective prophylactic medication, although weight gain may limit its use. A reasonable dose would be 500 micrograms three times a day.

Methysergide is also an effective prophylactic for classical migraine, but there is a real risk of retroperitoneal fibrosis developing, and this serious complication mitigates against the widespread use of this drug.

For acute attacks of headache that break through prophylactic medication, a simple and effective medication is aspirin combined with metoclopramide. Non-steroidal anti-inflammatory agents such as naproxen may also be useful. Ergotamine tartrate is much less in favour than it was 10 years ago, largely because of the problems of ergotamine intoxication, in which patients who have taken more than 10 mg or 12 mg of ergotamine each week for a period of some weeks then develop recurrent headaches which are relieved by increasing the dose of ergotamine. Unfortunately, attempts to withdraw ergotamine also exacerbate headaches. It may be necessary to tide the patient over a period of ergotamine withdrawal by hospital admission and carefully controlled analgesia.

Sumatriptan, a specific agonist of 5-HT$_{1D}$ receptors constricts cranial blood vessels, and also, in experimental animals, prevents extravasation of plasma from blood vessels in the dura mater, which may be important in the genesis of pain. Sumatriptan is of proven efficacy, but does not cross the blood–brain barrier, suggesting that its site of action is on extracerebral blood vessels. This drug is now available in tablet form. An initial dose of 100 mg aborts the attack in many cases. If headache returns, the dose may be repeated, but the total should not exceed 300 mg in one day. Unfortunately, Sumatriptan is very expensive. It is contraindicated in those with ischaemic heart disease and poorly controlled hypertension.

Leaving aside medication, other approaches include withdrawal of the contraceptive pill, and avoidance of precipitants that the patient has identified. If he or she has failed to identify any dietary precipitant, then it is reasonable to advise a period without cheese, alcohol, chocolate, or citrus fruits. However, knowledge about 'migraine' is so widespread amongst patients in developed countries, that few patients reach a neurologist without having already attempted a number of these strategies.

9.11.1 *Prognosis*

Few workers have had the patience to study patients with chronic recurrent headaches for any length of time. By and large, it seems that headaches continue in at least half the population studied very much as before, with attacks of equal frequency and severity. However, it appears that a visit to a doctor is effective in helping patients come to terms with their headaches, and to stop worrying about them.

A surprising finding in one study was that the relative mortality of women with recurrent non-specific headache is rather less than that of women without headaches. The excess mortality in the no-headache group was from vascular disease, and remained even when corrections were made for cigarette-smoking and analgesic consumption. It may be that women with headache attend their doctor more frequently and are therefore more likely to have any intercurrent disorder detected early.

9.12 Further reading

General

A series of papers in Supplement 1 to *Journal of Neurology* (1991), **238**.
A series of papers in Supplement 2 to *Neurology* (1992), **42**.
Barlow, C. F. (1984). *Headache and migraine in childhood*. Blackwell, Oxford.
Hopkins, A. (ed.) (1988). *Headache: problems in diagnosis and management*. W. B. Saunders, London.

Epidemiology

Linet, M. S., Stewart, W. F., Celantanou, D. D., *et al.* (1989). An epidemiologic study of headache among adolescents and young adults. *Journal of the American Medical Association* **261**, 2211–16.

Classification

The Headache Classification Committee (1988). Classification and diagnostic criteria for headache disorders, cranial neuralgias and facial pain. *Cephalalgia* **8**, (Suppl. 7), 1–96.

Pathophysiology

Editorial (1991). Migraine-related stroke in childhood. *Lancet* **337**, 825–6.
Iversen, H. K., Neilsen, T. H., Olesen, J., and Tfelt-Hansen, P. (1990). Arterial responses during migraine headaches. *Lancet* **336**, 837–9.
Lance, J. W. (1988). Fifty years of migraine research. *Australian and New Zealand Journal of Medicine* **18**, 311–17.

Treatment

Cady, R. K., Wendt, J. K., Kirchner, J. R., Sargent, J. D., Rothrock, J. F., and Skaggs, H. (1991). Treatment of acute migraine with subcutaneous sumatriptan. *Journal of the American Medical Association* **265**, 2831–5.
Friberg, L, Olesen, J., Iversen, H. K., and Sperling, B. (1991). Migraine pain associated with middle cerebral artery dilatation. Reversal by sumatriptan. *Lancet*, **338**, 13–17.
Winkler, R., *et al.* (1989). A clinical trial of a self care approach to the management of chronic headache in general practice. *Social Science and Medicine* **29**, 213–19.

Cluster headache

Sjaastad, O. (1991). *Cluster headache syndrome*. W. B. Saunders, London.

10 Vascular diseases of the nervous system

Most non-medical people think they know what is meant by a stroke. They think in terms of a sudden hemiplegia, and some perhaps in terms of a cerebral haemorrhage. But of course vascular events in the nervous system may result in syndromes other than hemiplegia, hemiplegia may be caused by non-vascular events such as a tumour, and cerebral haemorrhage itself is comparatively uncommon. The principal section of this chapter describes by far the commonest type of stroke, due to cerebral infarction or intracerebral haemorrhage as a result of atheromatous vascular disease, with or without associated hypertension. However, occlusions of cerebral arteries due to emboli arising from the heart, to arteritis, and to sickled red cells, for example, must also be considered. I also discuss the pathology and effects of haemorrhage outside the brain, in the subarachnoid space, and occlusions of the venous side of the cerebral circulation, and encephalopathy associated with accelerated hypertension.

Any ischaemic event, however transient, must be considered in four 'dimensions'—the clinical syndrome, the anatomical territory involved, the pathological basis, and the possible pathogenetic mechanism.

10.1 Atheromatous cerebrovascular disease

10.1.1 *Definitions*

A transient ischaemic attack (TIA) is a focal neurological deficit, such as a transient aphasia or weakness of one arm, due to a vascular cause, from which complete recovery of function and regression of neurological signs occurs within 24 hours. Most authorities accept that the persistence of an asymptomatic abnormal sign such as an extensor plantar response does not preclude the diagnosis of a TIA. If complete recovery occurs later than 24 hours, then the event is called by some a *reversible ischaemic neurological deficit (RIND)*, a 'minor' *completed stroke*. In the case of both TIAs and RINDs, investigation by CT scanning and MRI may show remaining anatomical changes, even though clinical recovery is complete. In practical terms, the significance of both these events is the same. The patient has made a full recovery, and investigation and treatment must be directed vigorously towards preventing a completed stroke. A *completed stroke* is one in which a neurological deficit remains, though virtually invariably there is some degree of recovery of function in the weeks following the event. The term '*stroke-in-evolution*' indicates neurological deficit that is advancing under the eye of the examiner, who has to consider whether any urgent intervention is indicated.

10.1.2 *Pathology*

There are four main types of pathological process underlying TIAs, RINDs, and strokes due to atheromatous vascular disease. The first is occlusion of small intracerebral arteries, either by a plaque of focal atheroma or by lipohyalinoid degeneration. At the site of lipohyalinoid degeneration, the arterial wall is swollen by the presence of fibrinoid necrotic material containing some macrophages, which react readily with stains for fat. Sometimes there is local extravasation of red cells. These changes lead to occlusion of these small vessels, and a small area of infarction occurs distal to the occlusion. Such small infarcts are known as 'lacunes'—the name given to the little lake or fluid-filled hole seen at autopsy after macrophages have carried off the necrotic material. They are particularly common in the territories of the lenticulo-striate, thalamo-geniculate and basilar perforating arteries, end-arteries which extend into the adjacent white matter of the internal capsule. They are visible in life on the cranial CT scan as areas of low attenuation and on MRI as zones of high signal. Such lacunar infarcts may result in a pure motor hemiplegia or, if in the posteroventral nucleus of the thalamus, a purely hemisensory syndrome. Although the concept of lacunar strokes has been clinically useful, it should be noted that not all pathologists believe that they have a distinct and individual pathology.

If lipohyalinoid necrosis and subsequent dilatation of small arteries is very prominent, then, in association with hypertension, microaneurysms may form. These are known as Charcot–Bouchard aneurysms after the French scientists who first described them in 1868. These aneurysms are only visible, by present techniques, post-mortem. They are only present in the brains of those with previous hypertension. They are quite different from the much larger berry aneurysms, which are associated with subarachnoid haemorrhage (Section 10.6.1). Many of these aneurysms are surrounded by small extravasations of red cells. It is believed that a rupture of one or more of the larger of a family of microaneurysms results in an intracerebral haemorrhage. These usually occur in the striatum or, less commonly, in the pons, at which sites lipohyalinoid necrosis and Charcot–Bouchard aneurysms also occur with particular frequency.

Atheromatous changes affect not only the small intracerebral vessels but also the larger extracranial vessels, particularly the internal carotid immediately above the bifurcation of the common carotid. Such atheroma may act as a source of embolism of aggregations of platelets, fragments of thrombus, and debris containing cholesterol, fibrin, and excessive collagen. The embolus is flushed downstream and impacts in a smaller vessel. The importance of these emboli was first realized when they were seen, with an ophthalmoscope, traversing the retinal arteries of patients suffering with episodes of transient monocular blindness ('amaurosis fugax') (Section 10.1.10.1). Once the retinal arterial emboli had been seen, it became clear that similar emboli could affect the cerebral circulation, though cerebral ischaemic events due to these are probably not as common as once thought—the importance of lacunar infarction being increasingly recognized in the past two decades.

Apart from acting as a seed-bed for embolism, an atheromatous plaque at the origin of an internal carotid or vertebral artery may reach sufficient size to stenose the artery. One possibility often considered is that, by purely mechanical means, the stenosis may be sufficient to reduce flow if mean arterial pressure falls for any reason. Although an attractive idea, there is little evidence that this often occurs, and the principal importance of such arterial stenoses is that they act as a source of emboli, or they proceed to total occlusion. Occlusion of such a larger artery may result in an infarction involving one- to two-thirds of a hemisphere. It is not uncommon, however, to find by chance during the course of neurological investigations a totally occluded internal carotid artery that was never associated with symptoms, as the anastomotic circulation was sufficient to prevent infarction.

Atheroma with or without associated hypertension is a diffuse arterial disease, so it is common to see a number of different types of event in the same patient. One classical example is recurrent monocular blindness due to retinal embolism from an ulcerated internal carotid, followed by subsequent hemisphere infarction and contralateral hemiplegia as the artery occludes. Another sequence of events is repeated lacunar infarction due to lipohyalinoid necrosis, terminating in pseudobulbar palsy (Section 6.4.2 and 10.1.11.3). Lipohyalinoid necrosis of small arteries and atheroma of large arteries often occur in the same patient.

10.1.3 *Epidemiology of atheromatous cerebrovascular disease*

Cerebrovascular disease is the third commonest cause of death, after heart disease and malignant disease.

The chances of suffering a stroke before the age of 70 are about 1 in 20. Twenty per cent of strokes occur in people younger than 65. In a White population with the usual distribution of ages, the annual incidence of completed stroke is about 195 per 100 000, and the prevalence of stroke survivors about 550 per 100 000. In other terms, a typical British general practice of three partners and a list of 6000 patients will see about 12 new cases of stroke each year, and look after about 33 survivors of stroke. Figure 10.1 illustrates the commonplace observation that the incidence of completed stroke increases with age. Note, however, that even young people can get athero-occlusive strokes, that some degree of female immunity extends only to the menopause, and that myocardial infarction is much commoner than stroke in men, but occurs with about the same frequency as stroke in women. The odds of a man sustaining a first stroke are, in Oxfordshire, about 26 per cent greater than for a woman. This, and much other useful epidemiological information about stroke, is based upon the long-term Framingham cohort study and the Oxford Community Stroke Project. Other community surveys indicate that the mortality of stroke is less than it was a few years ago. The decline is impressive, by 55 per cent in Rochester, Minnesota if the years 1975–79 are compared to 1950–54. The incidence of myocardial infarction is less, too, but only by about 14 per cent, possibly because the treatment of hypertension has a more important influence on cerebral rather than coronary arterial disease. Unfortunately, recent evidence from both Rochester and Sweden suggests that the incidence is beginning to rise again, suggesting that treatment of blood pressure is not the only important variable.

Surveys of transient ischaemic attacks are probably less reliable, as it seems likely that many brief episodes will never be reported to a physician. Based upon reviews of medical records in Rochester, Minnesota, the incidence was 70 per 100 000 for ages 55–64 and 220 per 100 000 for ages 65–74—less than it was a few years ago. Only about one patient in 10 has a TIA before a completed stroke, but as about one in three of all patients with a TIA will have a stroke in the next few years (most frequently within a few months of the TIA), energetic management of these warning events may be worthwhile for those who, at least in these circumstances, can be considered lucky enough to develop them. Figure 10.1 also shows the proportions of different types of cerebrovascular events found in men in the prospective Framingham survey. The numbers in women were not significantly different. The proportion of events

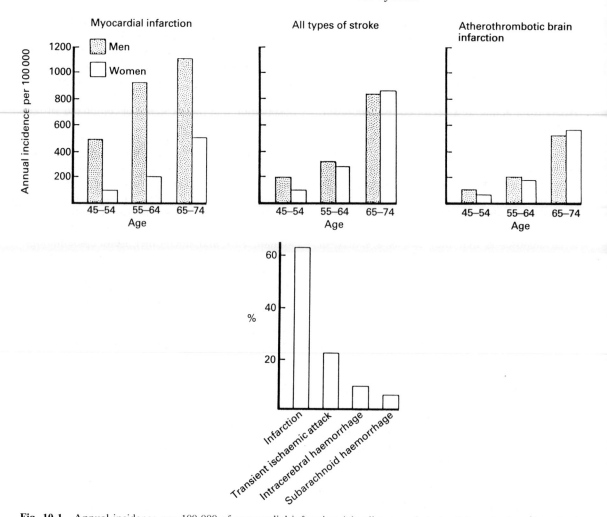

Fig. 10.1 Annual incidence per 100 000 of myocardial infarction (a), all types of stroke (b), and atherothrombotic cerebral infarction (c) for men and women (data redrawn with permission Kannel and Wolf 1983). The cerebrovascular syndrome at first presentation is shown in (d). Of those in the first column (infarction), about half are infarctions in the anterior circulation, a quarter in the posterior circulation, and a quarter are lacunes. About one-fifth will have a potential cardiac source of embolism. (Data from the Oxford Community Stroke Project, redrawn with permission.)

due to intracerebral haemorrhage is low, though it may be that the wider use of CT scanning in the future will detect a greater proportion of strokes due to this, as blood shows as a zone of high density on the scan (Fig. 10.2a).

From the foregoing paragraphs, it can be seen that a qualitative distinction in arterial pathology can be made between ischaemic lacunar and cortical strokes. However, the difference between a completed ischaemic stroke, a reversible ischaemic neurological deficit, and a transient ischaemic attack (Section 10.1.1) is quantitative, based on the duration of the patient's symptoms. Prospective studies have shown no major differences in terms of age, sex, prevalence of co-existing vascular disease, other risk factors, or prognosis. However, the immediate clinical actions that need be taken in response to a major event such as a stroke are different from those that should follow a tran-

Table 10.1   Classification of cerebral ischaemic events in association with atheroma

---

By time-course
  transient ischaemic attack
  reversible ischaemic neurological deficit
  stroke in progress
  completed stroke
By arterial territory
  for example, lenticulostriate artery
By underlying pathology
  atheromatous occlusion of large vessels
    resulting in large areas of infarction, involving
    cortex and underlying white matter
  athero-embolism
  lipohyalinoid necrosis or
    atheromatous occlusion of small vessels
    resulting in lacunar infarction
  atheromatous stenosis of large vessels
    resulting in insufficient flow (rare)
  Charcot–Bouchard aneurysms
    resulting in intracranial haemorrhage

---

sient ischaemic attack. The syndromes are therefore considered separately.

Table 10.1 indicates the framework within which a diagnosis of a cerebral ischaemic event should be made. Rather than referring to a patient with 'a stroke', it is far more informative in considering therapy, management and prognosis to record a longer diagnostic formulation. An example might be 'a man of 73 with a reversible ischaemic neurological deficit in the middle cerebral arterial territory, probably athero-embolic in nature'. Such a formulation can further be expanded to include risk factors, such as hypertension, which are considered next.

10.1.4   *Risk factors for transient ischaemic attacks and stroke*

Table 10.2 lists the factors that have, so far, been identified as predisposing to a greater than average risk of stroke in association with atheroma. These may be divided into those about which nothing can be done, such as increasing age, and those that are at least potentially modifiable. As there is little to encourage the hope that new methods of management of the acute phase of either cerebral infarction or haemorrhage (Section 10.1.7) will produce

substantial improvement in mortality and residual disability, there is considerable interest in the effects of modifying those factors that can be modified, such as hypertension (Section 10.1.4.1). Risk factors for transient ischaemic attacks and reversible ischaemic neurological deficits may be assumed to be the same as for stroke, although some surveys suggest small differences.

Of the non-modifiable risk factors, the effect of age and sex have already been considered (Fig. 10.1). In the UK, black people of Afro-Caribbean descent have about twice the risk of a stroke than Whites of the same age, though whether this increased risk is independent of the known propensity of Blacks to hypertension is not clear. Asian Indians in the UK have about one and a half times the risk of white people. Genetic factors are certainly important in the genesis of hypertension and stroke; the parents of patients with stroke are about four times more likely to have died of stroke than expected. For unexplained reasons, the risk is higher if the mother had the stroke.

The genetic predisposition to cerebrovascular

Table 10.2   Risk factors for stroke associated with atheroma

---

Non-modifiable
  increasing age
  male sex
  Black, Japanese or Asian Indian race
  family history
  previous TIA or stroke
  coronary heart disease, atrial fibrillation
  heterozygous or homozygous for homocystinuria
Potentially modifiable
  hypertension
  diabetes mellitus
  cigarette-smoking
  alcohol and drug abuse
  oral contraception
  elevated haematocrit
  symptomless carotid bruit

Notes:
1. In general, the effect of hypertension is greatest on the incidence of stroke, intermediate in its effect on coronary artery disease, and least on peripheral vascular disease. The effect of smoking is the reverse.
2. Obesity is also a risk factor, but probably only through its association with hypertension and alcohol consumption.
3. In contrast to coronary artery disease, hypercholesterolaemia does not seem to be an independent risk factor for stroke.

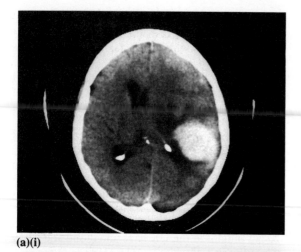

(a)(i)

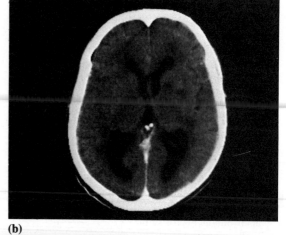

(b)

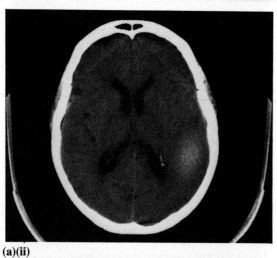

(a)(ii)

Fig. 10.2   (a) Cerebral haemorrhage. (i) Large left temporal haematoma. Note the surrounding oedema and shift of mid-line structures. (ii) Six weeks later: the haematoma and oedema have largely resolved. (iii) A further 17 weeks later: the haematoma is replaced by a low density cystic area overlying a moderately dilated lateral ventricle. (b) Lacunar infarctions.

(d) Another (unenhanced) cerebral infarction in the territory of the middle cerebral artery.

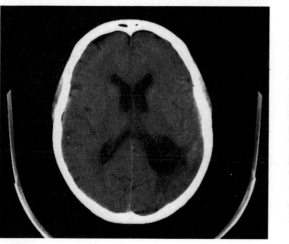

(a)(iii)

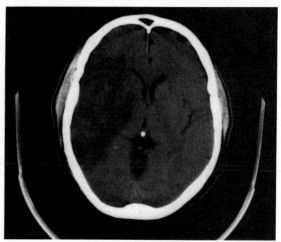

(d)

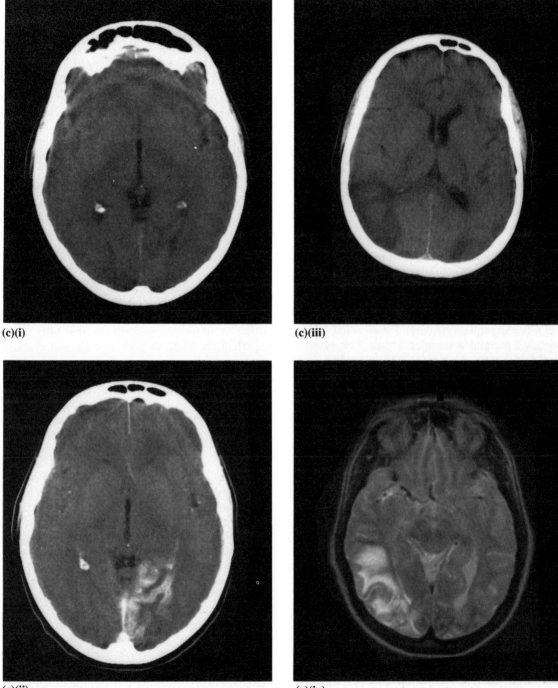

(c)(i)

(c)(iii)

(c)(ii)

(c)(iv)

(c) (i) Infarctions in left occipital lobe. Note that little abnormality can be seen until contrast enhancement as shown in ii. (ii) The same after contrast enhancement. (iii) Unenhanced CT scan of another patient with occipital infarction, in this case bilaterally—a large infarction on the right, a smaller one on the left. (iv) MRI of same patient as in iii.

disease is presumably multifactorial, the inheritance of hypertension being itself multifactorial. However, an interesting component of the genetic load has been uncovered recently. It has long been known that those with homocystinuria due to cystathionine β-synthase deficiency are particularly prone to premature atheromatous vascular disease. It has now been shown that those who are heterozygous for the gene, who number as many as 1 in 70 of the population, also have an increased risk of stroke and peripheral vascular disease. One type of cerebral amyloidosis, hereditary cystatin C amyloid angiopathy, is transmitted as an autosomal dominant. In this disorder death usually occurs before the age of 40 due to intracerebral haemorrhage. It may be that as hypertension is treated more and more effectively in the community, cerebral haemorrhage from these causes will become numerically more important than ruptured Charcot–Bouchard aneurysms.

A history of previous transient ischaemic attacks affecting the brain (but not the retina) is a risk factor for subsequent stroke and myocardial infarction, as is peripheral vascular disease. Left ventricular hypertrophy also is associated with subsequent stroke, as is coronary artery disease, whether judged by symptomatic or electrocardiographic criteria. The increased risk of stroke in the presence of coronary disease is independent of hypertension. Atrial fibrillation, if a manifestation of rheumatic heart disease, is strongly associated with stroke (Section 10.5.4), but even in the absence of valvular disease remains a strong association, presumably reflecting the nature of diffuse arterial disease affecting both coronary and cerebral arteries. This is one risk factor the influence of which can be modified by therapy (Section 10.5.4).

More relevant to therapeutic endeavour is the association of stroke with risk factors that are potentially modifiable.

10.1.4.1 *Hypertension*

Hypertension, both systolic and diastolic, is the most important risk factor. One disconcerting point that has emerged from the Framingham studies is that it seems as if there is no threshold value of blood pressure above which the incidence of stroke begins to increase. The rates of later stroke are higher for those with 'high normal' than

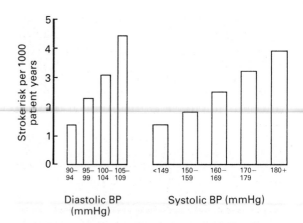

Fig. 10.3 Incidence of stroke in relation to diastolic and systolic blood pressure (Data from MRC trial, redrawn with permission from Ramsay and Walker 1986.)

for those with 'low normal' blood pressure. Figure 10.3 illustrates the rapidly increasing incidence of stroke in untreated patients in the MRC mild hypertension study as both systolic and diastolic pressures increase.

The Veterans' Administration Cooperative studies showed that the treatment of moderate and high levels of diastolic pressure substantially reduced the incidence of both fatal and non-fatal strokes. The effect of the treatment of mild hypertension (phase V diastolic between 90 and 109 mmHg) is more controversial. The MRC trial showed no reduction in mortality from all causes. There was, however, a significant reduction in the risk of stroke, a reduction that was greater in those patients taking a thiazide diuretic. Propranolol did not prevent strokes in smokers, but for non-smokers the reduction in risk was about the same as the benefit achieved by diuretic. However, the benefits of treatment have to be weighed in absolute rather than relative terms. It has been calculated that one would need to treat 31 patients with mild hypertension (diastolic <109 mmHg) for 20 years in order to prevent one cerebrovascular event, which might, in any event, be not very disabling, such as a transient ischaemic attack. Unfortunately, ischaemic heart disease dominates the prognosis of mild hypertension, and the treatment of mild hypertension does not prevent coronary events. It has been proposed that the difference is this: in the brain, oxygen extraction from the blood can be increased if blood pressure falls below the lower limit of autoregulation. However, in the coronary circulation, oxygen extraction is nearly maximal at rest, and a reduction in blood pressure can lead to myocardial ischaemia. It may, however, be that adverse effects on the lipids of diuretics and some beta blockers may keep up the rate of coronary disease, even though blood pressure is reduced.

As stroke is very much a disorder of older people, the question arises as to whether treatment of hypertension in the elderly is worthwhile, bearing in mind the presumably long duration of vascular disease. The European Working Party on Hypertension in the Elderly recruited patients over the age of 60 with diastolic pressures between 90 and 119 mmHg. Cardiovascular events were reduced by about a quarter, and non-fatal strokes by a half. There was, however, no difference in fatal stroke rate. An important point is that benefit was independent of entry blood pressure (within the defined limits) and the presence of previous cardiovascular events. No benefit could be observed in treating those over age 80.

Finally, at the end of this section on hypertension, it should be noted that there is anecdotal evidence that abrupt reduction of blood pressure, and circulatory blood volume (e.g. by frusemide) may precipitate cerebral infarction in the elderly.

10.1.4.2   Diabetes

Evidence from the Framingham survey, and a number of earlier surveys, has shown that patients with diabetes have a two-and-a-half to three times greater risk of stroke than the non-diabetic population (and an even greater risk of peripheral vascular disease and intermittent claudication). The risk is rather greater in women. The relative risk persists after adjusting for the effects of other risk factors, such as hypertension. The implication is that careful management of diabetes will reduce the risk of stroke.

10.1.4.3   Obesity, hyperlipidaemia, cigarette-smoking, and alcohol

Obesity itself is probably not a risk factor if considered independently of its association with hypertension and diabetes but, in view of the known beneficial effects of weight reduction on both,

obesity should be considered as relevant. It has been shown recently that snoring is a risk factor for stroke. Here, obesity, snoring, and hypertension secondary to the hypoxaemia and hypercapnia associated with snoring, are all inextricably linked.

The serum concentrations of lipids and cholesterol bear a less marked relation to stroke, in contrast to their importance in coronary artery disease. The importance of cigarette-smoking is also less than in coronary artery disease, although there is no doubt that it is an independent risk factor (Fig. 10.4). The relative risk of ischaemic stroke for smokers is about 5.7, but is not significantly raised for stroke due to cardiac emboli. Smoking and hypertension are multiplicative risk factors.

Alcohol has been shown to be a risk factor, independent of its effect upon generating hypertension, or the known association with smoking—men who drink heavily also smoke heavily. Strokes may follow 'binge drinking' even if the average daily consumption of alcohol is not high. Strokes are more common at weekends, when the consumption of alcohol is highest.

10.1.4.4   Cold weather

Deaths from stroke are distinctly higher in cold weather, particularly in older people. Whether this effect is distinct from the pressor effect of cold weather is not clear, but the relationship is circumstantial evidence for warm clothing and effective home heating for older people.

10.1.4.5   Oral contraceptives and post-menopausal oestrogens

The Collaborative Group for the Study of Stroke in Young Women found a risk of stroke for those on the pill to be about five times greater than for those not on the pill. However, further prospective studies, controlling for smoking and other variables, have failed to indicate such a substantial relative risk, although many feel that oral contraception is important in the genesis of many strokes in younger women. This is particularly so if the oestrogen content exceeds 50 μg.

At the end of reproductive life, it has been shown that oestrogen replacement therapy given to post-menopausal women protects against the

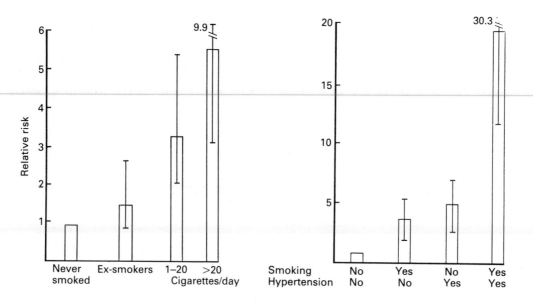

Fig. 10.4 Effect of cigarette-smoking (left) and smoking and hypertension (right) upon the risk of stroke. (Redrawn with permission from Bonita *et al.* 1986.)

risk of stroke. In one study, the relative risk was nearly halved.

10.1.4.6   *Polycythaemia*

The elevated blood viscosity associated with poly-cythaemia rubra vera predisposes to strokes. Even those with haematocrits in the high normal range are more at risk from stroke than those with 'low normal' haematocrits. However, the difference is insufficient to warrant venesection unless true polycythaemia exists.

10.1.4.7   *Anti-cardiolipin antibodies*

Circulating antibodies to cardiolipins are seen primarily in patients with systemic lupus erythematosus, and other related auto-immune diseases. However, younger patients are seen with a syndrome characterized by recurrent fetal loss, thrombocytopenia, and multiple cerebral infarctions with raised serum levels of anticardiolipin antibody. Recently, prospective studies have indicated that anticardiolipin antibodies may be found as a significantly greater concentration in unselected patients with stroke than in age-matched controls.

Furthermore, the prognosis with regard to functional outcome is distinctly less good in those older people with high levels of anticardiolipin antibody. The mechanism by which anticardiolipin antibodies may cause stroke is unknown, but it is thought that they may inhibit endothelial prostacyclin production or release, resulting in the loss of inhibition of platelet aggregation. Further work may well show that the presence of such antibodies will prove to be an independent risk factor and prognostic marker for first-ever strokes in the general population.

10.1.4.8   *Cervical bruits*

Symptomless cervical bruits may be found at screening examinations in 4 per cent of those over the age of 40. Prospective studies indicate that such a bruit, a marker of atheroma, does increase the risk of developing stroke or coronary artery disease in those aged less than 75, but the strokes that occur are not necessarily related to the affected carotid artery, and may be haemorrhagic or clearly embolic from the heart. The bruit appears only to be a marker (in some people) of vascular disease. In those aged over 75, the risk of stroke is not significantly increased if an asymptomatic bruit is found. There is insufficient evidence to warrant prophylactic endarterectomy if a bruit is found by chance (see Section 10.1.10.5). The increasing accuracy of non-invasive vascular testing may, in future, define a subgroup—those with advancing unilateral stenotic lesions—in whom surgery should be considered.

10.1.4.9 *Illicit drugs*

The widespread use of 'crack' (an adulterated alkaloidal form of cocaine) has been shown to be associated with an increased risk of cerebral infarction, intracerebral haemorrhage, and subarachnoid haemorrhage. The stroke is often preceded by a severe headache. Cocaine induces both transient hypertension and direct cerebral vasoconstriction, and both mechanisms may be important in crack-induced stroke.

10.1.4.10 *Interaction of risk factors*

Risk factors for stroke are multiplicative, as illustrated in Fig. 10.4. A major reduction in risk factors can be achieved by non-pharmacological means. Moderate exercise, avoidance of alcohol and reduction in salt intake result in significant falls in blood pressure. Smoking can be avoided.

10.1.5 *Clinical features of stroke*

10.1.5.1 *Ischaemic stroke*

Although transient ischaemic attacks often precede stroke, it is more convenient first to consider the fully developed syndromes and management of stroke. The management and prognosis of transient ischaemic attacks are considered in Section 10.1.10.

The predilection of atherothrombotic infarction

Table 10.3 Frequency of different types of ischaemic stroke

	per cent	chances of early death	chances of poor functional outcome	chances of recurrence of stroke
Total anterior circulation infarcts (TACI) (higher cortical dysfunction (eg. aphasia) plus homonymous field defect plus deficit of function of at least 2 of the 3 body areas (face, arm or leg)	17	high	high	moderate
Partial anterior circulation infarcts (PACI) (only two of the above three components—or a higher cortical dysfunction alone, or a more restricted dysfunction of face, arm or leg)	34	low	high	high
Lacunar infarcts (LACI) pure motor stroke pure sensory stroke sensori-motor stroke (without cortical dysfunction or a hemianopia) ataxic hemiparesis	25	low	moderate	moderate
Posterior circulation infarcts (POCI) ipsilateral cranial nerve nuclear palsy with contralateral motor and/or sensory deficit bilateral motor and/or sensory deficit disorder of conjugate eye-movement cerebellar dysfunction without ipsilateral long-tract deficit isolated homonymous hemianopia	24	low	moderate	moderate/high

(Data from Bamford *et al.* 1991)

for certain sites results in a limited number of principal syndromes (Table 10.3), though variations are infinite. Table 10.3 also shows one way of classifying the principal stroke syndromes based upon the Oxford Community Stroke Project.

There are four major syndromes due to lacunar infarctions. Patients may present with a pure motor stroke, a pure sensory stroke, a sensori-motor stroke, or an ataxic hemiparesis without much disturbance of consciousness. These syndromes are predictive of a small lacunar infarct which can be imaged in the basal ganglia or pons. As described in Section 10.1.2, most lacunar infarcts are thought to be caused by lipohyalinosis or by microatheroma of a single perforating artery. Because not much volume of tissue is involved by the ischaemic infarction, the immediate case-fatality rate is low. However, because the lacunes are in regions in which major fibre pathways descend from or ascend to the cortex, disability after a lacunar infarction can be prominent. However, the prognosis for recurrent strokes is reasonably good, insofar as lipohyalinosis or microatheroma has to develop or progress in another perforating artery before another stroke occurs. Lacunar infarcts are not associated with carotid artery disease, but with diffuse small vessel disease, and therefore with hypertension.

The next group of ischaemic strokes to be considered is those with total infarction in the territory of the anterior circulation. The CT scan or MRI will show evidence of ischaemia in both the deep and superficial territories of the middle cerebral artery, caused either by occlusion at the proximal stem of the middle cerebral artery, or by spread of thrombus into this vessel from a more proximal occlusion, usually of the internal carotid artery. The anterior cerebral artery may or may not be involved. Clinically, such patients have evidence of a major cortical dysfunction (such as aphasia or a disorder of visuo-spatial orientation), a field defect, and a hemiplegia, often with some impairment of consciousness in the acute stage. The chance of a good functional outcome after such a major volume of damaged tissue is poor, and there is a high mortality in the acute stage.

The Oxford workers also distinguish a partial anterior circulation infarct, in which the volume of tissue damage is smaller, and the arterial territory affected is usually due to occlusion of more distal divisions of the middle cerebral artery, or an isolated infarct in the anterior cerebral artery territory. The more distal branch occlusions are likely to be due to an embolus, either from the ipsilateral artery or from the heart. In support of this is the observation by the Oxford group that those with partial anterior circulation infarcts have a high risk of an early recurrence of a further ischaemic event, a pattern concordant with the observation that such strokes are commonly associated with evidence of carotid artery stenosis. Patients with partial anterior circulation infarcts do not tend to die in the acute stage, as the volume of infarcted tissue is less, but disability may progress due to the accrual of repeated strokes from an active embolic source.

The fourth principal type of ischaemic stroke is one in which the affected arterial territory lies in the posterior circulation. Ischaemic brain-stem strokes may produce neurological abnormalities of some apparent complexity, as many important tracts are tightly packed into its small diameter. As the trigeminal lemniscus decussates at a level at which strokes in the lower brain stem often occur, there may be impairment of sensation in the face on the same side or on the side opposite to impairment of sensation in the limbs. A number of syndromes of different arterial territories within the brain stem were described in the early days of neurological practice, of which the best known is the syndrome of lateral medullary infarction, illustrated in Fig. 10.5. However, most lacunar brain-stem strokes occur more rostrally in the pons. An occlusion in the posterior cerebral artery will result in an isolated homonymous hemianopia. In the posterior circulation, there is significant pathological evidence suggesting that in situ thrombosis is more common than in the anterior circulation. Non-embolic infarction may be due to atheroma in a parent artery circumferentially occluding the origin of a branch artery, or there may be thrombotic occlusion following failure of collateral supply after a more proximal occlusion. Patients with posterior circulation infarcts tend not to die in the acute stage unless the infarction involves vital brain-stem structures subserving respiration, but, at least in those admitted to hospital, substantial difficulties with double vision and in swallowing may continue.

A vertebral artery may be found to be occluded by chance in the course of angiography, without pre-existing relevant symptoms, adequate perfu-

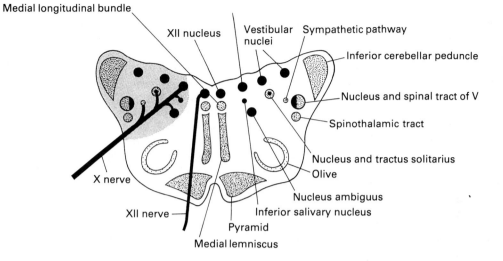

Fig. 10.5 The lateral medullary syndrome. Although classically caused by infarction in the territory of the posterior inferior cerebellar artery (shaded), more extensive lesions of a patchy nature may occur due to more widespread disease in the basilar arterial territory. In the pure lateral medullary syndrome (syndrome of Wallenberg) there is ipsilateral ataxia of the limbs due to damage to the inferior cerebellar peduncle, hoarseness and dysarthria due to damage to the vagus nucleus and fibres, ipsilateral facial numbness due to damage to the trigeminal nucleus, and contralateral hypoalgesia due to damage to the spinothalamic tract. If the lesion is more extensive rostrally, there is often an ipsilateral facial palsy. If it extends medially and anteriorly, there will be contralateral pyramidal signs, such as extensor plantar response.

sion of the brain stem taking place through the remaining vertebral and, from the anterior circulation, through the posterior communicating artery. Occlusion of one vertebral artery may, however, result in focal downstream infarction, sometimes in the territory of the posterior inferior cerebellar artery (Fig. 10.5). A major infarction in the basilar territory produces coma with pupillary abnormalities. The dorsal part of the pons, the tegmentum, may be relatively spared. If the patient then improves, it becomes clear that, although there is quadriplegia, and paralysis of horizontal eye and facial movements due to infarction of the ventral part of the pons, vertical eye movements and blinking remain. Such patients are conscious, but are said to be 'locked-in', their only possible communication with the outside world being through codes based upon blinking, or on vertical eye movements. (Section 7.3.3).

10.1.5.1   *Haemorrhagic stroke*

Just as there is a predeliction of atherothrombotic

infarction for certain anatomical sites, so intracerebral haemorrhage tends to be limited to comparatively few sites in the brain. As already mentioned in Section 10.1.2, hypertension is associated with the rupture of one or more micro-aneurysms sited on the deep penetrating arteries in the striatum, or, less commonly, in the pons. A haemorrhage in the striatum usually results in a major hemiplegia affecting face, arm, and leg, usually with depression of consciousness, and possible deviation of gaze to the side contralateral to the haemorrhage, due to interference with the pathways subserving eye movements descending from the frontal lobe. A pontine haemorrhage commonly results in abrupt loss of consciousness, with disturbance of the conjugate position of the eyes, and of pupillary and other brain-stem reflexes.

Intracerebellar haemorrhages are important, as early surgical evacuation may be life-saving. Large haemorrhages may be immediately fatal, but smaller haemorrhages present with dizziness and ipsilateral ataxia, followed by deepening unconsciousness due to compression of the brain stem, and herniation of the contents of the posterior fossa, either upwards through the tentorium, or downwards through the foramen magnum.

10.1.5.2 *Distinction of haemorrhagic stroke from cerebral infarction*

A reliable clinical distinction between cerebral infarction and supratentorial haemorrhage would be useful, in obviating the need for many cranial CT scans or MRI. Multivariate analysis of clinical variables affecting stroke patients in Thailand suggests that a simple score can predict whether a stroke is due to a haemorrhage or infarction with 90 per cent predictive accuracy. The Siriraj stroke score is calculated as

$(2.5 \times$ level of consciousness on a 0–2 point scale)
  $+ (2 \times$ vomiting on a 0–1 point scale)
  $+ (2 \times$ headache on a 0–1 point scale)
  $+ (0.1 \times$ diastolic pressure)
  $- (3 \times$ atheroma markers on a 0–1 point scale: these include diabetes, angina, or peripheral vascular disease) $- 12$.

If the score exceeds 1 a supratentorial haemorrhage is likely, if less than 1, an infarction. Such scales will need, for Western use, validating on a different population, but the method is certainly promising.

10.1.5.3 *Differential diagnosis of stroke*

The differential diagnosis of acute stroke from non-vascular lesions includes the distinction from a mass lesion. Occasionally a carotid occlusion can evolve sufficiently slowly to suggest that a tumour is the cause of a hemiparesis. The occurrence of seizures in association with a 'stroke' should raise suspicions that a tumour may be responsible, although seizures certainly may occur at the onset of a stroke. Occasionally a chronic subdural haematoma may cause a hemiplegia sufficiently acutely to cause diagnostic confusion (Section 15.6).

10.1.6 *Management and investigation of stroke*

The principles of initial management are much the same for hemiplegic strokes as for brain-stem and other types of stroke.

  The first decision to make is whether the patient needs to be admitted into hospital or not. In so far as this chapter will go on to point out that there is no major specific treatment required in the acute stage, it is right to question this. Factors that will predispose to admission include associated coma or confusion, the presence or absence of a potential carer at home, and the need for further investigations. It follows that there are two principal groups of patients who are admitted, the old and ill, who cannot be cared for at home, and a younger age-group in which it is believed that vigorous investigation may preclude further loss of function. If the patient is unconscious on admission, then the usual nursing practice outlined in Section 7.1 is instituted—attention to airway, position, pressure areas, bladder, eyes and, less urgently, hydration, nutrition, and passive movements of the limbs. It is particularly important to avoid hypoxia as there will be a compensatory fall in $P_{a\,CO_2}$, with a possible reduction in cerebral blood flow. If the patient is hemiplegic, and perhaps hemianopic, it makes sense to place him in a bed where his sound limbs and visual field are towards the open ward, and not against a wall. If the patient is aphasic, then immediate steps should be taken to establish what level of comprehension and expression remains, and to provide some sort of simple aid to communication (Section 26.5.2). If the patient cannot swallow but is conscious, as frequently occurs in brain-stem strokes, then hydration and nutrition should be maintained through a nasogastric tube. The level of neurological deficit should be recorded quickly, and explained to the nursing staff, so that any increasing deficit is noted rapidly (see stroke in evolution, Section 10.1.7). General physical examination should pay particular reference to the presence of vascular disease, as indicated by atrial fibrillation, left ventricular hypertrophy, occlusion of peripheral pulses, a mid-cervical bruit, or valvular murmurs. Although an elevated blood pressure on admission may not necessarily indicate pre-existing hypertension, records of continuing blood pressure should be kept. Neurological examination will be directed towards classifying patients into one of the principal syndromes of stroke listed in Table 10.3.

  It may well be appropriate not to investigate in any way some patients with stroke, for example the very elderly, in whom it is clear that therapeutic endeavour will, in any event, be limited.

Table 10.4   The investigation of stroke

Reasonable investigations for some patients with stroke
1. Haemoglobin and haematocrit
    for increased blood viscosity due to
    polycythaemia
2. Blood film
    for sickle-cell disease (confirmed by Hb
    electrophoresis)
3. Sedimentation rate
    for unusual forms of arteritis
4. Venereal Disease Research Laboratory (VDRL)
    test
    for arteritis due to *Treponema pallidum*
5. Blood sugar
    for hyperglycaemia, correlated with worse
    outcome
6. Electrocardiogram
    for assessment of associated vascular disease,
    e.g. left ventricular hypertrophy, coronary
    artery disease, atrial fibrillation
7. Serum lipids
    for modifiable risk factor for ischaemic heart
    disease
8. Chest X-ray
    for left ventricular hypertrophy; an unexpected

bronchial carcinoma with cerebral secondary
deposit may mimic a stroke

More complex investigations for some patients with
stroke
9. CT scanning or MRI
    for distinction from other causes of neurological
    signs, e.g. intracerebral tumour, subdural
    haematoma
10. Duplex ultrasonography of cervical vessels
11. Angiography of cervical vessels
    for carotid stenosis, or occlusion
12. Echocardiography
    for possible source of embolism

Investigations that have been largely superseded in the
investigation of stroke
    Lumbar puncture
    Mid-line echoencephalography
    Electroencephalography
    Isotope scanning

Research investigation
    Positron emission tomography

Reasonable investigations for those admitted to hospital will be directed towards improving the certainty of the diagnosis (see Section 10.1.5.1 for differential diagnosis), for improving the certainty of categorization of the vascular event, as a guide to prognosis (see Section 10.1.8), and for the ascertainment of risk factors, modification of which might prevent further strokes. Table 10.4 lists those investigations from which a choice may be made according to clinical circumstances. Those in the first section are cheap and, although very often not helpful (for example, the haematocrit, and the VDRL test), their cost-effectiveness is quite high. Those in the second group are more expensive, and will often be undertaken only after consultation with a physician or neurologist interested in stroke. These are now considered further.

Cranial CT scanning after cerebral infarction may be quite normal if the scan is undertaken in the early hours, or even in the early days, after a large infarct. A zone of low attenuation will usually become most prominent about 8–10 days after infarction. About two-thirds of infarcts will show enhancement of density after the injection of contrast media after some 2–3 weeks. The character and shape of the edge of the enhancing zone, and the appearance of the zone of low attenuation usually allows a distinction between infarct and tumour (compare Figs. 10.2c and 8.12).

CT scanning will show an intracerebral haemorrhage without difficulty as a zone of high density (Fig. 10.2a). In some patients the scan will also show that the haematoma has ruptured into the ventricles, a bad prognostic sign. If the scan is delayed for a week or two, clearance of the haemorrhage leaves a zone of low attenuation mimicking an infarct. However, often clearance takes longer than this. MRI results in similar information, but confers no special advantages over CT scanning.

The imaging and subsequent removal of an intracerebellar haemorrhage may be life-saving. In most other cases no therapeutic action follows scanning, but the accurate classification of the type of stroke reached by scanning allows more accurate prognosis.

Angiography is now seldom used in the assessment of a completed stroke, as even if an internal carotid artery or middle cerebral artery occlusion is demonstrated, no therapeutic action follows.

The importance of the heart as a potential source of cerebral emboli is outlined in Section 10.5. Although the yield of positive results on random echocardiography is low, this investigation should certainly be undertaken in patients aged less than 50, in those with cardiac murmurs, and in those with enlarged hearts on the chest X-ray.

The third section of Table 10.4 lists some investigations that are widely available, and therefore, until recently, widely used, particularly by non-neurologists. Lumbar puncture may show the presence of blood in the spinal fluid of patients with an intracerebral haematoma, but in those with small deep haemorrhages, none may be present. Conversely, some red cells may be found in the fluid after a large infarction. If there is a shift of intracranial contents following haemorrhage or infarction, then lumbar puncture may precipitate coning. Such shifts may be detected by mid-line echo studies, but although the necessary equipment is cheap, very little useful information emerges. Electroencephalography may help distinguish between large and lacunar infarcts, being more abnormal in the former, but the unit cost of this investigation is now not far removed from CT scanning and the amount of information obtained is far less. Isotope scanning may show up a small proportion of infarcts missed by CT scanning, but insufficient for this investigation to be worthwhile, except in cases of unusual clinical difficulty.

Measurements of cerebral blood flow, particularly if combined with positron emission tomography (PET) (Section 8.10.5), have given much useful information about the pathological physiology of stroke. The use of ^{15}O- and of ^{18}F-labelled glucose, in combination with measurements of flow, allows calculation of, and computer-generated images of oxygen and glucose consumption by the surviving brain. Around most areas of infarction is a zone of 'luxury' perfusion, in which flow is unnecessarily large for the amount of oxygen consumed. If greater amounts of oxygen are extracted per unit flow—the converse of luxury perfusion—then such

tissue can be considered to be suboptimally perfused, and at further risk. Unfortunately, the very short duration of half-life of the isotopes used means that such research investigations can only take place in the immediate proximity of a cyclotron.

10.1.7 *Medical treatment of acute stroke*

Faced with an acute disabling and often mortal illness, many active therapies have been tried, over the years, to save life and to diminish residual disability (Table 10.5). Unfortunately none has yet consistently been shown to be useful.

Table 10.5 Attempted treatments of acute stroke

None shown to be beneficial
1. Corticosteroid therapy
2. Hyperventilation with 5% P_{CO_2}
3. Infusion of low molecular weight dextran
4. Prolonged hypothermia +/− barbiturate anaesthesia
5. Immediate reduction in blood pressure
6. Calcium blockade
7. Blockade of excitatory neurotransmitters
8. Infusion of prostacyclin
9. Infusion of free-radical (peroxide, OH$^-$) scavengers
10. Anticoagulation

More appropriate treatment of acute stroke
1. Maintenance of airway
2. Attention to bladder
3. Attention to pressure areas
4. Attention to chest and joints
5. Attention to hydration and nutrition

Recent attention has been directed at abnormal events occurring at excitatory synapses following acute ischaemia, which release excessive amounts of glutamate into the extracellular space. This excites neurons and further depletes energy stores. Excitation of one subset of excitatory receptors, the *N*-methyl D-aspartate (NMDA) receptor, leads to excessive influx of sodium, chloride, and water into the neuron, which causes acute neuronal damage, and of calcium ions, which causes delayed and more permanent damage. There is, therefore, considerable experimental interest in using NMDA antagonists in stroke; candidates include dextrorphan and dextromethorphan and ketamine, all of which may block the NMDA channel at the phencyclidine-binding site. Non-competitive NMDA antagonists such as MK-801 reduce the size of ischaemic lesions in animals after experimental occlusion of the middle cerebral artery. Another approach is calcium-channel blockade. One trial of nimodipine after subarachnoid haemorrhage showed that it improved survival after stroke in men, and reduced the post-stroke residual neurological deficit. The dose used in this trial was 30 mg orally (if necessary by nasogastric tube) every 6 hours for 28 days. However, a more recent trial showed no benefit. It has been shown that acute β-blockade, as appears to be effective in subarachnoid haemorrhage (Section 10.6.4), does not benefit those with acute ischaemic stroke, but one study has shown that those previously on beta-blocking agents did have a better outcome.

Naftidrofuryl has been shown in two randomized trials to reduce time in hospital, and therefore, by implication, disability after stroke. However, no difference in functional recovery could be demonstrated and mortality was not affected. Furthermore, the number of patients recruited to the trials was so small that the confidence limits embraced the possibility that the drug increases mortality.

Corticosteroid therapy has a near miraculous effect on oedema associated with intracerebral tumours, and therefore numerous trials have been undertaken to assess the benefits of steroid therapy in large infarctions, in which the CT scan shows low attenuation and shift of mid-line structures. Unfortunately, no well-designed trial has shown improvements in outcome that could be attributed to treatment. Animal experiments suggest that the oedema around tumours is due to leakage of water and electrolytes through a damaged blood–brain barrier. Much of the oedema of ischaemic lesions is cytotoxic, a hypoxic failure of neurons and glia to maintain normal ion balances as just described. Such oedema responds poorly to steroids. It has also been shown that steroids do not reduce mortality or disability after intracranial haemorrhage. Other methods of reducing oedema, such as intravenous mannitol or urea, have also failed to show any benefit in the management of stroke. Glycerol may have some benefit on immediate mortality, but again an analysis of all trials shows that the confidence limits embrace the possibility that glycerol increases later mortality.

Attempts have been made to drive more oxygen into areas of ischaemic, but still viable, brain by hyperbaric oxygenation, but without proven benefit. An alternative approach is to attempt to improve blood flow to the same area. One technique used has been to ventilate patients with 5 per cent CO_2, but the viable ischaemic area around an infarct is already maximally vasodilated, and is maximally abstracting oxygen as PET scans show (Section 8.10.5), and no clinical benefit results. Another technique has been to lower blood viscosity by the infusion of low molecular weight dextran, but a controlled trial from Italy showed no benefit, even for those with the highest haematocrit. A further approach is to reduce oxygen consumption by either prolonged hypothermia or barbiturate anaesthesia. Although animal research shows clear benefit, the results in limited clinical research are not favourable—perhaps just as well, considering the enormous logistic difficulties that would arise.

Occasionally, a neurological deficit will increase during the first 24–48 hours after a stroke. In the great majority of patients this is due to brain-stem compression by herniation of intracranial contents—from above down in the case of a hemisphere lesion (usually a haemorrhage), from below up in the case of a cerebellar haematoma (Section 10.1.5.1). In some cases, however, progressive evolution of the deficit is due to progressive infarction, a so-called stroke in evolution. In a basilar artery occlusion, thrombus may be spreading distally, threatening the entry of anastomotic supply through the circle of Willis. Consideration of such cases is always fraught with anxiety, in case haemorrhage is precipitated but, if a CT scan confirms the absence of haemorrhage, such patients should be treated with intravenous heparin for a few days.

Anticoagulation may also be required for the few patients who develop clinical evidence of deep vein thrombosis after stroke. Pulmonary embolism is comparatively unusual, even though ^{131}I fibrinogen studies show some evidence of venous thrombosis in many more patients than have clinical evidence of this. Recent studies have shown an overall benefit from subcutaneous heparin after atheroembolic cerebral infarction without evidence of an increased rate of haemorrhage, but further research is needed to define the necessary criteria before this becomes a common practice.

Finally, a physician faced with a patient with

stroke with high blood pressure needs a policy about reducing it. A rapid reduction may result in reducing flow through the still viable but ischaemic zone around the infarct, and current practice is to lower pressure gradually. Blood pressure very often falls without treatment to normal or much nearer normal values in the days after a stroke, when a campaign for maintaining normal blood pressure can be planned for the minority with persistent hypertension. An exception to this policy is necessary in the management of hypertensive encephalopathy (Section 10.2.4).

Faced with this gloomy list of failed specific treatment in the acute phase of a stroke, the physician can spend his or her time usefully ensuring the best possible nursing management (Section 10.1.6) and physiotherapy (Section 10.1.9), the early treatment of complicating pulmonary infections, planning the active rehabilitation that the patient will surely need, and considering strategies for secondary prevention, such as the treatment of previously undiagnosed hypertension, and advice to the patient about smoking and alcohol consumption.

10.1.8   *Short- and long-term prognosis after stroke*

The mortality of all patients with strokes admitted to hospital is around 25 per cent—different results being found in different surveys according to the population admitted. In the Oxfordshire community study, the overall case fatality after a first-ever stroke at 30 days was 19 per cent, being 10 per cent for cerebral infarction and 52 per cent for primary intracerebral haemorrhage. Fatality rates are strongly linked to age, particularly for infarction, and to the degree of functional dependence before the first stroke. Over the past decade it has been realized that certain factors are particularly unfavourable. These are listed in Table 10.6. Apart from advanced age, which carries obvious implications for mortality, other factors in section (a)—depressed level of consciousness, deviation of the head and eyes away from the hemiplegic side (due to paralysis of tonic conjugate drive from the frontal eye fields of the damaged hemisphere), abnormal pupillary reflexes, Cheyne–Stokes ventilation, and neck stiffness—result from the effects of a very large supratentorial infarction with con-

Table 10.6   Unfavourable prognostic features of stroke

(a)   *For survival*
Depressed level of consciousness
Advanced age
History of previous stroke(s)
Deviation of head and eyes away from hemiplegic side
Abnormal pupillary reflexes
Cheyne–Stokes ventilation
Neck stiffness
Seizures
Hyperglycaemia
History of previous hypertension

(b)   *For recovery of functional independence*
All those factors listed above
Continuing incontinence of urine
Association of deficit of higher cerebral function and hemianopia with hemiplegia
Severity of motor paralysis
Depression
No spouse or other to care on discharge
Anterior circulation strokes carry worse prognosis than posterior
Right hemisphere strokes carry worse prognosis than left

sequent oedema and herniation and compression of the brain stem. Alternatively, coma and pupillary abnormalities can result from a major brain-stem infarction or haemorrhage, with an equally grave prognosis. Another factor that influences survival strongly is a history of previous strokes, which about doubles the chances of mortality from the current stroke.

A high blood pressure on admission is not a particularly unfavourable sign for survival, though known pre-existing hypertension is. Survival is less favourable in those with hyperglycaemia, even if true diabetes has not been present, possibly because the degree of hyperglycaemia is a marker of the extent of neural damage. There is, as yet, insufficient evidence to suggest that attempts should be made to reduce high blood sugars in the acute phase of stroke.

Fortunately, many of those who survive the first week after a stroke achieve a much greater level of independence than might at first sight seem probable. A complete hemiplegia, involving the face, arm and leg, with or without other deficits, is the commonest stroke syndrome, yet one can promise that 85 per cent of those who survive the first week will walk again without the aid of another person. The outcome of a hemiplegic hand, however, is less encouraging. Only about 30 per cent will regain useful function. If the hand remains without dexterous function at 28 days, further useful recovery is virtually unknown. Aphasia improves for up to six months, with only very limited gains thereafter. If a global aphasia (Section 6.1.1.1) persists for more than 28 days, then useful language is likely to be very limited indeed.

A number of research studies have now identified those factors that allow an early assessment of the likely recovery of functional independence. These are listed in the lower part of Table 10.6. Continuing incontinence of urine in the early days and weeks after a stroke might seem a surprising indicator, but this presumably reflects the size of an infarction, as do the next two factors in the

Table 10.7a   Guy's hospital prognostic score (prognostic score = 40 + total)

Clinical feature	Score
Complete paralysis of worst limb (MRC Grade 0 or 1)	−12
Higher cerebral dysfunction, and hemianopia and hemiplegia	−11
Drowsy or comatose after 24 hours	−10
Age (years)	(age ×−0.4)
Loss of consciousness at onset of stroke	−9
Uncomplicated hemiparesis (no higher cerebral dysfunction or hemianopia)	+8

table—the association of a focal deficit, higher cerebral function and hemianopia with hemiplegia, and the severity of the motor paralysis. A number of research studies use a prognostic score developed by Allen at Guy's Hospital, illustrated in Table 10.7a. Figure 10.6 illustrates its success at predicting outcome. The functional outcome of left hemisphere strokes is rather better, and a given level of function is achieved earlier, than for right hemisphere strokes, which at first sight is surprising, bearing in mind the handicap of deficit of language. However, large right hemisphere lesions may result in neglect of the left limbs and affect spatial orientation, praxis, and joint position sense

Table 10.7b   Yale–New Haven prognostic score

	Score
Age over 65	3 points
Diabetes	3 points
Hypertension (>180 systolic or >100 diastolic)	2 points
Stroke (rather than transient ischaemic attack)	2 points
Coronary heart disease	1 point

Outcomes using Yale–New Haven score
Risk of further stroke or death by 2 years

Risk group	Risk (per cent)
1 (points 0–2)	10
2 (points 3–6)	21
3 (points 7–11)	59

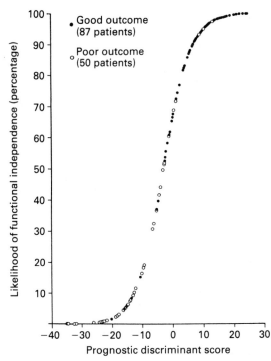

Fig. 10.6   A graph enabling the Guy's Hospital prognostic score for a patient (Table 10.7) to be converted into the likelihood of functional recovery (Allen 1984).

in such a way that a patient and the physiotherapist have a much more uphill task if the lesion is on this side rather than the left.

The Guy's Hospital prognostic score (Table 10.7a) is appropriate for a major hemiplegia, the score being dependent upon variables related to the stroke itself. Another prognostic system for outcome after a transient ischaemic attack or 'minor stroke' has been developed at Yale. Risk factors derived from multivariate analysis in a prospective cohort of patients at Yale were then tested against information available about another population in Canada. Table 10.7b shows the Yale score. Three points each are assigned for age of more than 65 years and diabetes, two points each for severe hypertension and stroke (compared with a transient ischaemic attack), and one point for coronary heart disease. Outcome rates (further stroke or death within two years) are, as shown in Table 7b, clearly related to the total number of 'points'. If all these unfavourable factors are present, the risk of a further stroke or death within two years is as high as 59 per cent.

Posterior circulation strokes have a good functional prognosis for those who survive the first week. Dysphagia, dysarthria, and diplopia may remain troublesome, but the former usually settles after a few weeks, during which a nasogastric tube is required. Patients and their relatives usually cope quite well with dysarthria and, if diplopia persists, within a limited range, the image from one eye can be suppressed by the use of an eye-patch, or frosted (Chevasse) lens.

The outcome of completed stroke in a community has been studied in the Oxfordshire Community Stroke Project, and Table 10.8 illustrates the survival at 30 days and 1 year, and the proportion of survivors who are functionally independent.

10.1.9 Rehabilitation after stroke

A considerable army of therapists may become involved in the rehabilitation of a patient after a stroke, and the effectiveness of their efforts has come under increasingly critical review in recent years. The principal question is this. Does active rehabilitation improve physical function, communication, and economic independence over and above that which occurs spontaneously in the weeks and months after a stroke?

It has been shown that patients admitted to a

stroke unit, receiving what may be considered to be the best modern care and active rehabilitation, do benefit in the short term over a control group admitted to general medical wards, in so far as a greater proportion become functionally independent. However, there are no significant differences in independence after 1 year, possibly because skills acquired during active rehabilitation are not practised in everyday life. The case for stroke units therefore depends more upon an economic deployment of rehabilitating staff rather than on long-term clinical gains.

The efficacy of speech therapy for aphasia after stroke has been assessed in a number of studies in recent years. The general conclusion is that there is no evidence that therapy offers gains over and above that which occurs spontaneously, or with the help of untrained volunteers. There may remain a place, however, for careful assessment of the type of aphasia (Section 6.1.1.1), so that the patient and his carer can concentrate on particular areas of difficulty.

No trial of physiotherapy versus no physiotherapy has as yet been undertaken, for the understandable ethical reason that existing empirical evidence suggests worthwhile benefit. Studies comparing the efficacy of intensive versus less intensive physiotherapy have shown modest benefits in functional recovery from the more intensive regimen, although social, financial, and administrative factors seem likely to prevent many patients from

Table 10.8 Survival and functional independence after a first-ever stroke (data based on community surveys)

Per cent survival	30 days	1 year	5 years
Infarction (Oxford)	90	77	–
Infarction (Rochester)	82	–	45
Infarction (Framingham)	85	–	60
Intracerebral haemorrhage (Oxford)	50	38	–
Subarachnoid haemorrhage	54	52	–

Percentage of survivors to 30 days who are functionally independent at 1 year (Oxford data)

Infarction	65
Intracerebral haemorrhage	68
Subarachnoid haemorrhage	76

receiving such intensive therapy as has been studied in the trials. Furthermore, many elderly patients are not capable of coping with 'intensive' physiotherapy.

All members of all caring professions should have some idea of the techniques used by the physiotherapist, as physiotherapists themselves can give only a limited time to each patient with stroke. In the acute stages of stroke, a physiotherapist will be principally concerned with putting all joints through a full range of passive movement, with particular attention to the shoulder of the paralysed side. Care should be taken not to sub-lux partially the shoulder joint of the weak side when lifting the patient. As soon as the patient's general condition allows, he or she should be sat up on the edge of the bed. Initially the patient will require support, as he or she will fall to the hemiplegic side. Gradually, however, sitting balance improves with practice, and truncal balancing reflexes return, even if the patient cannot prop himself or herself with a still paralysed arm. At a stage when the paresis of the limbs is still dense, the patient should practise sitting on a different variety of edges and surfaces, usually in the physiotherapy gymnasium. Righting responses of the trunk can also be retrained by helping the patient into an all-fours kneeling position, which the patient can practise holding. The next stage is to make use of the reflex extensor thrust of the paralysed lower limb, facilitated by pressure on the sole, inducing weightbearing first with assistance, and then only guidance. During this stage repeated passive movements of arm and leg will aid the reduction of spasticity, and may possibly facilitate the return of voluntary movement.

There is, of course, some way to go between using the extensor thrust to facilitate standing and the return of gait. Some hip flexion sufficient to move the lower limb forwards returns spontaneously, and the physiotherapist then concentrates on encouraging the patient to flex the knee and dorsiflex the foot as these movements return, avoiding, as far as possible, the development of what might be termed a neglected hemiplegic gait, with a spastic limb and stiffly plantar flexed foot. This has the effect of increasing the functional length of the lower limb, so the patient has to tilt to his sound side and circumduct the hip as he walks, so that his foot clears the floor. There is some evidence that some of the recovery after a

hemiplegia is due to the disclosure of ipsilateral corticospinal pathways.

The physiotherapist will also concentrate on helping the patient to transfer from bed to chair. The usual technique taught for rising from a chair is to clasp the hemiplegic hand in the sound hand and move both firmly in front, using the weight of both upper limbs to help bring the centre of gravity forwards to the edge of the chair. Usually sufficient strength returns in quadriceps and glutei to allow the patient to stand without aid, as long as the chair is high enough and firm enough—simple points often neglected.

Physical treatment of the hemiplegic upper limb is more disappointing, as judged by the level of functional recovery usually achieved. If the hand is going to recover dexterous function, it probably will in any event, without physiotherapy.

A major factor militating against better recovery of some patients is the onset of depression. Components of this depression undoubtedly reflect altered self-esteem, social withdrawal and apathy, economic circumstances, and impaired mobility. The Oxford Community Stroke Project has not found evidence of any focal brain lesion which predisposes to depression. Studies have shown that worthwhile improvements can be achieved with antidepressants such as nortriptyline. Most cases of depression settle within 1 year. The presence of an effective carer at home, usually the spouse, has a major effect upon the final level of independence achieved. It must also be remembered that caring relatives are also likely to be anxious, and may become depressed, particularly if the patient himself is severely depressed, aphasic, and immobile, although the carer's depression usually lifts in the second year.

10.1.9.1   *Risk of recurrent stroke*

The risk of subsequent stroke is substantially higher in stroke survivors than in the general population. One survey of stroke survivors has shown that about a third have had previous strokes. The Oxfordshire Community Stroke Project found that the risk of recurrent stroke after a lacunar infarction was 11.8 per cent after 1 year. Any treatment, yet to be found, which improves survival after acute stroke may well leave the community with a larger number of disabled stroke survivors at risk from a further stroke, which would have important socio-economic implications.

There is some evidence that, even in this late stage of the evolution of vascular disease, as evidenced by the occurrences of a stroke, attention to risk factors can reduce the probability of further strokes. Sequential arteriographic studies have shown that a significant proportion of atheromatous plaques regress.

10.1.10   *Transient ischaemic attacks*

10.1.10.1   *Clinical features*

Transient ischaemic attacks (TIAs) in the anterior (carotid) circulation are manifest by transient monocular blindness (amaurosis fugax), transient numbness, tingling and weakness of one side of the face and hand, or transient aphasia. The differential diagnosis of a TIA includes an episode of classical migraine. In this, teichopsia (scintillating lights in the visual field), nausea, and headache are more prominent (Section 9.4.1). Other possibilities include partial seizures; with the exception of the rare purely sensory or aphasic partial seizures, twitching of a limb or of the face will occur in these. Focal deficits can, surprisingly, occur in hypoglycaemia and hyponatraemia. The differential diagnosis of transient ischaemic events in the posterior circulation, which may result in dysarthria, vertigo, unsteadiness, diplopia, and circumoral parasthesiae largely involves the distinction of peripheral labyrinthine causes of vertigo (Table 6.7). Paroxysmal brain-stem events can occur in multiple sclerosis (Section 14.3.4), but the much younger age-group, and other evidence of multiple sclerosis, usually allow a ready distinction.

Drop attacks

A special point should be made about two types of transient symptom that are commonly attributed to transient cerebral ischaemia, albeit with very little evidence. The first is the syndrome of drop attacks. In this, the subject is usually a woman in middle age who complains of repeated falls on to her knees without warning. Such patients are usually quite specific about two things—that they have not tripped, and that there is no loss of consciousness. Drop attacks usually occur while walking, but can occur while standing still. Although traditionally attributed to vertebrobasilar ischaemia,

the sex and age distribution of those affected is quite unlike other patients with brain-stem vascular disease. Moreover, patients with drop attacks do not have symptoms suggestive of brain-stem involvement such as double vision or dysarthria in relation to the drop attacks. Very similar unexpected falls can occur in those with a myopathic weakness of the quadriceps, and it has been suggested, although there is no good evidence of this, that drop attacks in middle-aged and older women reflect some sort of 'menopausal myopathy.'

Transient global amnesia

The other transient neurological syndrome commonly stated to be due to transient cerebral ischaemia with not very good evidence is the syndrome of transient global amnesia. This syndrome is characterized by the abrupt onset of a strange state in which the patient, although alert and communicative, is amnesic for much of his or her life until the incident, and is unable to lay down new memories during the duration of the attack. This leads to repeated questioning of friends and relatives nearby. Consciousness is not disturbed, but as the patient comes out of the episode, usually gradually, it is clear that he or she is totally amnesic for the events of the previous few hours.

Occasionally episodes of transient global amnesia have been recorded in the course of cardiac catheterization in young people, suggesting that the episode can have a vascular origin. The concept of transient global amnesia as a variant of a more typical transient ischaemic attack rests on such observations, and also upon the fact that most people who suffer episodes of transient global amnesia are elderly. However, a case–control study has shown no significant differences in the prevalence of vascular risk factors between patients who have episodes of transient global amnesia and normal controls in the community. Vascular risk factors are substantially more frequent in patients with other evidence of transient cerebral ischaemia. Furthermore, whereas those with transient cerebral ischaemia may go on to have further episodes and stroke, the incidence of definite vascular events in those who have had transient global amnesia is low.

A proportion of patients with transient global amnesic attacks do go on to develop clear-cut epileptic seizures, suggesting that in a few patients, the episode of transient global amnesia was a type of complex partial seizure (see Section 12.4.1). However, a family or previous history of migraine is found in many patients with transient global amnesia, and it has been suggested that these episodes are migraine variants occurring in older people. Whatever the cause, the absence of vascular risk factors and the good prognosis for further vascular events makes it unlikely that episodes of transient global amnesia reflect transient cerebral ischaemia.

10.1.10.2 *Pathology*

Most TIAs have an embolic basis. The most direct evidence for this is the occasional observation of platelet–fibrin emboli, or cholesterol emboli, in retinal arteries during transient amaurosis, (amaurosis fugax), the retinal equivalent of a neurological TIA.

Sometimes transient amaurosis is accompanied by a contralateral transient hemiparesis, indicating that a shower of emboli have gone simultaneously into the retinal and ipsilateral hemisphere circulation. Such an event strongly implicates atheroma of the ipsilateral internal carotid artery. Pathological examination of the proximal part of the internal carotid artery may well show a ragged atheromatous ulcer or stenosis. Either excision of this region, or ligation (an uncommon treatment) may abolish the ischaemic episodes. TIAs are commonly stereotyped, similar symptoms occurring in each episode in an individual patient, and it might be thought unusual for emboli all to go to the same destination, but experiments in animals show that this often happens. A tight stenosis may imply that a reduction in blood flow is responsible for transient ischaemic events. However, it has been shown that a stenosis has to occlude nearly 90 per cent of the cross-sectional area of a large artery before flow is significantly reduced. Furthermore, it is difficult to reproduce the symptoms of TIAs by artificially reducing blood pressure. Some flow-related events certainly do occur (see the steal phenomenon in Section 10.1.11.2), most commonly in the posterior circulation, precipitated by exercise or a change in posture.

The investigation of transient ischaemic attacks follows similar lines to those listed in Table 10.4, with the exception that the principal objective is initially the anatomical localization of the source of thromboembolic events. After clinical assessment of the cardiovascular state, with special reference to blood pressure and cervical bruits, cardiac rhythm and murmurs, aided by electro- and echocardiography, a decision has to be made whether to proceed to investigate the extracranial circulation by angiography. Clearly, the presence of a localized mid-cervical bruit anterior to the sternomastoid will influence this decision. However, auscultation is not always of help. An atheromatous ulcer, a potent source of emboli, may be silent. Many bruits are due to tortuosity alone. If stenosis is severe, flow may be insufficient to generate a bruit.

Duplex ultrasound studies will give a good indication of reduced flow through a carotid stenosis, with reasonable definition obtained by combining B-mode images of the artery with range-gated pulsed-Doppler analysis of flowing blood at each point in the image. Hankey and Warlow have estimated the safest and most cost-effective way of investigating patients with transient ischaemic attacks in the carotid territory. To detect stenoses of 25 or 50 per cent, it is safer and more cost-effective to screen patients without an ipsilateral bruit by duplex ultrasonography, but if an ipsilateral bruit is present, proceed straight to angiography. If clinicians aim at detecting stenosis of 75 per cent or greater, then duplex ultrasonography is the preferred initial procedure, being less expensive, with associated occurrence of fewer strokes. However, the definitive investigation before surgery is likely to remain carotid angiography, although there is a significant risk of stroke related to the procedure. Unfortunately, intravenous digital subtraction angiography has not lived up to its early promise, and most neurologists believe that an arterial injection is necessary for adequate detail. Factors encouraging the neurologist to proceed to angiography include young age, presence of a localized bruit, and absence of hypertension. Conversely, arteriography is less often indicated in elderly patients, or those with hypertension, who are more likely to have lacunar infarction secondary to lipohyalinoid necrosis (Section 10.1.2).

Once a probable anatomical type and possible source of thromboembolism has been identified, other relevant investigations in Table 10.4 can be considered, as the presence or absence of abnormalities in, for example, glucose metabolism will influence management.

10.1.10.3   *Prognosis of transient ischaemic attacks*

There is an enormous variation in the prognosis for stroke after a transient ischaemic attack, depending upon the presence or absence of continuing risk factors (listed in Table 10.2). Overall, there is an annual risk of death from all vascular causes, or non-fatal completed stroke or non-fatal myocardial infarction of 7–12 per cent. The overall prognosis for those with normal arteriograms is only marginally better than for those with abnormal arteriograms, largely because of the occurrence of myocardial infarction. It has been shown that the treatment of hypertension after a transient ischaemic attack does reduce the risk of occurrence of a stroke.

10.1.10.4   *Medical management of transient ischaemic attacks*

It is against this uncertain background that the use of anticoagulants, aspirin, sulphinpyrazone, and ticlopidine have been studied. Anticoagulants were extensively used in the 1960s and early 1970s. Some of the trials showed a reduction in stroke rate, but not in mortality. In general, those neurologists who still favour anticoagulants do so for patients who have had recurrent transient ischaemic attacks in the carotid territory. As the risk of stroke is highest in the first few months after a transient ischaemic attack, anticoagulation is usually limited to this period, if undertaken at all. Anticoagulants are undoubtedly effective in preventing embolism from the heart (see Sections 10.5.1 and 10.5.4).

A single dose of aspirin, 325 mg, reduces human platelet cyclo-oxygenase activity by 90 per cent for at least 2 days, and the formation of thromboxane A_2, a prostaglandin that induces platelet aggregation. Aspirin has an opposing effect on arterial walls, reducing the production of the prostacyclin, an inhibitor of platelet aggregation, but the platelet system seems more sensitive in humans. The United Kingdom Transient Ischaemic Attack Trial showed that the chances of a non-fatal myocardial infarction, non-fatal major stroke, vascular death, or non-vascular death were 18 per cent less in those who took either 300 or 1200 mg of aspirin a day after a TIA. There was no difference in outcome between those who took the higher or the lower doses of aspirin. A subsequent trial from Holland has shown that 30 mg a day is as effective as 283 mg a day, with a smaller number of gastrointestinal bleeding episodes.

Sulphinpyrazone inhibits platelet cyclo-oxygenase, and therefore platelet aggregation. In spite of this, it has not been shown conclusively to be more or less effective than aspirin alone.

Dipyridamole inhibits platelet phosphodiesterase, increasing platelet cyclic adenine monophosphate, and reducing cytoplasmic calcium, thereby inhibiting prostaglandin synthesis. It has been shown to be of use, when combined with warfarin, in reducing embolism from prosthetic heart valves, but no study has shown a significant reduction in atheromatous thromboembolism to the brain over and above the reduction achieved by aspirin.

Ticlopidine inhibits neither cyclo-oxygenase or phosphodiesterase, but it inhibits platelet aggregation induced by adenosine diphosphate (ADP) and platelet adhesion, and prolongs the bleeding time. In a Canadian controlled trial, ticlopidine in a dose of 250 mg twice a day given to stroke survivors reduced the risk of stroke or myocardial infarction or other vascular death by about 30 per cent. Diarrhoea, skin rash, and neutropenia were quite common side-effects, causing 12 per cent to stop taking the drug.

Warlow has usefully summarized the available evidence about the effectiveness of anti-platelet drugs. He concludes that aspirin, 300 mg each day, has been shown to be effective. Since then, evidence from Sweden has shown that 75 mg/day is equally effective. Ticlopidine is probably about as effective as aspirin when the data from the different trials is analysed in a similar way. Sulphinpyrazone is not conclusively more or less effective than aspirin, but may be worth using if aspirin cannot be used.

Aspirin given prophylactically *before* any vascular event (to healthy physicians on a trial basis) may prevent a proportion of myocardial infarctions (the result of two trials were different), but has no effect upon the risk of stroke.

10.1.10.5   *Surgical management of transient ischaemic attacks*

If arteriography has shown a tight stenosis (70–99 per cent) of the internal carotid artery (Fig. 10.7a) and a patient in good general condition has experienced transient ischaemic attacks or reversible ischaemic neurological deficits in the hemisphere distal to that artery, then the evidence from the MRC European Carotid Surgery trial is that carotid endarterectomy should be undertaken. The trial showed that for nearly 800 patients the risks of surgery were significantly outweighed by later benefits. Although 7.5 per cent had a stroke or died within 30 days of surgery, during the next three years the risks of ischaemic stroke in the relevant hemisphere were only 2.8 per cent for those allocated to surgery, compared to nearly 17 per cent for those continuing on medical treatment. The total three-year risk of any disabling or fatal stroke or death in the perioperative period was 6 per cent for those allocated to surgery versus 11 per cent for those allocated to medical treatment. Conversely, for patients with mild stenosis (0–29 per cent), the risks of an ischaemic stroke occurring in the relevant hemisphere were very small in both the groups allocated to surgery and to continued medical treatment. From this study it is clear that non-stenosing atheromatous plaques do not warrant surgical intervention. The best policy for those with intermediate levels of stenosis (30–69 per cent) has not yet been elucidated. However, these and earlier results have not encouraged surgeons in the UK to advise endarterectomy for comparatively minor degrees of carotid stenosis.

Other studies indicate that perioperative morbidity and mortality are related to the experience of the surgical team. Advances in management include heparinization and, in some centres, intraoperative xenon measurements of cerebral blood-flow and electroencephalography, and postoperative observations on retinal artery pressure to ensure early diagnosis of postoperative occlusion.

The MRC European Carotid Surgery trial will undoubtedly have a major impact upon the current annual endarterectomy rates, which in the United States are about 430 per million per year, against 23 per million in the UK.

A troublesome problem is how to advise a patient who has an asymptomatic cervical bruit. These occur in about 4 per cent of patients over the age of 40. The first point is to exclude bruits conducted from the aortic valve, or venous hums. If attention is focused on those in whom the bruit is almost certainly arising from the carotid bifurca-

tion (heard only in the mid-cervical region anterior to the sternomastoid), a number of studies have shown that such a bruit is a marker of morbidity, as follow-up studies show an increased risk of stroke and myocardial infarction. However, strokes seldom occur without a warning TIA in these circumstances, and in any event are not particularly likely to occur in the hemisphere ipsilateral to the bruit. The consensus view is that there is insufficient evidence to warrant prophylactic endarterectomy. It must be remembered that the risk of perioperative stroke and death, even in the best centres, is each of the order of 2–4 per cent, and in the general population of those undergoing endarterectomy about 11 per cent. The increasing accuracy of non-invasive vascular testing may in future define a subgroup, those with advancing unilateral stenotic lesions, in whom surgery should be considered.

Another problem in these days of widespread coronary artery bypass surgery is what to do if a patient, under evaluation for such surgery, is found to have a carotid bruit. Some studies have shown that perioperative strokes are more frequent in those with bruits—in one study an odds ratio of 3.9 as compared with patients without bruit, and an absolute risk of 2.9 per cent. However, there is as yet no evidence that prophylactic endarterectomy reduces the overall risk.

The operation of extracranial–intracranial bypass, anastomosing a branch of the superficial temporal artery through a small craniectomy to a branch of the middle cerebral artery was developed in the 1980s. Postoperative angiograms show that the bypass hypertrophies and carries large volumes of blood. Unfortunately, the North American multicentre trial showed no benefit to any group of patients, even in those with bypassed stenoses of the internal carotid artery in the syphon, or focal middle cerebral artery stenoses. Although there have been criticisms of how patients were recruited for this trial, there seems to be no place at present for this operation.

Direct surgical procedures on stenosed vertebral arteries have not generally found favour, and, in general, good collateral circulation maintains flow. There are no grounds for undertaking carotid surgery for symptoms arising in the posterior circulation. There is no evidence that carotid surgery influences the course of multi-infarct dementia. Angioplasty, although highly successful in moulding

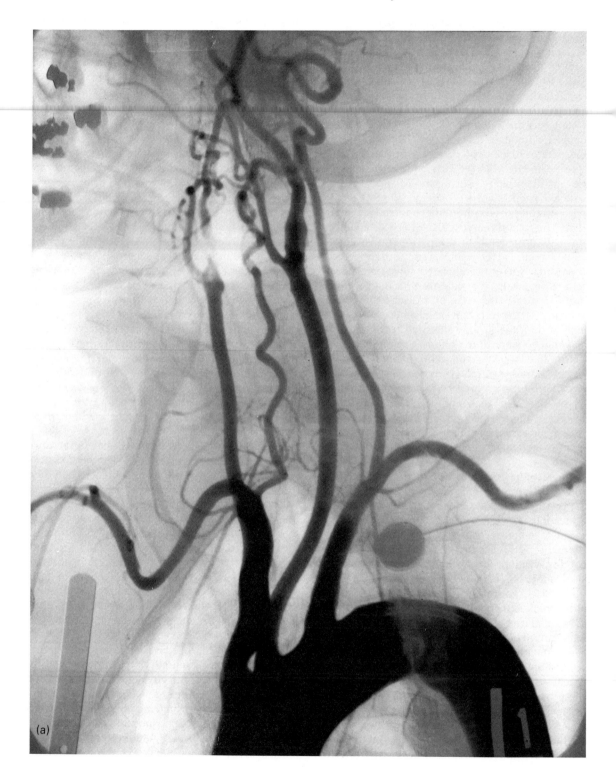

(a)

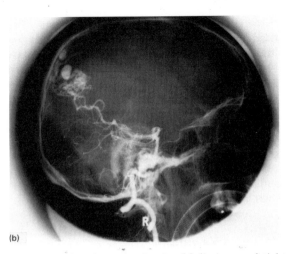

(b)

Fig. 10.7   Arteriography showing (a) (facing page) tight stenosis of the internal right carotid artery; a discontinuity in the contrast medium can be seen just above the carotid bifurcation. The wall of the left sided internal carotid at its origin has an irregular outline, indicating further atheroma. (b) angiomatous malformation on the posterior cerebral artery.

the stenoses of coronary artery disease, is not suitable for the more calcified plaques found in the carotid arteries.

10.1.11   *Other syndromes of atheromatous cerebrovascular disease*

10.1.11.1   *Ischaemic optic neuropathy*

The combination of acute impairment of vision, papilloedema, and subsequent optic atrophy is characteristic of occlusion of the posterior ciliary artery, resulting in partial or complete infarction of the pre-laminar optic nerve. The syndrome must be distinguished from a demyelinating or toxic optic neuritis (see Section 14.3.1). Ischaemic optic neuropathy can occur in giant-cell arteritis, diabetes mellitus, polycythaemia, and profound anaemia. Often no predisposing cause is found.

10.1.11.2   *Steal syndromes*

Occasionally the particular anatomy of stenotic arterial lesions may result in blood being diverted from a part of the brain, even though this is supplied by a patent vessel. The best example is of a stenotic lesion of the subclavian proximal to the

origin of the vertebral artery. Vigorous use of the muscles of that arm may result in diminished resistance in the muscular vascular bed. Blood then reaches the distal part of the stenosed subclavian by going up the contralateral vertebral artery and down the ipsilateral artery to the arm muscles, resulting in a transient ischaemic episode with brain-stem symptoms (Section 10.1.10.1). Screening (Doppler studies) of many patients with asymptomatic neck bruits has, however, shown that reversed flow down one vertebral artery is a comparatively common phenomenon, without inducing symptoms.

10.1.11.3   *Pseudobulbar palsy*

Pseudobulbar palsy, fully described in Section 6.4.2 is commonly due to bilateral lacunar infarction in the deep white matters of both hemispheres.

10.1.11.4   *Multi-infarct dementia*

Most patients with single large cerebral infarcts have no socially apparent dementia on recovery, though of course focal cognitive defects, such as aphasia, may remain. Psychometric assessment will, however, usually reveal some, albeit relatively minor, depression of global cognition and intellect. Patients who have multiple lacunar or cortical infarcts may develop what is termed multi-infarct dementia, considered fully in Section 11.5.5.

10.2   Other arterial diseases

10.2.1   *Atheromatous vascular disease affecting the spinal cord*

Considering the frequency of stroke, it is surprising how seldom the spinal cord is infarcted, although atheroma of the anterior spinal artery is quite frequently seen at post-mortem. Infarcts are most likely to occur at the lower dorsal level, in the border zone of perfusion between the territory of the contribution of the artery of Adamkiewicz, which joins the anterior spinal artery at about L2, and the contributions of intercostal arteries to the anterior spinal artery, usually at about T4 (see Section 18.5.2).

10.2.2 *Arterial dissection*

Dissection as a cause of stroke is comparatively rare, even in young adults. However, recent studies using ultrasound suggest that it is more common than previously diagnosed, and angiographic evidence of dissection may not remain apparent within a few days. Dissection may follow a wrenching injury to the neck, or direct trauma to the neck, or may be associated with deficiencies in the media. Pain in the territory of the dissecting artery, and a partial Horner's syndrome in the case of a dissecting carotid artery, are clues to the underlying pathology.

10.2.3 *Fibromuscular dysplasia*

This is an unusual condition often first noted as a chance finding on carotid arteriography, occurring more frequently in women. Hypertrophy of the media of the internal carotid artery alternates with zones of thinning of the media and disruption of the elastic lamina. When the vessel is filled with contrast medium, an appearance of alternating dilatations and constrictions, rather like a string of beads, is seen. Such arterial changes are more common in those with transient ischaemic attacks, either by causing thrombo-embolic events, or by restricting flow. Occasionally a dissecting aneurysm may arise in such an artery. However, in the great majority of cases the disorder appears relatively benign, and surgical treatment is rarely undertaken.

10.2.4 *Hypertensive encephalopathy*

Hypertensive encephalopathy is an acute event usually associated with severe hypertension in a previously normotensive patient. The usual clinical context is acute glomerulonephritis, or toxaemia of pregnancy. Less commonly, it occurs as part of an accelerated or malignant phase of previous hypertension. Clinical features include headache, seizures, visual disturbances, somnolence, or confusion. There are seldom focal neurological signs in the limbs. Inspection of the fundus will show retinal oedema, and maybe papilloedema, and retinal haemorrhages and soft 'cotton-wool' exudates. Whatever the cause, the severe hypertension results in focal arteriolar constriction, with hyaline necrosis of vessel walls, and increased permeability, resulting in cerebral oedema. The treatment of hypertensive encephalopathy is the urgent reduction of blood pressure, either by sodium nitroprusside administered by an infusion pump (0.5–0.8 micrograms/kg/min), or the rapid intravenous injection of diazoxide (50–150 mg). Cerebral oedema may be reduced by the concurrent administration of steroids and mannitol.

Malignant hypertension without encephalopathy should not be treated precipitously, as retinal, cerebral, or renal infarction may result. It is usually sufficient to reduce blood pressure over days rather than hours.

10.2.5 *Vasculitis*

10.2.5.1 *Giant-cell arteritis (cranial arteritis, temporal arteritis; polymyalgia rheumatica)*

This is an inflammatory disorder affecting arteries of medium diameter. As headache is such a prominent symptom, cranial arteritis is considered more fully in Section 9.7. Cerebral infarcts secondary to arteritis of the extracranial course of the vertebral or carotid arteries may occur, and visual loss due to optic nerve infarction is common.

The cause of cranial arteritis is not known. There is no consistent difference in human leucocyte antigen (HLA) types between patients and controls. It may be that the arteritis is due to some infectious agent triggering an auto-immune response.

10.2.5.2 *Other vasculitides*

Hypersensitivity vasculitis
This syndrome may be associated with systemic lupus erythematosus, rheumatoid arthritis, and polyarthritis. Characteristic pathological features include leucocyte infiltration of small blood vessels, particularly post-capillary venules, and fibrinoid necrosis. This syndrome may result in a confusional state or seizures rather than a focal overt ischaemic neurological deficit.

Polyarteritis nodosa
This is a disorder in which necrotizing vasculitis affects segments of small and medium-sized arteries. Major strokes may occur, but often there is a

general decline in cognitive function and alertness, sometimes accompanied by focal seizures, all secondary to multiple small infarcts. A more frequent neurological presentation of polyarteritis nodosa is as a mononeuritis multiplex (see Section 19.6).

Granulomatous angiitis

This is an uncommon disorder of older people, affecting segments of arterioles or venules. The disorder may occur in association with lymphoma and with varicella infection. Headache is a prominent feature together with evidence of ischaemic events. The diagnosis is not always made on angiography, sometimes only being made on meningeal biopsy or biopsy of an apparent mass lesion, which is found to contain mononuclear cells, multinucleated giant cells, and plasma cells with granuloma formation. The CSF may contain many lymphocytes; the ESR is often elevated. Patients may respond to treatment with cyclophosphamide or corticosteroids.

Takayasu's arteritis

This type of arteritis affects the adventitia and vasa vasorum of the aorta and its major branches. Secondary thickening of the intima may result in occlusion of major cerebral vessels. The aetiology is unknown. The disorder may respond in part to medication with corticosteroids.

Cerebral amyloid angiopathy

This rare disorder found in elderly people usually presents as repeated multiple large haemorrhages or infarctions secondary to deposition of amyloid in vessel walls. It is frequently associated with Alzheimer's disease. The amyloid is similar to that found in Alzheimer's disease (Section 11.5.1.4).

Syphilitic arteritis

Meningovascular syphilis may result in cerebral infarcts secondary to arteritis. Uncommon in recent years, it now appears that concurrent infection with human immunodeficiency virus (HIV) may accelerate the development of neurosyphilis.

Other bacterial arteritis

Basal meningitis due to tuberculosis can cause an inflammatory arteritis and occlusion of major vessels. The septicaemia of subacute bacterial endocarditis may cause an arteritis and the formation of mycotic aneurysms (see Section 10.6.7).

Wegener's granulomatosis

This is a systemic granulomatous vasculitis that affects the upper and lower respiratory tract, with or without associated glomerulonephritis. The nervous system may be involved by direct spread of granulomatous lesions from the paranasal sinuses, or by vasculitis. The diagnosis is supported by the finding of neutrophil cytoplasmic autoantibodies, or by biopsy. The disease responds well to treatment with cyclophosphamide.

Behçet's syndrome

This is a syndrome primarily of recurrent genital and oral ulceration, associated with iritis. Less common features include a vasculitis, particularly in the retinal vessels and cerebral circulation. Cerebral venous sinuses may become occluded by the inflammatory process. Other features sometimes present are a meningoencephalitis, bowel ulceration, and vasculitic aneurysmal formation in the systemic and pulmonary circulation. Neurological involvement occurs in about 20 per cent of cases. Syndromes include episodes of sudden dysfunction affecting a cerebral hemisphere or the brain stem, with subsequent improvement. The course of the disorder therefore often resembles multiple sclerosis. The cause of the disorder, found principally around the eastern Mediterranean, is obscure, but probably reflects an immunological attack on vascular endothelium. There is a significant association with certain tissue haplotypes, notably DR7. Treatment with azathioprine is effective in suppressing disease activity. Acute exacerbations can be treated with corticosteroids.

Moya-moya

The arteriographic appearance of this disorder is a fine leash of abnormal vessels arising from the terminal part of bilaterally occluded internal carotid arteries. The cause of this anomaly is not known.

10.3   Cerebral venous thrombosis

No community-based studies of the incidence of cerebral venous thrombosis have been reported, but certain conditions clearly predispose to thrombosis, either in the cortical draining veins, or in the great dural sinuses. These are listed in Table 10.9.

Table 10.9   Factors predisposing to cerebral venous thrombosis

---

Pregnancy and the puerperium
Oral contraception
Local infection
     of face or paranasal sinuses, leading to cavernous
         sinus thrombosis
     of ears and mastoid cavity, leading to transverse sinus
         thrombosis
Systemic infection, septicaemia
Metabolic disturbances, including diabetes mellitus and
     extreme dehydration
Haematological disorders
     sickle-cell disease
     polycythaemia
     leukaemia

The presentation of thrombosis of the draining cortical veins and of dural sinuses is rather different. In the first case there will be headache and drowsiness, or confusion. Often seizures occur, sometimes in association with a hemiparesis, raised intracranial pressure, and papilloedema. If a transverse sinus becomes thrombosed, the presentation is more insidious. The reduction in absorption of cerebrospinal fluid results in raised intracranial pressure.

A cavernous sinus thrombosis may follow an orbital injury or infection in the paranasal sinuses. Impaired venous return from the eye results in proptosis and conjuctival oedema, and papilloedema. As cranial nerves III, IV, and VI lie in the lateral wall of the infected sinus, there is usually a complete ophthalmoplegia, including pupillary paralysis. Although infection may begin on one side, as there are small bridging veins between the two cavernous sinuses, infection, and the physical signs, soon become bilateral. An important differential diagnosis of cavernous sinus thrombosis is paranasal infection with the fungus Mucor. Zygomycosis occurs in diabetic or immunocompromised patients and may well prove fatal (see Section 17.11.6).

The cerebrospinal fluid may be under raised pressure, and may contain some red blood cells and a few polymorphs. Cranial CT scanning shows patchy areas of low attenuation due to oedema, or high attenuation due to haemorrhagic infarction.

Arteriography may confirm the diagnosis of dural sinus thrombosis. Particular attention needs to be directed to the venous phase of the arteriogram. The superior sagittal sinus will show best on oblique films. A smaller cortical venous thrombosis may not be seen. MR angiography may well become the investigation of choice.

The best hopes for treatment of this hazardous condition lie in vigorous antibiotic treatment, if infection is clearly a causal factor. Adequate hydration to minimize blood viscosity may be important, particularly in infants. Finally, although it might seem hazardous to heparinize the patient to prevent further thrombus formation, because of the risk of turning a haemorrhagic infarct into a frank intracranial haemorrhage, recent studies show no excess incidence of haemorrhage and a significantly better outcome.

10.4   Sickle-cell disease

The sickle-cell gene affects people of African, Afro-Caribbean, and, to a lesser extent, of Middle Eastern, Indian, and Mediterranean descent. The abnormal gene codes for the β-chain of adult haemoglobin, which in sickle-cell disease is termed HbS. The synthesis of fetal haemoglobin (HbF) is normal, so homozygotes for HbS do not usually declare themselves clinically until HbF synthesis declines to adult levels at about 6 months of age.

Sickling of red cells is caused by the polymerization of deoxygenated HbS. The sickled cells increase blood viscosity and this is associated with infarction of bone marrow (resulting in painful sickle crises), renal damage, and, from the neurological point of view, stroke. Stroke affects about 6 per cent of those homozygous for HbS, often at an early age. At least two-thirds of those who have a stroke will have a further stroke within 1 year. Transfusion or exchange transfusion, by reducing the proportion of HbS, may reduce the risk.

10.5   Cardiac disease and the nervous system

Atheromatous vascular disease accounts for a high proportion of strokes, but a number of studies have shown that, with careful investigation, the heart is probably the source of embolism in about 20 per cent of events.

10.5.1   *Valvular disease*

Rheumatic mitral stenosis is associated with embolism in about 10 per cent of cases when the heart is in sinus rhythm, but as soon as atrial fibrillation begins the risk rises about threefold. Unfortunately, mitral valve replacement does not terminate this risk, and it is necessary to continue lifelong anticoagulation for those with mechanical valves. The risks of embolism from biological (allograft) valves is substantially less, but most surgeons continue to think that anticoagulation is necessary. Rheumatic mitral incompetence in association with atrial fibrillation is also associated with a substantial risk of embolism. In recent years, interest has centred upon the association of mitral valve prolapse with transient ischaemic attacks and stroke. Mitral valve prolapse is very common, affecting perhaps 5 per cent of the normal population, as judged by echocardiography, and the risk of any individual suffering cerebral embolism is low. The risk of an embolus is higher in older males who have redundant or thickened valve leaflets. However, as valve prolapse is so common, the number of events *in toto* may be considerable. Patients who have had embolic events have a shortened platelet survival time, but it is not clear why the ballooning cusp should be particularly liable to result in the formation of thrombus.

Atheromatous, rheumatic, or congenital aortic valve disease seem rarely to be associated with thrombo-embolic events, at least in younger people. In older age-groups, with widespread atheroma, it is often difficult to be sure that the embolus has arisen from the valve or some more distal site of atheroma.

Both aortic and mitral valves, however, are potent sources of thrombo-embolism in those with bacterial endocarditis. Nearly 40 per cent of patients with subacute bacterial endocarditis have neurological complications, and the prognosis is particularly unfavourable in this group. It is not unusual for the disease to present to the neurologist with a transient ischaemic attack or stroke as the first manifestation. A story of general malaise and weight loss, and fever, and a cardiac murmur on examination will be important clues as to the correct diagnosis, as will anaemia and a raised ESR. Sometimes the infected valve will be a prosthetic one, and emergency valve replacement may be necessary.

10.5.2   *Congenital heart disease*

Cyanotic heart disease with right-to-left shunting of venous blood makes it possible for thrombus from the systemic circulation (e.g. the leg or pelvic veins) to gain access to the left side of the heart and cerebral circulation. Such 'paradoxical emboli' can also occur through a patent foramen ovale, and there is a much increased prevalence of foramen ovale in young adults with unexplained stroke. Patency of the foramen ovale can be demonstrated by contrast echocardiography while the patient undertakes the Valsalva manoeuvre.

Congenital heart disease with right-to-left shunting is also a major risk factor for cerebral abscess—microemboli from an area of peripheral sepsis gaining easy access to the cerebral circulation (Section 17.2.1).

10.5.3   *Myocardial infarction*

A partial thickness myocardial infarct may have no effect on the intraventricular endocardium, but as the thickness of the infarct increases, the endocardium is likely to be damaged, and become a sticky surface on which thrombus can form, and from which embolic fragments may arise. However, probably less than 1 per cent of myocardial infarcts give rise to clinically detected cerebral embolism. Left ventricular thrombi usually overlie areas of ventricular wall malfunction, and are consequently more frequently associated with anterior myocardial infarctions. Although the incidence of cerebral haemorrhage is slightly increased by the use of thrombolytic therapy, this gives some protection against later ischaemic events, and overall the use of thrombolytic therapy (at least with strepokinase in one big trial) does not increase the incidence of cerebrovascular events.

10.5.4   *Disorders of cardiac rhythm*

Atrial fibrillation is an important cause of thrombo-embolism, even in the absence of mitral valve disease. The prevalence of non-rheumatic atrial fibrillation in the UK population rises from about 0.5 per cent in middle age to 5 per cent in the over 75s. About 13 per cent of patients with stroke have atrial fibrillation, but very probably this high rate reflects only diffuse vascular disease, not a causal relationship. Prospective studies of those with thyrotoxicosis and atrial fibrillation suggest that the risk of stroke is not greater than in a control population if age is taken into account as a variable. In non-rheumatic atrial fibrillation, congestive cardiac failure, a history of hypertension and previous arterial thrombo-embolism are risk factors for subsequent stroke. There has, for a long time, been concern as to whether such patients should receive aspirin or warfarin. Two recent controlled trials indicate that low-dose aspirin (75 mg/day) is of no benefit, but a higher dose (325 mg/day) may be. Warfarin does significantly reduce the risk of cerebral embolism. Low-dose warfarin, sufficient to maintain an International Normalized Ratio (INR) of 1.5–2.7 is effective; adverse effects such as haemorrhage were quite frequent in one trial, but not in the other. The cardiomyopathies associated with alcohol and with late pregnancy are particularly likely to be associated with atrial fibrillation and thrombo-embolism.

Paroxysmal atrial fibrillation may be associated more frequently with cerebral embolism than is sustained atrial fibrillation, presumably because sudden changes in rhythm may dislodge atrial thrombus. This, too, is the danger of cardioversion.

Although cardiac dysrhythmias may be associated with non-specific neurological symptoms such as dizziness and blackouts, presumably due to a fall in cardiac output, there is no good evidence that a dysrhythmia *per se* can cause *focal* neurological events.

10.5.5 *Atrial myxoma*

This rare benign atrial tumour is frequently associated with cerebral embolism.

10.5.6 *Cerebral events in association with cardiopulmonary bypass surgery*

Coronary artery bypass surgery is associated with a high incidence of neurological injury. Although major focal infarctions can occur, the most usual syndrome is transient confusion, accompanied by neurological signs such as extensor plantar responses. The extracorporeal circuit during bypass generates gaseous microbubbles and platelet–fibrin microaggregates. The affects of these can be visualized directly by fluorescein retinal angiography during bypass; multiple occlusions can be visualized, and presumably similar events occur within the cerebral circulation. Fortunately, the clinical outcome after such multiple microvascular occlusions is good.

In a prospective study, Shaw and colleagues have shown that certain clinical factors are more likely to be associated with post-operative neurological deficit. These include the duration and severity of heart disease before surgery, the presence of extracoronary vascular disease, a history of cardiac failure, and a history of diabetes. A number of intra-operative factors are also predictors of increased risk, such as hypotension and a large drop in haemoglobin during surgery.

Although they may follow any period of profound hypotension, such as following blood loss, *border zone infarctions* are seen today most commonly after cardiac surgery or brief cardiac arrest. The border zones of perfusion lie between the territories of anterior, middle, and posterior cerebral arteries. The common border zone between all three lies in the parieto-occipital region and, if infarcted bilaterally, produces a syndrome of visual disorientation, with defective visual judgment of size, distance and motion. Bilateral lesions in the territory between anterior and middle cerebral arteries produce weakness and cortical sensory impairment of both hands, often with a temporary loss of conjugate gaze. Lesions in the middle–posterior border zones produce dyslexia, constructional dyspraxia, and impairment of memory.

10.6   Subarachnoid haemorrhage

Haemorrhage into the subarachnoid space may occur as a result of cranial trauma, but the term 'subarachnoid haemorrhage' usually implies spontaneous subarachnoid haemorrhage. Subarachnoid haemorrhage is a grave disorder. In the UK, about 5000 patients bleed from a cerebral aneurysm each year, of whom it is estimated 700 die before they reach hospital.

10.6.1 *Epidemiology and pathology*

Population-based studies, such as those at Oxford, show that subarachnoid haemorrhage is responsible for about 5 per cent of all cerebrovascular events, including TIAs (Fig. 10.1). The average annual incidence is about 15–25 per 100 000.

Table 10.10 shows the source of haemorrhage identified in a large co-operative study in the USA. The figures shown demonstrate that a source of bleeding often cannot be identified with certainty. In many of the 22 per cent of patients in whom the cause remained unidentified, a small aneurysm or angioma was probably destroyed beyond recognition when rupturing; in others the leak may have occurred from a local area of arteriosclerotic disease, and in others from occult angiomas lying principally in the dura, with rupture into the subarachnoid space. Aneurysms are rather more common in men under the age of 40, but overall there is a 3 : 2 preponderance of women. Aneurysms by no means always rupture; they may be found in as many as 5 per cent of routine autopsies in which special attention is paid to the cerebral circulation. Aneurysms are found more commonly than would be expected in those with co-arctation of the aorta, an asymmetrical circle of Willis, polycystic kidney disease, and the Ehlers–Danlos syndrome, in which there is a defect of collagen metabolism. Sometimes there is a family history of subarachnoid haemorrhage due to ruptured aneurysms.

Table 10.10 Sources of subarachnoid haemorrhage

	%
Intracranial aneurysms	51
Hypertensive and/or arteriosclerotic vascular disease	15
Arteriovenous malformations	6
Miscellaneous or multiple causes	6
Causes undetermined even after angiography or autopsy	22

Notes:
(1) trauma excluded;
(2) extent of angiography variable;
(3) Arteriovenous malformations are much commoner in the South-East Asian population
Source: total 5431 cases with angiographic or autopsy study (Sahs *et al.* 1969).

If an unruptured aneurysm is found in the course of investigation and if its diameter is greater than 4 mm, then elective neurosurgery is probably indicated, as the risk of rupture of aneurysms of this size is considerable.

Modifiable risk factors for aneurysmal rupture include hypertension, alcohol, smoking, and oral contraception. Concurrent smoking and oral contraception synergistically raise the relative risk of subarachnoid haemorrhage more than twentyfold. Other risk factors identified include pregnancy-induced hypertension, and the long-term use of alcohol. Apparent precipitants of rupture include lifting, bending, defaecation, coughing, and coitus, but the great majority occur during no special activity, and at least one-third of aneurysms rupture during sleep.

10.6.2 *Clinical features*

The patient's story is one of the classical histories of neurology—the abrupt onset of an excruciating headache, associated with nausea and vomiting. If the haemorrhage is large, consciousness may be depressed or lost. Often a story may be obtained of a preceding vague malaise or 'dizziness', or a sudden milder occipital or vertical headache insufficient to cause the patient to seek medical advice. Such prodromal symptoms are almost certainly due, with the benefit of hindsight, to warning leaks from the aneurysm, which then partially heals by fibrotic repair. Unfortunately such prodromal headaches are insufficiently characteristic to give one much hope that they will, in future, be correctly diagnosed in advance of a major bleed. Those with subarachnoid haemorrhage who have had sentinel headaches have a worse prognosis.

On examination, neck stiffness is present, and Kernig's sign positive, although both these signs may take a few hours to develop if the bleed is small. At an early stage, there are no focal neurological signs, but there may be a hemiparesis if an aneurysm in the middle cerebral artery ruptures into the sylvian fissure, with a haematoma spreading into the temporal lobe. There may be unilateral ptosis and pupillary dilatation if the aneurysm lies on a posterior communicating artery, in the neighbourhood of the third cranial nerve. The sudden increase in intracranial pressure may cause pre-retinal (subhyaloid) haemorrhages, which are sometimes sufficiently large to interfere with vision. There may also be papilloedema.

There is usually little doubt about the differential diagnosis in a 'full-blown case.' If the onset of headache is less abrupt, meningitis (Section 17.1.2) should be suspected. More commonly, the distinction lies between subarachnoid haemorrhage and a severe migrainous episode, acute exertional headache, or coital headache (Section 9.5.1). An unfortunate category of patients is that of patients who are brought to the emergency room with what, in fact, is nothing more than a severe migraine or a sudden exacerbation of tension headache, who undergo an ill-timed and traumatic haemorrhagic lumbar puncture by young and eager physicians. They are then subsequently transferred to a specialized unit for angiography, and they are finally told that 'the weak spot in one of their brain vessels has probably healed, but that they would be wise to take things a bit easier in the future.' (Vermeulen and van Gijn 1990).

10.6.3   Investigation

As blood has a high attenuation coefficient, it can readily be visualized on CT scanning, and this is the investigation of choice. However, whether or not blood is imaged in the subarachnoid space depends upon the quantity released, and the interval between the haemorrhage and the scan. About 30 per cent of scans will be falsely negative. As Fig. 10.2e shows, blood may collect in the sylvian fissures and basal cisterns, but it is often seen in the ventricles as well. Red blood cells may readily be detected by microscopy of spinal fluid obtained by lumbar puncture. The presence of red cells in the spinal fluid may, of course, indicate no more than a traumatic tap, but in this latter case the numbers of red cells will decrease as the fluid is collected serially into different numbered containers as the needle is flushed clear. Within a few hours of a true subarachnoid haemorrhage, some red cells will lyse, leading to yellow staining (xanthochromia) of the supernatant of the centrifuged spinal fluid. The degree of xanthochromia may be slight, but pigments can sometimes be demonstrated spectroscopically, and this should certainly be undertaken if the diagnosis is seriously entertained in spite of a fluid that appears clear to the naked eye. Haem pigments persist in the fluid for

more than 3 weeks in the majority of cases, but intact cells disappear within a few days.

The sudden rush of blood into the subarachnoid space is soon followed by cerebral oedema and raised intracranial pressure. Lumbar puncture in these circumstances may cause a dangerous downward herniation of cerebral contents (coning). It is for this reason that CT scanning has largely replaced lumbar puncture. Furthermore, CT scanning may give some clue as to the origin of the bleeding, if the blood is seen to be most prominent at one of the classical sites for an aneurysm. However, lumbar puncture should never be omitted if fulminant meningitis or a small haemorrhage likely to be below the sensitivity of CT scanning remains a diagnostic possibility.

Having confirmed the diagnosis of subarachnoid haemorrhage, an attempt should be made, in patients who are fully conscious, or only a little drowsy, to identify the bleeding site by angiography (Fig. 8.25). About half the patients will prove to have intracranial aneurysms. Table 10.11 lists the sites at which an aneurysm is likely to be found.

10.6.4   Management

The further management of proven subarachnoid haemorrhage remains one of the controversies of neurology and neurosurgery.

The first problem is that the initial haemorrhage itself carries a high mortality which, in most published series from neurosurgical units, is underestimated, as an uncertain number of patients die before reaching one—perhaps 10–15 per cent of the total. A further 30–40 per cent die in the early days following the initial haemorrhage. Numerous studies have shown that early operative intervention on a bleeding aneurysm in an obtunded patient carries a high mortality. A principal factor in this is spasm of cerebral arteries in the neighbourhood of the bleeding vessel. This is particularly likely if blood collects in the basal cisterns. The substances causing vasospasm have not yet been identified, but may prove to be serotonin and some prostaglandins. Vasospasm usually begins about 4 days after an initial bleed, and may significantly reduce flow to the areas of brain supplied by the constricted arteries, producing focal neurological signs.

Deterioration due to spasm between the fourth

and around the tenth day is often misinterpreted as a second haemorrhage. Many surgeons are interested in exploiting this 'window' before the fourth day by investigating and operating very early on patients in good condition, using an operating microscope to place a clip across the neck of the aneurysm. This then protects the patient against a further haemorrhage, and hopefully spasm, and shortens the time spent in hospital. Once the aneurysm has been safely clipped, some surgeons will attempt to increase flow through the artery in spasm by inducing hypertension, or by increasing plasma volume with low molecular weight dextran. It has been shown that early surgery in alert patients lessens overall mortality significantly. Unfortunately, the logistic difficulties of transferring patients, arranging arteriography and then surgery, prevent early operation in many cases. Investigation and then operation appear to be best postponed until patients who have a focal neurological deficit (without impairment of consciousness) stabilize. Those whose consciousness remains impaired are probably best treated conservatively with bed rest for 6 weeks. Many physicians also believe that, as operative mortality and morbidity rise so sharply in patients over the age of 60, older patients should not be transferred to a neurosurgical centre as the results of conservative management are better than those of operation.

Table 10.11 Probability of site of single aneurysm, which has bled (all ages) (Sahs *et al.* 1969)

	Male	Female
Anterior communicating region	0.41	0.22
Posterior communicating/internal carotid region	0.18	0.29
Middle cerebral at main branches	0.12	0.14
All posterior circulation sites	0.06	0.05

One decision the neurologist or neurosurgeon has to make is the extent of his angiographic investigation. As Table 10.11 shows, about 5 per cent of all aneurysms will lie on the posterior cerebral circulation, which is much less accessible to surgery. Even if both internal carotid arteries are injected, and the posterior circulation filled by injection of one vertebral artery, a small number of aneurysms will be missed, lying on the contralateral vertebral artery before its fusion to form the basilar artery. Of those patients with aneurysms, about one patient in seven has more than one (Table 10.12); the surgeon then has to decide which has leaked. Usually neighbouring spasm gives a good indication.

Table 10.12 Frequency of multiple aneurysms (Sahs *et al.* 1969)

	%
One aneurysm	81
Two aneurysms	14
Three aneurysms	3
Four or more aneurysms	1

Using all data—angiography, surgical exploration, autopsy; $n = 3321$.

Apart from recurrent haemorrhage and vasospasm, other problems may arise in the acute stage of the illness. The electrocardiogram often appears very abnormal, with prolonged Q–T intervals, depressed ST segments and inverted T waves across the chest leads. This is due to subendocardial myonecrosis, associated with the release of an enormous amount of noradrenaline secondary to the haemorrhage. β-Adrenergic blocking drugs may be used to prevent these changes. It is true that there are usually no clinical concomitants of the electrocardiographic abnormalities, though some workers believe that the prolonged Q–T interval may favour the occurrence of arrhythmias, and contribute to mortality.

What steps can the neurologist take if conservative treatment is adopted? Although not formally submitted to trial, all believe that strict bed rest and adequate analgesia is essential. Straining at stool should be avoided with laxatives and enemas if necessary. Sedation with a benzodiazepine may well be needed, as some patients are confused and obstreperous. Activity associated with this confusion may elevate arterial pressure and precipitate a further bleed, the mortality from which approaches 60 per cent.

Interest in recent years has centred on the possibilities of reducing fibrinolysis, so that the chances of a rebleed due to dissolution of a fine fibrin meshwork over the leak are lessened, and on reducing spasm. Both ε-aminocaproic acid and tranexamic acid have been used to inhibit fibrinolysis, but the design and power of the trials has been inadequate. It has been calculated that, if the mortality in the control group was 33 per cent, nearly 1000 patients would have to be studied to have an 80 per cent chance of detecting a 25 per cent difference in mortality. None of the studies approach these numbers. All that can be said is, although the chances of rebleeding may be lessened by antifibrinolytic agents, there is no obvious effect upon morbidity and mortality—possibly because any improvement in rebleeding is matched by an increased occurrence of intracerebral infarction and systemic venous thrombosis. The other principal approach has been to relieve spasm. A recent trial showed that nimodipine significantly reduced the incidence of cerebral infarction and ischaemic deficits, from 33 per cent in controls to 22 per cent in those who received the drug. Nimodipine, a calcium-channel blocker, should be given as soon as possible after the haemorrhage, by intravenous infusion in a dose of 0.5–1.0 mg/hr initially, increasing after 2 hours to 2 mg/hr if there is no major drop in blood pressure. The infusion should be continued for 5 days, and may be followed by oral nimodipine, 60 mg every 4 hours for a further few days. Another compound under active investigation is calcitonin-gene-related peptide, a powerful vasodilator found in the perivascular neural network of cerebral blood vessels.

If a patient with an aneurysm survives the hazardous first 14 days after a subarachnoid haemorrhage and leaves hospital after 5–6 weeks, he remains at risk from late rebleeding if treated conservatively. The risk of a further bleed is about 3 per cent per year for the first decade and rather less thereafter. This may not sound a high risk, but a moment's calculation will show that after 10 years nearly one-third of the survivors of a first aneurysmal bleed will have had a further late haemorrhage. Such late haemorrhages are often particularly catastrophic, with a mortality of about 75 per cent. The prognosis of patients with subarachnoid haemorrhage who have had no aneurysm of arteriovenous malformation demonstrated on angiography (about 15–20 per cent) is very much better—the annual risk of rebleeding being only 0.3 per cent a year in one study, a tenth of that if the original bleed had been due to an aneurysm.

Communicating hydrocephalus (Section 11.5.9) may occur as an acute, subacute, or late complication of subarachnoid haemorrhage, and shunting after appropriate investigation may greatly improve the clinical state of a patient whose progress appears to have halted or reversed. Features suggestive of a communicating hydrocephalus include dilatation of the lateral ventricles on CT scanning or MRI (Section 7.1.1.1). Older age, a low Glasgow score on admission, previous hypertension, an aneurysm on the posterior circulation, and blood in the ventricles are all factors that predispose to subsequent hydrocephalus. Another delayed complication of a subarachnoid haemorrhage is inappropriate secretion of anti-diuretic hormone, hyponatraemia, and resulting confusion (Section 23.2.2).

10.6.5 *Giant aneurysms*

Not all aneurysms present to a neurologist as a subarachnoid haemorrhage. Giant aneurysms may arise on the supraclinoid portion of the internal carotid artery, and, by the compression of adjacent optic nerve and chiasma, present with gradual impairment of visual acuity and field. Alternatively, severe retro-ocular pain, accompanied by ptosis and other evidence of a third nerve palsy, may be the presentation of a large infraclinoid aneurysm. Giant aneurysms at the termination of the basilar artery may project into the floor of the third ventricle and present as hydrocephalus. Advances in neurosurgical techniques over the past 15 years have meant that many such lesions have become operable, or manageable by interventional radiology (Section 8.11.1).

10.6.6 *Arteriovenous malformations*

These may lie either predominantly on the surface of the brain or they may be deep-seated in white matter. An example is shown in Fig. 10.7(b). If the latter rupture, then an intracerebral haemorrhage results. The rupture of a more superficially placed lesion will spill blood into the subarachnoid space, with symptoms identical to those of a ruptured aneurysm. However, there is often also some parenchymatous disruption, so focal neurological signs may be more prominent. As the ruptured vessel is often a vein carrying blood at comparatively low pressure, the early mortality and rate of both early and late recurrent haemorrhage is less than with a ruptured aneurysm. A careful study of the arteriographic findings is necessary to decide whether it is better to attempt to remove abnormal vessels, or to follow the patient without operating. It may look simple to tie off one or more vessels feeding the malformation, but experience shows that other smaller vessels soon dilate and continue to supply the angioma. Alternative treatment approaches include embolization of the angioma, through a transfemoral catheter, with particulate material or a cyanoacrylate plastic which polymerizes rapidly *in situ*, and intensely focused radiation by a so-called 'gamma knife'—highly collimated γ-rays from a cobalt source, which induce a fibrosing and thrombotic occlusion of the angioma over the next 1–2 years. Both procedures may result in a neurological deficit such as a hemiplegia, and the option of no active treatment, particularly in the elderly, should always be considered first.

Angiomas often declare themselves by seizures rather than by subarachnoid haemorrhage. There seems to be a tendency for such angiomas to continue without haemorrhage, and therefore conservative treatment is usually advised. Occasionally an angioma may increase formidably in size over the years and, by shunting oxygenated blood away from normal brain, may produce progressive ischaemic neurological deterioration. The right moment to intervene surgically can therefore never be certain.

10.6.7 *Rare causes of subarachnoid haemorrhage*

In subacute bacterial endocarditis, a septic embolus may lodge in a distal cerebral artery, and then, over the next days, result in an infective weakening of the arterial wall, with subsequent rupture. Such so-called mycotic aneurysms should be suspected in any patient with neurological symptoms that are not explained by systemic illness. They are usually silent before rupture, but they may be associated with headache, an aseptic meningitis, and transient neurological signs, including cranial nerve palsies. Early detection by angiography, if there are symptoms, and early excision of accessible aneurysms are recommended, as there may be progressive increase in size despite antibiotic treatment. Subarachnoid haemorrhage may also result from a hypertensive crisis, for example, after

abusing amphetamines, or combining a monoamine oxidase inhibitor with inappropriate aminergic drugs or cheese. Finally, anticoagulant drugs, or disorders of coagulation associated with leukaemia or other myeloproliferative disorders, can result in a subarachnoid haemorrhage.

10.7 Further reading

General

Allen, C. M. C., Harrison, M. J. G., and Wade, D. T. (1989). *The management of acute stroke*. Castle House Publications, Tunbridge Wells.

Dale, S. H. (1988). *Stroke*. Office of Health Economics, London.

Mendelow, A. D. (1991). Spontaneous intracerebral haemorrhage. *Journal of Neurology, Neurosurgery and Psychiatry* **54**, 193–5.

Sandercock, P. A. G. (1991). Recent developments in the diagnosis and management of transient ischaemic attacks and minor strokes. *Quarterly Journal of Medicine, New Series* **78**, 101–12.

Toole, J. F. (ed.) (1990). *Cerebrovascular disorders*. Raven Press, New York.

Yatsu, F. M. and Fisher, M. (1989). Atherosclerosis: current concepts on pathogenesis and interventional therapies. *Annals of Neurology* **26**, 3–12.

Epidemiology

Incidence and prevalence

Bamford, J., Sandercock, P., Dennis, M., Warlow, C., Jones, L., McPherson, K., *et al.* (1988). A prospective study of acute cerebrovascular disease in the community: the Oxfordshire Community Stroke Project. 1 Methodology, demography and incident cases of first ever stroke. *Journal of Neurology, Neurosurgery and Psychiatry* **51**, 1373–80.

Garraway, W. M., Connolly, D. C. C., Elveback, L. R. and Whisnant, J. P. (1983). The dichotomy of myocardial and cerebral infarction. *Lancet* **2**, 1332–5.

Kannel, W. B. and Wolf, P. A. (1983). Epidemiology of cerebrovascular disease. In *Vascular disease of the central nervous system*, (ed. R. W. Ross Russell), pp. 1–24. Churchill Livingstone, Edinburgh.

Risk factors

General

Sandercock, P. A. G., Warlow, C. P., Jones, L. N., and Starkey, I. R. (1989). Predisposing factors for cerebral infarction: the Oxfordshire Community Stroke Project. *British Medical Journal* **298**, 75–80.

Shaper, A. G., Phillips, A. N., Pocock, S. J., Walker, M., and Macfarlane, P. W. (1991). Risk factors for stroke in middle-aged British men. *British Medical Journal* **302**, 1111–15.

Ethnicity

Balarajan, R. (1991). Ethnic differences in mortality from ischaemic heart disease and cerebrovascular disease in England and Wales. *British Medical Journal* **302**, 560–4.

Hypertension

Amery, A., *et al.* (1986). Efficacy of anti-hypertensive drug treatment according to age, sex, blood pressure, and previous cardiovascular disease in patients over the age of 60. *Lancet* **2**, 589–92.
Medical Research Council Working Party (1985). MRC trial of mild hypertension: principal results. *British Medical Journal* **291**, 97–104.
Ramsay, L. E. and Walker, P. C. (1986). Strokes in mild hypertension: diastolic rules. *Lancet* **2**, 854–5.
Wilcox, R. G., Mitchell, J. R. A., and Hampton, J. R. (1986). Treatment of high blood pressure: should clinical practice be based on results of clinical trials? *British Medical Journal* **293**, 433–7.

Hyperglycaemia

Stout, R. W. (1989). Hyperglycaemia and stroke. *Quarterly Journal of Medicine (NS)* **73**, 997–1004.

Smoking

Bonita, R., *et al.* (1986). Cigarette smoking and risk of premature stroke in men and women. *British Medical Journal* **293**, 6–8.
Donnan, G. A., *et al.* (1989). Smoking as a risk factor for cerebral ischaemia. *Lancet* **2**, 643–6.

Alcohol

Gill, J. S., Zezulka, A. V., Shipley, M. J. *et al.* (1986). Stroke and alcohol consumption. *New England Journal of Medicine* **315**, 1041–6.

Oral contraceptives

Paganini-Hill, A., Ross, R. K., and Henderson, B. E. (1988). Postmenopausal oestrogen treatment and stroke: a prospective study. *British Medical Journal* **297**, 519–22.
Vessey, M. P., Lawless, M., and Yeates, D. (1984). Oral contraceptives and stroke: findings in a large prospective study. *British Medical Journal* **289**, 530–1.

Anti-cardiolipin antibodies

Chakravarty, K. K., Byron, M. A., Webley, M., Durkin, C. J., al-Hillawi, A. H., Bodley, R., and Wozniak, J. (1991). Antibodies to cardiolipin in stroke: association with mortality and functional recovery in patients without systemic lupus erythematosus. *Quarterly Journal of Medicine, New Series* **79**, 397–405.

Hyperhomocysteinaemia

Clarke, R., Daly, L., Robinson, K., Naughten, E., Cahalane, S., Fowler, B., and Graham, I. (1991). Hyperhomocysteinaemia: an independent risk factor for vascular disease. *New England Journal of Medicine* **324**, 1149–55.

Cervical bruits

Chambers, B. R. and Norns, J. W. (1986). Outcome in patients with asymptomatic neck bruits. *New England Journal of Medicine* **315**, 860–5.

General factors

Boers, G. H. J., *et al.* (1985). Heterozygosity for homocystinuria in premature peripheral and cerebral occlusive arterial disease. *New England Journal of Medicine* **313**, 709–15.

Stroke syndromes

Allen, C. M. C. (1983). Clinical diagnosis of the acute stroke syndrome. *Quarterly Journal of Medicine, New Series* **52**, 515–23.
Bamford, J., Sandercock, P., Dennis, M., Burn, J., and Warlow, C. (1991). Classification and natural history of clinically identifiable subtypes of cerebral infarction. *Lancet* **337**, 1521–6.
Bornstein, N. M. and Norns, J. W. (1986). Subclavian steal: a harmless haemodynamic phenomenon. *Lancet* **2**, 303–5.
Editorial (1988). Cerebellar stroke. *Lancet* **1**, 1030–1.
Glass, J. D., Levey, A. I., and Rothstein, J. D. (1990). The dysarthria-clumsy hand syndrome. *Annals of Neurology* **27**, 487–94.
Hankey, G. J. and Warlow, C. P. (1991). Lacunar transient ischaemic attacks: a clinically useful concept? *Lancet* **337**, 335–8.
Landau, W. M. (1989). Au clair de la lacune: holy, wholly, holey logic. *Neurology* **39**, 725–30.
Pearce, J. M. S. (1987). The locked in syndrome. *British Medical Journal* **1**, 198–9.
Poungvarin, N., Viriyavejakul, A., and Komotri, C. (1991). Siriraj stroke score and validation study to distinguish supratentorial haemorrhage from infarction. *British Medical Journal* **302**, 1565–7.

Medical treatment of acute stroke

Barer, D. H., Cruikshank, J. M., Ebrahim, S. B., and Mitchell, J. R. A. (1988). Low dose beta blockade in acute stroke ('BEST' trial): an evaluation. *British Medical Journal* **296**, 737–42.

Barsan, W. G., Brott, T. G., Olinger, C. P., and Marler, J. R. (1989). Early treatment for acute ischaemic stroke. *Annals of Internal Medicine* **111**, 449–51.

Collins, R. C., Dobkin, B. H., and Choi, D. W. (1989). Selective vulnerability of the brain: new insight into the pathophysiology of stroke. *Annals of Internal Medicine* **110**, 992–1000.

Editorial (1991). Treatment for stroke? *Lancet* **337**, 1129–31.

Trust Study Group (1990). Randomised, double blind, placebo-controlled trial of nimodipine in acute stroke. *Lancet* **336**, 1205–9.

Prognosis after stroke

Allen, C. M. C. (1984). Predicting the outcome of acute stroke: a prognostic score. *Journal of Neurology, Neurosurgery and Psychiatry* **47**, 475–80.

Bamford, J., Sandercock, P., Jones, L., and Warlow, C. (1987). The natural history of lacunar infarction: the Oxfordshire Community Stroke Project. *Stroke* **18**, 545–51.

Bamford, J., Sandercock, P., Dennis, M., Burn, J., and Warlow, C. (1990). A prospective study of acute cerebrovascular disease in the community: the Oxfordshire Community Stroke Project 1981–1986. 2 Incidence, case fatality rates and overall outcome at one year of cerebral infarction, primary intracerebral and subarachnoid haemorrhage. *Journal of Neurology, Neurosurgery and Psychiatry* **53**, 16–22.

Bamford, J., Dennis, M., Sandercock, P., Burn, J., and Warlow, C. (1990). The frequency, causes, and timing of death within 30 days of a first ever stroke: the Oxfordshire Community Stroke Project. *Journal of Neurology, Neurosurgery and Psychiatry* **53**, 824–9.

Kernan, W. N., Horwitz, R. I., Brass, L. M., Viscoli, C. M., and Taylor, J. W. (1991). A prognostic system for transient ischaemic attack or stroke. *Annals of Internal Medicine* **114**, 552–7.

Rehabilitation after stroke

A series of papers in *Archives of Neurology* (1989) **46**, 700–3.

Flicker, L. F. (1989). Rehabilitation for stroke survivors – a review. *Australian and New Zealand Journal of Medicine* **19**, 400–6.

Hewer, R. L. (1990). Rehabilitation after stroke. *Quarterly Journal of Medicine, New Series* **76**, 659–74.

House, A., Dennis, M., and Mogridge, L. (1991). Mood disorders in the year after first stroke. *British Journal of Psychiatry* **158**, 83–92.

Young, J. B. and Forster, A. (1992). The Bradford

community stroke trial: results at six months. *British Medical Journal* **304**, 1085–9.

Carotid artery disease and stroke

Brook, R. H., Pask, R. E., Chassin, M. R. *et al.* (1990). Carotid endarterectomy for elderly patients: predicting complications. *Annals of Internal Medicine* **113**, 747–53.

Brown, M. M., Butler, P., Gibbs, J., Swash, M., and Waterston, J. (1990). Feasibility of percutaneous transluminal angioplasty for carotid artery stenosis. *Journal of Neurology, Neurosurgery and Psychiatry* **53**, 238–43.

European carotid surgery trialists' collaborative group (1991). MRC European carotid surgery trial: interim results for symptomatic patients with severe (70–99 per cent) or with mild (0–29 per cent) carotid stenosis. *Lancet* **337**, 1235–43.

Grotta, J. C. (1987). Current medical and surgical therapy for cerebrovascular disease. *New England Journal of Medicine* **317**, 1505–16.

Hodges, J. R. and Warlow, C. P. (1990). The aetiology of transient global amnesia. A case–control study of 114 cases with prospective follow up. *Brain* **113**, 639–658.

Hankey, G. J. and Warlow, C. P. (1990). Symptomatic carotid ischaemic events: safest and most cost effective way of selecting patients for angiography, before carotid endarterectomy. *British Medical Journal* **300**, 1485–91.

Hart, R. G. and Easton, J. D. (1985). Dissections. *Stroke* **16**, 925–7.

Mayberg, M. R., Wilson, S. E., Yatsu, F., Weiss, D. G., Messina, L., Hershey, L. A. *et al.* (1991). Carotid endarterectomy and prevention of cerebral ischemia in symptomatic carotid stenosis. *Journal of the American Medical Association*, **266**, 3289–94.

Anti-platelet agents

Antiplatelet Trialists' Collaboration (1988). Secondary prevention of vascular disease by prolonged antiplatelet treatment. *British Medical Journal* **296**, 320–31.

Editorial (1991). Ticlopidine. *Lancet* **337**, 459–60.

The Dutch TIA trial study group (1991). A comparison of two doses of aspirin (30 mg vs. 283 mg a day) in patients after a transient ischemic attack or minor ischemic stroke. *New England Journal of Medicine* **325**, 1261–6.

Hennekens, C. H., Peto, R., Hutchinson, G. B., and Doll, R. (1988). An overview of the British and American aspirin studies. *New England Journal of Medicine* **318**, 923–4.

Peto, R., Gray, R., Collins, R., *et al.* (1988). Randomised trial of prophylactic daily aspirin in British male doctors. *British Medical Journal* **296**, 313–16.

UK-TIA Study Group (1988). United Kingdom transient

ischaemic attack (UK-TIA) aspirin trial: interim results. *British Medical Journal* **296**, 316–20.

Warlow, C. (1990). Ticlopidine, a new anti-thrombotic drug: but is it better than aspirin for long term use? *Journal of Neurology, Neurosurgery and Psychiatry* **53**, 185–7.

Cerebral venous thrombosis

Einhäupl, K. M., Villringer, A., Meister, W., *et al.* (1991). Heparin treatment in sinus venous thrombosis. *British Medical Journal* **338**, 597–600.

Sickle cell disease

Adams, R., McKie, V., Nichols, F. *et al.* (1992). The use of transcranial ultrasonography to predict stroke in sickle cell disease. *New England Journal of Medicine* **326**, 605–10.

Cardiac disease and stroke

Albers, G. W. (1991). Stroke prevention in non-valvular atrial fibrillation. *Annals of Internal Medicine* **115**, 727–36.

Chesebro, J. H., Fuster, V., and Halperin, J. L. (1990). Atrial fibrillation – risk marker for stroke. *New England Journal of Medicine* **323**, 1556–8.

Editorial (1989). Mitral valve prolapse. *Lancet* **1**, 1173–4.

Lechat, P., Mas, J. L., Lascault, G. *et al.* (1988). Prevalence of patent foramen ovale in patients with stroke. *New England Journal of Medicine* **318**, 1148–52.

Maggioni, A. P., Franzosi, M. G., Farina, M. L., Santoro, E., Celani, M. G., Ricci, S., and Tognoni, G. (1991). Cerebrovascular events after myocardial infarction: analysis of the GISSI trial. *British Medical Journal* **302**, 1428–31.

Shaw, P. J., Bates, D., Cartilidge, N. E. F., *et al.* (1989). An analysis of factors predisposing to neurological injury in patients undergoing coronary bypass operations. *Quarterly Journal of Medicine (NS)* **72**, 633–46.

The Stroke Prevention in Atrial Fibrillation Investigators. (1992). Predictors of thromboembolism in atrial fibrillation: I. Clinical features of patients at risk. *Annals of Internal Medicine* **116**, 1–5.

Arteritis

Allison, M. C. (1988). Temporal artery biopsy. *British Medical Journal* **297**, 933–4.

Case records of the Massachusetts General Hospital (1991). *New England Journal of Medicine* **325**, 42–54.

Wegner's granulomatosis

Hoffman, G. S., Kerr, G. S., Leavitt, R. Y. *et al.* (1992). Wegener granulomatosis: an analysis of 158 patients. *Annals of Internal Medicine* **116**, 488–98.

Behçet's syndrome

Wechsler, B. and Piette, J. C. (1992). Behçet's disease. *Lancet* **304**, 1199–200.

Subarachnoid haemorrhage

Adams, H. P. (1991). Non-aneurysmal subarachnoid haemorrhage. *Annals of Neurology* **29**, 461–2.

Briggs, M. (1984). When should ruptured aneurysms be operated upon? In *Dilemmas in the management of the neurological patient*, (ed. C. Warlow and J. Garfield.) Churchill Livingstone, Edinburgh.

Brust, J. C. M., Dickinson, P. C. T., Hughes, J. E. D., and Holtzman, R. N. N. (1990). The diagnosis and treatment of cerebral mycotic aneurysms. *Annals of Neurology* **27**, 238–46.

Heros, R. C. and Korosue, K. (1990). Radiation treatment of cerebral arteriovenous malformations. *New England Journal of Medicine* **323**, 127–9.

Maurice Williams, R. S. (1987). *Subarachnoid haemorrhage: aneurysms and vascular malformations of the nervous system.* Wright, Bristol.

Nishioka, H., Torner, I. C., Grod, C. J., *et al.* (1984). Cooperative study of intracranial aneurysms and subarachnoid haemorrhage: a long term prognostic study. *Archives of Neurology* **41**, 1142–51.

Ostergard, J. R. (1990). Warning leak in subarachnoid haemorrhage. *British Medical Journal* **301**, 190–1.

Pickard, J. D., Murray, J. D., Illingworth, R. *et al.* (1989). Effect of oral nimodipine in cerebral infarction and outcome after subarachnoid haemorrhage. *British Medical Journal* **298**, 636–42.

Radford, N. R., Torner, J., Adams, H. P., and Kassell, N. F. (1989). Factors associated with hydrocephalus after subarachnoid haemorrhage. *Archives of Neurology* **46**, 744–52.

Sahs, A. L., Perret, G., Locksley, H.B B., *et al.* (1969). *Intracranial aneurysms and sub-arachnoid haemorrhage: a cooperative study.* J. B. Lippincott, Philadelphia.

Solomon, R. A. and Fink, M. E. (1987). Current strategies for the management of aneurysmal subarachnoid haemorrage. *Archives of Neurology* **44**, 769–74.

Stein, B. M. and Mohr, J. P. (1988). Vascular malformations of the brain. *New England Journal of Medicine* **319**, 368–70.

Vermeulen, M. and van Gijn, J. (1990). The diagnosis of subarachnoid haemorrhage. *Journal of Neurology, Neurosurgery and Psychiatry* **53**, 365–72.

11 Dementia

11.1 Definition

Dementia can be defined as an acquired persistent impairment of intellectual function sufficient to interfere with social or occupational function, without impairment of consciousness. The word 'acquired' distinguishes dementia from developmental impairment of intellect, mental retardation. The word 'persistent' distinguishes dementia from the transient impairment of organic confusional states. However, 'persistent' implies only a longer time-course and does not exclude the possibility of successful treatment if dementia is due to certain causes, unfortunately rare. For the diagnosis of dementia. intellectual function must be impaired in at least two of the spheres of activity listed in Table 11.1. A purely focal deficit of one sphere of activity, such as language or memory, is not considered to be sufficient evidence of dementia, although in some cases global deterioration of all skills may begin with a particularly marked deficit in one of these areas.

11.2 Epidemiology

There are considerable difficulties in defining a level of function in community surveys below which people might, at different ages, be considered to be demented. A number of different studies suggests that the incidence derived from case register studies (first *referrals* for problems associated with dementia) is of the order of 2–3 per 1000 per year over the age of 60, in the UK, but this low rate probably reflects awareness that

Table 11.1   Diagnosis of dementia

For diagnosis of dementia, intellectual function must be impaired in at least two of these spheres:
    language
    memory
    spatial orientation
    personality and social skills
    abstract reasoning and judgment

little can be done rather than a true incidence figure.

The prevalence rates are of course much higher, as illustrated in Fig. 11.1. A community study from the USA showed even higher rates—for those aged 75–84 the rate was 19 per cent and for those aged 85 years or older 47 per cent (95 per cent confidence limits 37–66 per cent). The very steep increase in prevalence rates of dementia as age increases will be of increasing economic importance as the numbers in this age-group increase for demographic reasons. The numbers illustrated in Fig. 11.1 show that the average general practitioner in the UK will care for about 25 patients with dementia, of whom half will be severely demented. Some of the more gravely demented will be in permanent institutional care. A number of longitudinal studies of the 'healthy elderly' are in progress. In a population of 80-year-olds, studied for 4–5 years, new cases of dementia were as common as myocardial infarction and twice as common as stroke.

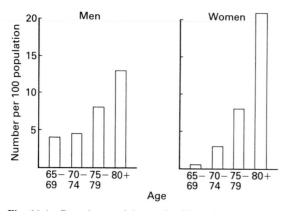

Fig. 11.1 Prevalence of dementia. (Data from a report of the Royal College of Physicians by the College Committee on Geriatrics; reproduced by permission.)

The current direct and indirect annual cost of Alzheimer's disease in the USA has been established to lie between 24 and 48 billion dollars.

11.3 The differential diagnosis of dementia

Before considering the causes of dementia, two related questions must first be considered: Is the patient really demented or not? If not demented, can the initial impression of dementia be due to some other illness, such as a depressive illness? (Table 11.2).

Table 11.2 The differential diagnosis of dementia

Benign senescent forgetfulness
Depression
Drug-induced confusional states
Other neurological illnesses, e.g. stroke, tumour, Parkinson's disease
Psychotic illnesses of old age

11.3.1 *Is the patient really demented?*

Some patients bring themselves to the family doctor or neurologist complaining of failing memory. Usually they are reacting badly to the normal increasing forgetfulness of middle age. They are not coping as well as before with a busy working or domestic life. As age advances, memory further declines. A woman of, say, 75, may be functioning perfectly well, but cannot remember reliably the names of all 10 grandchildren. This is sometimes called benign senile forgetfulness; it usually does not worry the subject very much, although it may annoy the family. On the other hand, a spouse, workmates, or business friends may each or all successfully conceal for months or years a progressive dementing illness, by gradually taking over the domestic or working functions of the affected person.

Some objective measurement of cognitive function is therefore required. The most widely used standard is the Weschler Adult Intelligence Scale, which examines language, reasoning, spatial orientation, calculation, and memory. Those who are becoming globally demented usually retain relatively higher scores on verbal subtests of the scale. The scores on the individual subtests of the performance scale tend to be widely scattered, the patient performing near normally in some subtests, but at a defective level on others. This scatter and the disparity between scaled verbal and performance intelligence quotients are the hallmarks of early dementia. The drawback to the general use of the scale is that it takes 1–1.5 hours to administer. Such an assessment of the patient is usually

Table 11.3   Abbreviated mental test (Hodkinson, 1972)

1.   Age
2.   Time (to nearest hour)
3.   Address for recall at end of test—this should be repeated by the patient to ensure it has been heard correctly: e.g. 42 West Street, Edinburgh
3.   Year
5.   Name of institution
6.   Recognition of two persons (doctor, nurse etc.)
7.   Date of birth (day and month sufficient)
8.   Years of First World War
9.   Name of present monarch
10. Count backwards 20 to 1

One point scored for each correct answer.
A score of 0–3 indicates severe impairment, 4–7 moderate impairment, and 8–10 normal cognitive function.

considered to be within the domain of a clinical psychologist. In recent years, the construction of various mini-mental state examinations of which the 'Abbreviated Mental Test' is one example (Table 11.3) have been of considerable help to neurologists. This only takes 5 minutes to administer, and a number of studies have shown that scores on the Abbreviated Mental Test correlate well with scores on the Weschler Adult Intelligence Scale, although the test has a bias towards detecting left hemisphere or bilateral impairment. A score summing tests of recall and orientation is almost as sensitive and specific as a full mini-mental state test. In the longitudinal study of 80-year-olds already mentioned, those who made a small number of errors on a mini-mental state examination were much less likely to develop dementia in the next 5 years than those who made rather more errors.

11.3.2   *Is the initial impression of dementia due to some other process?*

Depression in elderly people often mimics dementia. Apathy, psychomotor retardation, impaired concentration, and inability to follow the thread of a discussion are all features common to both illnesses. Clearly, it is of the utmost importance to think of this possible diagnosis, as such depression

may be readily reversible by antidepressants.

Reversible toxic confusional states in the elderly can be caused by a number of drugs; the most frequent offenders are listed in Table 11.4. Less commonly, other psychiatric illnesses in the elderly may mimic some features of dementia, notably the paranoid delusional symptoms of paraphrenia of late onset. Such patients usually have intact personalities apart from their delusional life.

Table 11.4   Some of the drugs that cause toxic confusional states in the elderly

CNS depressants
  alcohol
  hypnotics, especially barbiturates
Anticholinergic drugs
  benzhexol, benztropine, hyoscine, atropine
Antihistamines
Antidepressants
Beta-blockers, especially propranolol, oxprenolol, pindolol
Digoxin
Cimetidine
Lithium
Methyldopa
Phenytoin
Clonidine

Diagnostic difficulty is sometimes increased by the coexistence of depression and dementia. Patients with brain infarcts may be depressed before the onset of multi-infarct dementia but, once dementia is established, patients with Alzheimer's disease are more likely than those with multi-infarct dementia to be depressed.

11.4   The concept of cortical and subcortical dementias

Cortical and subcortical dementias are the two main syndromes of 'brain failure'. Although the distinction is a little artificial, clinical practice supports the division. Furthermore, neuropsychological studies demonstrate that lesions in specific subcortical structures produce identifiable cognitive deficits. The principal differences are listed in Table 11.5. In cortical dementia, of which Alz-

Table 11.5   Cortical and subcortical dementias (based on Cummings 1990)

	Cortical	Subcortical
Examples	Alzheimer's disease Creutzfeldt–Jakob disease	Progressive supranuclear palsy Huntington's disease Parkinson's disease Spinocerebellar degenerations Vascular disease
Anatomy and metabolism on PET scan	Cortex involved; basal ganglia, thalamus, mesencephalon largely spared	Cortex largely spared; involvement of basal ganglia, thalamus, and mesencephalon
Neurotransmitters involved	Acetylcholine	Dopamine, γ-aminobutyric acid
Mental status		
language	Aphasia	No aphasia
memory	Difficulty in learning new material	Difficulty in retrieving learned material
cognition	Severely disturbed: aphasia, agnosia, alcalculia, but relatively normal response time	Impaired problem-solving produced by slowness and forgetfulness
personality	Unconcerned	Apathetic
mood	May be depressed	Often depressed
Motor system		
speech	Normal	Dysarthria, impaired fluency
posture	Normal upright	Flexed
gait	Normal	Abnormal
motor system	Normal	Slow movements; rigidity, tremor, chorea, or ataxia may occur

heimer's disease is the prototype (although the primary metabolic defect may lie in deeply lying neurons; Section 11.5.1.2), the principal defects are cognitive—aphasia, agnosia, and apraxia—and in learning new material. The defects in subcortical dementias (for example, progressive supranuclear palsy; Section 13.4) involve more forgetfulness, slowing of mental processes, apathy, more prominent motor disturbances, and milder intellectual impairment.

11.5   The causes of dementia

Table 11.6 lists some of the causes, assigned to 'common' and 'rare' groups. Not every physician would agree with this arbitrary distinction. In developing countries, for instance, dementia due to the late effects of inadequately treated purulent and tuberculous meningitis must be vastly more common than, for example, dementia due to long-term overadministration of barbiturates. Nevertheless, the table gives some idea of what pathological causes should be considered when confronted by a patient who is demented. Some causes, such as the static dementia following a severe head injury, are immediately obvious. In others, dementia occurs as part of a pre-existing neurological illness, such as Parkinson's disease. A policy for appropriate investigation of the remainder is outlined in Section 11.6.

11.5.1   *Alzheimer's disease*

11.5.1.1.   *Epidemiology and clinical features*

Alzheimer first described this disease in 1906. It is by far the commonest cause of dementia. It accounts for about 50 per cent of all cases of dementia in hospital surveys, and, if those in the

Table 11.6   Some causes of dementia

Common	Rare
'Degenerative' disorders	
Alzheimer's disease	Huntington's disease
Parkinson's disease	Progressive supranuclear palsy
	Pick's disease
	Spinocerebellar degenerations
Vascular causes	
Multi-infarct dementia	Disseminated lupus erythematosus
After subarachnoid haemorrhage	
The effects of trauma	
After major head injury	Cumulative effects of minor head injuries—boxing
Subdural haematoma	
Intracranial tumours	
Particularly frontal, and in the corpus callosum	
Infective causes	
AIDS	Bacterial, e.g. syphilis, post-meningitic dementia
	Fungal, e.g. *Cryptococcus*
	Viral, e.g. subacute sclerosing panencephalitis, progressive multifocal leucoencephalopathy, post-encephalitic dementia
	Other infective agents, e.g. Creutzfeldt–Jakob disease
Hydrostatic causes	
	Communicating or obstructive hydrocephalus
Toxic and metabolic causes	
Chronic alcoholism	Hypothyroidism
Long-term drug intoxication, especially barbiturates	B_{12} and folate deficiency
	Hepatic and renal failure
	Aluminium poisoning
	Wilson's disease
	Remote effects of cancer
	Adult onset of metabolic disorders usually seen in childhood, e.g. metachromatic leucodystrophy
Anoxic causes	
After cardiac arrest	Carbon monoxide poisoning
Other causes	
	Multiple sclerosis

community were included, probably nearer 80 per cent. The arbitrary separation of pre-senile and senile dementia at age 65 has been abandoned. The disease is three times more common in women, but this difference is largely, if not wholly, accounted for by the longer survival of women into the age-groups in which Alzheimer's disease is very common.

Impairment of memory is the usual first symptom. However, patients in the early stages are often brought to the family doctor or neurologist by the family as, although a fair amount of insight into social and cognitive difficulties is usually maintained in the early stages, organizing a complex occasion such as an independent visit to the doctor is just the sort of problem with which the patient will have difficulty coping. If the patient does come independently, he or she may report vague non-specific symptoms, such as tiredness. If the doctor knows the patient well, he will be aware that a certain sharpness of previous personality is lost; the patient seems vague and perhaps less well-dressed than before. As dementia progresses, memory for events of personal life declines further. Domestic skills such as shopping, cooking, and housework are neglected. Those engaged in office life are no longer able to function as judgment declines. Spatial disorientation occurs, so that the patient may find himself lost in familiar surroundings, even within his own home. The patient becomes indifferent to his personal appearance and increasingly apathetic. Later, apathy may give way to incomprehensible verbal ramblings, rest-

lessness, and nocturnal wanderings. Eventually the patient will be unable to wash or dress himself, and ends his life mute, bedfast, and incontinent.

Very occasionally patients are seen with a progressive aphasia or hemiparesis, which eventually turns out to be the initial manifestation of more widespread neuropathological changes of the Alzheimer type.

11.5.1.2 *Pathological changes*

Post-mortem examination of the brains of those dying from Alzheimer's disease will show consider-

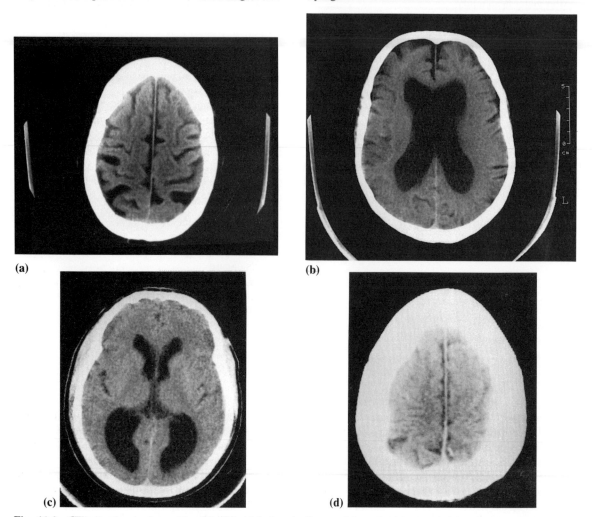

(a)

(b)

(c)

(d)

Fig. 11.2 CT scanning in dementia. (a), (b) Alzheimer's disease. Note the large ventricles, insular atrophy, and dilated sulci over the vertex. (c), (d) Communicating hydrocephalus. The ventricles are dilated, but the sulci over the vertex are not.

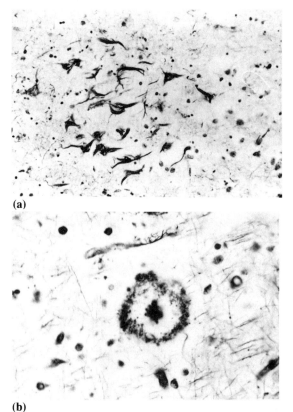

(a)

(b)

Fig. 11.3 (a) Neurofibrillary tangle and (b) argyrophilic plaque in Alzheimer's disease. (Reproduced by permission from Dr M. Esiri and the editor of *MRC News*.)

able atrophy of the brain, particularly in the temporoparietal regions and at the frontal poles of the hemispheres. The gyri are flattened, the sulci widened, and the ventricles dilated. These changes are reflected on the cranial CT scan (Fig. 11.2a,b) and on MRI.

The characteristic microscopical findings in the brain are the presence of neurofibrillary tangles, senile plaques, granulovacuolar degeneration, and loss of neurons from specific areas.

Neurofibrillary tangles

These tangles within neurons stain densely with silver (Fig. 11.3a). Tangles are particularly common in neurons in the hippocampus and amygdala, and pyramidal neurons. Tangles consist of structures called paired helical filaments. The fila-

ments consist of a core, which is extremely resistant to protease digestion, surrounded by an easily stripped 'fuzzy coat'. It has been shown that a protein called tau is an important constituent of the filaments. Tau is one of the proteins making up microtubules, the fine cylindrical structures concerned with intraneuronal and intra-axonal transport.

Senile or neuritic plaques

These are areas of degenerating neuronal processes surrounding an extracellular central core which stains with Congo red (amyloid) (Fig. 11.3b). Plaques are usually disposed fairly close to blood vessels. Electron microscopy shows a fibrillary appearance of the core, which is largely composed of a highly insoluble 42-amino-acid protein fragment. This is known as β-amyloid; it is derived by proteolysis from one of a larger group of proteins of about 700 amino acids known as amyloid precursor protein, the gene of which maps to chromosome 21. At least four forms of this precursor protein exist, and many cell types, both within and outside the nervous sytem, produce it. It is not yet known whether deposition of β-amyloid reflects overexpression of the amyloid precursor gene, or abnormal post-translational processing of the product.

Granulovacuolar degeneration

This is a term used to describe vacuoles within the cytoplasm of neurons, particularly within the hippocampus. Some of the vacuoles contain granules of unknown constitution.

Loss of neurons from specific areas

The enzyme choline acetyltransferase identifies cholinergic neurons. There is a widespread reduction in the enzyme, and therefore presumably loss of neuronal processes, in the cerebral cortex of people with Alzheimer's disease. This reflects loss of the neurons in the medial septal nucleus, the horizontal nucleus of the diagonal band of Broca, and the basal nucleus of Meynert (Fig. 11.4). These neurons lie underneath the globus pallidus and project widely to the cortex. CSF levels of acetylcholinesterase tend to be lower in patients with Alzheimer's disease, but there is considerable overlap with the levels found in normal patients. However, the CSF of affected patients may contain an anomalous form of the enzyme, as identified by

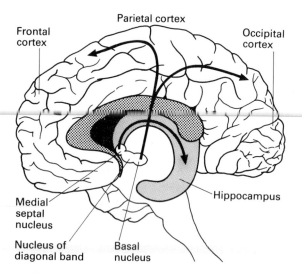

Fig. 11.4 Cholinergic pathways in the brain. (Reproduced from *Scientific American*, with permission).

Table 11.7   Is Alzheimer's disease different from normal ageing?

In favour
    Loss of some cognitive function and memory in most very aged people
    Neurofibrillary tangles and plaques found in most aged brains
Against
    Specific areas of brain affected by neuronal loss in Alzheimer's disease
    Numbers of plaques and tangles distributed bimodally, suggesting distinct populations
    EEG changes in aged patients and in those with Alzheimer's disease are different
    Specific losses of neurotransmitter are found in Alzheimer's disease
    choline acetyltransferase
    somatostatin
    High incidence of Alzheimer's-like disease in Down syndrome suggests a specific abnormality
    Undoubted genetic cause in some families with Alzheimer's disease

isoelectric focusing. The loss of cholinergic neurons in some cases is not great, and degeneration of nerve endings of these neurons rather than their cell bodies may be important in Alzheimer's disease. Neurites that contribute to senile plaque formation are, however, derived from the cell bodies of many different neurotransmitter systems. Loss of neurons is more profound and widespread in younger patients: in older patients the loss may be confined to the temporal lobe, particularly the hippocampus. There is also in younger patients a marked loss of noradrenergic projections to the cortex from the locus coeruleus. A reduction in somatostatin has also been demonstrated in the temporal lobes of those with Alzheimer's disease, particularly those with a younger age of onset. Cells making up neurofibrillary tangles stain for somatostatin.

11.5.1.3   *Is Alzheimer's disease different from normal ageing?*

Although superficially there appears to be some overlap between the cognitive disabilities of demented patients and those considered to be part of normal ageing, there is evidence that the quality and accurancy of long-term recall is very much more impaired in the demented patient (Table 11.7). Furthermore, although neurofibrillary tan-

gles and senile plaques are found in the brains of 'normal' aged patients, their number and distribution is quite different from those with Alzheimer's disease. It has been shown that the density of senile plaques correlates reasonably well with the degree of dementia at death, so on this ground it could be argued that those with Alzheimer's disease are only one end of a continuum of normal ageing. However, the most convincing evidence that Alzheimer's disease is 'different' comes from the enzyme studies described above, and the genetic studies in the next section. The losses of noradrenergic neurons and somatostatin are not features of normal ageing, and there are relatively few changes in the distribution of choline acetyltransferase in normal aged brains.

11.5.1.4   *The cause of Alzheimer's disease*

The cause or causes have not yet been identified, although the area is one of vigorous research. Clues as to the aetiology include the occasional occurrence of Alzheimer's disease in families. It may be that the genetic component of Alzheimer's disease is much more important than at first sight appears from epidemiological studies. Most people with a genetic predisposition to Alzheimer's disease may die before they reach the age of expression of the gene, but the 90-year lifetime risk among first-degree relatives of patients with Alzheimer's disease is close to 50 per cent, suggesting an autosomal dominant pattern of inheritance.

Another piece of evidence suggesting a genetic contribution to the cause of Alzheimer's disease comes from Down syndrome—chromosome 21 trisomy. Patients with Down syndrome almost invariably show neurofibrillary tangles and neuritic plaques indistinguishable from those found in Alzheimer's disease if they survive beyond the age of about 40.

The gene that encodes amyloid precursor protein (APP), precursor of β-amyloid (see Section 11.5.1.2) also lies on chromosome 21. It is present in all normal individuals. APP is normally inserted into the cell membrane and cleaved outside releasing a soluble form of the precursor protein. The fact that the normal cleavage site lies within the β fragment suggests that β-amyloid is not normally generated, and that there is some fault in APP metabolism. A number of families have been described in which the pedigree indicates autosomal dominant transmission of the gene, the genetic defect being on the proximal part of chromosome 21q. However, this gene and the gene for APP do not segregate exclusively in the reported pedigrees, and there appear to be some families without any chromosome 21 markers. However, in two large families with early onset Alzheimer's disease linked to chromosome 21, gene sequencing has shown a valine to isoleucine substitution within exon 17 in those family members with the disease, not found in unaffected older members or normal individuals.

There has also been speculation that amyloid plaques do not represent waste collections of macromolecules secondary to neuronal degeneration, but aggregations of a proteinaceous infective agent, a 'prion', of the same class as that which causes scrapie in sheep. The prion of scrapie, and of kuru and Creutzfeldt–Jakob disease (Section 17.15.1), clearly replicate, and can be transmitted between animals, but so far it has not been possible to induce the histological changes of Alzheimer's disease in animals after inoculations with brains of patients with Alzheimer's disease. Furthermore, amyloid plaques differ in molecular weight, amino-acid composition, and amino-acid sequences from the fibrils associated with scrapie.

Other suggested hypotheses for the cause of Alzheimer's disease have included an environmental toxin, stimulated by the occurrence of dementia in patients with renal failure dialysed in areas in which the water used for the dialysate has a high aluminium content. However, although neurofibrillary tangles can be produced in animals by the intracerebral injection of aluminium salts, they are different from the tangles of Alzheimer's disease. Although aluminium can be identified at the core of senile plaques, this probably represents no more than the abnormal accumulation of the metal in association with damaged cytoskeletal elements. One recent study has shown a slowing in the rate of progress of dementia by the use of the ion-specific chelating agent desferrioxamine. However, the study was not double blind, and, even if the results are confirmed, the effect could be due to other actions such as inhibition of free radical formations.

Head injury has also been implicated as a possible cause for Alzheimer's disease. Case–control studies show an increased incidence of prior head trauma. Histological examination of brains soon after cranial injury shows β-amyloid deposits even in young people, though the distribution of these is not that seen, in Alzheimer's disease.

One hypothesis that ties many observations together is the suggestion that APP cleavage products containing amyloid β-protein are neurotoxic and lead to cell death, possibly by rendering neurons more sensitive to calcium-mediated damage, possibly by phosphorylation of the tau protein. By this hypothesis, a number of factors—genetic, infective, or toxic, could precipitate β-amyloid deposition.

11.5.1.5   Prognosis and treatment of Alzheimer's disease

It is difficult to obtain reliable figures for life expectancy of Alzheimer's disease as symptoms are of such insidious onset. The enrolment of a large panel of healthy older people who will be followed prospectively offers the prospect of much better epidemiological information in the future. However, one recent study on demented patients seen in outpatient practice showed that the three-year survival rate for patients with Alzheimer's disease was just under 70 per cent, compared to 84 per cent for control non-demented patients attending the same geriatric assessment centre. Median survival in one cohort study was 9.3 years from onset of symptoms and 5.3 years from time of first evaluation. Patients with psychotic or extrapyramidal features soon after onset have a distinctly worse prognosis, as do those who wander or who have repeated falls or who have behavioural problems at the time of evaluation, all factors probably representing the extent of neuronal loss at this time. Much of the increased mortality appears to be due to associated physical incapacity. After admission to institutional care, however, 50 per cent of demented patients will be dead within 6 months, and 90 per cent within 2 years. Patients in the last stages of the disease are mute, bed-fast, and incontinent, and may be fixed in a flexed posture with rigid limbs.

The general care of the dementing patient is considered in Section 11.7. Specific treatment has included attempts to correct the defect in cholinergic mechanisms by administering precursors of acetylcholine, such as lecithin or choline, without benefit. Short-term experiments with physostigmine underline the importance of cholinergic mechanisms in memory, as this drug improves recall in normal subjects, and reverses impairment of memory induced artificially by scopolamine. It also increases regional cerebral blood flow in patients with Alzheimer's disease, but not in control patients. Tetrahydroaminoacridine, a centrally acting anticholinesterase inhibitor, with or without the addition of lecithin, has been shown to be ineffective in recent trials, despite initial promise. Other pharmacological leads include the demonstrated short-term effects on memory of vasopressin and of procaine. Of the drugs at present marketed for the treatment of dementia, physicians remain sceptical of the benefits of piracetam, a cyclic derivative of γ-aminobutyric acid. In 1984, Hydergine (a proprietary brand of ergoloid mesylates) was the eleventh most commonly prescribed drug in the world, as early, largely unsatisfactory, trials showed apparent evidence of benefit. However, a recent, carefully controlled, double-blind trial failed to show any evidence of benefit. There is, therefore, no good evidence at present of any specific beneficial effect of any drug upon Alzheimer's disease. Potential interventions include, in theory, the use of inhibitors of the proteases that break down APP at the abnormal site.

11.5.2 *Parkinson's disease*

There is no doubt that some patients with Parkinson's disease become demented, but the number is not as great as previously thought. The main reason for earlier overestimates is the confusion of 'arteriosclerotic parkinsonism' (Section 10.1.11.3) with the true illness. The former is due to multiple bilateral lacunar infarctions, and is associated with multi-infarct dementia (Section 11.5.5). True parkinsonian dementia is presumably associated in some way with the widespread loss of dopaminergic neurons but, as Alzheimer's disease and Parkinson's disease are both so frequent in the elderly population, some patients may have both. Finally, as depression is a frequent association with Parkinson's disease, doctors must be careful to avoid overlooking a depressive pseudodementia in those patients. When all these factors are taken into account, probably only about 10–15 per cent of patients with true Parkinson's disease become demented.

11.5.3 *Diffuse Lewy body disease*

Diffuse Lewy body disease is an entity in which rounded eosinophilic inclusion bodies (Lewy bodies) are found within the brain-stem nuclei and throughout the cerebral cortex. It is characteristic of this syndrome that cognitive function may fluctuate markedly in the early stages of the disease, often resulting in a diagnosis of multi-infarct dementia. Either an extrapyramidal syndrome may precede dementia, or dementia precede an extrapyramidal Parkinson-like syndrome. Diffuse Lewy body disease may therefore be a significant cause of dementia in those usually regarded as having idiopathic Parkinson's disease.

11.5.4 *Rarer 'degenerative' disorders*

The dementias associated with Huntington's disease (Section 13.6.2.2), progressive supranuclear palsy (Section 13.4), and multiple sclerosis (Section 14.3.4.) are discussed elsewhere. *Pick's disease* shares many clinical features with Alzheimer's disease, but changes in personality and aberrant behaviour occur rather earlier in the course of the illness. Atrophy of the brain affects the frontal and temporal lobes, rather than, as in Alzheimer's disease, primarily the parietal lobes. The histological findings, however, are quite distinct. Neurons inflated with an abundance of cytoplasm are seen. Pyramidal neurons lose their dendrites. Many cells show dense intracellular structures known as Pick bodies, constituted of neurotubules and neurofilaments. The cause of Pick's disease is unknown.

11.5.5   *Multi-infarct dementia*

A cortical infarct (Section 10.12) due to occlusion of, for example, an internal carotid artery, may result in hemiplegia and focal deficits such as aphasia, without important degrees of cognitive impairment, until the mass of infarcted tissue exceeds about 50 ml. A lacunar infarction (Section 10.12) may result in a pure hemiplegia, again without significant cognitive impairment. However, repetitive infarctions, particularly lacunar infarctions, do cause an accumulation of physical and cognitive deficits, and very often the latter predominate. Because of the frequency of vascular disease, multi-infarct dementia is the second commonest cause of dementia. Table 11.8 lists those features noted by Hachinski and his colleagues to

Table 11.8   Hachinski score for dementia

Abrupt onset	2
Fluctuating course	2
History of strokes	2
Focal neurological symptoms	2
Focal neurological signs	2
History of hypertension	1
Evidence of associated atherosclerosis	1
Stepwise deterioration	1
Nocturnal confusion	1
Relative preservation of personality	1
Depression	1
Somatic complaints	1
Emotional incontinence	1

If points total more than 7, the patient is likely to have multi-infarct dementia; if less than 4, Alzheimer's disease.

distinguish between Alzheimer's disease and multi-infarct dementia. However, prospective studies supported by post-mortem examination have shown that multi-infarct dementia is often misdiagnosed as Alzheimer's disease, even in the presence of a moderately high Hachinski score.

Many patients with multi-infarct dementia show a constellation of neurological signs, which makes reference to a Hachinski score unnecessary. The bilateral lacunar infarctions result in bilateral pyramidal lesions which induce a shuffling short-stepped gait, often known as *marche à petit pas* (Section 10.1.11.3). There may be an apraxia of truncal movements so that the patient has difficulty in organizing his body into a chair or out of bed, even in the absence of overt muscular weakness. There may be some degree of dysarthria. This clinical syndrome is quite distinct from, though vaguely reminiscent of, the difficulties experienced by people with Parkinson's disease, and for some time confusion reigned as the diagnosis of 'arteriosclerotic Parkinson's disease' was made. The lack of response of such patients to L-dopa clearly distinguishes the two clinical syndromes.

Other clinical features of those with multi-lacunar infarctions, not all of whom are demented, include inappropriate weeping or laughter, often stimulated by trivial events such as a sentimental movie on the television. This results from the release of primitive brain-stem reflexes (an anencephalic baby can cry). Other primitive reflexes, such as a pout or sucking reflex, or a brisk jaw jerk (Section 10.1.11.3) may be found. There may also be a palmomental reflex (Section 6.1.5).

Cerebral blood-flow studies associated with positron emission tomography (Section 8.10.5) have shown that there is a decline in cerebral blood flow and metabolism in patients with both Alzheimer's disease and multi-infarct dementia. However, there is no increase in the oxygen extraction ratio in those with multi-infarct dementia, supporting the view that the dementia is due to infarction, and not to chronic hypoperfusion through arteriosclerotic arteries. This supports the clinical experience that the so-called cerebral vasodilators such as cyclandelate have no place in the management of this illness. All that can be done is to treat appropriately any associated hypertension, diabetes, or cardiac disease, and help the patient and his family in the manner outlined in Section 11.7.

11.5.5.1   *Other vascular causes of dementia*

Some patients who survive a subarachnoid haemorrhage are left demented. This is particularly likely if a bleeding aneurysm lies on the anterior communicating artery, so that its rupture destroys the adjacent medial parts of both frontal lobes. Another mechanism is the clogging of arachnoid villi by degenerating red cells, which may result in a communicating hydrocephalus (Section 11.5.9). Other rare vascular causes of dementia include cranial arteritis and arteritis in association with collagen diseases.

11.5.6   Traumatic dementia

Patients who survive severe closed head injuries, usually sustained in road traffic accidents or in construction work, form by far the largest number of younger demented patients. Unfavourable prognostic features for recovery of cognitive function after trauma include older age, and a prolonged period of post-traumatic amnesia. In addition to defects in cognitive function, irritability and social disinhibition are important factors. The dementia of such patients may advance with increasing age on account of increasing neuronal loss. There is also evidence of β-amyloid deposition (Section 11.5.1.4). Some patients may develop super-added communicating hydrocephalus (Section 11.5.9).

Repeated cranial trauma is sustained by boxers, at whatever level of skill. Impairment of memory and cognitive function is often then accompanied by dysarthria, unsteadiness and, in severe cases, an extrapyramidal syndrome. Rupture of the septum pellucidum and degeneration of the fornices and mamillary bodies are frequent findings at autopsy. Even relatively minor cranial injuries may, if repeated, result in impairment of intellect and memory, as shown by a study on jockeys (Section 15.8.2).

After a head injury, blood may slowly collect in the subdural space, and the resulting subdural haematoma may result in significant distortion of the intracranial contents, with fluctuating confusion, irritability, and impaired memory (Section 15.6). This can readily be confused with a irreversible dementia, particularly if, as is often the case in older people, the rupture of subdural veins from which the haematoma forms occurs without a history of any significant head injury.

11.5.7   Intracranial tumours causing dementia

Intracranial tumours are particularly likely to cause a dementia if they arise in or adjacent to the frontal lobes, and if they are large. Meningiomas arising from the sphenoidal wing, olfactory groove, or frontal convexity, and gliomas of the anterior corpus callosum are particularly likely to present in this way. A tumour in or adjacent to the third ventricle may produce a predominantly amnesic syndrome that may be mistaken for dementia.

11.5.8   Infective causes

Dementia due to the HIV virus and to the acquired immunodeficiency syndrome (AIDS), unconventional viruses such as the Creutzfeldt–Jakob agent, syphilis ('general paralysis of the insane'), and chronic fungal and chronic viral infections such as subacute sclerosing panencephalitis are considered in Chapter 17. Dementia due to delayed or inadequate treatment of meningococcal, pneumococcal, and tuberculous meningitis occurs particularly in Third World countries. Dementia may also follow herpes encephalitis (Section 17.12.3).

11.5.9   Hydrostatic causes

Obstructive hydrocephalus in childhood is associated with mental retardation. In adult life a new obstruction—caused by, for example, a colloid cyst of the third ventricle—can occasionally cause dementia without focal signs. Sometimes a previously compensated hydrocephalus, such as may be caused by stenosis of the aqueduct, becomes decompensated, the intracranial pressure rises, and mental impairment follows. Usually, however, the presence of headache, drowsiness, vomiting, and unsteadiness in these examples draws attention to the need for neurosurgical investigation.

Much more difficult to elucidate, however, is so-called normal pressure (communicating) hydrocephalus which, although not common, is important to recognize as it is potentially reversible. In these circumstances there is a defect in absorption of cerebrospinal fluid due to meningeal thickening at the base of the brain, or in the cortical channels over the convexity, and around the arachnoid villi. These changes follow subarachnoid haemorrhage, head injury, or meningitis. The ventricles dilate, but the pressure within them is only intermittently high. The clinical syndrome is characterized by ataxia of gait, intermittent incontinence, and impairment of cognitive function. Some patients develop a similar clinical picture and ventricular dilatation without evidence of any predisposing cause.

Shunting the dilated ventricles with an appropriate low-pressure valve to the peritoneum or left atrium may result in a dramatic improvement in cognitive function, continence, and gait. However, the selection of suitable patients remains difficult, as no single method of investigation reliably predicts those who are likely to improve.

11.5.10   Toxic and metabolic causes

11.5.10.1   Toxic causes

The commonest toxic cause of dementia is *alcohol* which, taken in excess over years, does produce a mild dementia. In many patients with alcoholism, the dementia is due, at least in part, to repeated head injuries while drunk, and the possibility of a subdural haematoma complicating the issue must be borne in mind. In others, the picture is complicated by hepatic encephalopathy. It may be that alcohol itself produces specific changes in cholinergic neurons as are found in Alzheimer's disease (Section 11.5.1.2). On this hypothesis, alcoholic dementia and Korsakoff's psychosis, an amnesic syndrome associated with alcohol and thiamine deficiency (Section 23.4.2.4), are more closely related than previously thought. Some alcoholics may also develop dementia due to demyelination of the corpus callosum and other areas of central white matter—the Marchiafava–Bignami syndrome.

Intoxication with some *heavy metals*, such as manganese, lead, and mercury, may produce some degree of intellectual impairment, though only manganese does this to any significant extent. Interest in metallic intoxication has recently centred on the probability that a dementia associated with chronic renal dialysis was associated with high levels of aluminium in the dialysate. Since deionized water has been used to make up the dialysate, the incidence of dialysis dementia has fallen markedly.

Drug intoxication is an important cause of organic confusional states (Table 11.4). Stopping the administration of barbiturates may not, however, necessarily reverse a dementia that seems to have been induced by their injudicious long-term use. Indeed, it can be said that the first stage of the investigation of any demented older patient is to stop all medication, if possible, and review the situation after a few weeks.

11.5.10.2   Metabolic causes

Hypothyroidism is an important treatable cause of dementia, though it seldom presents in this way. Severe hypothyroidism can also result in a psychotic state with hallucinations and paranoia—'myxoedema madness'. Occasionally *hyperthyroidism* in the elderly may present in the so-called apathetic form, with prominent psychomotor retardation.

Deficiency of vitamin B$_{12}$ may present to neurologists as a neuropathy or as a cord lesion (Section 23.2.4.4), and occasionally as a dementia. Any of these syndromes may precede overt anaemia, but macrocytosis will be apparent. *Deficiency of folate* has also been reported to cause a dementing illness in the elderly, and replacement of folic acid may, at least in part, reverse this. *Deficiency of thiamine* produces the amnesic syndrome of Wernicke–Korsakoff (Section 23.4.2.4), rather than a global dementia. The mental changes of *hepatic and renal failure* and of *porphyria* and *hyponatraemia* present more often as confusional states. *Remote effects of some malignancies*—particularly oat cell carcinoma of the bronchus—may cause a rapidly advancing dementia distinct from any effects mediated through hyponatraemia in association with inappropriate secretion of antidiuretic hormone. Characteristically, the patient is particularly anxious, depressed, or disturbed, in addition to being amnesic or demented. Histological examination shows loss of neurons and perivascular inflammatory infiltrates, most marked in the medial temporal areas. It is not certain whether these changes are metabolic, or induced by reactivation of a dormant virus by immunological changes associated with the tumour. The latter seems more likely as the syndrome is not reversed by removal of the tumour.

11.5.11   Anoxic causes

Patients who just survive a cardiac arrest may persist in a persistent vegetative state (Section 7.3.1) or may survive with a substantial degree of dementia, sometimes associated with myoclonus. Dementia following partial recovery from carbon monoxide poisoning is particularly likely to be associated with extrapyramidal signs.

11.6 The investigation of the patient with dementia

The great majority of older demented patients in clinical practice will have Alzheimer's disease, multi-infarct dementia, or an immediately recognized cause, such as dementia following head injury or cardiac arrest. Some will become demented as part of some already recognized neurological illness, such as Parkinson's disease. Investigation should be directed towards the recognition of potentially treatable causes of dementia and, within economic limits, sufficient categorization of the exact type of non-treatable dementia.

The first step, undoubtedly, is to review all drug medication, in case the patient is chronically intoxicated by unnecessary polypharmacy (Table 11.4).

The next step is to arrange for investigations that are sufficiently easy to perform and cheap that every demented patient ought to have them performed, as it would be intolerable to overlook an easily treatable cause (Table 11.9). Tests of thyroid

Table 11.9 Investigation of dementia

1. For nearly all patients
    full blood count, ESR
    B_{12}, folate
    thyroid function tests
    liver function tests
    calcium, urea
    VDRL
    chest X-ray

2. For many patients
    HIV titre
    cranial CT scan

3. For occasional patients
    electroencephalography
    isotope scan or cisternogram
    lumbar puncture

and liver function, and estimations of haemoglobin, serum B_{12}, calcium, urea, erythrocyte sedimentation rate, and a VDRL test fall into this group. A chest X-ray may demonstrate a relevant neoplasm of the bronchus or secondary deposits. Younger patients will require testing for human immunodeficiency virus. Lumbar puncture seldom

adds any useful information unless a chronic fungal or other unusual meningeal infection is suspected.

The final step should be to consider what specialized investigations are appropriate, bearing in mind the age of the patient, and suspicions raised by clinical examination. For example, most would agree that it would not be appropriate to scan a chronically demented 90-year-old patient. On the other hand, a cranial CT scan or MRI is a crucial investigation in the analysis of dementias due to hydrostatic causes, and in the investigation of tumours and suspected subdural haematomas. Some subdural haematomas can be difficult to image on CT scanning as they may have the same Hounsfield number as underlying brain. An isotope scan may be useful in this particular circumstance, showing increased uptake of isotope over the haematoma. In richer societies, CT scanning will be used more often to demonstrate to patients' relatives that all possible has been done. Electroencephalography is usually of little help, except in the analysis of patients with Creutzfeldt–Jakob disease, or subacute sclerosing panencephalitis, when characteristic periodic complexes occur, or in hepatic encephalopathy, with its typical triphasic frontal slow waves.

Of all patients investigated, those that cause the most anxiety are those with ventricular dilatation, without wide cortical sulci, who might conceivably have communicating hydrocephalus (Fig. 11.2c,d). A number of investigations have been suggested that might predict reliably those who would benefit from ventriculo-peritoneal or ventriculo-atrial shunting. One is the injection of radio-iodinated human serum albumin into the lumbar subarachnoid space, subsequently tracking the isotope into the skull. In the normal subject, or in a patient with Alzheimer's disease, the isotope rapidly rises towards the vertex, and is absorbed through the arachnoid villi. In patients with communicating hydrocephalus, the isotope diffuses into the ventricles, and remains there for the next 2–3 days. Another test is to measure the rate of absorption of cerebrospinal fluid by infusion of Ringer's–lactate solution at a rate such that the pressure remains constant. It has been shown that if the outflow resistance is less than 11 mmHg/ml/min, then the patient is unlikely to benefit from shunting. Others have monitored intracranial pressure by the insertion of extradural monitors. In the final analysis, however, the decision to operate rests upon the presence of the clinical triad of dementia, disturbance of gait, and incontinence. The results of shunting are better in those who have a defined cause for ventricular enlargement, such as previous subarachnoid haemorrhage, than in those in whom the hydrocephalus has arisen without any known preceding event. It must be remembered that the insertion of a shunt is by no means a benign procedure. Complications such as shunt infection, subdural haematoma, and epilepsy occur in about one-third of patients.

11.7   The general care of the dementing patient

The previous sections of this chapter have indicated those causes of dementia for which specific treatment is needed. For the vast majority, only care and support is available. A quiet domestic life—getting dressed, eating, simple expeditions with other members of the family, and sitting in front of the television set—can continue for some time as long as a caring spouse is available at home to organize the infrastructure of the household. Depression may coexist with Alzheimer's disease, and some benefit in the early stages may result from treating this, often with monoamine oxidase inhibitors, as tricyclic antidepressants may add to confusion.

As apathy and social disorganization increase, a spouse is increasingly unable to take the patient out, and the house becomes a prison for both. By this stage the carer will certainly be requiring increasing support from other members of the family, and from social and voluntary agencies. Avenues that should be explored include getting the patient to a day centre, arranging a roster of 'granny-sitters', or brief admission to hospital so that the carer can have a well-earned rest. Appropriate financial support, such as the Attendance Allowance (Section 26.9) should be mobilized. The relatives of those with Alzheimer's disease often value being put in touch with an Alzheimer's Disease Society. Attention should be given to physical safety within the home, particularly in regard to gas (left on, but unlit), and open front doors which may allow distressing wanderings. Dementing patients may resist their relatives' wishes, and be aggressive towards a previously loved spouse. The situation may be made easier

for all by the judicious use of a phenothiazine, such as thioridazine or chlorpromazine. If begun in small doses, say 10–25 mg of chlorpromazine or 25–50 mg of thioridazine, and the dose titrated against the response, there may be a useful suppressant of agitation and other behavioural disturbance without undue drowsiness. Haloperidol, at first sight an attractive alternative, very frequently produces an extrapyramidal syndrome in elderly people. Benzodiazepines and barbiturates should certainly be avoided as they will almost certainly precipitate further confusion.

Many elderly people cannot cope with the advanced stages of their spouse's illness, and hospital or hospice care is then required. Unfortunately the protracted nature of the illness and the extent of support required may lead to exhaustion of financial savings carefully tended for a lifetime, and this, and the strains within different generations of a family caring for a demented patient, may exacerbate family feuds.

In late stages of the illness, difficult ethical decisions need to be made about how much pharmacological and nutritional support should be given to a patient whose life is, in any event, so limited.

11.8   Further reading

General reviews

Cummings, J. L. (ed.) (1990). *Subcortical dementia.* Oxford University Press, New York.

Wurtzman, R. J., Corkin, S., Ritter-Walker, E., and Growdon, J. H. (eds) (1990). *Alzheimer's disease. Advances in Neurology*, Vol. 51. Raven Press, New York.

Epidemiology of dementia

Berg, L. (1985). Does Alzheimer's disease represent an exaggeration of normal aging? *Archives of Neurology* **42**, 737–9.

Brayne, C. and Calloway, P. (1988). Normal ageing, impaired cognitive function and senile dementia of the Alzheimer's type: a continuum. *Lancet* **1**, 1265–6.

Evans, D. A., Funkenstein, H., Albert, M. S., *et al.* (1989). Prevalence of Alzheimer's disease in a community population of older persons: higher than previously reported. *Journal of the American Medical Association* **262**, 2551–6.

Galasko, D., Klauber, M. R., Hofstetter, R., *et al.*

(1990). The mini-mental state examination in the early diagnosis of dementia. *Archives of Neurology* **47**, 49–52.

Hodkinson, M. M. and Quereschi, A. N. (1974). Evaluation of a ten question mental test in the institutionalized elderly. *Age and Ageing* **3**, 152–7.

Katzman, R., Aronson, M., Fuld, P., *et al.* (1989). Development of dementing illnesses in an 80-year-old volunteer cohort. *Annals of Neurology* **25** 317–24.

O'Brien, J. T. and Levy, R. (1992). Age associated memory impairment. *British Medical Journal* **304**, 5–6.

Royal College of Physicians (1981). A report of the Royal College of Physicians by the College Committee on Geriatrics. Organic mental impairment in the elderly. Implications for research, education and the provision of services. *Journal of the Royal College of Physicians of London* **15**, 141–68.

Differential diagnosis

Arie, T. (1983). Pseudodementia. *British Medical Journal* **286**, 1301–2.

Burns, A., Luthert, P., and Levy, R. (1990). Accuracy of clinical diagnosis of Alzheimer's disease. *British Medical Journal* **301**: 1206.

Byrne, E. J., Lennox, G., Lowe, J., and Godwin-Austen, R. B. (1989). Diffuse Lewy body disease: clinical features in 15 cases. *Journal of Neurology, Neurosurgery and Psychiatry* **52**, 709–17.

Homer, A. C., Honavar, M., Lantos, P. L., *et al.* (1988). Diagnosing dementia: do we get it right? *British Medical Journal* **297**, 892–6.

MRC (UK) Alzheimer's disease Workshop Steering Committee (1989). Recommended minimum data to be collected on research studies on Alzheimer's disease. *Journal of Neurology, Neurosurgery and Psychiatry* **52**, 693–700.

Mulley, G. P. (1986). Differential diagnosis of dementia. *British Medical Journal* **292**, 1416–18.

Genetics

Goate, A. M., Chartier-Harlin, M. C., Mullan, M., *et al.* (1991). A missense mutation in the amyloid precursor protein gene segregates with familial Alzheimer's disease. *Nature* **349**, 704–6.

Harrison, P. J. (1991). Alzheimer's disease and the β amyloid gene. *British Medical Journal* **302**, 1478–9.

Types of dementia

Cummings, J. L. and Benson, D. F. (1984). Subcortical dementia; review of an emerging concept. *Archives of Neurology* **41**, 874–9.

Hachinski, V. C., Illif, L. D., Zipkha, E., *et al.* (1975). Cerebral blood flow in dementia. *Archives of Neurology* **32**, 632–7.

Whitehouse, P. J. (1986). The concept of subcortical and cortical dementia: another look. *Annals of Neurology* **19**, 1–6.

Causes of dementia

Calne, D. B., Eisen, A., McGeer, E., and Spencer, P. (1986). Alzheimer's disease, Parkinson's disease and motor neurone disease: abiotrophic interaction between ageing and environment? *Lancet* **2**, 1067–70.

Crapper McLaclan, D. R., Dalton, A. J., Kruck, T. P. A., Bell, M. Y., Smith, W. L., Kalow, W., and Andrews, D. F. (1991). Intramuscular desferrioxamine in patients with Alzheimer's disease. *Lancet* **337**, 1304–8.

Editorial (1990). Normal pressure hydrocephalus. *Lancet* **1**, 22.

Evenhuis, H. M. (1990). The natural history of dementia in Down's syndrome. *Archives of Neurology* **47**, 263–7.

Hardy, J. A. and Higgins, G. A. (1992). Alzheimer's disease: the amyloid cascade hypothesis. *Science* **256**, 184–5.

Lishman, W. A. (1986). Alcoholic dementia: a hypothesis. *Lancet* **314**, 1101–11.

Navaratnam, D. S., Priddle, J. D., McDonald, B., Esiri, M. M., Robinson, J. R., and Smith, A. D. (1991). Anomalous molecular form of acetylcholine esterase in cerebrospinal fluid in histologically diagnosed Alzheimer's disease. *Lancet* **337**, 447–50.

Roberts, G. W., Gentleman, S. M., Lynch, A. and Graham, D. I. (1991). βA4 amyloid protein deposition in brain after head trauma. *Lancet* **338**, 1422–3.

Sherrard, D. J. (1991). Aluminium—much ado about something. *New England Journal of Medicine*. **324**, 558—9.

Vascular dementia. A series of short papers in *Archives of Neurology* (1988) **45**, 497–801.

Yanknere, B. A. and Marsel-Mesulam, M., (1991) β-amyloid and the pathogenesis of Alzheimer's disease. *New England Journal of Medicine* **325**, 1849–57.

Treatment of dementia

Byrne, E. J. and Arie, T. (1990). Are drugs targeted at Alzheimer's disease useful? 2. Insufficient evidence of worthwhile benefit. *British Medical Journal* **300**, 1132–3.

Gauthier, S., Bouchard, R., Lamontagne, A., *et al.* (1990). Tetrahydroaminoacridine-lecithin combination treatment in patients with intermediate stage Alzheimer's disease. *New England Journal of Medicine* **322**, 1272–6.

Levy, R. (1990). Are drugs targeted at Alzheimer's disease useful? 1. Useful for what? *British Medical Journal* **300**, 1131–2.

Thompson, T. L., Filley, C. M., Mitchell, W. D., *et al.* (1990). Lack of efficacy of hydergine in patients with Alzheimer's disease. *New England Journal of Medicine* **323**, 445–8.

Prognosis

Drachman, D. A., O'Donnell, B. F., Law, R. A., and Swearer, J. M. (1990). The prognosis in Alzheimer's disease: 'how far' rather than 'how fast' best predicts course. *Archives of Neurology* **47** 851–6.

Martin, D. C., Miller, J. K., Kapvor, W., *et al.* (1987). A controlled study of survival with dementia. *Archives of Neurology* **44**, 1122–26.

Stern, Y., Hesdorffer, D., Sano, M., and Mayeux, R. (1990). Measurement and prediction of functional capacity in Alzheimer's disease. *Neurology* **40**, 8–14.

Walsh, J. S., Welch, H. G., and Larson, E. B. (1990). Survival of outpatients with Alzheimer's-type dementia. *Annals of Internal Medicine* **113**, 429–34.

Care of patients with dementia

Curran, W. J. (1985). Defining appropriate medical care: providing nutrients and hydration for the dying. *New England Journal of Medicine* **313**, 940–2.

Emanuel, E. J. (1988). Should physicians withhold life-sustaining care from patients who are not terminally ill? *Lancet* **1**, 106–8.

Mace, N. L. (ed.) (1990). Dementia care: patient, family and community. Johns Hopkins University Press, Baltimore.

Mace, N. L. and Rabins, P. V. (1985). The 36-hour day, (adapted for the UK by B. A. Castleton, C. Cloke, and E. McEwen). Edward Arnold, London.

Miner, G. D., Winters-Miner, A., Blass, J. P., Richter, R. W., and Valentine, J. L. (ed.) (1989). *Caring for Alzheimer's patients: a guide for family and health care providers*. Plenum Press New York.

12 Epilepsy

12.1   Definitions

An *epileptic seizure* may be defined as *a paroxysmal discharge of cerebral neurons sufficient to cause clinically detectable events that are apparent either to the subject or an observer*. This definition is designed to exclude clinical events such as a transient hemiparesis caused by depression of neuronal activity resulting from, for example, migraine or ischaemia.

Events resulting from a paroxysmal neuronal discharge may be apparent only to the subject, as in some distorted perception resulting from a seizure beginning in the mesial temporal lobe. Alternatively, events may be apparent only to the observer, for example someone who has a generalized convulsion during sleep may have no recollection of the event whatsoever.

The use of the words '*clinically detectable*' in the foregoing definition is necessary so that paroxysmal discharges in the electroencephalogram (EEG), without clinical concomitants, are not called seizures. There are difficulties here, however, as sophisticated analysis of performance shows that cognitive function is impaired during brief seizure discharges, even though such events are not detectable by usual clinical observation.

The adjective '*epileptic*' also causes some difficulty. Febrile convulsions, considered in Section 12.11, are certainly seizures, but as they are not usually followed by epileptic attacks in adult life, it is helpful to distinguish them clearly from epileptic seizures. Many observers also maintain that the first seizure should not be considered as epileptic. However, as the majority of initial seizures are followed by others, this is a rather arbitrary exclusion. Finally, anoxic seizures, considered in Section 12.7.1, are clearly not epileptic.

Epilepsy itself is best defined as *a condition in which more than one non-febrile seizure of any type has occurred*. This rather begs the question of when someone stops being an epileptic, having had, for example, three or four seizures in adolescence. It is clearly not very fruitful to refer to someone as 'an epileptic' if he has not had an attack for two or three decades. However, such a subject may have a further attack after a long interval when some provoking event occurs, for example the prescription of amitriptyline, an epileptogenic agent, for a mid-life depression.

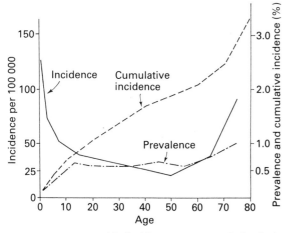

Fig. 12.1 Age-specific incidence rate, cumulative incidence rate, and prevalence rate of epilepsy (data from Rochester, Minnesota. (Reproduced by kind permission from Hauser *et al* 1983.)

A convenient way of looking at the problem is to think in terms of a seizure threshold, which tends to be low between the ages of about 18 months and 4 years, allowing febrile convulsions to break through. Later in life, a subject with a lower than average seizure threshold may have a seizure provoked by an external agent, such as amitriptyline or alcohol, and is more likely to have a seizure following cranial trauma than someone with a higher seizure threshold.

In older life, areas of minor cortical damage due to ischaemic events, or more diffuse cortical damage in the case of dementing illnesses, become fairly frequent, and the incidence of new cases of epilepsy is higher in the last two decades of life than it is in mid-life.

12.2   Incidence and prevalence

The incidence and prevalence of epilepsy is best summed up in Fig. 12.1. This shows a higher annual incidence at the extremes of life. The prevalence of epilepsy at different ages is a reflection of the balance between the age at onset and the duration of illness before remission, or, in a few cases, death. The prevalence is more or less steady through the greater part of life, at about 0.6–0.7 per cent. This prevalence figure is based upon an assessment of those patients who have had at least two non-febrile seizures in the past 2 years, or who are on anticonvulsants for previous seizures.

The most interesting curve in Fig 12.1. is the *cumulative* incidence rate of epilepsy—that is to say the number of subjects who, at *any* time in their life, have had more than one non-febrile seizure. On this basis, a lifetime (cumulative) incidence of *ever* having been considered as an epileptic is as high as 3.2 per cent. It has been shown, by the same workers whose results are illustrated in Fig. 12.1, that nearly 6 per cent of the total population may be expected to experience at least one non-febrile seizure in their lifetime.

It is useful to remember these high figures for incidence when patients are urgently referred for consideration of their initial seizure. Epilepsy is not a rare or unusual condition. Seizures involve one or more members of many families.

Most studies record a slight excess of males with epilepsy. Epilepsy is more likely to occur in economically deprived groups, possibly because of the greater incidence of pre-term birth, and of subsequent occupational cranial trauma. Epilepsy is also proportionately more frequent in the elderly, secondary to vascular disease and Alzheimer's disease.

12.3 Pathophysiology

Substances such as strychnine and penicillin applied to the cortex produce epilepsy in experimental animals, and much of our understanding of the pathophysiology of epilepsy comes from such observations. In recent years, interest has shifted from experiments on intact animals to cortical brain slices.

Neurons exposed to convulsant agents such as penicillin or picrotoxin discharge with brief rapid bursts of action potentials, arising from abrupt,

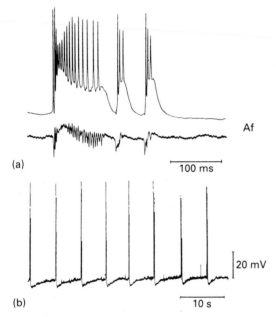

(a)

100 ms

(b)

10 s

20 mV

Fig. 12.2 Intracellular recording of a brain slice made 'epileptic' by adding picrotoxin to the bathing solution. Note the massive depolarization shift, which triggers a burst of high-frequency action potentials (a) Neurons in epileptic tissue are abnormally synchronous, as revealed by the simultaneous extracellular field recording (Af). The slower time-base (b) shows that each paroxysmal depolarization shift terminates in a hyperpolarization. (Figure provided by courtesy of J. G. R. Jefferys.)

large depolarizations on the resting membrane potential, known as paroxysmal depolarization shifts (Fig. 12.2). It is possible to induce such changes by disrupting inhibition with antagonists to the inhibitory transmitter, γ-aminobutyric acid, such as picrotoxin and bicuculline. However, a burst discharge pattern in individual neurons does not constitute epileptic activity; it is necessary that the discharges of many neurons be synchronized to generate the electro-encephalographic and clinical features of a seizure. It is possible to show in brain slices, and also in computer models, that synchronization can occur if powerful monosynaptic divergent pathways go from neuron to neuron. There may well be other mechanisms of synchronization, such as non-synaptic electric field effects, and the diffuse effects of changes in extracellular ion concentrations.

In addition to models of acute epilepsy, caused by the topical application of a drug such as bicuculline, experiments have also been carried out on chronic partial epilepsies. For example, a small dose of tetanus toxin injected into the rat hippocampus will result in chronically recurring generalized seizures. Brain slices of the injected hippocampus can be examined. Of interest during the past few years has been the phenomenon known as kindling, a progressive reduction in seizure threshold resulting from repeated stimulation. A typical kindling stimulus, for example, to the amygdala initially causes little or no response from the animal. As the stimulus is repeated every few hours to days, the response increases progressively through local myoclonus to partial and then to generalized seizures. Whether this is due to the prolonged enhancement of synaptic efficacy known as long-term potentiation is not clear, and, in any event, it is not certain whether kindling occurs in the human brain.

There are, of course, structural changes in many chronic epileptic foci, both in experimental animals and in humans. It is possible that some seizures arise from the selective loss of inhibitory neurons. Many of the surviving neurons in chronic epileptogenic lesions have short dendritic spines, receiving fewer than normal synaptic inputs.

Epileptiform discharges are usually spatially limited, partly by surviving inhibitory pathways, and partly by, presumably, changes in external ion concentrations. Seizure discharges may, however, spread through subcortical pathways and to the other hemisphere through commissures, resulting in secondary generalization.

Any model of epilepsy has also to take into account the primary generalized epilepsies, considered in Section 12.4.2. There are some animal models of primary generalized epilepsy—some baboons develop myoclonic seizures after exposure to flashing light, and some strains of mice in response to loud sounds. The genetic transmission of primary epilepsies in humans and in experimental animals suggests a primary metabolic disturbance. Epileptic photosensitivity, both in the baboon and in humans, can be blocked by dopamine agonists.

12.4   Different types of epileptic seizure

During the past 20 years, there have been repeated attempts to classify the different types of epileptic seizures. The full International Classification of Epileptic Seizures extends to many pages, but a simplified classification, based on the framework of the International Classification is presented in Table 12.1.

12.4.1   *Partial (focal, local) seizures*

These are seizures in which the first clinical or EEG changes indicate initial activation of a group of neurons in part of one cerebral hemisphere. With the exception of benign childhood epilepsy with centro-temporal spikes (see Section 12.5), all partial seizures can be considered to arise from a local structural abnormality of the brain. Depending on the area of the brain involved, partial seizures may be motor or sensory. For example, a partial seizure affecting the lower part of the pre-Rolandic motor strip results in jactitation of the contralateral finger and thumb, and the muscles of the contralateral side of the face. As the muscles of the upper part of the face are innervated from each cerebral cortex, there may also be some limited jactitation of the ipsilateral frontalis muscle.

A partial seizure in which consciousness is not disturbed is said to be a simple partial seizure. If there is disturbance of consciousness, so that the subject is unable to comprehend what is going on,

Table 12.1   Classification of epileptic seizures

1. Partial seizures
   A. Simple partial—consciousness not disturbed, e.g. simple motor seizure
   B. Complex partial—consciousness disturbed, e.g. with a sense of distortion of time or reality; such seizures used to be called 'temporal lobe' seizures
   C. Either simple or complex partial seizures may evolve to a secondary generalized tonic–clonic seizure
2. Generalized seizures
   A. Absence seizure—with 3 c/s spike–wave EEG
   B. Primarily generalized tonic–clonic seizure
   C. Other types:
      myoclonic seizures
      tonic seizures
      clonic seizures
      atypical absences
      atonic seizures

or is unable to respond, even if there is not total loss of consciousness, then the seizure is called a complex partial seizure.

A seizure that arises in the mesial part of one temporal lobe may produce, as the initial symptom, some sort of disturbance of special senses and perception. For example, there may be a perception of an unpleasant or distorted smell. There may be complex visual hallucinations, or states in which there is a sense of the distortion of time, of which the phenomenon of *déjà vu* is the best known. Such temporal lobe seizures are particularly likely to be associated with impairment of consciousness. Although not an exact equivalent, in general, patients who were previously described as having temporal lobe epilepsy have, in the modern classification, complex partial seizures.

All partial seizure discharges can spread. A simple partial motor seizure, for example, may spread to contiguous areas of the motor strip, resulting in what is called a march (of clinical events), a so-called Jacksonian seizure. For example, a seizure beginning in the foot area of the left motor strip, perhaps due to a small parasagittal meningioma in that region, may spread from the big toe of the right foot, to the finger and thumb on the same side, and finally to the facial muscles on the same side, resulting in an arrest of

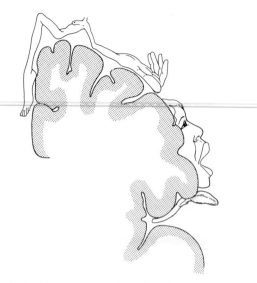

Fig. 12.3 The representation of various parts of the body on a coronal section through the precentral gyrus (redrawn, with permission, from Wilder and Penfield 1950).

speech if, as in this case, the lesion is in the dominant hemisphere. Figure 12.3 illustrates the cortical representation of various parts of the body, from which the reader can visualize how the march may occur.

Any type of partial seizure may evolve to a generalized tonic–clonic (grand mal) seizure. A common clinical story is of a subject who has quite frequent complex partial seizures with phenomena, perhaps, of *déjà vu* and a sense of unreality, and occasional tonic–clonic seizures. Some of these tonic–clonic seizures will be preceded by a warning

along the same lines as the complex partial seizures. Not infrequently, however, the secondary generalization is so abrupt that the initial warning is not experienced.

Partial seizures commonly occur in clusters, with several occurring over a few days, and then perhaps none for several weeks. They are commonly followed by 'neuronal exhaustion'. This is most obvious if the partial seizure has affected the motor strip, when there may be a contralateral hemiparesis lasting for a few minutes to an hour or two. This is known as a Todd's paralysis. Post-ictal aphasia and post-ictal hemianopia are also seen.

12.4.2 *Generalized seizures*

So far, we have considered partial seizures, and partial seizures that may become secondarily generalized. The remaining principal group of seizures is that in which the first clinical or EEG changes indicate initial simultaneous involvement of both hemispheres. Such primary generalized seizures frequently have their onset in childhood or adolescence, and genetic factors are important (see Section 12.6.1).

One such primary generalized seizure is an absence seizure. These are also known as petit mal seizures. The hallmark of a typical absence attack is the sudden interruption of ongoing activities, a blank stare, and possibly some fluttering of the eyelids, or a brief upward rotation of the eyes. If walking, the patient stops in his or her tracks. The attacks are of brief duration, from a few seconds to half a minute or so.

The EEG during a typical absence seizure consists of 3 c/s spike and wave, as seen in Fig. 12.4.

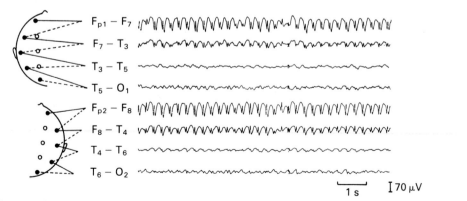

Fig. 12.4 Absence seizure. Typical spike–wave discharge at 3 c/s. (Figure provided by courtesy of Dr H. Luders).

Video-recordings of patients with such seizure discharges have shown that motor behaviour during absence attacks may be more complex than just described. There may be some sort of fumbling with the clothes, or turning of the head, licking of the lips, and some sort of attempt at responding to a command. Visual inspection of the seizure may be insufficient to distinguish such an attack from a seizure arising in one temporal lobe. Simultaneous video- and EEG recording will clarify the point. An example is shown in Fig. 12.5. Many patients with typical absences have also had myoclonic jerks, particularly on waking in the morning. Brief shock-like muscle contractions affect particularly the arms, and may usher in a tonic–clonic seizure.

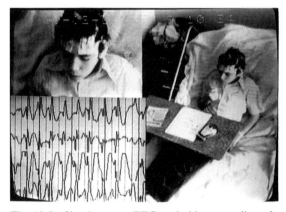

Fig. 12.5 Simultaneous EEG and video-recording of a typical absence seizure. The 3 c/s seizure discharge is best illustrated in the third channel from the top. (Figure provided by courtesy of Dr Fritz Dreifuss.)

It has already been noted (p. 190) that partial seizures may become secondarily generalized. Patients with absence attacks or myoclonic jerks may also have tonic–clonic seizures. Figure 12.6 elaborates on this point. If a young person is seen with a tonic–clonic seizure, unless there is clear clinical evidence of a partial onset, it is impossible to tell whether the tonic–clonic seizure is secondarily generalized from a partial seizure, or whether the tonic–clonic seizure is a manifestation of primary generalized epilepsy. Video-monitoring and electroencephalography usually help to distinguish between the two possibilities.

Other variants of primarily generalized seizures include tonic seizures, clonic seizures, and atonic seizures. In these last, the sudden loss of muscular

Types of epilepsy
a + b = Symptomatic epilepsy
c + = Cryptogenic epilepsy
d + e = Idiopathic epilepsy (primary generalized or constitutional epilepsy)

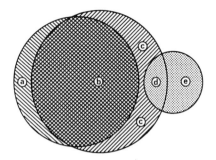

a) Partial seizures alone
b) Partial seizures evolving to tonic–clonic seizures
c) Tonic–clonic seizures of uncertain origin
d) Tonic–clonic seizures in association with
   typical absences
e) Typical absences alone

Fig. 12.6 The relationship between the different types of seizure. The areas of the sets represent very approximately the proportion of patients with different types of epilepsy.

tone may result in the patient dropping objects, and occasionally falling. Some of the most troublesome seizures in childhood are of this type. A child with such seizures may suffer repeated head injuries. Another variant of seizures in childhood is the so-called infantile spasm, or salaam attack. In these episodes, further considered in Section 12.5, there is an abrupt flexion of the head and limbs, the whole seizure lasting only a few seconds. This type of attack occurs in the early months of life.

12.5 Different types of epileptic syndromes ('epilepsies')

During the past 15 years, neurologists have found it helpful not only to distinguish the different types of epileptic seizures, but also different epileptic syndromes, best defined as disorders characterized by clusters of signs and symptoms customarily occurring together. The signs and symptoms may be not only clinical; ancillary investigations such as electroencephalography are invoked in the International Classification of Epilepsies (Table 12.2).

Table 12.2   Classification of epilepsy syndromes

1. Localization-related epilepsies
    A. Idiopathic, e.g. benign focal epilepsy of childhood
    B. Symptomatic, e.g. seizures due to a temporal lobe lesion
2. Generalized epilepsies
    A. Idiopathic, e.g. absence epilepsy of childhood
    B. Sometimes idiopathic, sometimes symptomatic, e.g. infantile spasms, Lennox–Gastaut syndrome
    C. Symptomatic, e.g. epilepsy complicating recessively inherited metabolic disorders of childhood
3. Epilepsies undetermined, whether focal or generalized, e.g. grand mal occurring during sleep, without evidence for more accurate classification
4. Special syndromes
    A. Febrile convulsions
        NB *Although inserted here in the International Classification, most clinicians do not refer to these as 'epileptic' (see Section 12.11)*
    B. Epilepsies characterized by specific modes of precipitation, e.g. photosensitive epilepsy, reading epilepsy
    C. Epilepsies characterized by status-like EEG activity, e.g. epilepsia partialis continua

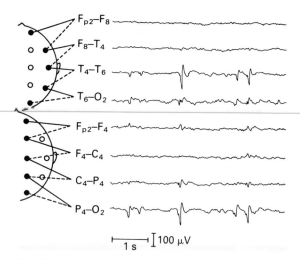

Fig. 12.7   Benign focal epilepsy of childhood. Note the location of spikes over the Rolandic region. (Figure provided by courtesy of Dr H. Luders.)

Most clinicians have found this less useful than the classification of seizures (Table 12.1).

The first heading in the International Classification is 'Localization-related epilepsies and syndromes'. Of these, by far the commonest is the example already given, seizures arising from a structural lesion in, for example, one temporal lobe. There is, however, an important variant in childhood known as benign childhood epilepsy with centro-temporal spikes. In this syndrome, the affected child or teenager has brief simple partial motor seizures, often evolving into tonic–clonic seizures, and often occurring at night. The EEG looks rather somewhat alarming, with high-voltage centro-temporal spikes (see Fig. 12.7), but the prognosis is very good, and such seizures are not associated with structural lesions. Genetic factors are important.

The next heading in the Classification is 'Generalized epilepsies', of which the best-known examples are epilepsies with absence seizures and myoclonic seizures, as mentioned above. Primary generalized seizures may be symptomatic of underlying diffuse encephalopathies, and the infantile spasm mentioned earlier is one such syndrome. For example, infantile spasms may be a manifestation of a severe perinatal anoxic episode, or an inherited disorder such as tuberous sclerosis or of infection with Cytomegalovirus (Section 17.12.9).

An important generalized epilepsy of childhood is the Lennox–Gastaut syndrome. This, like infantile spasms, is a heterogeneous group of disorders with myoclonic seizures, occurring in early childhood, often associated with intellectual deterioration. The EEG is characterized by slow spike–wave discharges. Atonic seizures, falls, and injuries are common. This syndrome probably represents no more than a stereotyped reaction of the immature nervous system to diffuse insults of various cause. Generalized seizures may also be a manifestation of known metabolic disorders, such as the gangliosidoses.

A particular variety of primary generalized epilepsy is known as juvenile myoclonic epilepsy of Janz. Occasional tonic–clonic seizures are associated with matutinal myoclonic jerks. Although seizures are often rare, they may continue throughout life.

The International Classification of Epileptic Syndromes also includes a group of so-called 'special syndromes' under which heading are included seizures precipitated by alcohol, drugs, deprivation of sleep, and the bizarre syndromes in which attacks are precipitated by specific events such as reading, or hearing particular strains of music. The most common variant of these so-called reflex epilepsies are photosensitive epilepsies. Finally, there are two rare syndromes of childhood characterized by continuous epileptiform activity in the EEG—epilepsia partialis continua of childhood (Kojewnikow syndrome) and acquired epileptic aphasia (Landau–Kleffner syndrome).

12.6   The causes and precipitation of seizures

12.6.1   *Causes of epilepsy*

It is helpful to distinguish *causes* of epilepsy and *precipitation* of seizures. By *cause* is meant more-or-less steady-state background factors. An example is the scarring of brain following head injury. By *precipitation* is meant the effects of short-term stimuli, such as seizures precipitated by exposure to television screens in susceptible people. Table 12.3 lists some of the causes of seizures. It must be said, however, that a number of community surveys have shown that even when the most careful analysis has been made, a cause can be identified in only about 25–40 per cent of all patients with epilepsy. If a definite cause is found, the epilepsy is sometimes said to be *symptomatic* (Fig. 12.6).

Both absence epilepsy and benign childhood epilepsy with centro-temporal spikes are probably inherited as autosomal dominants, at least as judged by EEG recording from relatives. The expression of the gene in overt seizures does not, however, always occur, so only a small proportion of siblings of patients with absence attacks and centro-temporal spikes will be affected, even though the EEGs of the unaffected siblings may show the EEG abnormality. Epilepsy with a clear genetic cause such as this is said to be *idiopathic*.

The threshold at which seizures occur in response to a variety of extrinsic and intrinsic

Table 12.3   The 'causes' of epilepsy

Genetic propensity
  recessively inherited disorders of lipid and amino-acid metabolism
  recessively inherited 'developmental' disorders—tuberous sclerosis; neurofibromatosis
  dominantly inherited disorders—primary generalized epilepsy
  polygenic inherited propensity (probable)
Congenital abnormalities
  microgyria
  focal cortical dysplasia
  megaloencephaly
Ante- and perinatal injury
  anoxia
  intracerebral haemorrhage
  infarction; porencephalic cyst
Effects consequent to prolonged febrile convulsions
Trauma
  accidental
  following elective neurosurgery
Infections
  bacterial meningitis
  cerebral abscess
  viral encephalitis
  parasitic infections
Immunization
  pertussis vaccine
Vascular causes
  infarction
  hyptertensive encephalopathy
  cerebral venous thrombosis
  arteriovenous malformations
  post-anoxic encephalopathy
Toxic causes
  alcohol ingestion and withdrawal; chronic alcoholic encephalopathy
  heavy metals, particularly lead
Metabolic causes

hypoglycaemia	hyperglycaemia
hypoxia	hyperbaric oxygenation
hypocalcaemia	hypercalcaemia
hyponatraemia	hypernatraemia
	uraemia

  deficiency of pyridoxine
Degenerative causes
  Alzheimer's disease

factors is probably inherited through the interaction of a number of genes. Consequently, if a patient has epilepsy due to a clear-cut structural cause, such as a tumour, his or her children have a slightly greater risk of epilepsy than the population as a whole. On empirical grounds, if the cause of epilepsy is not known, a patient can be told that his or her children's cumulative risk of epilepsy to the age of 20 is about 4 per cent, compared to 1 per cent at the same age for the population as a whole (see Fig. 12.1).

Perinatal injury, trauma, tumours, stroke, vascular disease, and degenerative disorders such as Alzheimer's disease all cause epilepsy through what is immediately intuitively apparent, that is to say, in each condition there are one or more zones of neuronal damage. Why that neuronal damage results in seizures in some but not others is not known, but may reflect variations in inherited seizure threshold. It is clear that neurons in the hippocampus of the temporal lobe are particularly prone to damage from ischaemic or hypoxic events, and such sclerotic areas of damage are often foci from which partial seizures subsequently arise (see Section 12.9.1).

If no clear-cut cause of epilepsy is found, and yet the type of epilepsy is not clearly primary generalized, the epilepsy is sometimes said to be *cryptogenic* (Fig. 12.6).

12.6.2   *Precipitation of seizures*

Patients often have firm views about what causes or precipitates their seizures, and yet the following example shows just how difficult it may be to be sure. Take a man with a moderate genetic predisposition to seizures. Add the effects of a moderate cranial injury some 2 years before. Add also the effect of stress at the office during the preceding month, and then also the effects of amitriptyline prescribed to help the depression associated with this stress. If this man then has a seizure after consuming a moderate amount of alcohol the night before, what caused it—the genetic propensity, the cranial injury, the stress, the alcohol, the disturbance of sleep associated with the depression, or the amitriptyline? In spite of the force of this point, there is good evidence that all the factors listed in Table 12.4 are important precipitants. Seizures are particularly likely to occur in certain phases of sleep, approximately 2 hours

after going to bed, and shortly before and shortly after waking. Seizures around the time of waking are particularly likely to occur in those with juvenile myoclonic epilepsy (Section 12.5). Deprivation of sleep is undoubtedly an important seizure precipitant, and indeed may be used to evoke abnormal paroxysmal discharges in the electroencephalogram as part of an investigation into seizure type. Seizures of all types also may occur more often than would be expected by chance shortly before or around menstruation.

Alcohol is associated with seizures in a number of ways. First, acute intoxication may precipitate seizures. Secondly, withdrawal after a period of chronic alcohol abuse may also precipitate seizures. Finally, seizures may occur after some years of alcohol abuse as a feature of alcohol-induced brain damage. Alcohol taken within social limits does not seem to affect the frequency of seizures in those with epilepsy due to other causes.

A number of drugs precipitate seizures. Antidepressants such as imipramine and amitriptyline are the most frequent, but chlorpromazine, haloperidol, izoniazid, lignocaine, and lidocaine, and bronchodilators such as theophylline and aminophylline have all been reported to cause seizures.

Metabolic precipitants for seizures are not

Table 12.4   Suggested precipitants of seizures

Sleep
Waking
Deprivation of sleep
Menstrual cycle
Toxic and metabolic causes
acute alcohol intoxication
withdrawal from alcohol
drugs
hypoglycaemia
hypoxia
Reflex causes
glare, flashing lights, television
reading
sounds
thinking
startle
movement
Stressful life events

common, but hypoglycaemia and uraemia may precipitate seizures. An abrupt rise in blood pressure in accelerated hypertension may also result in seizures.

Amongst the most interesting precipitants of seizures are the reflex precipitants. About 3 per cent of patients with epilepsy have seizures induced by viewing intermittent light, patterns, or television. Most of the subjects are young, and girls are more commonly affected than boys. During electroencephalography, the neurophysiological recordist will study the effects of flashing lights at different frequencies. It is common to detect the normal evoked occipital response to flash which follows the flash frequency at slow rates of flash. However, in about 5 per cent of those with seizure disorders, and some relatives of those with seizure disorders, the photic following response is replaced or followed by a photoconvulsive response, consisting of regular or irregular spikes interspersed with slow waves. The discharges may outlast the photic stimulation and be associated with myoclonic jerks, and even a tonic–clonic seizure.

In day-to-day life, epilepsy in such subjects is most likely to be induced by television. The evocative stimulus is the pattern of interlacing lines formed by the flying spot from the elcctron gun. It has been shown that it is safer to use a small screen, or a large screen viewed from a considerable distance, in order that the visual angle subtended by the lines is below the threshold that evokes paroxysmal discharges.

Other interesting reflex epilepsies include seizures induced by reading, hearing particular sounds or sequence of sounds, startle, movement, and even thinking about specific tasks, such as playing chess or cards. It is assumed that the neuronal activity associated with these psychological activities in some way recruits other neurons into an epileptic discharge.

Finally, most physicians and their patients believe that stress precipitates seizures, but it is understandably difficult to quantify stress. What may be seen as a trivial life event to a doctor may have caused considerable anxiety and stress to a subject.

12.7 The first seizure and the diagnosis of epilepsy

12.7.1 *The differential diagnosis of seizures*

The distinction between a first seizure due to paroxysmal neuronal discharge and some other event is primarily a clinical one. It is practically always necessary to obtain a first-hand account from a witness of the event, as many patients with 'blackouts' can understandably give no description of what transpired during the attack.

Some common differential diagnoses of seizures are shown in Table 12.5. The most frequent distinction that needs to be made is between a seizure and syncope. By syncope is meant an impairment or loss of consciousness due to transient failure of global cerebral perfusion. Causes of syncope include the sudden cardiac slowing associated with emotional factors, such as the sight of blood (vasovagal syncope), or transient cardiac tachyarrhythmias, or bradyarrhythmias (Stokes–Adams attacks). Other cardiac causes include aortic stenosis, aortic obstructive cardiomyopathy, and failure of left atrial output due to an atrial myxoma or a tight mitral stenosis.

Postural hypotension may in itself result in vasovagal syncope, for example in soldiers standing to attention for a longer period. Postural hypotension and syncope may occur in those on hypotensive medication, or in patients with an autonomic neu-

Table 12.5 Differential diagnosis of epilepsy

Syncope
    vasovagal episodes
    postural hypotension
    micturition syncope
    cardiac causes
        brady- or tachyarrhythmias
        aortic or mitral stenosis, atrial myxoma
        obstructive cardiomyopathy
Panic attacks
Migraine
Transient ischaemic attacks
Cataplexy
Drop attacks
Hypoglycaemia

Pseudoseizures

In childhood, the differential diagnosis includes:
    breath-holding attacks
    night terrors

ropathy, such as occurs in diabetes (Table 19.8 and Section 19.7.2.1) or in the Shy–Drager syndrome (Section 13.2.1).

A common story is of a man who gets out of bed at night to pass urine, and loses consciousness after doing so. Part of the fall in blood pressure is due to getting out of a warm bed with peripheral vasodilatation, but there is also further reflex vaso-dilatation during the act of micturition. This is called micturition syncope.

The distinction between syncope and a seizure is usually fairly straightforward. Most patients are aware of pre-syncopal symptoms, such as a feeling of coldness, and the greying out or blacking out of vision due to a failure of retinal perfusion. Bystanders will notice extreme pallor, as intense vasoconstriction occurs through baro-receptor reflexes as the blood pressure falls. Many subjects also notice that they feel cold and are sweaty.

Sometimes a patient who is about to faint will report a sensation along the lines that 'voices sounded distorted and far away'. This commonly occurs in syncope, but the history may be misinter-preted as a distortion of consciousness of the type seen in a complex partial seizure.

Other difficulties occur if the reduction in cere-bral perfusion is so intense that one or two anoxic myoclonic jerks occur ('anoxic seizures'). It is important not to leap to the conclusion that such jerks indicate an epileptic seizure. Other differen-tial diagnoses of epilepsy are considered in Table 12.5. Panic attacks may be manifest by the sudden onset of a feeling of intense apprehension or terror, associated with paraesthesiae and a sense of unreality. Unless the diagnosis is thought of, again it is possible to confuse these with complex partial seizures. The periodic disturbances of neurological function associated with classical migraine may be confused with epilepsy, but scin-tillating scotoma are common in migraine, and such visual disturbances are rare in epilepsy. A slow evolution over a period of minutes suggests migraine rather than a seizure discharge.

Transient ischaemic attacks affecting the motor cortex produce a sudden focal impairment of func-tion, but the clinical distinction is that ischaemic events are *negative* phenomena. Epileptic events in the same territory have the positive effects of jactitation. Another type of attack is transient global amnesia which may be confused with com-plex partial seizures. The pathophysiological nature of these is obscure (Section 10.1.10.1).

In childhood, the differential diagnosis extends to breath-holding attacks and night terrors. A history of these, and also the history of narcolepsy (Section 22.2.4.1), cataplexy (Section 24.2.4.2), and hypoglycaemia (Section 23.2.4) is usually suf-ficiently characteristic once the diagnosis has been considered.

The distinction between an epileptic seizure and one of the other events listed in Table 12.5 is usually easy enough, but if not, it may be necessary to proceed to electroencephalography and electro-cardiography. Depending upon the frequency of the episodes, it may be justifiable to try to capture one or more attacks by long-term monitoring with magnetic recording of ECG and EEG signals. Best of all is to have a video-recording of the attack, with simultaneous EEG and ECG (Fig. 12.5). It must be remembered that prolonged cardiac arrhythmias may produce secondary EEG abnormalities; conversely, some temporal lobe seizures are associated with secondary cardiac dysrhythmias.

In older patients, syncope due to some sort of cardiac dysrhythmia is common, and more inten-sive electrophysiological monitoring may prove its nature, particularly if associated with a head-up tilt test, either alone or in association with isoproter-enol infused at a rate sufficient to achieve an increase in heart rate of at least 20 per cent. In those with cardiac disease, as judged by a reduced left ventricular ejection fraction, a sustained mono-morphic ventricular tachycardia occurs in a sub-stantial number of patients during such studies, in association with syncope. A few patients have inducible supraventricular tachycardias elicited and others have developed marked bradycardias. These patients may be helped with β-blockade with metoprolol, and those with tachyarrhyth-mias may be helped with appropriate treatment such as an automatic implantable cardioverter defibrillator.

Finally, it must be remembered that up to 20 per cent of those referred for the evaluation of intract-able epilepsy turn out not to have epileptic seizures at all, but simulated seizures, or so-called pseudo-seizures. A not uncommon complicating factor, however, is that patients with real epilepsy may simulate a few seizures when they are experiencing particular social or emotional difficulties (p. 206).

12.7.2   *The risk of recurrence after an initial seizure*

A first seizure is a common clinical event, and patients understandably wish to know their chances of recurrence, and the likely cause. The questions arise as to what investigations should be done that allow the determination of a serious cause such as a tumour, and of what help are investigations in predicting the risk of recurrence.

The risk of recurrence after an initial seizure in adult life is about 40 per cent by the end of the first year, and over 50 per cent by the end of 3 years (Fig. 12.8). Similar figures have been reported for children. In practice, the great majority of the recurrences occur in the first few weeks. Indeed, recurrences often occur during the course of out-patient investigation. It has been shown that clinical factors particularly associated with recurrence include younger age and a family history of epilepsy or of febrile convulsions. Seizures occurring between midnight and breakfast time are more likely to recur than those occurring later in the day.

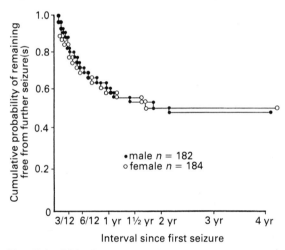

Fig. 12.8   Risk of recurrence after a first seizure in adult life. (Data from Hopkins, Garman, and Clarke 1988.)

12.7.3   *The investigation of seizures*

In adults, approximately half of those who have had a seizure have an abnormal EEG, but the abnormality is very often a non-specific one, such as an excess of theta activity over one or both temporal lobes. A focal paroxysmal discharge in some studies does predict that seizures are more likely to recur, as do spike–wave discharges in children.

It must be remembered that a normal EEG does not disprove the diagnosis of an epileptic seizure. It has been shown that the longer the EEG is recorded, the greater the possibility of picking up some sort of paroxysmal discharge. However, for practical purposes, when using a 1 hour recording with the usual activating techniques of hyperventilation and photic stimulation, approximately half those who have had an undoubted tonic–clonic seizure will have a normal inter-ictal EEG. The EEG does, however, come into its own when one is investigating multiple seizures with a view to treatment, as a clear guide may be given to the origin or type of seizure, and thence to further investigation or treatment.

In adults, CT scans or MRI will reveal an unsuspected tumour in only about 3 per cent of all patients with first seizures. Although tumour cases are more likely to have early relapses, other types of imaging abnormality, such as small infarcts or areas of atrophy, are not helpful in predicting recurrence. It is clear that those with physical signs not accounted for by a known prior neurological insult, such as a head injury, require imaging, as do those with simple partial seizures. The yield of significant abnormalities on scanning those with other types of seizures is so low that the decision rests on economic rather than clinical grounds.

It has been shown that MRI is more sensitive than CT scanning at picking up small tumours. However, in the UK at least, it is unlikely that resources will be available for early MRI of those with seizures unless they are being investigated with a view to surgery (see Section 12.9.1).

Other imaging procedures are of limited use in epilepsy. Plain X-ray has really been overtaken by CT scanning and MRI, though abnormal calcification or abnormal vascular markings or cranial hemiatrophy may give clues to an underlying lesion. Cerebral angiography may be useful to investigate further angiomas, which sometimes cause epilepsy, but many angiomas will be shown by CT or MRI.

Research techniques include positron emission tomography, using ^{18}F or ^{15}O, which reveals areas of focal hypometabolism around partial seizure foci.

12.8 The treatment of epilepsy by anticonvulsant drugs

At present, few neurologists treat initial seizures, but as the high rate of relapse becomes more widely acknowledged, it is probable that more patients will be advised to have drugs after the first episode. Leaving aside the social disadvantages of recurrent epileptic seizures (Section 12.12), there is some evidence that neuronal damage may occur as a result of repeated seizures, and it may be that each seizure makes subsequent ones more likely. Most neurologists will therefore recommend treatment after two or three epileptic attacks, unless these are separated by intervals of many years.

The choice of drug depends largely on seizure type (Table 12.6). Absence attacks are best treated with sodium valproate, or ethosuximide. Phenobarbitone and phenytoin may exacerbate absence seizures.

Partial seizures, whether or not secondarily generalized, are best treated by carbamazepine and phenytoin. Although other drugs may be used for resistant seizures, there are seldom indications for starting patients on drugs other than carbamazepine, phenytoin, or sodium valproate. These drugs are next considered in detail.

Carbamazepine is in some ways the easiest drug to use, as the relationship between oral dose and serum level is linear. A common adult maintenance dose is between 600 and 1200 mg each day, although it is wise to start on no more than 100 mg twice a day. The optimal therapeutic range is 15–50 μmol/l (3.5–11.5 μg/ml). The principal drawback to the drug is its relatively short half-life (5–20 hours). This means that the drug needs to be given at least three and preferably four times a day in order to avoid wide fluctuations in serum level. A formulation known as Tegretol-Retard diminishes the extent of fluctuations in serum concentrations. Good seizure control can be achieved by twice daily dosage with this.

Carbamazepine is probably the best drug from the point of view of the relative absence of unwanted effects on alertness and cognitive function. Nausea and dizziness are occasional problems, and some patients complain of double vision as they begin the drug. Depression of the bone marrow has been reported very rarely.

Phenytoin is also an effective drug for the treatment of partial and tonic–clonic seizures. An average daily dose for an adult is 250–400 mg/day. The therapeutic range lies between 30 and 80 μmol/l (7–20 μg/ml). Some patients seem to be well controlled by blood levels even lower than 30 μmol/l.

Phenytoin is easier to use than carbamazepine in one sense—the half-life is sufficiently long that all the drug may be given in a single dose, most practically on going to bed at night. One major drawback is that there is considerable variability in absorption and metabolism, so that, in adults at least, there is little correlation between dosage requirement and weight. Phenytoin is hydroxylated in the liver by an enzyme system that the drug can induce but then saturate. A small increase in dose may then produce a large increase in serum level, and precipitate intoxication characterized by drowsiness, ataxia, and nystagmus. Other unwanted side-effects include hypertrophy of the gums, coarsening of the features and hirsutism in young people, drug eruptions, and, rarely, a peripheral neuropathy and chronic cerebellar degeneration. Phenytoin may also result in an effective vitamin D deficiency, producing rickets or osteomalacia.

Table 12.6   Anticonvulsant therapy

Seizure type	First-line drug	Average adult daily dose (mg)	Therapeutic level in serum (μmol/l)
Absences	Sodium valproate	2000	See text
Partial seizures	Carbamazepine	600	15–50
	Phenytoin	350	30–80
Tonic–clonic seizures	use valproate if associated with absences or 3 c/s spike–wave activity, otherwise carbamazepine or phenytoin		

One particular unwanted effect of phenytoin, and to a lesser extent of carbamazepine, deserves special mention, and that is their effect on oral contraception. Induction of hydroxylating enzymes in the liver results not only in increased hydroxylation of the anticonvulsant drugs, but also of steroid hormones, including those contained in the contraceptive pill. Consequently, less than adequate contraceptive protection is given by the pill in epileptic patients taking these drugs. Women must be warned of this, and, if they are not prepared to take the risk of pregnancy, use an alternative method of contraception.

Sodium valproate, the drug of choice for absence seizures, is usually given on a twice-daily regimen. There is some evidence that the drug is tissue bound, and therefore serum levels do not reflect biological activity. The usual maintenance dose is 600–2000 mg/day. Unwanted effects include transient hair loss, or changes in the hair so that it becomes curly, some impairment of cognitive function and alertness (less than with phenytoin but more than with carbamazepine), weight gain, and tremor. Very rarely, acute hepatic failure occurs, but this is virtually only seen in young children with pre-existing neurological abnormalities.

It is now standard practice to treat all new patients with epilepsy with one drug, using one of the three drugs just mentioned. The chances of achieving seizure control by adding a second drug once the first has failed are probably no more than 5–10 per cent. The chances seem to be no better if two drugs are given in combination than sequentially. There are also interactions between anticonvulsant drugs. For example, carbamazepine levels are often lowered by the simultaneous use of phenytoin. It should also be remembered that other drugs being used for other medical conditions may influence markedly the serum levels of anticonvulsant drugs. For example, denzimol, isoniazid, cimetidine, verapamil, erythromycin, and dextropropoxyphene may all elevate the serum level of carbamazepine. Conversely, the introduction of carbamazepine may reduce the phenytoin level, and phenobarbitone, primidone, tolbutamide, diazepam, and other drugs have a similar effect. Ethosuximide, propranolol, and warfarin may all raise serum phenytoin levels.

If one of the three front-line drugs fails, other anticonvulsants can be considered. Phenobarbitone is an effect anticonvulsant but makes children grizzly and miserable, and adults are often depressed and complain of impaired cognitive function. An average daily dose is 120 mg. Primidone, the principal metabolite of which is phenobarbitone, has similar effects. An average daily dose is 750 mg.

For absence seizures, ethosuximide is undoubtedly effective, but sodium valproate is probably superior. There are other suxinimide drugs, such as methsuximide and phensuximide, available.

Most benzodiazepines are not effective chronic anticonvulsants (although diazepam is one of the treatments of choice for the management of status epilepticus, see Section 12.10). However, both clonazepam and clobazam are useful adjunctive drugs occasionally. Unfortunately, the first of these has frequent sedative effects, and tolerance often develops to the second.

12.8.1   *Newer anticonvulsant drugs*

Gabapentin, an analogue of γ-aminobutyric acid (GABA) has been shown to be effective when added to the existing anticonvulsant therapy of patients with drug-resistant partial epilepsy. Although a quarter of the patients in one study had the number of partial seizures at least halved, no patient became free of seizures, and adverse events such as somnolence, fatigue, and dizziness were common.

Vigabatrin (γ-vinyl GABA) is an irreversible inhibitor of GABA aminotransferase. As with gabapentin, when added to existing anticonvulsant therapy this drug diminishes the frequency of partial seizures; there is less effect upon secondarily generalized seizures. Side-effects are similar to gabapentin but, in addition, intramyelinic oedema has been observed in animals. The significance of this is uncertain, and it has not yet been seen in humans. Most patients require, after a lower initial dose, 2–3 g daily. Measurement of serum levels is not appropriate, as the drug action is through its binding to GABA aminotransferase. Adverse reactions include drowsiness, fatigue, dizziness, irritability, depression, and headache. There may be an increase in seizure frequency in those with myoclonic seizures.

Lamotrigine is unrelated chemically to other anticonvulsants. It may exert its anticonvulsant effect by inhibiting the release of excitatory amino-acid neurotransmitters. The usual maintenance dose is 200–400 mg per day in two divided doses after initial lower dosage. As an add-on drug, it has proved useful in reducing the number of partial seizures and secondarily generalized seizures, but it is unlikely to render the patient free of seizures. Adverse effects are common and include diplopia, tiredness, ataxia, headache and skin rashes.

Oxcarbazepine is the 10-keto analogue of carbamazepine. Its 10-hydroxymetabolite is responsible for its anticonvulsant effect. Possible advantages of this drug over carbamazepine include the fact that it does not induce enzymes, nor does it have an active epoxide metabolite. It may therefore be more predictable in use, and be better tolerated.

12.8.2 Prevention of post-traumatic epilepsy

Post-traumatic epilepsy is common after penetrating injuries which result in cortical damage. It is therefore frequent after missile injuries in wartime, and civilian head injuries associated with a depressed fracture, particularly if the dura is torn. If these last two features are present, and if there is an intracerebral haematoma, then the risk of post-traumatic epilepsy reaches 60 per cent. It is not surprising, therefore, that anticonvulsants are often prescribed after head injury in an attempt to reduce this high incidence. However, a controlled trial has shown that although an intravenous loading dose of phenytoin is effective in reducing the incidence of seizures in the first week, continuing phenytoin thereafter does not prevent the occurrence of seizures subsequently.

It is probable that these results can be extrapolated to epilepsy induced by neurosurgical trauma. For example, a subfrontal approach to a pituitary tumour is followed by a significant risk for the development of post-traumatic epilepsy.

12.8.3 Teratogenecity of anticonvulsant drugs

Mothers with epilepsy have a slightly higher risk of having an abnormal baby than the population at large. The risk is probably not genetic, as children of epileptic fathers do not have an increased risk of fetal abnormality. Furthermore, most studies have shown that epileptic mothers taking anticonvulsant drugs during pregnancy are more likely to have an abnormal fetus than those not taking anticonvulsant drugs.

The commonest abnormality found is cleft lip and palate, congenital heart disease, hypoplasia of nails and of optic nerve, and general dysmorphic features affecting the ears and epicanthic folds. Phenytoin and phenobarbitone have the worst reputation for such abnormalities. Sodium valproate and carbamazepine are associated with an increased risk of spina bifida.

In an ideal world, a remission of seizures should be achieved, and anticonvulsants withdrawn, before a woman with epilepsy conceives. However, all too often this is not practical. Furthermore, many women have been taking anticonvulsant drugs during the first three or four weeks of pregnancy before they realize that they are pregnant. The risks of fetal abnormality have to be balanced against the risks to the mother and fetus of allowing seizures to continue during pregnancy. Indeed, the frequency of seizures increases in about a third of epileptic women during pregnancy, partly due to alterations in metabolism of anticonvulsant drugs. Furthermore, the risk of anticonvulsant medication has to be put into perspective. Even if the risk of fetal abnormality is increased threefold, about 95 per cent of all epileptic mothers will have a normal child, and of the remainder, many of the abnormalities are relatively minor.

In general, the present practice is to suggest that epileptic women of childbearing age who need anticonvulsant drugs should take carbamazepine, if they require anticonvulsant medication, as the reports of fetal abnormality appear to be fewer with this drug than with others.

12.8.4 Withdrawal of anticonvulsant drugs

When a patient has been free from seizures for 2 or 3 years, withdrawal of anticonvulsant medication should be considered. Although apparently very safe drugs when used carefully, the very long term effects (>30 years) are not really known. There is some evidence of hepatic and Purkinje cell damage with prolonged use.

The Medical Research Council (MRC) trial has shown that the risk of recurrent seizures within two years is about 40 per cent, but this should be contrasted with a risk of about 20 per cent of further seizures occurring even if drugs are not withdrawn. A decision to withdraw drugs will be influenced by social factors, such as the effect of a recurrent seizure upon a patient's livelihood and desire to drive a motor car. The MRC trial has demonstrated a number of variables associated with recurrence on withdrawal of drugs. Unfavourable factors include the duration of previous anticonvulsant treatment, and the number of drugs being prescribed at the time of the decision to withdraw (both reflecting perhaps the 'severity' of

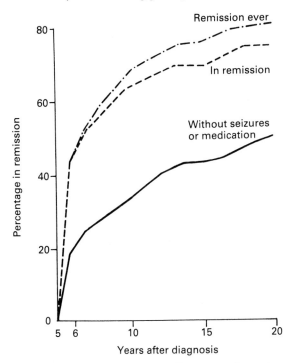

Fig. 12.9 Remission of seizures. Top curve: the probability of completing a period of 5 consecutive years without seizures. For example, 6 years after diagnosis 42 per cent of subjects have been seizure-free for 5 years. Middle curve: the probability of being in remission for at least the past 5 years. The difference between the top and middle curves is due to relapse after achievement of a five-year remission. For example, at 20 years after diagnosis 70 per cent are currently free from seizures, and have been for 5 years, and a further 6 per cent have had at least one seizure-free period of at least 5 years duration but have subsequently relapsed. Lowest curve: the probability of being free of seizures for at least 5 years while not taking anticonvulsant drugs. In summary, 20 years after diagnosis, 50 per cent have been free from seizures without anticonvulsants for at least 5 years. A further 20 per cent continue to take anticonvulsant medication and have also been free of seizures for at least 5 years. Seizures continue, in spite of medication, in 30 per cent. (Reproduced with kind permission from Annegers *et al*, 1979.)

the epilepsy), and a history of tonic–clonic seizures, particularly if associated with a generalized spike–wave discharge on the electroencephalogram. In this and other studies, a few seizures that responded rapidly to treatment indicate a good prognosis on withdrawal. Conversely, complex partial seizures with secondary generalization, the presence of identified focal cerebral disease, or neurological signs, or psychiatric disturbances, have all been identified as unfavourable prognostic features. The juvenile myoclonic epilepsy of Janz (p. 192) is particularly likely to recur. An abnormal EEG before treatment, if associated with continuing abnormalities during treatment, is also an unfavourable feature. It is usual practice to withdraw anticonvulsants over a period of many months, in order to avoid the possibility of withdrawal seizures, particularly if phenobarbitone has been used. The risk of recurrent seizures is highest in the early months following withdrawal.

12.8.5   *Factors indicating a poor prognosis for epilepsy*

The general prognosis of epilepsy in the community is illustrated in Fig. 12.9, but it is worth noting at this point those factors that predict that epilepsy will respond poorly to treatment. The outlook for children with infantile spasms and the Lennox–Gastaut syndrome is poor, not only for seizure control, but also for cognitive development. In adult life, patients with frequent seizures, especially of partial origin, who have already proved resistant to treatment are likely to remain resistant to treatment whatever adjustments to medication are made. Other unfavourable features include a tendency for seizures to cluster over short periods of time, a combination of different types of seizure, psychiatric abnormalities, cognitive impairment, and the presence of focal neurological signs.

12.9   Treatments other than drugs for intractable epilepsy

12.9.1   *Surgery*

For those patients just considered, treatment other than anticonvulsant drugs needs to be considered. Experience has shown that surgical removal of an epileptogenic lesion in one or other temporal lobe is highly effective. Pre-conditions for surgery include intractability of epilepsy, after an energetic trial of all appropriate anticonvulsant drugs, with evidence of satisfactory compliance as judged by serum levels, and the identification of seizure onset consistently within one temporal lobe. This is particularly important, as scalp EEG recordings may show confusing 'mirror foci' over the opposite temporal lobe. Many surgical centres use evidence from long-term depth recording—fine insulated wires inserted deep in the temporal lobe through burr holes—or from sheets of electrodes mounted in plastic sheets and left to lie over the cortex for a week or two, having been inserted through burr holes or a preliminary craniotomy. A recent intriguing possibility is the localization and activation of a seizure focus by transcranial magnetic stimulation (Section 8.6).

Other pre-conditions include the absence of evidence of any diffuse cerebral disease, which might be indicated by a globally low intellect, bilateral clinical neurological signs, diffuse EEG abnormalities, or a severe psychological abnormality. Even if all these conditions are satisfied, it is still necessary to work out what are likely to be the psychological effects of removing a temporal lobe. Language is usually situated in the left temporal lobe, but significant aphasia does not occur unless the resection extends more than 6 cm posteriorly from the tip. Many patients with long-standing temporal lobe epilepsy have mixed handedness, and it may be necessary to sort out in which hemisphere language and verbal memory lie. This is achieved by temporarily subduing one hemisphere by the intracarotid injection of amylobarbitone. The dose is adjusted so that a contralateral hemiplegia is induced, without significant impairment of consciousness, and psychological function in the remaining active hemisphere is then assessed. This procedure is known as the Wada test. In general, a left temporal lobectomy may have significant effects upon verbal memory, which may be of crucial importance in some professions such as the law.

Sophisticated imaging procedures may also be useful. MRI has shown that a number of patients who have been thought to have non-progressive lesions in the temporal lobe are actually harbouring small tumours. Single-photon emission computerized tomography may also be useful. Other

pathological abnormalities giving rise to temporal lobe epilepsy include small hamartomas—areas of non-neoplastic but abnormal tissue development—and, most importantly, mesial temporal sclerosis, which follows anoxic events in early childhood.

If the patients are carefully chosen, temporal lobe surgery can produce complete control of previously intractable epilepsy in 60–70 per cent of cases.

Other operations are occasionally done. In young children with an infantile hemiplegia and severe epilepsy, the whole hemisphere may be removed, as it is an origin for seizures and yet no use to the child. The corpus callosum in other patients can be divided to prevent seizure discharges spreading contralaterally. Focal cortical scars, particularly in the frontal region, may occasionally be excised, but the results are not nearly as good as operations on the temporal lobe.

12.9.2 Other methods of treatment of intractable epilepsy

There is, at present, increasing interest in behavioural and other psychological methods of controlling seizures. Biofeedback was in fashion a few years ago, but controlled studies failed to show benefit. A ketogenic diet controls seizures in a significant number of children, although the diet, rich either in cream or medium-chain triglycerides, is relatively unpalatable. Unfortunately, after an initial 'honeymoon' period, relapse often occurs even if the diet is continued.

12.10 Status epilepticus

Status epilepticus is defined as serial seizures without recovery of full consciousness between them. In practice, serial seizures—several each day with reasonable recovery of consciousness—present the same urgent problem of management.

The most worrying form of status epilepticus is tonic–clonic (grand mal) status epilepticus, as the frequent tonic–clonic seizures, during which there are long periods of hypoxia, lead to cardiorespiratory problems. Even in modern hospital settings, the mortality of status epilepticus of this type may reach 30 per cent. Specialist advice is often not sought early enough.

Absence status, and complex partial status, give rise to peculiar twilight clinical states of confusion and partial responsiveness, which may unfortunately be misdiagnosed as of psychological origin until the EEG reveals the continuing seizure discharge.

Status epilepticus may be the first manifestation of epilepsy, as a result of cranial trauma or after a cranial operation. A frontal tumour may present with status. More commonly, however, status epilepticus supervenes in someone with chronic epilepsy, not infrequently because of the intentional or inadvertent withdrawal of appropriate anticonvulsant medication. Other precipitating factors include withdrawal from alcohol, and intercurrent infection.

Unless the patient is already known to have epilepsy, which has appropriately been investigated, the first steps in management should include appropriate investigation to elucidate the cause of the status, in which case clinical examination may give some clues, and a CT scan, MRI, and a lumbar puncture may also be necessary.

Even while these procedures are taking place, however, urgent steps should be taken to treat status. An intravenous line should be inserted. Blood is then withdrawn for estimation of the serum level of any previously given anticonvulsants, and estimation of serum glucose, electrolytes, and urea. It may be appropriate to set up blood cultures. Treatment should be given through the same intravenous line, using diazepam, 2 mg/min to a total of 20 mg. This often proves to be sufficient in someone whose epilepsy has previously been well managed, and who is running reasonable serum anticonvulsant levels. If the patient is a new patient in status, then phenytoin should also be infused at a rate not exceeding 50 mg/min to a total of 18 mg/kg. The best way of infusing phenytoin is to use the solution (50 mg/ml) in propylene glycol, diluted with normal saline in a 100 ml volume control set.

If seizures recur in spite of one bolus injection of diazepam and the infusion of phenytoin, the two next best options are to give, through the intravenous line, diazepam as follows: 50–100 mg of diazepam diluted in 500 ml of dextrose saline and run in at 40 ml/h. Alternatively, thiopentone, 2 mg/min in normal saline, may be given through a micro-infusion pump.

As will be judged from these last statements, the management of status should take place in the intensive care ward with facilities for full monitoring of ventilation and perfusion. In resistant cases, it may be necessary to increase the dosage of thiopentone to anaesthetizing doses and ventilate the patient.

12.11   Febrile convulsions

Children with cerebral palsy and other chronic neurological disorders can have seizures when febrile and not at other times. This can be regarded as epilepsy precipitated by fever. However, convulsions frequently occur in the course of a febrile illness in otherwise healthy young children between the ages of 18 months and 5 years, most often occurring towards the lower end of this age-range. Simple febrile convulsions may be defined as brief generalized seizures, seldom lasting for more than a few minutes, occurring soon after a rise in body temperature, in children in whom there is no clinical or laboratory evidence of overt cerebral infection or intoxication. The incidence of such convulsions is between 20 and 40 per 100 000. That is to say, about 1 in 25 children will have a convulsion. Boys are rather more likely to have a convulsion than girls, the sex ratio being about 1.2 : 1. Girls tend to have their first seizure in association with a fever at a rather younger age than boys.

12.11.1   *Cause of febrile convulsions*

The 'cause' of febrile convulsions can be divided into three components—the genetic background, the neurological development before the first convulsion, and the precipitating event in association with the fever.

All studies show that first-degree relatives of children with febrile convulsions have a higher than expected incidence of convulsive disorders. Between 10 and 20 per cent of the parents of children with febrile convulsions have had some sort of convulsive disorder, either febrile convulsions or epilepsy. It is not yet certain whether one or more genes are responsible for this transmission of risk.

The neurodevelopmental status of the child prior to the first convulsion is also helpful in understanding the significance of febrile convulsions. The mothers of children who have febrile convulsions have a greater than expected incidence of chronic ill health, suggesting that the potential for sub-optimal neurological development is present even before conception. During the course of the pregnancy, threatened abortion or ante-partum haemorrhage are also present in a greater proportion of histories of children with febrile convulsions than would be expected by chance. Although earlier studies suggested that the incidence of breech delivery and Caesarean section is also greater in those mothers whose babies subsequently go on to convulse, the consensus view is that no perinatal factors are important if neurological development is normal.

If neurological development after birth is clearly delayed, and a child then convulses with fever, the prognosis for further seizures in later childhood and adult life is significantly higher than for those who have simple febrile convulsions on a background of normal early development. If the neurological defect is obvious, then the general rule is to consider that seizure as a precipitation of epilepsy by fever. However, minor neurological abnormalities before the first seizure may well be overlooked, so there is a 'grey area' in definition here.

A child does not become febrile without some specific cause, and when a vigorous search is made for an infectious agent, evidence of a viral infection can be found in up to 85 per cent of cases. Examination of the spinal fluid in children with febrile convulsions will often reveal a few lymphocytes as evidence of a viral infection of the nervous system, and a few children will have a frank viral meningitis.

12.11.2 Investigation

One of the difficulties in assessing a child with a febrile convulsion is to be sure that the child has not got a bacterial meningitic illness. As it is difficult to be certain of the signs of neck stiffness and minor alterations in conscious level in very young children, especially in the post-ictal state, the general view is that, if recovery from a convulsion appears to be delayed, and if there is any suspicion of meningitis whatsoever, then examination of the spinal fluid is essential. Some authorities recommend that all children who convulse in association with fever before the age of 18 months should also have a lumbar puncture.

12.11.3 Management of febrile convulsions

Most febrile convulsions terminate by the time that a doctor arrives on the scene, but if the convulsion is still continuing, then diazepam, 0.5 mg/kg body weight, should be given rectally. If the seizure continues after this, the dose should be repeated after 15 minutes and the child admitted to hospital. There is no evidence that rapid cooling by sponging influences whether or not further seizures occur but immersion in warm water will lower temperature faster than simple exposure.

Over the past decade there have been a number of trials of anticonvulsants used as prophylaxis against recurrent febrile convulsions. However, phenobarbitone has been shown to cause unacceptable overactivity in 20 per cent of children, even though it is an effective drug in preventing recurrences, as is sodium valproate. Phenytoin and carbamazepine have been shown to be ineffective. However, few parents, or doctors, are entirely happy about continuous prophylactic medication at this stage of development, and most authorities now recommend giving intermittent prophylactic rectal diazepam at times of high fever in children who have shown a predisposition to febrile convulsions. Diazepam, 5 mg rectally, given at times of fever, will reduce the recurrence rate to about 10 per cent if the parents have appreciated early enough that the child is not well.

12.11.4 Prognosis of febrile convulsions

The actuarial cumulative risk of subsequent epilepsy is 2 per cent at the age of five, 5.5 per cent at the age of 15, and 7 per cent by the age of 25. Reference to Fig. 12.1 shows that this is about a fivefold risk compared to the risk of epilepsy in the general population. Risk factors significantly related to later epilepsy include abnormal cognitive and motor development prior to the initial febrile convulsion, prolonged repeated or asymmetrical convulsions, and a history of afebrile seizures in parents or siblings. Virtually all the excess risk of epilepsy over that sustained by the general population is accounted for by these risk factors and, if none of these factors is present, the risk of subsequent epilepsy in a child who has had a febrile convulsion is barely greater than that of the population as a whole.

12.12   Sociological aspects of epilepsy

Having epilepsy does not just mean the unpleasantness of recurrent seizures, and coping with long-term drug therapy, but coping also with some degree of public antipathy and disadvantage at work. It is clear that there are some occupations that are totally inappropriate for someone with recurrent disturbances of consciousness, for example any occupation that includes driving. People with epilepsy should not work at heights from which they might fall if consciousness were disturbed. Heavy moving machinery is also a risk. More contentious, however, are those employers who refuse to employ people with epilepsy even if the seizure is no more than a temporary inconvenience in the course of their employment. Many education authorities, for example, discourage people with epilepsy from applying for jobs as teachers.

Perhaps because they feel stigmatized, even if they themselves have not actually encountered overt prejudice, many people with epilepsy conceal their seizures when seeking employment. Even within the family circle, children with epilepsy grow up perceiving that epilepsy is something 'bad' through their parents' frequent concealment of seizures from those outside the family circle.

The difference between epilepsy and many of the other physical disabilities considered in this book is that for 99.9 per cent of the time someone with epilepsy is entirely normal, compared to someone with an overt disability such as, for example, a patient with muscular dystrophy. It has been suggested that when an apparently normal person suddenly has a seizure in front of his friends who are 'not in the know', then these friends feel let down and deceived. Someone with infrequent recurrent seizures, therefore, has the great stress of deciding how much of his disability he should reveal to others. Such stresses may themselves result in anxiety and tension.

All the anticonvulsant drugs have some effect on cognitive function. Phenobarbitone is probably the worst offender, follwed by phenytoin, sodium valproate, and carbamazepine in decreasing importance. Even when taking this last drug, however, many people feel somewhat slowed in their mental abilities. Their own perceptions are supported by quantitative psychometric tests.

12.13   Psychiatric aspects of epilepsy

The difficulties mentioned in the preceding paragraphs may be associated with a frank depressive illness. Some workers have found that depression is more likely to occur in people with temporal lobe epilepsy, but this has not been the case in all studies. The risk of suicide is approximately five times greater in those with epilepsy than in the general population.

The areas of focal brain damage causing epilepsy, particularly if in the temporal lobe, may occasionally give rise to a schizophreniform psychosis. Any of the phenomena of schizophrenia can occur in such patients, although there is often little flattening of affect. There are interesting case reports of so-called 'forced normalization'. These words have been used of subjects with temporal lobe epilepsy whose seizures improve as their psychosis gets worse, and vice versa.

Arguments continue in the neurological literature about whether or not patients with epilepsy have a specific type of personality. It is not uncommon in outpatient practice to meet patients with temporal lobe epilepsy who have an undue preoccupation with religious and philosophical concerns, mild depression and irritability, and obsessionality about their epilepsy and their medication. The present view is that many of these concerns arise as an understandable reaction to the effect of epilepsy upon such patients' lives, and the onset, in some people, of clear-cut psychiatric illness. If these are excluded, then most of the measured differences in personality between those with temporal lobe epilepsy and the general population disappear.

Unfortunately, some patients with epilepsy commit criminal acts, sometimes aggressive acts. If relevant at all, it is probable that aggression is related to the underlying brain damage of which the epilepsy is a symptom, rather than epilepsy *per se* resulting in aggression. Very rarely, aggression may occur during a seizure or immediately afterwards in the confused post-ictal state.

Sexual function may be disturbed in those with temporal lobe epilepsy. Studies have shown low levels of free serum testosterone in men. It appears that women with seizures arising from the right temporal lobe are particularly likely to lack sexual interest. Although these specific points are interesting, it must not be overlooked that some patients with epilepsy secondary to structural lesions within the brain are relatively dependent people with poor social skills and poor self-image. It is probably these factors that contribute principally to any sexual problems that they encounter.

Finally, there is the interesting condition of pseudoseizures. Patients with true epilepsy, and occasionally people who have never had a truly epileptic seizure may sometimes simulate a seizure when they are under particular stress, or when they are dissatisfied with aspects of their life or medical management. It is necessary to avoid the trap of overprescribing anticonvulsant drugs in an attempt to gain control of seizures that are not epileptic.

After a true epileptic seizure, the serum prolactin rises to more than 800 micro-units/ml. This is true not only of tonic–clonic seizures, but also of those partial seizures in which the seizure discharge spreads to mesial limbic structures. An elevation of this order is not seen after pseudoseizures. Apart from this biochemical pointer, close observation, preferably by video-recording and simultaneous EEG, may show features that are anomalous for true epileptic attacks.

12.14 Epilepsy and driving

It is obvious that if a seizure occurs while driving, then, even if the seizure only partially disturbs consciousness, an accident is very likely. All developed countries, therefore, have some restrictions on issuing drivers' licences to people with epilepsy. In the UK, an applicant for a licence suffering from epilepsy has to satisfy the conditions that he shall have been free from any epileptic attack during the period of 2 years immediately preceding the date when the licence is to come into effect.

The current regulations in the UK also contain a statement to the effect that the '. . . driving of a vehicle by [an applicant suffering from epilepsy] . . . is not likely to be a source of danger to the public.' This last statement can override other statements, and is sometimes invoked in those with undoubted neurosurgical causes for their epilepsy, such as a glioma, even though they have not had a seizure in the last 2 years.

Other aspects not covered by the UK regulations, but included in the formal practice of the

Drivers' and Vehicle Licencing Agency, include restrictions on those who have suffered a single seizure (one year without a licence), and on those who, even though they have remained seizure-free, have recently altered their anticonvulsant medication. It is not surprising, therefore, that many patients with epilepsy do not declare their seizures to the licencing authorities. In some of the United States, it is the responsibility of the physician to inform the licencing authority of his patient's epilepsy, but this is not the case in the UK. A physician must, however, remind his patient of his responsibility to inform the Drivers' and Vehicle Licencing Agency in Swansea of their seizures. If there is doubt about what should be done, medical advisers at that centre can refer the papers to a Specialist Advisory Panel.

12.15 Further reading

General

Dam, M. and Gram, L. (eds.) (1990). *Comprehensive epileptology*. Raven Press, New York.
Epilepsy: a *Lancet* review (1990). Lancet Publications, London.
Hauser, W. A., Annegers, J. F., and Anderson, V. F. (1983). Epidemiology and the genetics of epilepsy. In *Epilepsy* (ed. A. A. Ward *et al*). Raven Press, New York.
Hopkins, A. (ed.) (1987). *Epilepsy*. Chapman and Hall, London.
Penfield, W. and Rasmussen, T. (1968). *The cerebral cortex of Man: a clinical study of localisation of function*. Macmillan, New York.
Porter, R. J. (1989). *Epilepsy: 100 elementary principles*, (2nd edn). W. B. Saunders, London.
Resor, S. R. and Kutt H. (eds) (1991). *The medical treatment of epilepsy*. Marcel Dekker, New York and Basel.
Scheuer, M. L. and Pedley, T. A. (1990). The evaluation and treatment of seizures. *New England Journal of Medicine* **323**, 1468–74.

Epidemiology

Sander, J. W. A. S. and Shorvon, S. D. (1987). Incidence and prevalence in epilepsy and their methodological problems: a review. *Journal of Neurology, Neurosurgery and Psychiatry* **50**, 829–39.
Sander, J. W. A. S., Hart, Y. M., Johnson, A. L., and Shorvon, S. D. (1990). National General Practice

Study of Epilepsy: newly diagnosed epileptic seizures in a general population. *Lancet* **336**, 1267–71.

First seizures and the investigation of epilepsy

Chadwick, D. (1991). Epilepsy after first seizures: risks and implications. *Journal of Neurology, Neurosurgery and Psychiatry* **54**, 385–7.

Hauser, W. A., Rich, S. S., Annegers, J. F., and Anderson, V. E. (1990). Seizure recurrence after a first unprovoked seizure: an extended follow up. *Neurology* **40**, 1163–70.

Hopkins, A., Clarke, C. R. A., and Garman, A. (1988). Recurrence rates after first seizures in adults: predictive value of EEG and CT scanning. *Lancet* **i**, 721–7.

Differential diagnosis

Manolis, A. S., Linzer, M., Salem, D., and Estes, N. A. M. (1990). Syncope: current diagnostic evaluation and management. *Annals of Internal Medicine* **112**, 850–63.

Sra, J. S., Anderson, A. J., Sheikh, S. H., *et al.* (1991). Unexplained syncope evaluated by electrophysiological studies and head up tilt-testing. *Annals of Internal Medicine* **114**, 1013–19.

Stephenson, J. P. (1991). *Fits and faints*. MacKeith Press, London.

Van Lieshout, J. J., Wieling, W., Karemaker, J. M., and Eckberg, D. L. (1991). The vasovagal response. *Clinical Science* **81**, 575–86.

Treatment

Dasheiff, R. M. and Porter, R. J. (1989). Epilepsy surgery: is it an effective treatment? *Annals of Neurology* **25**, 506–10.

Engel, J. (ed.) (1987). *Surgical treatment of the epilepsies*. Raven Press, New York.

Levy, R. H., Dreifuss, F. E., Mattson, R. H., *et al* (ed) (1989). *Anti-epileptic drugs*, (3rd edn). Raven Press, New York.

Report of a Working Group (1990). Standards of care for patients with neurological disease: a consensus. *Journal of the Royal College of Physicians of London* **24**, 90–7.

Prognosis

Annegers, J. F., Hauser, W. A., and Elveback, L. R. (1979). Remission of seizures and relapse in patients with epilepsy. *Epilepsia* **20**, 729–37.

Elwes, R. D. C., Johnson, A. L., and Reynolds, E. H. (1988). The course of untreated epilepsy. *British Medical Journal* **297**, 948–51.

Stopping anticonvulsant treatment

Medical Research Council Antiepileptic Drug Withdrawal Study Group (1991). Randomised study of antiepileptic drug withdrawal in patients in remission. *Lancet* **337**, 1175–80.

Febrile convulsions

Annegers, J. F., Hauser, W. A., Shirts, S. B., and Kurland, L. T. (1987). Factors prognostic of unprovoked seizures after febrile convulsions. *New England Journal of Medicine* **316**, 493–5.

Joint Working Group of the Research Unit of the Royal College of Physicians of London and the British Paediatric Association (1991). Guidelines for the management of convulsions with fever. *British Medical Journal* **303**, 634–6.

Verity, C.M. and Golding, J. (1991). Risk of epilepsy after febrile convulsions: a national cohort study. *British Medical Journal* **303**, 1373–6.

Post-traumatic epilepsy

Hauser, W. A. (1990). Prevention of post-traumatic epilepsy. *New England Journal of Medicine* **323**, 540–1.

Driving and epilepsy

Hansotia, P. and Broste, S. K. (1991). The effect of epilepsy or diabetes mellitus on the risk of automobile accidents. *New England Journal of Medicine* **324**, 22–6.

Psychiatric complications

Trimble, M. R. (1991). *The psychoses of epilepsy*. Raven Press, New York.

Surgery for intractable epilepsy

Spencer, S. S. and Spencer, D. D. (1990). *Surgery for epilepsy: contemporary issues in neurological surgery*; Vol. 2. Blackwell, Oxford.

13 Movement disorders

The term 'movement disorders' is given to a group of conditions of which many involve the basal ganglia. Obviously, disorders of movement in the sense of paralysis occur in, for example, strokes and paraplegia, but discussion in this chapter is limited to those conditions listed in Table 13.1. The general term movement disorders is increasingly preferred, as for many patients the difficulty lies in the execution of a normal temporal or spatial pattern of movement, without weakness. In some of the disorders, these difficulties are accompanied by involuntary movements, such as chorea or tremor. This forms the basis for the classification in Table 13.1. There are, of course, considerable

Table 13.1 Classification of movement disorders

Syndromes with poverty of movement
   Parkinson's disease
   parkinsonism secondary to encephalitis
   parkinsonism secondary to drugs
   parkinsonism secondary to toxins
   parkinsonism secondary to trauma
   parkinsonism secondary to hypoxia
   multisystem atrophy
   Shy–Drager syndrome
   olivopontocerebellar degeneration
   progressive supranuclear palsy
Syndromes with dystonia (see Table 13.3)
   examples: Wilson's disease, spasmodic torticollis
Syndromes with chorea (see Table 13.4)
   examples: Huntington's disease, rheumatic chorea
Syndromes with tics
   example: Gilles de la Tourette syndrome
Syndromes with myoclonus (see Tables 13.5 and 13.6)
   examples: essential myoclonus, metabolic
   encephalopathies
Syndromes with tremor
   example: essential tremor

difficulties in this classification. For example, although chorea (Section 13.6) is a feature of both Huntington's and Sydenham's diseases, there is nothing to suggest a common aetiology, and there is little likelihood of diagnostic confusion. Other members of the list, however, do have a close relationship, for example the depletion of striatal dopamine in both Parkinson's disease and parkinsonism secondary to the use of some drugs, such as reserpine.

13.1 Parkinson's disease

13.1.1 *Definition and history*

This is the name given to 'idiopathic' parkinsonism—that is to say, a gradually progressive disorder in which slowness and poverty of voluntary movement are accompanied by tremor and by muscular rigidity. The first description, by James Parkinson, a physician of Hoxton in London, in 1817, was so accurate and succinct that it is worth quoting here, as it effectively defines the disease

and is a tribute to the effectiveness of clinical observation.

'So slight and nearly imperceptible are the first inroads of this malady, and so extremely slow is its progress, that it rarely happens that the patient can form any recollection of the precise period of its commencement. The first symptoms perceived are a slight sense of weakness, with a proneness to trembling in some particular part; sometimes in the head, but most commonly in one of the hands and arms. These symptoms gradually increase in the part affected; and at an uncertain period, but seldom in less than twelvemonths or more, the morbid influence is felt in some other part. Thus assuming one of the hands and arms to be first attacked, the other, at this period becomes similarly affected. After a few more months the patient is found to be less strict than usual in preserving an upright posture: this being most observable whilst walking, but sometimes whilst sitting or standing. Sometime after the appearance of this symptom, and during its slow increase, one of the legs is discovered slightly to tremble, and is also found to suffer fatigue sooner than the leg of the other side: in a few months this limb becomes agitated by similar tremblings, and suffers a similar loss of power.

Hitherto the patient will have experienced but little inconvenience; and befriended by the strong influence of habitual endurance, would perhaps seldom think of his being the subject of disease, except when reminded of it by the unsteadiness of his hand, whilst writing or employing himself in any nicer kind of manipulation. But as the disease proceeds, similar employments are accomplished with considerable difficulty, the hand failing to answer with exactness to the dictates of the will. Walking becomes a task which cannot be performed without considerable attention. The legs are not raised to that height, or with that promptitude which the will directs, so that the utmost care is necessary to prevent frequent falls.

At this period the patient experiences much inconvenience, which unhappily is found daily to increase. The submission of the limbs to the directions of the will can hardly ever be obtained in the performance of the most ordinary offices of life. The fingers cannot be disposed of in the proposed directions, and applied with certainty to any proposed point. As time and the disease proceed, difficulties increase: writing can now be hardly at all accomplished; and reading, from the tremulous motion, is accomplished with some difficulty. Whilst at meals the fork not being duly directed frequently fails to raise the morsel from the plate: which, when seized, is with much difficulty conveyed to the mouth. At this period the patient seldom experiences a suspension of the agitation of his limbs. Commencing, for instance in one arm, the wearisome agitation is borne until beyond sufference, when by suddenly changing the posture it is for a time stopped in that limb, to commence, generally, in less than a minute in one of the legs, or in the arm of the other side. Harassed by this tormenting round, the patient has recourse to walking, a mode of exercise to which the sufferers from this malady are in general partial; owing to their attention being thereby somewhat diverted from their unpleasant feelings, by the care and exertion required to ensure its safe performance.

But as the malady proceeds, even this temporary mitigation of suffering from the agitation of the limbs is denied. The propensity to lean forward becomes invincible, and the patient is thereby forced to step on the toes and fore part of the feet, whilst the upper part of the body is thrown so far forward as to render it difficult to avoid falling on the face. In some cases, when this state of the malady is attained, the patient can no longer exercise himself by walking in his usual manner, but is thrown on the toes and forepart of the feet; being, at the same time, irresistibly impelled to take much quicker and shorter steps, and thereby to adopt unwillingly a running pace. In some cases it is found necessary entirely to substitute running for walking: since otherwise the patient, on proceeding only a very few paces, would inevitably fall.

In this stage, the sleep becomes much disturbed. The tremulous motions of the limbs occur during sleep, and augment until they awaken the patient, and frequently with much agitation and alarm. The power of conveying the food to the mouth is at length so much impeded that he is obliged to consent to be fed by others. The bowels, which had been all along torpid, now, in most cases, demand stimulating medicines of very considerable power: the expulsion of the faeces from the rectum sometimes requiring mechanical aid. As the disease proceeds towards its last stage, the trunk is almost permanently bowed, the muscular power is more decidedly diminished, and the tremulous agitation becomes violent. The patient walks now with great difficulty, and unable any longer to support himself with his stick, he dares not venture on this exercise, unless assisted by an attendant, who walking backwards before him, prevents his falling forwards, by the pressure of his hands against the fore part of his shoulders. His words are now scarcely intelligible; and he is not only no longer able to feed himself, but when the food is conveyed to the mouth, so much are the actions of the muscles of the tongue, pharynx, &c. impeded by impaired action and perpetual agitation, that the food is with difficulty retained in the mouth until masticated; and then with difficulty swallowed. Now also, from the same cause, another very unpleasant circumstance occurs: saliva fails of being directed to the back part of the fauces, and hence is continually draining from the mouth, mixed with the particles of food, which he is no longer able to clear from the inside of the mouth.

As the debility increases and the influence of the will over the muscles fades away, the tremulous agitation becomes more vehement. It now seldom leaves him for a moment; but even when exhausted nature seizes a small portion of sleep, the motion becomes so violent as not only to shake the bed-hangings, but even the floor and sashes of the room. The chin is now almost immoveably bent down upon the sternum. The slops with which he is attempted to be fed, with the saliva, are continually trickling from the mouth. The power of articulation is lost. The urine and faeces are passed involuntarily; and at the last, constant sleepiness, with slight delirium, and other marks of extreme exhaustion, announce the wished-for release.'

Other landmarks in the understanding of Parkinson's disease were the description of Lewy bodies (Section 13.1.3) in 1913, confirmation that the disease was associated with lesions of the substantia nigra by Tretiakoff in 1919, observations of the gross reduction in striatal dopamine levels in patients with Parkinson's disease by Ehringer and Hornykiewicz in 1960, the subsequent beneficial effects of infused L-dopa by Birkmayer and Hornykiewicz in 1961, and the later effective trials of large oral doses of L-dopa by Cotzias and colleagues in 1967.

13.1.2 *Incidence and prevalence*

The overall annual incidence of Parkinson's disease is about 20 per 100 000. This means that the average UK general practitioner will see about two new cases in 5 years. The prevalence is about 165 per 100 000, the average duration of the disease from onset to death being about 11 years, so that the general practitioner will be looking after about four cases of Parkinson's disease at any one time. Figure 13.1 shows the age-specific incidence and prevalence of the disease, underlining the marked increase of its occurrence in older age-groups.

Parkinson's disease may be slightly commoner in males at any age, but as women live longer, and the incidence increases with age, there are more affected older women.

13.1.3 *The pathology of Parkinson's disease*

The hallmark of the disease is degeneration of the dopaminergic pathway, the melanin-containing cell bodies of which lie in the substantia nigra, the axons projecting to the striatum. Naked-eye exam-

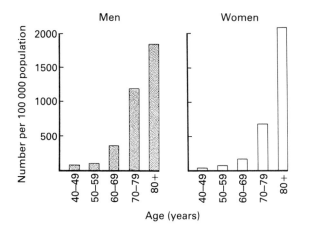

Fig. 13.1 Prevalence of Parkinson's disease at different ages. (Data from Mutch *et al.* 1986.)

ination of the brains of advanced cases of Parkinson's disease shows loss of melanin from the pars compacta of the substantia nigra. Quantitative histochemical examination confirms loss of nigrostriatal dopaminergic neurons in the substantia nigra. There is also a marked loss of serotonin-synthesizing neurons in the median raphe, and loss also of noradrenergic cells containing substance P in the pons and medulla. Surviving neurons contain eosinophilic Lewy bodies. Electron microscopic and histochemical observation of these bodies show an electron-dense, amorphous, proteinaceous core surrounded by radiating filaments. The overall appearance has been compared to the head of a sunflower. Lewy bodies and degeneration of dopinergic neurons are also found in the locus coeruleus and dorsal nucleus of the vagus, and outside the central nervous system in sympathetic ganglia. Lewy bodies are highly characteristic of Parkinson's disease, but they are occasionally found at routine autopsy in 'normal' brains and in a few patients with Alzheimer's disease. It is conceivable that such incidental findings in 'normal' brains may represent early undiagnosed parkinsonism.

Lewy bodies are not found in post-encephalitic parkinsonism, nor in chemically induced parkinsonism (Section 13.1.4). If we knew exactly what caused Lewy bodies to form, our understanding of Parkinson's disease would probably be much increased.

13.1.4 *The cause of Parkinson's disease*

There are no geographical variations in the incidence of Parkinson's disease to suggest a disorder acquired from the environment; however, recent research suggests that the cause must be sought there. The reasons are as follows.

First of all, although earlier reports suggested a familial incidence of Parkinson's disease, the late age of onset has always meant that a proband's account of an affected parent had to be taken on trust, as the latter was nearly always dead from advanced age. It was possible that parental benign essential tremor (Section 13.9.1) or diffuse arteriosclerotic cerebrovascular disease (Section 10.1.11.3) had been mistaken for true Parkinson's disease. If familial studies are confined to siblings and twins, then there is no evidence of a hereditary factor in the genesis of Parkinson's disease. Particularly striking is the almost total lack of concordance amongst the monozygotic twins of patients affected by the disease.

The second reason suggesting an environmental factor is the outbreak of post-encephalitic parkinsonism. A severe parkinsonian syndrome occurred in many patients previously affected by the epidemic of encephalitis lethargica that occurred throughout the world in the years 1915 to 1926. Although post-mortem studies at the time left no doubt that this was an inflammatory encephalitic illness, no infectious agent was ever isolated. After a brief prodromal syndrome suggestive of an upper respiratory tract infection, patients developed a state of hypersomnolence associated with ocular and bulbar palsies and generalized rigidity. About 40 per cent of patients died in the acute stage, and about one third of the survivors developed a parkinsonian illness within a few months or years of the onset. The clinical picture is quite distinct from that of idiopathic Parkinson's disease, often with an onset in the second or third decade of life. Cranial nerve palsies, dystonia, choreo-athetosis, disturbances of behaviour and oculogyric crises are characteristic. In these last, the eyes are turned, usually strongly upwards, and maintained in that position for several minutes or hours, the patient being unable to deviate the eyes downwards. Tics, particularly affecting the respiratory muscles, were also frequent.

Post-mortem examinations of the brains of those dying of postencephalitic parkinsonism showed bilateral diffuse degeneration and gliosis of the substantia nigra and locus coeruleus in the brain stem, but no Lewy bodies. There were also more widespread neurofibrillary filament tangles in the brain stems and mesencephalic tegmentum.

The cohort of patients afflicted by this severe disorder is now virtually extinct, but the disorder is of historical interest as some of these patients were first partly liberated from their disability by large doses of L-dopa in early trials of this drug in 1966.

The understandable feeling amongst neurologists has been that if one infective agent caused an illness with many of the features of Parkinson's disease, then it was reasonable to believe that other agents might be responsible for the true 'idiopathic' disorder. However, extensive serological and epidemiological research has failed to incriminate any known virus. Neither is there any evidence incriminating an unconventional 'slow' virus. The disorder has not been successfully transmitted to animals by inoculation of affected brain, as has Creutzfeldt–Jakob disease and kuru (Section 17.15). Furthermore, the histological changes in the brains of those with Parkinson's disease are quite unlike the spongiform change seen in astrocytes in slow virus infections.

The third reason why researchers are seeking an environmental cause for Parkinson's disease is the finding in some epidemiological studies that the prevalence of the disease is less in smokers than in those who have never smoked. The significance of this observation might be that nicotine, or some other constituent of cigarettes, protects against the development of Parkinson's disease. An alternative view is based upon the pre-morbid personalities of those with Parkinson's disease who appear, in some studies, to have been rather unadventurous and obsessional in their conduct long before the onset of the illness. Such people are less likely to acquire the habit of smoking. In this view, then, non-smoking is only a behavioural marker of a brain predisposed, on biochemical grounds, to demonstrate Parkinson's disease later in life.

The fourth and most potent reason for seeking an environmental factor is the occurrence of an intense parkinsonian syndrome amongst those exposed to 1-methyl-4-phenyl-1,2,3,6-tetrahydropyridine (MPTP). An American addict manufacturing his own pethidine analogue in 1976 unwittingly produced some related by-products, one of which was subsequently proved to be MPTP. Three days after injecting the mixture he developed a severe parkinsonian syndrome, which responded partially to treatment with L-dopa until his suicide 18 months later. At autopsy there was a loss of dopaminergic neurons within the substantia nigra. This is not an isolated occurrence. A further seven addicts who administered MPTP intravenously, under the impression that it was synthetic heroin, have developed a parkinsonian syndrome, as has a chemist working in the laboratory on the product. Intravenous infusion of MPTP produces a parkinsonian syndrome in rhesus and squirrel monkeys (but not in rodents, which, interestingly, do not have neurons that contain melanin) with akinesia, rigidity, tremor, a flexed posture, and impaired righting reflexes. Histological examination of the brains of these monkeys shows a loss of pigmented neurons in the pars compacta of the substantia nigra, and a marked reduction in the dopamine content of the striatum.

There are histological differences between experimental MPTP parkinsonism and the idiopathic disease. In MPTP parkinsonism, degeneration in dopaminergic neurons does not occur outside the substantia nigra, and Lewy bodies have not, with one exception, been found.

Although the toxic agent was initially identified as MPTP, it has been shown that it requires conversion to the 1-methyl-4-phenylpyridinium ion (MPP+). MPP+ induces dopaminergic cell death by the inhibition of NADH coenzyme Q_1 reductase. This first protein of the mitochondrial respiratory chain has recently been shown to be reduced in some patients with idiopathic Parkinson's disease.

13.1.5 *The biochemistry of dopamine*

Figure 13.2 shows the main metabolic pathways of dopamine. Infusion of radiolabelled dopamine has shown that most is metabolized to homovanillic acid, and a lesser proportion through the catecholamine pathway to noradrenaline and homovanillic acid.

Ehringer and Hornykiewicz first discovered the depletion of dopamine in the substantia nigra and striatum of patients with Parkinson's disease. Correlations between clinical, biochemical, and postmortem evidence show that symptoms and signs of Parkinson's disease do not appear until the sub-

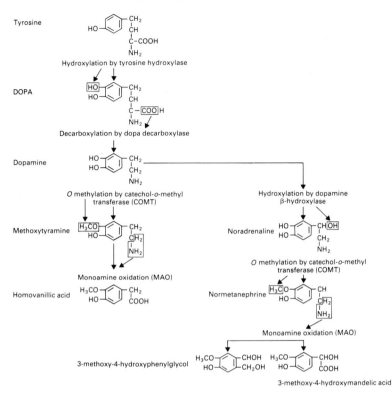

Fig. 13.2   The metabolic pathways of dopamine.

stantia nigra has lost more than 80 per cent of its pigmented neurons, and until the striatum is depleted of 80 per cent of its dopamine content. There is evidence that the surviving neurons are working harder to compensate, as the ratio between brain dopamine and its metabolite homovanillic acid—a measure of dopamine turnover—increases, although the absolute values of these substances decrease. Compensation also occurs at a post-synaptic level, as the number of dopamine receptors in the striatum increases in the early stages of the illness. Consequently, dopamine liberated by surviving nigrostriatal neurons has an enhanced effect due to denervation supersensitivity. Eventually, further loss of neurons occurs, possibly due not to any further exposure to an environmental agent (be it toxic or infective) but as a consequence of normal ageing. Compensation then fails, and the severity of the untreated illness follows the degree of striatal dopamine deficiency.

13.1.6   Clinical features of Parkinson's disease

Parkinson's original description is quoted in Section 13.1.1. The principal features of the disease are tremor, slowness and poverty of voluntary movement, rigidity of muscles, and impairment of postural reflexes. Each of these is described below, but before obvious disturbances occur there is what might be termed a 'pre-neurological' phase, dominated by loss of previous energies, obscure muscular aches, pains and tinglings, cramps, and sometimes depression.

13.1.6.1   Tremor

This is the symptom presenting to a physician in about 70 per cent of cases, although examination at this time will usually show other signs of Parkinson's disease to be already present. Tremor with a frequency of 4–5 c/s commonly begins in one hand, with rhythmic movements of the thumb across the index and middle fingers (or vice versa). This is the movement that pre-industrial pharmacists used to roll pastes into 'pills', hence the description of a 'pill-rolling tremor'. Later the tremor spreads to the foot on the same side, or to the other hand. In the early stages a patient can usually briefly control the tremor by an effort of will. The tremor persists when the limb is fully supported, and disappears, at least in the early stages, during the course of a voluntary movement. In these characteristics it is quite distinct from an intention tremor (Section 6.2.5). The tremor of Parkinson's disease may be brought out by asking the patient to walk. It is also often exacerbated by tension or excitement. It disappears during sleep. (This is one observation about which James Parkinson was incorrect.)

The operation of stereotactic thalamotomy (Section 13.1.8.8) has allowed considerable research on the tremor of Parkinson's disease. Microelectrode recordings have shown the presence of neurons in the ventral nuclei of the thalamus which fire bursts of activity, synchronous with and time-locked to tremor in a particular part of the contralateral hand or leg. The discharge of these thalamic neurons can be modified by stretching the muscles involved in that tremor, but not by tactile stimuli. This is concordant with the observations made by patients (and by James Parkinson) that they can briefly inhibit the tremor by shifting their position.

Electromyographic observations on tremor reveal that there is reciprocal excitation of muscles with opposing actions. The frequency of tremor tends to be the same in closely related muscle groups, but varies a little from one limb, or one part of a limb to another—that is to say, there is no evidence of a single 'tremogenic clock', driving all muscles synchronously.

13.1.6.2 Slowness and poverty of voluntary movement

These disabilities are often known as bradykinesia and hypo- or akinesia. There is no muscular weakness as such, nor is the slowness of movement necessarily associated with muscular rigidity. There is slowness in initiating a movement in response to a stimulus. The patient activates the appropriate muscles, but cannot drive his anterior horn cells fast enough to generate sufficient muscle force rapidly enough for a planned fast voluntary

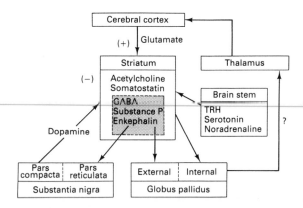

Fig. 13.3 Some interconnections of the basal ganglia. (Reproduced with kind permission from Martin 1984.)

movement. Instead, the limb is jerkily dragged to the required position by a series of small bursts of muscle activity.

It has been suggested that the function of the basal ganglia is to initiate and then automatically and subconsciously to run a sequence of motor programmes that comprise a planned action. Some of the interconnections of the basal ganglia are shown in Fig. 13.3. Patients with Parkinson's disease can learn and store motor programmes, but the initiating and running of the programmes is impaired. The more complex the activity, the greater the impairment. A striking example of this is the inability of many patients with Parkinson's disease to perform two simple motor acts simultaneously, although they can often perform either individually.

A further aspect is fatigue—patients find it impossible to sustain repetitive motor programmes, such as alternating pronation and supination of one hand. The difficulty in executing and sustaining complex motor tasks leads to one of the most characteristic features of the illness—impairment of handwriting, which characteristically becomes smaller, slower and shakier, and gradually less legible. The first few letters may be well formed, but then legibility tails away. Similar difficulties may be encountered in other repetitive movements, such as cleaning the teeth.

In addition to these impairments of voluntary movements, major clinical points are the relative absence of normal spontaneous movements, particularly blinking, changes in facial expression, and the small shifts in the sitting position which we all make from time to time. There may also be a defect in relevant associated movements, such as swinging the arms on walking. This is an action to which no conscious thought is given during normal gait, but it disappears early in the course of Parkinson's disease.

Speech is impaired in Parkinson's disease; the voice is soft and monotonous. There may be a hesitation in starting to speak and, like the gait, an impression of hurrying.

The eye movements in Parkinson's disease are not normal. Convergence is impaired, and lateral movements jerky and broken up. The blink reflex elicited by tapping the glabella does not fatigue, as it normally does, after two or three trials, but continues indefinitely. Involuntary fluttering of the eyelids—blepharoclonus—may occur.

13.1.6.3 *Gait*

It is impossible to better the description given by Parkinson, and quoted in Section 13.1.1. The disturbance of gait can sometimes be remarkably improved by afferent input; for example, a friend walking arm-in-arm with an affected person can cause a considerable lengthening of the stride. Conversely, perceived obstacles, as trivial as a line painted on the floor, may cause the patient's feet to freeze to the ground, and he or she may be unable to start walking again until light assistance is provided. 'Freezing' may also affect arm movements, trunk movements such as turning over in bed, and speech.

13.1.6.4 *Impaired postural control*

Patients with advanced Parkinson's disease lose their righting reflexes, so if pushed or jostled they fall easily. This impairment extends to the sitting posture; patients may topple sideways or forwards in their chairs. In advanced cases, there is a disturbance of the normal erect posture, the patient becoming increasingly flexed.

13.1.6.5 *Rigidity*

Parkinson himself did not mention rigidity—that is to say, increased resistance of limbs to passive stretch—but it is an early finding on clinical examination and is independent of bradykinesia and

tremor. There is uniform resistance in flexor and extensor muscle groups, this distinguishing the pattern of increased tone from that of spasticity (Section 6.2.3.2). Slow rates of stretch of a muscle induce vigorous anterior horn cell discharges to the same muscle in patients with Parkinson's disease, whatever the amount of ongoing background electromyographic abnormality. In contrast, a much faster rate of stretch is necessary in normal subjects. There is good evidence that a long-loop cortical pathway is involved in this response, and presumably the gain of this reflex is enhanced, in Parkinson's disease, by some abnormality of basal ganglia drive.

If there is clinical doubt about the presence of rigidity in any patient, then two manoeuvres may exaggerate it: either increasing the rate of stretch of the muscle by, for example, more rapid flexion and extension of the wrist, or asking the patient to raise the contralateral arm at the shoulder. This alteration in posture, and hence, presumably, modification in the output of the basal ganglia, facilitates the stretch reflex in the limb under examination.

Whether or not the patient has a tremor, as the wrist is flexed and extended an increased resistance will be felt to fluctuate in a jerky way—so-called 'cogwheeling'. Analysis of the cogging shows that it has a frequency of 6 c/s, quite distinct from that of the resting tremor of Parkinson's disease. It has been suggested that the afferent input to the thalamus resulting from muscle stretch precipitates burst activity in some thalamic neurons which were previously inactive. An alternative view, based upon the fact that clonus in pyramidal lesions also has a frequency of 6 c/s, is that abnormal function in the basal ganglia alters spinal activity, and muscle stretch elicits clonic movements. The tendon reflexes in Parkinson's disease are not usually brisk, which militates against this explanation.

13.1.6.6 *Mental changes in Parkinson's disease*

Depression may precede or coexist with Parkinson's disease. Although undoubtedly some elements of that depression are due to the physical limitations and reduced expectations in life, the impression is that depression in Parkinson's disease is more common and of greater intensity than in other disabling physical illnesses. Treatment with imipramine, an antidepressant drug, without L-dopa, does modestly improve rigidity and akinesia in addition to depression, and there are reports of electroconvulsive therapy (ECT), given for depression, also improving parkinsonian symptoms. Dopaminergic pathways are certainly of importance in animal experiments in which, although mood cannot be judged, behaviour in response to 'pleasurable' stimuli can be assessed. For example, the dopamine-receptor antagonist, haloperidol, will prevent animals from choosing an environment in which D-amphetamine is readily available. The relationship between dopamine and mood is, however, not straightforward. It appears that the increased mobility following L-dopa treatment may help any component of depression that is reactive to the physical disability, but L-dopa may *exacerbate* any underlying depression.

Dementia occurs in about 10–15 per cent of patients with Parkinson's disease (Section 11.5.2). The brains of some patients with Parkinson's disease show degeneration of cholinergic neurons in the substantia innominata. Anticholinergic agents used in treatment may exacerbate the confusion of demented patients.

13.1.6.7 *Other clinical features of Parkinson's disease*

Infrequency of normal swallowing gives the appearance of increased salivation, and patients with advanced disease may drool. The skin often appears greasy. Constipation may be prominent. Muscular aches and pains, and painful limitations of movements of joints secondary to disuse, particularly the shoulder, are very common. Unexplained uncomfortable paraesthesiae are also described by patients.

13.1.7 *Differential diagnosis of Parkinson's disease*

Parkinson's disease is one of those medical conditions that are usually diagnosed on sight, rather as one might have little doubt of the nature of a measles rash. It is particularly helpful to see patients walk, preferably without them realizing that they are under observation. The flexed posture, tremor, and failure to swing one or other arm

Table 13.2 The differential diagnosis of Parkinson's disease

Post-encephalitic parkinsonism
Drug-induced parkinsonism
Benign essential tremor
Depression with motor retardation
Normal pressure hydrocephalus, with abnormal gait
Degenerative disorders
Steele–Richardson–Olszewski syndrome
Shy–Drager syndrome
Alzheimer's disease
diffuse Lewy body disease
Cranial trauma
dementia pugilistica
Intoxications
carbon monoxide
manganese
MPTP
Diffuse cerebrovascular disease, with abnormal gait

are then often very obvious. Inspection of the seated patient may show a fixity of gaze, facial expression, and immobile position that suggest the diagnosis. Increased tone in the limbs usually clinches it.

There are, however, other neurological conditions which may be confused with Parkinson's disease. First of all, there are the other causes of parkinsonism, listed in Table 13.2, from which 'idiopathic' Parkinson's disease must be distinguished. By far the commonest member of this group is drug-induced parkinsonism (Section 13.10.1), and a careful drug history should be taken. Tremor is perhaps less prominent in patients with drug-induced parkinsonism than in Parkinson's disease.

There are other conditions that must be clearly distinguished from parkinsonism or Parkinson's disease, as the pathology, natural history, therapy, and prognosis are so different. Foremost among these is benign essential tremor (Section 13.9.1). This is surprisingly frequently mistaken for the tremor of Parkinson's disease, yet an essential tremor will always cease if the limb is fully supported.

The symptoms of Parkinson's disease may be much more prominent on one side, so much so that it initially appears that the patient has a hemiplegia and is investigated on that basis. The

immobility of a severe depressive illness may sometimes cause confusion. Sometimes those with Alzheimer's disease are rigid and immobile, but of
course depression, dementia, and Parkinson's disease can all coexist. Other degenerative disorders
with major extrapyramidal features are listed in
Table 13.2. The Shy–Drager syndrome (Section
13.2.1) is distinguished from Parkinson's disease
by the features of prominent autonomic failure,
and the Steele–Richardson–Olszewski syndrome
(Section 13.4) largely by the distinct abnormalities
of eye movements. Patients with normal pressure
hydrocephalus (Section 11.5.9) may have apparently parkinsonian features, with bradykinesia, rigidity, and an abnormal gait. The posture and gait
of diffuse multi-infarct cerebrovascular disease
(Sections 10.1.11.3 and 10.1.11.4) is rather reminiscent of parkinsonism, but there is no depletion
of dopamine, and it is not helpful to speak of
'arteriosclerotic parkinsonism'. Finally, diffuse
neuronal atrophy following repeated cranial injuries (dementia pugilistica) and carbon monoxide
poisoning result in a disability with many extrapyramidal features. Manganese poisoning is not
really seen outside the mines of South America.
The story of MPTP is considered in Section 13.1.4.

13.1.7.1 *Investigations*

There are no laboratory or radiological investigations in routine use for the diagnosis of Parkinson's
disease. The diagnosis is a clinical one, and attention to the points outlined in Sections 13.1.6 and
13.1.7 will usually allow the diagnosis to be made
with confidence. If there is doubt, there is everything to be gained by further examination after an
interval of 2–3 months. An infusion with apomorphine, a short-acting dopamine agonist, will help
distinguish patients with true Parkinson's disease
from other striatal syndromes (see Sections 13.2.3,
13.3, and 13.4), in so far as it will predict the
response to L-dopa. A cranial CT scan will be
required if any other diagnosis, such as normal
pressure hydrocephalus, is seriously entertained.

13.1.8 *The treatment of Parkinson's disease*

13.1.8.1 *The use of L-dopa and dopa*
          decarboxylase inhibitors

The principal drug now used for the treatment of

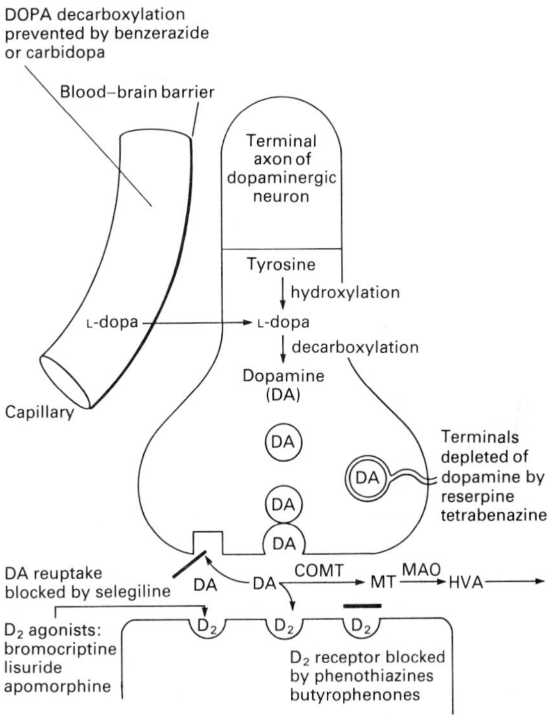

Fig. 13.4 L-dopa therapy and the dopaminergic synapse. DA, dopamine; COMT, cathechol-*o*-methyl transferase; MT, methoxytyramine; MAO, monoamine
oxidation; HVA, homovanillic acid.

Parkinson's disease is L-dopa, which is decarboxylated to dopamine (Fig. 13.2). The principal intracerebral effect of dopamine is to stimulate directly
striatal receptors which, by virtue of the death of
nigrostriatal neurons, show denervation supersensitivity (Fig. 13.4). Indeed, severely affected
patients respond more to a test of L-dopa than less
severely affected patients, presumably as they have
a greater degree of denervation supersensitivity.
Dopamine agonists, such as bromocriptine, have
the same function. However, surviving nigrostriatal neurons may be driven, by the L-dopa
administered, to take up more L-dopa and increase
their own transmitter output. Finally, dopamine
may exert a background neuromodulatory effect in
addition to acting as a neurotransmitter.

The first successful trial of oral L-dopa therapy
used very large doses (up to 8 g/day), as dopa
decarboxylase is present in many tissues outside
the brain. These large doses were necessary to

surmount peripheral decarboxylation so that sufficient L-dopa, having crossed the blood–brain barrier, was available to be converted to dopamine
within the brain. Dopa decarboxylase inhibitors
had already been synthesized, in the early 1960s,
in an (unsuccessful) attempt to treat hypertension.
Fortunately, two are available which do not cross
the blood–brain barrier. This means that the total
daily dose of L-dopa can be reduced by a factor of
about 10, and the adverse peripheral effects of
dopamine (Section 13.1.8.3) are largely prevented.

13.1.8.2 Beginning therapy with L-dopa

Two pharmaceutical preparations of L-dopa plus a
suitable dopa decarboxylase inhibitor are available. Co-beneldopa (Madopar) contains L-dopa
plus benserazide, and co-careldopa (Sinemet), L-
dopa plus carbidopa. There is no evidence that one
combination is better than the other. Treatment is
instituted with one of these combinations so that
the patient initially receives not more than 200 mg
of L-dopa a day, gradually increasing the dose over
the next 3 or 4 weeks until adequate clinical benefit
is obtained, adverse effects occur, or until a daily
dose of 750–800 mg L-dopa is reached. Using this
regime, most patients gain worthwhile relief of
symptoms in the short term, although tremor is
relatively resistant to therapy.

Some physicians use a single larger dose of
L-dopa initially; for example, co-careldopa 275, 1
tablet. The overall longer term response to L-dopa
can be predicted by the initial response in most
cases. A significant proportion of those who fail to
respond well to a single dose of co-careldopa
develop atypical features, suggesting multi-system
atrophy or some other extrapyramidal disorder in
the next two years.

There are, however, many continuing problems
with the treatment of Parkinson's disease, which
are considered next.

13.1.8.3 Early adverse effects of L-dopa

Unpleasant nausea and vomiting were frequent
limiting factors when L-dopa was used alone. Dopa
decarboxylase inhibitors have greatly reduced the
incidence of these effects. Postural hypotension is
also much less frequent now as dopa decarboxylase
inhibition prevents the peripheral vasodilator
action of dopamine.

Psychological effects may be prominent.
Increased energy is often noted, which is all to the
good, but abnormal elevation of mood may occur
so that the patient is unduly active, excited, and
occasionally confused. Conversely, a severe
depression may be precipitated. Sleep may be
disturbed by vivid dreams. Sexual drive may
increase.

Acute glaucoma may be precipitated in those
with narrow angles of ocular drainage. A few cases
of acceleration of growth in or apparent precipitation of malignancy in melanomas have been
reported. Occasionally, cardiac arrhythmias may
be precipitated.

Dyskinesia may occur. This is the principal limiting factor in the successful use of co-beneldopa
and co-careldopa. Common dystonic involuntary
movements induced by L-dopa include turning of
the head, shrugging of a shoulder, involuntary
movements of the limb, interruption of speech,
and a distorted dystonic gait. In the early stages of
treatment, such dyskinesias clearly indicate excessive treatment, but by the end of 6 years of
treatment nearly 80 per cent of patients will have
some dyskinesia at some time during the day.

13.1.8.4 Management of L-dopa therapy in the longer term

There are undoubted problems with L-dopa therapy. There are good arguments for suggesting that
management should be shared between neurologist
and general practitioner, the latter initiating and
managing this common disorder during a 'honeymoon' period of 3–4 years, when the benefits of L-
dopa are unmistakable (Fig. 13.5a) and the problems confined to those noted above. Unfortunately
problems then usually supervene. The most frequent, affecting about two-thirds of patients after
5 years, is the 'wearing-off effect' or end-of-dose
deterioration (Fig. 13.5b) in which patients complain of a progressive reduction in the duration of
benefit from each dose. If the dose is increased in
an attempt to overcome this, then dyskinesias may
supervene an hour or so after taking the dose (Fig.
13.5c). These peak-dose dyskinesias may be
avoided, at least for a time, by dividing the existing
daily dose, or a slight increment, into frequent
small doses, say two-hourly, in an attempt to
achieve reasonably stable plasma levels of L-dopa
(Fig. 13.5d). Problems may continue to mount,

however, with 'off'-periods that are resistant to L-dopa (Fig. 13.5e). Most difficult of all are sudden brief unexplained off-periods ('freezing') (Fig. 13.5f), which may be associated with 'yo-yoing' to dyskinesia. Such fluctuations are invariably aggravated by increasing the dose of L-dopa, and only occasionally relieved by reducing it.

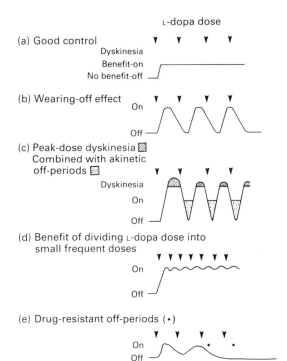

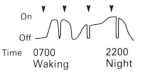

Fig. 13.5 Problems with L-dopa therapy. (a) Good control; intermittent dosage of L-dopa results in smooth control. (b) Wearing-off effect; clinical benefit wears off some hours after a dose. (c) Peak-dose dyskinesia combined with akinetic off-periods; fluctuations in brain dopamine levels result in dyskinesia 1–2 hours after a dose of L-dopa, then a period of reasonable control, then a wearing-off effect. (d) Repeated small doses of L-dopa may smooth out the fluctuations seen in (c). (e) Drug-resistant off-periods; note no benefit from third and fourth doses illustrated. (f) Late stage of treated Parkinson's disease; unexplained off-and on-periods are not reliably related to the timing of the dose.

The pathophysiology of the events illustrated in Fig. 13.5 is not at all clear. The basis of 'wearing-off' is probably due to the progressive loss of nigrostriatal neurons and their dopaminergic terminals as Parkinson's disease progresses. The resulting decline in striatal dopamine decarboxylase activity means that, even if plasma levels of dopa remain as before, less dopamine is formed in the striatum. The reduced number of dopaminergic terminals also results in less available storage for dopamine. This view is supported by the fact that the administration of apomorphine, a dopamine agonist, will reverse end-of-dose deterioration. It is more difficult to explain the abrupt fluctuations illustrated in Fig. 13.5f, but almost certainly part of the cause is fluctuations in plasma levels of dopa, as continuous intravenous L-dopa can reduce fluctuations. It is now recognized that dietary factors are important in achieving reasonably steady-state plasma levels of L-dopa. Variations in the rate of gastric emptying are important, and a large protein meal will reduce plasma levels of L-dopa as large neutral amino acids (e.g. valine, leucine, etc.) actively compete with L-dopa for transport across the cell membranes of the bowel wall. However, this phenomenon is not likely to be important with diets containing average amounts of protein unless the patient is at a 'brittle' stage of his Parkinson's disease. Metabolic changes of an uncertain nature in post-synaptic receptor mechanisms are probably also important in the genesis of sudden fluctuations of function.

13.1.8.5 *When should treatment with L-dopa be started?*

The question, of course, arises as to when treatment with L-dopa should begin. Does L-dopa prevent natural progression of the disease? Or does L-dopa cause a decline in dopamine receptor sensitivity and contribute to progressive failure of treatment? The evidence is controversial, some believing that the incidence of troublesome dyskinesia is proportional to the length of treatment and to the dose. Even with low-dose therapy (500 mg of L-dopa a day), 15 per cent of patients develop dyskinesia after 1 year, and 25 per cent after 3 years. Apart from dyskinesia, the on–off effect and psychiatric complications have, by some, been related to the cumulative dose of L-dopa. However, studies suggest that there is benefit from early treatment with L-dopa. For example, the observed to expected mortality ratio of patients in a number of early experimental trials of L-dopa is smaller in those who began treatment with L-dopa early in the course of the disease. It may be that the favourable effect is simply to keep patients active for longer as they approach old age, or it may be that in some way L-dopa has some specific action in slowing further nigrostriatal death. The evidence from one very large series is that it is youthful age of onset rather than early treatment which predisposes to dyskinesias.

There has been considerable discussion as to whether patients in the long term do better on submaximal doses. It appears that there is a trade-off between a lesser incidence of dyskinesias (and the later onset of on–off effects) and a lesser therapeutic benefit. The consensus view is to begin with a low dose of L-dopa and increase this gradually according to clinical need.

13.1.8.6   Other pharmacological methods of treatment.

Dopamine agonists

As already noted, dopamine agonists such as bromocriptine, apomorphine, pergolide, and lysuride directly interact with dopamine receptors on the post-synaptic neurons in the striatum (Fig. 13.4). The greatest experience has been with the use of oral bromocriptine, which may sometimes be useful in smoothing out fluctuations later in the disease. When starting this, it is necessary to reduce the oral dose of L-dopa by about a third. There is also increasing evidence that there is some advantage in using bromocriptine or lysuride de novo in the management of Parkinson's disease in combination with L-dopa. With this approach, the evolution of dyskinesias and fluctuations is less when reviewed 4 years after starting treatment. A suitable starting dose of bromocriptine is 1.25 mg twice a day, with subsequent small increments, and of lysuride 200 μg. A limiting factor in the use of bromocriptine and lysuride is nausea and vomiting, but this can be reduced by the concurrent administration of domperidone, which blocks dopaminergic receptors in the chemoreceptors in the area postrema, which lie outside the blood–brain barrier. A suitable dose is 10 mg by mouth, or a suppository of 30 mg. The manufacturers suggest

that the use of the drug is limited to a period of 12 weeks.

Pergolide and lysuride are structurally related to bromocriptine, but act directly at striatal receptors and, unlike bromocriptine, do not require the release of pre-synaptic dopamine. Pergolide often successfully reduces the requirements for L-dopa, with a reduction in disability and time spent 'off', but it is not very successful as therapy on its own without L-dopa. Some patients who have failed to respond to bromocriptine may respond to pergolide. Unfortunately, adverse effects such as nausea and vomiting are common, but slow upward adjustment of dose may avoid these. Treatment should begin with as little as 0.05 mg per day, increasing by increments of 0.05 mg to 0.1 mg a day every few days. Usual daily maintenance doses are around 2.5 mg.

A further approach is the constant subcutaneous infusion by microdrive pump of dopaminergic agonists such as lysuride and apomorphine. Some patients with brittle yo-yoing between on- and off-periods may be able to smooth out their fluctuations in this way. With careful adjustment of dose, psychotoxic complications are relatively infrequent. Alternatively, a small subcutaneous injection of apomorphine may be used on an ad hoc basis by patients, as the control of their Parkinson's disease turns 'off'.

Dopamine potentiators

There are other ways of manipulating the biochemistry of the dopaminergic synapse to the advantage of patients with Parkinson's disease (Fig. 13.4). Selegiline is a potent selective inhibitor of monoamine oxidase B isoenzyme. It was introduced with the idea that such enzyme inhibition might prolong the action of dopamine but, independent of this action, selegiline inhibits the re-uptake of dopamine into nerve terminals. Both effects prolong the 'life expectancy' of a dopamine molecule in the synaptic cleft. Selegiline hydrochloride (deprenyl) has proved useful in smoothing out the clinical control of patients with Parkinson's disease in its later stages. A suitable initial dose is 5 mg in the morning.

Monoamine oxidase inhibitors

Of greater potential importance is the fact that MPTP is converted to MPP+ (Section 13.1.4) by monoamine oxidase B, which mediates other oxidative mechanisms, leading to the production of free radicals which damage nigrostriatal neurons. If the cause of Parkinson's disease is related to free-radical formation, or the production of a compound analogous to MPP+, then selegiline may prevent its progression. For example, a redox reaction between MPDP+ and MPP+ generates free radicals through the formation of superoxide; this reaction is blocked by selegiline.

Trials have shown that selegiline, 10 mg/day, given to patients early in the disease delays the onset of the need for L-dopa for about a year, compared to placebo. Although the results are consistent with delaying the progress of the disease, by protecting neurons against the effects of some 'toxin' analogous to MPP+, they are also consistent with a direct action of selegiline on symptoms, perhaps by increasing the availability of nigrostriatal dopamine through the inhibition of monoamine oxidase, or by an antidepressant effect, postponing the need for L-dopa therapy. These results therefore require validation with respect to the progression of the disease as demonstrated by other end-points, such as survival to death, and neuropathological changes. Earlier uncontrolled studies have suggested that survival is prolonged by selegiline.

Amantadine has also been shown to be of benefit in Parkinson's disease. It probably does so by increasing the rate of liberation of dopamine from granule stores. A suitable dose is 100 mg twice a day.

Anticholinergic drugs

Long before the advent of L-dopa, moderate successes in the treatment of Parkinson's disease were obtained by the use of anticholinergic agents, and these certainly still have a place in the management of the disease. Physostigmine, an anticholinesterase which penetrates the blood–brain barrier, exacerbates Parkinson's disease, and, conversely, benzhexol, orphenadrine, and benztropine, all anticholinergic agents, reduce tremor and appear also to have a modest effect on rigidity. Some neurologists prefer to use one of these drugs in the early management of the illness, in view of the incidence of dyskinesias and other adverse effects with L-dopa therapy (see Section 13.1.8.4). However, many patients find that the dry mouth produced by the atropine-like effects of these drugs is a significant handicap, and older people may well become confused, and older men may develop retention of urine. Benzhexol is probably the easiest of this group to use. A suitable starting dose is 2 mg twice a day.

13.1.8.7 Cell implantation

The last few years have seen great interest in attempting to reverse the progression of Parkinson's disease by implanting cells that may take on some of the functions of the missing dopaminergic neurons. These ventures began when it was shown in 1979 that tissue rich in dopamine taken from the ventral mesencephalic region of embryonic donor rats could be transplanted into adult rat striatum. Such transplantation would correct behavioural abnormalities induced by an experimental denervating lesion of the dopamine system. Electron microscopic observations showed the development of some appropriate synaptic junctions. Adrenal grafts also work in rodents, and some transplanted adrenal cells switch some metabolism towards dopamine. In 1985 minor improvements were noted in patients with Parkinson's disease who had adrenal autografts implanted into the putamen, and a more dramatic improvement 2 years later in operations from Mexico. These were uncontrolled observations, as have been other observations, although in more recent publications efforts have been made to use the patient as his own control, scoring disability in a number of domains before and after operation. An overview of the results from 13 centres in the USA and Canada reports a slightly longer time 'on', and improved function in 'off' periods (Section 13.1.8.4). However, there was a significant perioperative morbidity and mortality, and significant late psychiatric morbidity. More recently, human embryonic grafts have been used, using nigral cells harvested from 8–10 week embryos, obtained at termination of pregnancy. Again there have been reports of modest improvement, but it is clear that there are enormous ethical and practical difficulties involved. Although of considerable biological interest, it seems unlikely that cell implantation will prove an important advance in the management of Parkinson's disease.

13.1.8.8 Surgical treatment

Twenty-five years ago a large number of stereotactic thalamotomies were performed. A lesion placed in the ventrolateral nucleus of the thalamus successfully abolished tremor in a large proportion of patients. However, the operation did nothing for bradykinesia and rigidity, and many patients remarked that they found the hand no more useful, even though the tremor was abolished. There remains an occasional need for the operation, however, if the tremor itself is very disabling, and not relieved by pharmacological therapy.

13.1.8.9 *Other management of Parkinson's disease*

Physiotherapy

Many patients with Parkinson's disease are 'stiff', not only because of their rigidity and akinesia, but also because of secondary change in the joints, particularly the shoulders. All should be taught exercises to mobilize these joints. A physiotherapist can also aid patients by instructing them to sit up straight, to adopt consciously an erect posture, and to aim for heel strike while walking. Although clearly not influencing the progress of the disease, there are clear benefits in morale for the patient and his relatives. Group work with exercises to music, or relaxation exercises may be useful. At later stages of the disease, provision of aids such as a Zimmer frame or a stable heavy frame with wheels may be useful. Speech therapy may help patients develop better vocal strategies for communication. Modifications to the kitchen and bathroom may be necessary (Section 26.6.1.6). Many patients with advanced Parkinson's disease find it particularly difficult to turn over in bed. Patients can be helped by being advised to flex the hips fully, take one foot to the opposite knee and drop it over, clasp their hands together and swing them over, and then work the leg over. Moving the bed close to a (turned off) radiator, for example, upon which the patient can get a grip, may also be a useful strategy.

Constipation is often a feature, and may be helped by bran or other bulking agents, such as sterculia.

13.1.9 *The natural history and prognosis of Parkinson's disease*

There are good studies of the prognosis of Parkinson's disease before the advent of L-dopa. Fifty per cent of patients were either incapable of employment or completely disabled 4 years after onset, and the mean duration of disease before death was 9 years. Fortunately, modern treatment has considerably altered this. More than 6 years after starting treatment, more than half the patients are fitter than before treatment. The mean duration of the disease to death has been increased from 9 to 14 years.

Life table analysis shows that those who are early failures to treatment continue to have a relatively high mortality, but those who have a good response to L-dopa therapy enjoy a longer expectancy of life. This approaches, but by no means reaches, the expectancy of life for the population as a whole.

13.2 Multiple system atrophies

This is one of the most confusing areas of neurology, as the name becomes a convenient dumping ground for a number of degenerative disorders affecting different groups of neurons and nerve processes. Some of the multiple system atrophies, however, do have prominent extrapyramidal features. The syndromes to be described are sometimes familial, and sometimes not. Their very heterogeneity defies description. It is probably best to stick to the use of 'multiple system atrophy' as a diagnosis, using the following terms as a shorthand description of the dominant clinical features.

Most are accompanied not only by a deficiency of striatal dopamine, but also by a loss of noradrenaline in the nucleus accumbens, septal nuclei, and locus coeruleus.

13.2.1 *The Shy–Drager syndrome*

In this condition, there is a severe loss of cells from the intermediolateral cell column of the spinal cord, the origin of the sympathetic and parasympathetic outflow. In addition to parkinsonian features, impotence is a common feature, and the patients fail to sweat in response to a thermal challenge. The most important feature, however, is usually postural hypotension, which may be profound and lead to death. Expansion of plasma volume by fludrocortisone may be helpful. Some patients are still able to release renin, and for these tilting the bed head up at night may be useful.

Patients with the Shy–Drager syndrome often have marked bradykinesia and rigidity. Unfortunately, they are not responsive to L-dopa.

13.2.2 *Autonomic failure due to dopamine β-hydroxylase deficiency*

Postural hypotension characterizes the multisystem atrophies, particularly the Shy–Drager variant described above. Of great interest is a rare syndrome characterized by orthostatic hypotension, ptosis, nasal stuffiness, and impotence. Noradrenaline and adrenaline are virtually absent in the plasma and CSF, but dopamine is increased. The disorder has been shown to be due to dopamine β-hydroxylase deficiency (Fig. 13.2). Cases have been reported in which the metabolic defect has been successfully bypassed by giving DL-dihydroxyphenylserine orally, which is decarboxylated to noradrenaline. This resulted in a useful rise in blood pressure and relief of some symptoms.

13.2.3 *Striatonigral degeneration*

The characteristic pathological feature of this condition is pigmentation of the putamen by haematin and lipofuscin in the astroglia, and degeneration of the substantia nigra. The rigidity and akinesia of such patients does not respond, or responds only poorly, to L-dopa, presumably due to loss of striatal neurons that carry dopamine receptors. Patients are often misdiagnosed as having Parkinson's disease, but onset with tremor is less frequent, and falling early in the disease is an important clue. Orthostatic hypotension and other clinical evidence of autonomic failure is frequent, as is excessive snoring due to partial paralysis of the laryngeal abductors.

13.2.3.1 *Olivopontocerebellar atrophy*

Some of the patients with striatonigral degeneration also have atrophy of the pons, olive, and cerebellum, and minor cerebellar clinical features. In other patients with olivopontocerebellar atrophy, the dominant clinical features are ataxia, dysarthria, and a cerebellar tremor, but other features, such as autonomic failure and pyramidal signs, coexist. In some patients with this combination of signs, a deficiency of glutamate dehydro-

genase has been demonstrated in fibroblasts, platelets, and leucocytes.

13.3 Diffuse Lewy body disease

This extrapyramidal disorder is described briefly in the chapter on dementia (Section 11.5.3).

13.4 Progressive supranuclear palsy (synonym: Steele–Richardson–Olszewski syndrome)

This is a progressive, degenerative, non-familial movement disorder, beginning in adult life. The cardinal feature is a disturbance of voluntary downward gaze, although vestibulo-ocular doll's eye movements are preserved. Upward gaze is also affected, but this is often somewhat limited in any event in older people and in those with Parkinson's disease. Lateral gaze is also affected in about 50 per cent of patients. Eyelid retraction and fixity of gaze give a curious staring appearance to the expression.

Other principal features include axial rigidity and dystonia, features reminiscent of pseudobulbar palsy (Section 10.1.11.3), bradykinesia, postural instability with frequent backward falls, and evidence of lobe dysfunction—forced grasping, utilization behaviour, and perseveration (Section 6.1.5).

Pathological studies show loss of nerve cells and neurofibrillary tangles in the zona compacta of the substantia nigra (the basis, presumably, of the parkinsonian features described above), in the superior colliculus, periaqueductal grey matter and pretectal areas (concerned with control of ocular movements), and in the pallidum at the origin of the pallidothalamic frontal pathway. The frontal lobes remain histologically unaffected, although partially disconnected by changes in the pallidothalamic frontal system. The neurofibrillary tangles represent clusters of straight filaments arranged in interlacing bundles. Antibodies that bind to the paired helical filaments of Alzheimer's disease also bind to the straight filaments found in progressive supranuclear palsy.

A number of biochemical abnormalities have

been described. Dopamine levels are certainly reduced in the striatum, as are numbers of D_2 receptors, but it seems probable that striatal cholinergic pathways are also impaired. Unfortunately, with rare exceptions, L-dopa has no effect upon the course of this disorder, which proceeds to death in about 6 years. Although dementia is not so profound as in Alzheimer's disease, care is very much along the general lines as outlined in Section 11.7.

13.5 Syndromes with dystonia

Dystonia is a name given to a syndrome in which sustained muscle contractions cause twisting and repetitive movements, or abnormal postures. As twisting of axial and limb muscles is prominent, the word 'torsion' often precedes the word dystonia.

Dystonic movements may be rapid, or so slow that one abnormal posture slowly changes to another. They are influenced by placing the body, or part of the body, into specific postures. They can be modified by sensory input. For example, the twisting neck of spasmodic torticollis (Section 13.5.2) may be influenced by a light finger touch on the chin.

Muscles that go into dystonic spasm during the execution of some movements may function entirely normally in others. An extreme example is a patient with generalized dystonia whose attempts to walk forward are inhibited by gross torsion spasm, yet who can walk backwards with ease. A similar dysjunction between different movements occurs in writer's cramp (Section 13.5.3). These anomalies suggest that dystonic movements must be organized at the highest levels of the nervous system.

In the absence of clear pathophysiological change, dystonia is best classified according to the dimensions shown in Table 13.3. Age of onset is important in so far as the earlier the onset of dystonic posturing, the more likely it is that dystonia will become more severe and spread to other areas of the body.

In focal dystonia, only a single body part is affected. Examples include blepharospasm (Section 13.5.4), spasmodic torticollis (Section 13.5.2), and occupational cramps (Section 13.5.3). These are three of the commoner types of dystonia. By

segmental dystonia is meant the combination of dystonia affecting contiguous parts of the body, e.g. one leg and trunk. The other terms in Table 13.3 are self-explanatory.

In idiopathic dystonia, by definition, no pathological or biochemical abnormality has been found as yet. In some families, torsion dystonia, sometimes leading to progressive deformity ('dystonia musculorum deformans') is inherited through a gene, now known to lie on chromosome 9. Other cases are probably new mutations or non-genetic phenocopies, but clinically indistinguishable. The earlier the age of onset, the greater is likely to be the degree of severity.

A hemidystonia is more likely to be symptomatic, but symmetrical symptomatic dystonias occur in Wilson's disease (Section 13.5.5), Huntington's disease (Section 13.6.2), and some of the lipidoses and other inherited disorders considered in Chapter 23. Dystonia may follow a perinatal birth injury, encephalitis, cranial trauma, and cerebral infarction. It may result from a cerebral tumour and may occur in Parkinson's disease. Brief tonic 'spasms' occur in multiple sclerosis. Dystonia may be induced by drugs, including L-dopa, dopamine receptor antagonists, and anticonvulsants.

Table 13.3 Classification of dystonia

1. By age of onset
    childhood, until age 12 years
    adolescence, 12–20 years
    adult, >20 years
2. By distribution
    focal
    segmental
    multifocal
    generalized
    hemidystonia
3. By cause
    idiopathic
      sporadic
      familial
    symptomatic
      associated with other inherited neurological disorders (e.g. Wilson's disease)
      due to known environmental or acquired cause (e.g. perinatal injury, cranial trauma, drug intoxication)

Many of the unusual structural causes of dystonia, such as a tumour, are too diffuse to allow an accurate understanding of the pathological anatomy and physiology. However, in some cases of symptomatic hemidystonia, a structural defect in the contralateral putamen, or its afferent or efferent connections, has been found, with sparing of the globus pallidus.

13.5.1 *The treatment of dystonia*

Existing drug therapy should be reviewed, in case the dystonia is drug induced. Reversible causes such as Wilson's disease (Section 13.5.5) should be considered. About 10 per cent of children with torsion dystonia respond well to a small dose of L-dopa, and continue to benefit for years without increasing the dosage. These children are particularly likely to have dystonia affecting the legs, and may have sudden falls. They may also show some features suggestive of Parkinson's disease. It is, however, difficult to predict the responders, so it is worth trying L-dopa first. If this fails, or in older people, anticholinergic drugs such as benzhexol may be used. Although the initial dose may be low (e.g. benzhexol 2 mg twice daily), it may be gradually increased, especially in younger people, to levels higher than those used in Parkinson's disease. A dose of benzhexol reaching 30 mg/day for young people is not unusually given with benefit, and tolerance to side-effects usually develops. Older people will almost certainly be confused on such doses. Tetrabenazine, a dopamine-depleting drug is also sometimes useful, and can be given in doses of up to 25 mg three times a day. Higher doses may cause depression. Diazepam in high dosages or carbamazepine are occasionally useful.

Some of the dystonias deserve special mention.

13.5.2 *Spasmodic torticollis*

Not all patients with a torticollis necessarily have dystonia. An important differential diagnosis in childhood is of a head turned and tilted due to an oculomotor imbalance. The abnormal head posture is adopted to gain fused ocular images, of which, in this case, the ocular muscles themselves are incapable.

True spasmodic torticollis is one of the commoner forms of focal or segmental dystonia. The patient's head rotates to one side in either a rhythmic jerking way, or as a maintained posture. As noted above, the movement can sometimes be inhibited if the subject rests one finger lightly on his chin. The neck may also be held hyperextended (retrocollis). If occurring in childhood, torticollis may be the presenting symptom of a dystonia that later becomes generalized. About 10 per cent of cases undergo an unexplained spontaneous remission. Some patients respond to anticholinergic medication such as benzhexol, but carbamazepine, benzodiazepines, and tetrabenazine have all been reported to benefit a few cases.

Numerous surgical attempts have been made to improve torticollis. However, the movements appear to be organized bilaterally centrally, and involve so many nerve roots peripherally, that either a bilateral thalamotomy or a very extensive cervical denervation would have to be performed. The former may result in severe dysphonia, and the latter in a floppy neck, which is still moving abnormally, albeit to a lesser extent. Surgery has now largely been replaced by the selective blockade of those muscles identified as being responsible for the principal movements, using botulinum toxin. For example, for a torticollis that was primarily rotational, the contralateral sternomastoid and ipsilateral splenius capitis would be injected. The toxin prevents the pre-synaptic calcium-dependent release of acetyl choline (Section 17.7.2.1). Terminal axonal sprouting restores neuromuscular transmission after 3 months or so, so further injections are always required.

13.5.3 *Writer's cramp*

This is one example of an occupationally induced dystonia. Other examples include violinist's cramp and telegraphist's (Morse key) cramp. Common to all occupational cramps is an overuse of a skilled movement. In writer's cramp, attempts to write are inhibited by dystonic posturing of the hand and arm. The pen is gripped tightly. In an attempt to overcome this, the patient may hold the pen in an unusual way, but the tonic spasm again soon supervenes. The hand can still be used for all other movements; for example, patients with writer's cramp can use a keyboard with ease. It appears that the act of holding the pen, or the mental act of preparing to write, calls forth an erroneous, dystonic, motor programme. If the subject learns to write with his non-dominant hand, cramp may supervene in that too.

In spite of the similarity between the arm movements in idiopathic torsion dystonia and writer's cramp, the latter never proceeds to a full-blown progressive dystonic syndrome, although dystonia may involve the limb as far proximally as the shoulder.

No drug treatment has been shown to be of great benefit in writer's cramp. It is necessary to limit severely writing, perhaps merely to signing cheques, and to rely on dictation and/or keyboard skills. Curiously, typists and word-processor operators do not seem to get occupational cramps. Occasionally, anticholinergic drugs, such as benzhexol, help. Botulinum toxin (see above) is occasionally successful if the muscle(s) primarily responsible for the induction of the cramp can be recognized.

13.5.4   *Blepharospasm*

This is a focal dystonia affecting the orbicularis oculi and neighbouring facial muscles. This is often combined with an oromandibular dystonia; this is then known as Meige's syndrome. By blepharospasm is meant an involuntary sustained and forced closure of the eyelids, which may occur spontaneously, or be precipitated by bright light. Sensory or other 'tricks', such as shaking the head may, at least in the earlier stages of this dystonia, block a spasm.

The best treatment of this condition is the local injection of botulinum toxin. Controlled local injection of toxin at levels insufficient to cause diffuse facial weakness is very successful at controlling blepharospasm, although there may be some degree of paralytic ptosis thereafter. Repeated injections are almost always necessary at intervals of several months.

13.5.5   *Wilson's disease (synonym: hepatolenticular degeneration)*

This is a rare disorder of copper metabolism inherited on an autosomal recessive basis, the gene lying on chromosome 13. The prevalence is about 30 per million. The basic lesion is a hepatic defect in biliary copper excretion, leading to copper deposition in the liver and cirrhosis, with episodes of recurrent jaundice, escape of copper from hepato-

cytes into the blood, and eventual deposition of copper in the brain. (See also Section 23.1.3.5).

13.5.5.1   *Clinical features*

Hepatic compensation may be such that in about 40 per cent of cases the first symptoms are neurological. Other presentations include haematological disturbances, and syndromes due to renal tubular defects. Other patients present in hepatic failure.

Neurological disabilities include dysarthria, clumsiness, dystonic postures, tremors, intellectual retardation, and disturbance of gait. The dysarthria is of a dystonic type; the speech sounds characteristically strained. This may progress to anarthria. Automatic swallowing of saliva may fail, so the patient may drool. Rigidity and hypokinesia may superficially mimic Parkinson's disease; another variant, in which tremor and ataxia are prominent, may mimic multiple sclerosis. Psychiatric presentations with psychosis, socially unacceptable behaviour or dementia are also common.

In all patients with Wilson's disease, copper deposits are visible in Descemet's membrane near the limbus on slit-lamp examination. The appearance is known as Kayser–Fleischer rings.

13.5.5.2   *Pathology*

The pathological changes of Wilson's disease in the brain include atrophy and softening of the basal ganglia, particularly of the putamen. More generalized atrophic changes are also seen in the cerebral white matter. Initially, the liver shows nonspecific changes with fatty infiltration and increased fibrosis, and subsequently a macronodular or micronodular cirrhosis.

13.5.5.3   *Investigation*

The crucial investigation is measurement of caeruloplasmin, the copper-containing protein of plasma. Levels below 200 mg/litre strongly suggest Wilson's disease. Urinary copper excretion is increased above 100 micrograms/24 h. Plasma copper levels may be misleading. Hepatic biopsy and measurement of copper content may sometimes be necessary (reference level less than 250 μg/g on needle biopsy). Alternatively, the rate of incorporation of ^{64}Cu into caeruloplasmin can be measured.

13.5.5.4   *Treatment*

Wilson's disease is eminently treatable. The most widely used drug at present is penicillamine, which chelates copper and increases urinary excretion. The dose is 250 mg four times a day. There may be an initial exacerbation of symptoms during chelation therapy. Sometimes allergic reactions, the occurrence of proteinuria, or a lupus-like syndrome limits the use of penicillamine. An alternative chelating agent is triethylene tetramine. In recent years oral zinc sulphate has been used. This compound prevents copper absorption from the bowel and increases faecal copper excretion.

Unfortunately, some patients with Wilson's disease have psychiatric syndromes which interfere with their compliance with therapy, and late relapses due to this are quite common. If chelating agents are reliably used, the results can be quite dramatic. Clearly, however, the earlier the diagnosis, the less time there has been for copper-induced irreversible neurological damage to have taken place.

13.6   Syndromes with chorea

Chorea is the name given to rapid, irregular, involuntary, jerky movements which flow randomly from muscle to muscle. These movements are never integrated into a co-ordinated movement, although they may be followed by a voluntary movement involving the same part of the body, in an attempt to disguise it. The major disorders causing chorea are listed in Table 13.4.

13.6.1   *Rheumatic chorea (synonym: Sydenham's chorea, St Vitus' dance)*

This is now a rare disease, as it used to be associated with acute rheumatic fever and carditis, now themselves rare. Diagnosis is largely clinical, as the sedimentation rate is often normal and the antistreptolysin titre is not usually raised. In severely affected cases, now not seen in developed countries, a vasculitis in the basal ganglia is found at post-mortem. Some of the young people with Sydenham's chorea develop associated psycho-

logical symptoms, even a confusional state. The choreic movements can usually be controlled with benzodiazepines. Penicillin should be given to eradicate any underlying infection, but the movements may remain present for months.

Table 13.4   Causes of chorea

Rheumatic chorea (Sydenham's chorea)
(may relapse during pregnancy (chorea gravidarum),
or in relation to oral contraception)
Inherited chorea
Huntington's disease
neuroacanthocytosis
benign hereditary chorea
Symptomatic chorea
systemic lupus erythematosus
thyrotoxicosis
polycythaemia rubra vera
Drug-induced chorea
oral contraceptives
neuroleptics
phenytoin
Hemichorea (hemiballismus)
vascular disease
tumour
trauma

Girls who have suffered rheumatic chorea in childhood or adolescence may suffer a return of movements when taking the contraceptive pill in adult life, or when pregnant (chorea gravidarum).

13.6.1.1   *Other choreic syndromes*

Other choreic syndromes include the inherited disorders of Huntington's disease (Section 13.6.2), benign hereditary chorea, and neuroacanthocytosis (Section 13.6.3).

Chorea may complicate the other disorders listed in Table 13.4. Hemichorea (hemiballismus) is a rare disorder usually caused by a small infarct in the subthalamic nucleus of Luys, although a tumour in the same site may be the cause. Wild, irregular, jerky movements of one side of the body may continue explosively for some weeks after an infarct in this region. Fortunately, they usually fade to a more tolerable level, or cease entirely.

13.6.2 *Huntington's disease*

Huntington's disease is an autosomal dominantly inherited disorder that usually begins in middle life, and is characterized by involuntary choreic movements and dementia. It was first described by George Huntington in 1872, who had observed cases in his general practice in Long Island.

13.6.2.1 *Epidemiology*

Huntington's disease has been found in all races and countries of the world. Many cases can be traced back to a single progenitor. For example, cases in Tasmania have been traced to a family from Somerset, and many US cases have been traced back to a family from Suffolk. Analysis with restriction-fragment-length polymorphisms has located the gene to 4p.

The autosomal dominant inheritance of Huntington's disease means that each son or daughter of an affected parent has a 50 per cent risk of inheriting the gene. It is believed that all carriers will express the disease if they live long enough. As the first symptoms do not appear until middle life, usually several years after the next generation has been born, the disease has continued. Epidemiological studies indicate that new mutations are very rare; exceptions can usually be explained by incorrect diagnosis or paternal uncertainty. Those advising a grandchild of an affected grandparent can calculate out the residual risk of his carrying the gene, depending on the age that his parent has reached without yet showing symptoms.

The prevalence of overt disease is of the order of 8 per 100 000. That is to say, only one in six family doctors are likely to have a case registered with them. The incidence and prevalence of the disease depends to some extent upon geographical clustering of descendants of the progenitor.

13.6.2.2 *Clinical features*

Although involuntary jerky (choreic) movements are considered to be the cardinal feature, the illness usually begins with psychological features. Depression, change in behaviour, and increased irritability are common, followed by early signs of impairment of cognitive function—inability to concentrate and loss of social skills.

Such insidious symptoms make it difficult to define the age of onset, but this is usually in the late thirties, with involuntary movements occurring a few years later. In about 3 per cent of cases, the disease begins in adolescence, and then rigidity and dystonia may replace the usual chorea. This variant was described by Westphal. In such cases, transmission from the father is more likely. It has been suggested that maternally transmitted factors such as mitochrondrial DNA or other extrachromosomal organelles may influence the expression and age of onset of the disease. In other cases, the onset of dementia and abnormal movements may not occur until the late fifties or even later, at which stage it may be impossible, due to death of aged relatives and family dispersion, to obtain a family history of a similar disorder.

The choreic movements are difficult to describe, but once seen are seldom forgotten. An impression of restlessness and fidgeting may be initially all that is seen. Many of the movements can be incorporated into apparently purposeful movements, such as repeatedly crossing and uncrossing the legs. It may become difficult to hold a knife and fork. The choreic movements may be brought out by asking the subject to walk or to do some skilled action with his hands. They disappear during sleep. Speech becomes slurred, and the gait unsteady. Physical examination shows not only the abnormal movements and dementia, but also generally brisk reflexes and often impaired saccadic eye movements and impaired optokinetic nystagmus. Dementia advances as the movements become more prominent, so that supportive care is necessary for the last years of the patient's life. The mean duration of the illness from onset to death is about 13–15 years.

13.6.2.3 *Differential diagnosis*

The principal differential diagnosis is an involuntary movement disorder induced by drugs in patients with primary psychiatric disease. Rarely, confusion may arise with Wilson's disease (Section 13.5.5), which usually presents in younger patients. Other diagnoses to be considered include myoclonic movements in association with other forms of dementia including Creutzfeldt–Jakob disease (Section 17.15.1), and involuntary movements associated with striatal infarcts. Neuroacanthocytosis should also be considered (Section 13.6.3).

13.6.2.4   *Genetics*

The identification of a restriction-fragment-length polymorphism mapped to chromosome 4p, and linked to the Huntington's disease gene, now means that predictive testing can be offered to families, although, as the marker is not immediately adjacent to the gene, some errors in prediction will occasionally arise, due to variable recombination between the marker and gene.

It is obvious that there are extreme ethical difficulties in counselling young, clinically normal members of an affected family. The general view is that children at risk should not be tested. Many of those at risk decide not to be tested when informed of its availability. Of those who come forward, neurological examination shows that some already have minor clinical evidence of the disease. These, and those not clinically affected but who have to be informed that they carry the gene, may become significantly depressed as they have to face the remainder of their lives with that knowledge, often informed by the insights gained first hand from caring for an affected parent. There are enormous implications for marriage, procreation, and employment.

Considerable criticism has been directed at the failure of neurologists to communicate the diagnosis to all those potentially affected, or at least to their general practitioners. The disease is, *par excellence*, one in which a national register of those affected and those at risk could be maintained, should considerations of privacy allow. The ethical considerations are, however, enormous.

13.6.2.5   *Neuropathology*

Whatever the abnormal gene product proves to be, the prominent histological abnormalities lie in the corpus striatum. The earliest histological change is in medium-sized neurons, with many spiny processes which become curled and branched. Striatal neurons are reduced in number, but there is relative sparing of axons *en passage* and afferent axons, and relative sparing of striatal neurons containing somatostatin or neuropeptide Y. There is early loss of striatal enkephalinergic neurons projecting to the external globus pallidus, and neurons containing substance P projecting to the substantia nigra. Striatal *N*-methyl-D-aspartate receptors are reduced in number. This subtype of glutamate receptor may be concerned with excessive excitatory neuronal action and premature neuronal death (Section 10.1.7).

By analogy with the role of dopamine in Parkinson's disease, it has been hoped that a specific neurotransmitter deficit may be identified in Huntington's disease. Unfortunately, this has not proved to be the case. The activity of glutamic acid decarboxylase is reduced by about 85 per cent in the striatum, and the levels of acetylcholine and choline acetyltransferase by about 50 per cent. The dopaminergic projection from the substantia nigra remains intact. Levels of somatostatin are increased but, as yet, these changes have not been synthesized to form a coherent hypothesis of how the striatum fails in Huntington's disease.

13.6.2.6   *Investigations*

The CT scans and MRI images of patients with advanced Huntington's disease show atrophy of the caudate nuclei, with corresponding enlargement of the frontal horns. Positron emission tomography using ^{18}F fluorodeoxyglucose shows reduced glucose metabolism. The alpha rhythm on the EEG tends to be of low amplitude. All these indirect investigations are likely to give way to recombinant DNA techniques.

13.6.2.7   *Treatment*

No treatment is known to halt the progress of the disease. It may be possible to suppress partially the chorea with tetrabenazine. This depletes monoamines and blocks both pre- and post-synaptic dopamine receptors. A dose of up to 200 mg/day may be used. However, the chorea is usually the least of the patient's own problems and, as tetrabenazine may add to or precipitate depression, there is often no point in using it. Support to both patient and carer, along the lines indicated in Section 11.7 are really all that can be offered.

13.6.3   *Neuroacanthocytosis*

Acanthocytosis is the name given to the presence of abnormal red blood cells bearing spiky projections in peripheral blood. The association of a neurological disorder with acanthocytosis was first described in inherited abetalipoproteinaemia. However, there is a non-inherited syndrome of a movement disorder, personality change, and progressive intellectual deterioration rather similar to that seen in Huntington's disease. The syndrome also includes seizures, tic-like vocalizations, biting of the lips and tongue, areflexia and wasting of the muscles due to an axonal peripheral neuropathy. The principal importance of the syndrome is in its distinction from Huntington's disease, in order to provide accurate genetic counselling for the latter.

13.6.4   Athetosis

This is a slow, irregular, sinuous movement seen in the limbs, particularly after severe perinatal brain injury involving the striatum or kernicterus. If the movements are rather more jerky, they may be called choreo-athetosis. Athetosis was also used to describe some of the movements now more commonly called dystonic.

Pseudo-athetosis is a quite different disorder. This is the name given to abnormal posturings of the outstretched hands due to a disturbed sense of finger position in severe peripheral neuropathies (Section 6.3.1.3). The same abnormal movements may occur in one hand after a contralateral parietal lesion.

13.7   Syndromes with tics

A tic is an abrupt, jerky movement, repeated at intervals that are usually short. Tics mimic a normal co-ordinated movement. Attempts may be made to conceal a tic by allowing a voluntary movement to flow from it. Tics can be suppressed by voluntary effort for a minute or so, during which time the subject—sometimes known as a tiqueur—feels an increasing desire to tic. When the tiqueur has made his or her movement, there is a brief period of relief of tension.

Simple tics are found in about 4 per cent of all children, as a temporary phenomenon, with a peak incidence at around the age of 6 or 7 years. The vast majority settle spontaneously by the age of 12, but a few continue to tic in adult life. Tics most commonly involve the periocular muscles, but all muscles of the face, neck, and shoulders may be affected. Occasionally trunk and lower limb muscles may tic.

Simple idiopathic tics of this type are distinguished from other compulsive patterns of behaviour such as nail-biting or picking. However, the feeling of tension relieved by the act of biting or picking suggests some common ground between tics and what have been called socially offensive manipulations of the body. These are particularly likely to occur at times of boredom or anxiety. Tics are also exacerbated by stress.

Although few would classify such bodily manipulations as anything other than aberrant behaviour, and basically curable if sufficient 'will' is brought to bear, the status of tics is less clear cut. Numerous hypotheses have been advanced that rest on a psychodynamic formulation, but even if some tics have a psychological basis, others do not. The principal evidence for this is the occurrence of typical tics after encephalitis lethargica (see Section 13.1.4). Furthermore, some observers, but by no means all, find evidence of so-called 'soft' neurological signs in tiqueurs, and an increased incidence of left-handedness, suggesting that tics arise in association with minimal brain damage.

13.7.1   Gilles de la Tourette syndrome

Some children with tics do not improve in adolescence, and carry on with tics in adult life. In a small proportion, the tics become more severe and involve many more muscle groups. Some of these patients develop respiratory tics, with sniffs and grunts, and a few develop the syndrome first described by Gilles de la Tourette, in which the respiratory and vocal tics are replaced by the compulsive utterance of improper four-letter words. This is called coprolalia. Sufferers may also have a desire to repeat the last words in any conversation—echolalia. Other compulsive acts such as touching potentially dangerous objects, and obscene gestures (e.g. V signs) are commonly seen.

The bizarre use of four-letter words and obscene gestures is at first sight difficult to associate with an organic state, but it has been shown that computers programmed to create words of four letters often create phonemes that we regard as obscene. It has been suggested, therefore, that coprolalia represents no more than the production of phonemes that in any event have a high probability of occurrence. Against this hypothesis, however, is the rarity of coprolalia in patients with Gilles de la Tourette syndrome in Japan.

No clear-cut pathological abnormality or biochemical abnormality has as yet been found, but there is suggestion of low levels of homovanillic acid and 5-hydroxy-indole-acetic acid in the CSF, suggestive of a reduced turnover of dopamine metabolism in the spinal fluid.

The syndrome of Gilles de la Tourette may occur in more than one family member. If simple tics are regarded as a more benign variant of the condition, then nearly 50 per cent of those with Gilles de la Tourette syndrome have a family history of tics.

13.7.1.1   *Treatment*

Deciding when to start pharmacological treatment in a youngster with tics is always difficult. The effects of the tic on emotional and personal development have to be balanced against the uncertain long-term effects of drugs which are certainly useful in the short term. Dopamine receptor blockade by haloperidol (beginning with 0.25 mg two or three times a day) or pimozide (starting with 1 mg once or twice a day) reduces the frequency and amplitude of tics. Sulpiride, a selective D_2 dopamine receptor antagonist, has also been used. The evidence that dopamine blockade is beneficial is supported by the fact that dopamine agonists such as bromocriptine exacerbate tics, as do methylphenidate and amphetamine, which promote the synaptic release of dopamine.

Most children who tic become free of tics in adolescence. Vocal tics have a worse prognosis, and boys fare less well than girls. The prognosis for the fully developed syndrome of Gilles de la Tourette is much worse, and tics usually continue. Spontaneous remissions do, however, occasionally occur.

13.8   Syndromes with myoclonus

Myoclonus is the word used to describe quick muscle contractions—jerks—arising from neural activity in the central nervous system. Muscle twitching due to lower motor neuron lesions is called fasciculation (Section 6.2.2). Myoclonic jerks are not under voluntary control, unlike tics, which can be briefly suppressed (Section 13.7). They do not possess the random flow of movement typical of chorea (Section 13.6).

Myoclonus, like an epileptic seizure, is just one type of clinically evident neural behaviour, and,

like epilepsy, can be classified on the basis of clinical, electrophysiological, or pathological features (Tables 13.5 and 13.6).

Table 13.5   Classification of myoclonus

Clinical
physiological
essential
related to epilepsy
Physiological
cortical, time-locked to EEG discharge
subcortical, not time-locked
Anatomical
focal or segmental
generalized
Pathological
nature of underlying encephalopathy, e.g. postanoxic damage, viral origin

13.8.1   *Physiological myoclonus (synonym: hypnic jerks)*

This occurs in about 60–70 per cent of healthy subjects during the early stages of falling asleep. The brief jerk is probably an arousal response to some minimal stimulus. Sleep myoclonus occurs after sleep onset, usually in the legs, and usually in older people. The jerks occur every 30 seconds or so for hours at a time, but are inhibited during rapid eye movement sleep (Sections 24.2.1.1 and 24.2.1.2).

13.8.2   *Essential myoclonus*

This term is applied to myoclonus without other evidence of neurological disease. It occurs in families, inherited as an autosomal dominant trait. Another name given to this condition is paramyoclonus multiplex.

13.8.3   *Epileptic myoclonus*

Myoclonus is also a feature of many of the epilepsies, occurring in absence epilepsy, in juvenile myoclonic epilepsy, photosensitive epilepsy, infantile spasms, and the Lennox–Gastaut syndrome (Sections 12.4.2 and 12.5).

Table 13.6   Causes of myoclonus

Generalized	Metabolic
Physiological	e.g. uraemia, hepatic failure
hypnic jerks	Drug-induced
Essential	e.g. amitriptyline
inherited, but no other neurological abnormality	Infective
Inherited	e.g. Subacute sclerosing panencephalitis,
as part of idiopathic generalized epilepsy	Creutzfeldt–Jakob disease
(juvenile myoclonic epilepsy)	Degenerative
as part of other myoclonic epilepsies	e.g. Alzheimer's disease
infantile spasms	Postanoxic
Lennox–Gastaut syndrome	e.g. after cardiac arrest
as part of a progressive myoclonic encephalopathy	
storage disorders	Segmental
lipid (e.g. Gaucher's disease)	Palatal
lipopigment (e.g. Batten's disease)	Spinal
mucopolysaccharide (e.g. Lafora body)	Cortical
spinocerebellar degenerations	cortical reflex myoclonus
	epilepsia partialis continua

13.8.4   *Symptomatic myoclonus*

Myoclonus may also be symptomatic of a great number of generalized static or progressive encephalopathies. Examples include lipid storage disorders (e.g. G_{M2} gangliosidosis), epileptic myoclonus (Baltic or 21 q), dementias (e.g. Creutzfeldt–Jakob disease), viral encephalitis (e.g. subacute sclerosing panencephalitis), metabolic encephalopathies (e.g. hepatic failure), and postanoxic encephalopathies (e.g. after cardiac arrest).

13.8.5   *Physiology of myoclonus*

Physiological exploration of patients with myoclonus indicates that in some the jerk may be time-locked to a preceding cortical event in the EEG. One example is the myoclonic jerks of epilepsis partialis continua. A brief delay between the cortical discharge and the onset of a focal jerk (about 20 ms to the arm) suggests a powerful monosynaptic pathway from the cortex to a group of anterior horn cells. This is sometimes called *cortical* or *pyramidal myoclonus*. The EMG activity resulting in a jerk is of brief duration, 30 ms or so. In some subjects with cortical myoclonus, jerks can be precipitated by touching an appropriate area of skin, or stretching the jerking muscle. It appears that the cortex has become 'over-sensitive' to such peripheral stimulation. In many such patients cortical sensory evoked potentials are much larger than normal. These large potentials, and the cortical discharge, may result from a loss of cerebellar inhibitory input to the cortex.

Subcortical myoclonus is distinguished by a generalized jerk. There may or may not be a cortical EEG correlate, but if this is present it is not time-locked to the jerk. Indeed, the first myoclonic response, in muscles innervated by the lower brain-stem nuclei, may *precede* the cortical discharge, suggesting that the origin of the events lies in the brain-stem reticular formation. In subcortical myoclonus, the EMG discharge continues for up to 90 ms, giving a rather slower appearance to the jerk than that seen in cortical myoclonus.

Postanoxic myoclonus is one variety that has attracted particular interest. It may occur after cardiac arrest from which resuscitation has been less than fully successful, resulting in some cerebral damage. Myoclonus is particularly likely to be precipitated by movement in this condition. This variety of myoclonus may be relieved by 5-hydroxytryptophan, which is of considerable theoretical interest, but in practice sodium valproate or clonazepam are easier drugs to use, and also effective.

A final type of myoclonus is *focal* or *segmental myoclonus*. Rarely, a spinal cord tumour may result in myoclonic jerks affecting the limb muscles innervated by the affected segment. Such myoclonus is unaffected by sleep. A diffuse inflammatory disorder of the spinal cord may cause widespread segmental myoclonus, so-called spinal myoclonus. A bizarre example of segmental myoclonus is palatal myoclonus, in which the palate jerks at a rate of about 1.5–3 c/s, and may produce an audible clicking sound. This occurs in disorders affecting the connecting pathways between the dentate nucleus, red nucleus, and olive. In post-mortem studies the olive has been found to be hypertrophied. Carbamazepine and trihexyphenidyl may occasionally be effective in reducing or controlling palatal myoclonus.

13.9   Syndromes with tremor

A tremor is defined as a rhythmic oscillation of a body part about one or more joints. A tremor of the head on the trunk is called a titubation.

13.9.1   *Essential tremor (synonym: benign essential tremor)*

This is probably the most common disorder of movement, affecting about 500 per 100 000 over the age of 40. A general practitioner in the UK will have about five patients with essential tremor on his list. The prevalence of essential tremor rises steeply in older age-groups.

About 30 per cent of patients give a family history of this disorder. It is probable that the disorder is dominantly inherited, with variable penetrance, and expression influenced by advancing age. A subject with tremor may not have a positive family history simply because a parent carrying the gene died before the onset of tremor.

Essential tremor is a postural tremor, principally affecting the distal upper limbs. The tremor disappears when the limb is fully supported against gravity, so in this regard it is easily distinguished from the tremor of Parkinson's disease. Although the tremor attenuates during movement, it becomes more obvious as the target is reached. A mild tremor of the outstretched hands may not look very much to the examining neurologist, but

proves incapacitating when the subject attempts to pick up a cup of tea.

The frequency with which the hand shakes initially lies in the range of 7–11 c/s, and looks like an enhanced physiological tremor. As the tremor becomes of coarser amplitude, the frequency usually declines below 6.5 c/s. Tremor may spread from the upper limbs to the cervical muscles, producing a titubation of the head, or to the jaw.

The only real differential diagnosis is from Parkinson's disease, and all too often a misdiagnosis occurs. The characteristics of the tremor described above are quite different from Parkinson's disease (Section 13.1.6.1), and if any doubt remains, some of the procedures described in Section 13.1.6.5 can be used to exaggerate the underlying increase in tone present in Parkinson's disease, and not present in patients with essential tremor. The latter also retain a full range of facial expression.

Occasionally patients are seen who have characteristics of both Parkinson's disease and essential tremor. This arises more frequently than chance would allow. A tremor that looks like essential tremor may be associated with spasmodic torticollis or torsion dystonia, but the nosology of such combinations remains confused.

13.9.1.1   *Treatment*

Many patients discover for themselves that their tremor is improved by one or two alcoholic drinks, which is fortunate as essential tremor is usually exacerbated by stress and excitement, such as may occur at a party. Exacerbation by stress and anxiety suggests that an adrenergic mechanism plays some part in the modulation, if not the genesis, of essential tremor. The treatment of choice has proved to be a β-adrenoreceptor antagonist. No beta-blocker has as yet been shown to be superior to propranolol, which blocks both β-1 and β-2 adrenoreceptors, but experiments with highly selective receptor blockade indicate that the β-2 adrenoreceptor is the site of major importance in the control of essential tremor.

Propranolol also reduces the amplitude of physiological tremor. Hence it tends to be used, or rather abused, by competitors in snooker (pool), shooting, and archery.

Early experiments by Owen (later leader of the Social Democrat Party in the UK) and Marsden showed that infusion of propranolol into a brachial artery reduced the tremor in the ipsilateral hand. Hence the beneficial effect of the drug occurred through blockade of peripheral receptors in muscles, and not by any action within the central nervous system. β-2 receptors are located on both intrafusal and extrafusal muscle fibres. Presumably blockade of either of these receptors alters the gain in the feedback loops, oscillations in which produce tremor. These neural circuits are illustrated schematically in Fig. 13.6.

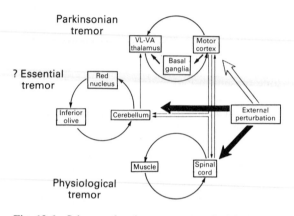

Fig. 13.6 Scheme of pathways concerned with the genesis of tremor (reproduced by kind permission, from Lee and Stein 1981).

A single oral dose of 120 mg propranolol will be very effective in about half the patients. This means that they do not have to take the drug on a regular basis (though many choose to do so), but rather take a single dose about 1–3 hours before an important social event. If taken on a regular basis, 80 mg three times a day is a suitable dose. Propranolol must be avoided in those with congestive cardiac failure and asthma, and in patients with atrioventricular block. In many patients, the common unwanted effects of tired legs, cold feet, and sexual dysfunction in men limit its use. In such patients it is worth trying the effect of primidone or phenobarbitone, both of which have been shown to help some patients when used in doses similar to those used for epilepsy (Section 12.8).

Occasionally an essential tremor may be of such large amplitude, and so disabling, that surgical treatment is necessary. A stereotactically placed lesion is made in the ventral intermediate nucleus

of the thalamus. Neurophysiological recordings from this site reveal burst discharges synchronous with tremor, which are modulated by passive movements of the tremulous limb.

13.10   Drug-induced movement disorders

Since the introduction of potent neuroleptic drugs, an increasing number of drug-induced movement disorders have been recognized (Table 13.7). These are best classified along the lines of the spontaneous disorders they mimic.

13.10.1   *Drug-induced parkinsonism*

It is probable that drug-induced parkinsonism will occur in anyone given sufficient doses of dopamine receptor antagonist drugs such as those shown in Table 13.7 (haloperidol, chlorpromazine, prochlorperazine, trifluoperazine, sulpiride, and metoclopramide). Drugs that deplete nerve terminals of dopamine (e.g. reserpine) have the same clinical effect.

The clinical features of drug-induced parkinsonism are virtually identical with the spontaneous disease, although some observers believe that tremor is less prominent. Elderly patients are particularly prone to drug-induced parkinsonism, possibly because the numbers of dopaminergic neurons in the substantia nigra are already depleted by age. Some patients relieved of their drug-induced parkinsonism by withdrawal of the neuroleptic drug may return, months or years later, with spontaneous Parkinson's disease, suggesting that in some elderly patients drug-induced parkinsonism is an unmasking of latent Parkinson's disease.

It usually takes about 8 weeks for the symptoms and signs to disappear after stopping the drug, but it may be much longer. If it is necessary to continue the neuroleptic or other medication, then anticholinergic drugs, such as benzhexol, can be used. L-dopa is of no value.

13.10.2   *Akathisia*

Akathisia is a state of motor restlessness induced by antipsychotic drugs. It is characterized by a

Table 13.7 Drug-induced movement disorders

Movement disorders	Drug	Age at risk	Incidence	Time of onset after beginning drug	Effect of drug withdrawal	Treatment
Parkinsonism	Dopamine receptor antagonists, e.g. chlorpromazine prochlorperazine trifluoperazine	Any age, but elderly at risk	Dose dependent; may be as high as 50%	Weeks	Relieved	Anticholinergics (e.g. benzhexol)
	Dopamine terminal depleters, e.g. butyrophenones reserpine tetrabenazine					
	Mechanism uncertain, flunarizine					
Akathisia	As for parkinsonism (see above)	Any age, but elderly at risk	20%	Weeks	Relieved	Propranolol
Tardive dyskinesia	Dopamine receptor antagonists (see above) but not dopamine depleters	Elderly	20–40%	1–2 years	Continues in at least a third, may get worse	Reserpine, combined with α-methyl paratyrosine
Acute dystonia	As for parkinsonism (see above) diazoxide	Young	Rare	A few minutes	Relieved	Anticholinergics (e.g. benztropine)
Neuroleptic malignant syndrome	Dopamine receptor antagonists and terminal depleters; risk is probably higher if lithium taken at same time	Any age	Rare, but high mortality	Days to weeks	Relieved gradually	Bromocriptine, dantrolene
Tremor	β-adrenergic agonists, these exacerbate physiological tremor caffeine amphetamine methyl phenidate pemoline isoprenaline diethylpropion ergotamine	Any age	Dose-dependent	Days–weeks	Relieved	Propranol
	Other drugs, usually inducing an action tremor lithium phenobarbitone phenytoin carbamazepine primidone sodium valproate alcohol (and alcohol withdrawal) vidarabine tricyclic antidepressants					

feeling of tension and inability to tolerate inactivity, a feeling briefly relieved by tapping the feet, shifting the position of the body on a chair, or getting out of the chair and walking around. As the condition often occurs in schizophrenics under treatment, the disorder may mimic an exacerbation of the original psychiatric disorder, particularly as the inner tension may give rise to considerable mental agitation.

Akathisia affects between 20 and 30 per cent of patients on phenothiazines or butyrophenones. It usually begins within the first few months of treatment. Dopamine receptor blockade is postulated as the mechanism of akathisia, but dopamine depleters, such as reserpine and tetrabenazine, have also been reported to cause akathisia. Experimental prefrontal lesions in rats may induce increased motor activity, and it is believed that the responsible receptors that are blocked by medication lie in the prefrontal mesocortical dopamine receptor system.

Fortunately, unlike tardive dyskinesia, akathisia usually settles on withdrawal of the offending drug. However, this may be an unrealistic strategy in patients with severe psychotic illnesses. Some patients respond to propranolol, presumably by central β-2 adrenergic receptor blockade.

13.10.3 *Drug-induced tardive dyskinesia*

Tardive dyskinesia is the name given to persistent repetitive choreiform movements of voluntary muscles, most often affecting the face and tongue. They disappear during sleep, and may be exacerbated by emotion. Oral dyskinesias may interfere with speech and swallowing. Although orofacial tardive dyskinesia may arise spontaneously, most are drug-induced by phenothiazines and butyrophenones (see Table 13.7). Older people are at greater risk, presumably due to age-related striatal neuronal depletion.

Tardive dyskinesia usually appears after 1–2 years on a neuroleptic drug or metaclopramide, but onset may occasionally be earlier. It is believed that dopamine receptor blockade leads to the development of a functional dopamine receptor supersensitivity. This explains why tardive dyskinesia induced by metoclopramide may improve, temporarily, if the dose of metoclopramide is increased, and the supersensitive receptors further blocked. Such a course is not recommended, as a

vicious circle may well be induced. This model also accounts for a temporary exaggeration of the dyskinesias as the offending drug is withdrawn. Unfortunately, tardive dyskinesia may well continue even when the drug is stopped. The primary method of avoiding tardive dyskinesia is to avoid the use of dopamine antagonists for relatively mild symptoms, for example metaclopramide for gastric symptoms, and prochlorperazine for migraine and non-specific 'dizziness'.

The pharmacological treatment of tardive dyskinesia is disappointing. Although it is well-recognized that anticholinergic drugs may exacerbate dyskinesia, cholinergic drugs, such as physostigmine, are seldom effective. Long-term neuroleptic agents have been reported to reduce serotoninergic activity, and for this reason L-tryptophan, a precursor of serotonin, has been used with some success. Probably the most effective treatment is reserpine, combined with another presynaptic dopamine depletor, α-methyl-paratyrosine.

13.10.4 *Drug-induced acute dystonia*

A dystonic reaction may occur as an acute reaction to phenothiazines, (particularly to fluphenazine), to butyrophenones (particularly metoclopramide), and to diazoxide, a benzothiadiazine used in the management of severe hypertension. The dystonic reaction may be very frightening for the patient— and for the doctor who has just given the injection. Oculogyric crises may occur. The reaction is usually readily aborted by the intravenous injection of an anticholinergic drug, such as 1–2 mg benztropine.

Acute dystonias are also seen in patients with Parkinson's disease treated with L-dopa (see Section 13.1.8.3.).

13.10.5 *The neuroleptic malignant syndrome*

This rare syndrome is characterized by akinesia, which may be so severe as to appear catatonic, extreme muscular rigidity, hyperthermia, autonomic instability (labile blood pressure, tachycardia, and sweating), and altered consciousness. It occurs usually within a few days of beginning treatment with a phenothiazine or butyrophenone drug, most commonly haloperidol, chlorpromazine, or fluphenazine. The coincident prescription of lithium may be a factor. It is presumed that dopamine receptor blockade in the basal ganglia and hypothalamus is responsible. Controlling hyperpyrexia, cooling, maintaining the circulation, and other supportive treatment is necessary. Benefit has been reported using bromocriptine, a dopamine agonist, and dantrolene, which reduces muscular rigidity and hyperpyrexia.

13.10.6   *Drug-induced tremor*

Some drugs have a direct agonist action on β-2 adrenergic receptors in muscle, and so may exaggerate physiological or essential tremor. The anticonvulsants listed in Table 13.7 often induce an action tremor when serum levels are above their therapeutic range, but sodium valproate may induce a rather finer amplitude action tremor in therapeutic dosage. The mechanism of action of these and the other drugs listed in the table is uncertain.

13.11   Further reading

General

A series of papers in *Journal of Neurology, Neurosurgery and Psychiatry, Special Supplement*, (June 1989), pp. 1–118.

Quinn, N. and Jenner, P. (eds.) (1989). *Disorders of movement: clinical, pharmacological and physiological aspects*. Academic Press, London.

Parkinson's disease

General

Agid, Y. (1991). Parkinson's disease: pathophysiology. *Lancet* 337, 1321–4.

Lee, R. G. and Stein, R. B. (1981), Resetting of tremor by mechanical perturbation: a comparison of essential tremor and parkinsonian tremor. *Annals of Neurology* 10, 523–31.

Marsden, C. D. (1990). Parkinson's disease. *Lancet* 335, 948–52.

Parkinson, J. (1817). *The shaking palsy*. Sherwood, Neely and Jones, London. Facsimile edition prepared by Roche Products.

Report of a Working Group (1990). Standards of care for patients with neurological disease: a consensus. *Journal of the Royal College of Physicians of London* 24, 90–7.

Stern, G. M. (1990). *Parkinson's disease*. Chapman and Hall, London.

Epidemiology and causation

Langston, J. W. (1985). Mechanism of MPTP toxicity: more answers, more questions. *Trends in Pharmacological Science* 6, 375–8.

Mutch, W. J. *et al*. (1986). Parkinson's disease in a Scottish city. *British Medical Journal* 292, 534–6.

Pathology

Halliday, G. M., *et al*. (1990). Neuropathology of immunohistochemically identified brain stem lesions in Parkinson's disease. *Annals of Neurology* 27, 373–85.

Diagnosis

Hughes, A. J., Lees, A. J., and Stern, G. M. (1990). Apomorphine test to predict dopaminergic responsiveness in parkinsonian syndromes. *Lancet* 336, 32–4.

Treatment

A series of papers in *Neurology, Supplement 2* (November 1989), pp. 4–106.

Cederbaum, J. M., Gandy, S. E., and McDowell, F. H. (1991). Early initiation of levodopa treatment does not promote the development of motor response fluctuations, dyskinesias or dementia in Parkinson's disease. *Neurology* 41, 622–9.

Clough, C. G. (1991). Parkinson's disease: management. *Lancet* 337, 1324–7.

Diamond, S. G., *et al*. (1987). Multi-center study of Parkinson mortality with early versus later dopa treatment. *Annals of Neurology* 22, 8–12.

Dunnett, S. B. (1991). Transplantation of embryonic dopamine neurons: what we know from rats. *Journal of Neurology* 238, 65–74.

Goetz, C. G., Stebbins, G. T., Klawans, H. L., *et al*. (1991). United Parkinson Foundation Neurotransplantation Registry on adrenal medullary transplants: presurgical, and 1- and 2-year follow-up. *Neurology* 41, 1719–22.

Frankel, J. P., Lees, A. J., Kempster, P. A., and Stern, G. M. (1990). Subcutaneous apomorphine in the treatment of Parkinson's disease. *Journal of Neurology, Neurosurgery and Psychiatry* 53, 96–101.

Nutt, J. G. (1990). Levodopa-induced dyskinesia: review, observations and speculations. *Neurology* 40, 340–5.

The Parkinson Study Group (1989). Effect of deprenyl on the progression of disability in early Parkinson's disease. *New England Journal of Medicine* **321**, 1364–71.

Quinn, N. (1990). The modern management of Parkinson's disease. *Journal of Neurology, Neurosurgery and Psychiatry* **53**, 93–5.

Williams, A. (1990). Cell implantation in Parkinson's disease: more patients have probably been harmed than helped so far. *British Medical Journal* **301**, 301–2.

Wooten, G. F. (1988). Progress in understanding the pathophysiology of treatment-related fluctuations in Parkinson's disease. *Annals of Neurology* **24**, 363–5.

Multiple system atrophies

General

Biaggioni, I. and Robertson, D. (1987). Endogenous restoration of nor-adrenaline by precursor therapy in dopamine-beta-hydroxylase deficiency. *Lancet* **1**, 1170–2.

Quinn, N. (1989). Multiple system atrophy—the nature of the beast. *Journal of Neurology, Neurosurgery and Psychiatry, Special Supplement*, pp. 78–89.

Striatonigral degeneration

Fearnley, F. M. and Lees, A. J. (1990). Striato-nigral degeneration: a clinicopathological study. *Brain* **113**, 1823–42.

Progressive supranuclear palsy

Lees, A. J. (1987). The Steele–Richardson–Olszewski syndrome (progressive supranuclear palsy). In *Movement Disorders 2* (ed. C. D. Marsden and S. Fahn), pp 272–287. Butterworths, London.

Maher, E. R. and Lees, A. J. (1986). The clinical features and natural history of the Steele–Richardson–Olszewski syndrome (progressive supranuclear palsy). *Neurology* **36**, 1005–8.

Diffuse Lewy body disease

Editorial (1989). Diffuse Lewy body disease. *Lancet* **2**, 310–11.

Syndromes with dystonia

Jankovic, J. and Brin, M. F. (1991). Therapeutic uses of botulinum toxin. *New England Journal of Medicine* **324**, 1186–94.

Lees, A. J., Turjanski, N., Rivest, J., Whurr, R., Lorch, M., and Brookes, G. (1992). Treatment of cervical dystonia hand spasms and laryngeal dystonia with

botulinum toxin. *Journal of Neurology* **23**, 1–4.

Marsden, C. D. and Quinn, N. P. (1990). The dystonias. *British Medical Journal* **300**, 139–44.

Writer's cramp

Hudgson, P. (1983). Writer's cramp. *British Medical Journal* **286**, 585.

Blepharospasm

Grandas, F., Elston, J., Quinn, N., and Marsden, C. D. (1988). Blepharospasm: a review of 264 patients. *Journal of Neurology, Neurosurgery and Psychiatry* **51**, 767–72.

Wilson's disease

Editorial (1989). Homing in on Wilson's disease. *Lancet* **1**, 822–3.

Oder, W., Grimm, G., Kollegger, W., Ferenci, P., Schreider, B., and Decote, L. (1991). Neurological and neuropsychiatric spectrum of Wilson's disease: a prospective study of 45 cases. *Journal of Neurology* **238**, 281–7.

Myoclonus

Fahn, S., Marsden, C. D., and van Woert, M. (eds.) (1986). Myoclonus. *Advances in Neurology*, Vol. 43. Raven Press, New York.

Essential tremor

Findley, L. J. and Koller, W. C. (1987). Essential tremor: a review. *Neurology* **37**, 1194–7.

Huntington's disease

Albin, R. L., Young, A. B., Penney, J. B., *et al.* (1990). Abnormalities of striatal projection neurons and N-methyl-D-aspartate receptors in presymptomatic Huntington's disease. *New England Journal of Medicine* **322**, 1293–8

Harper, P. S., Morris, M. J. and Tyler, A. (1990). Genetic testing for Huntington's disease. *British Medical Journal* **300**, 1089–90.

Harper, P. S. (ed.) (1991). *Huntington's disease*. W. B. Saunders, London.

Martin, J. B. (1984). Huntington's disease: new approaches to an old problem. *Neurology* **34**, 1059–72.

Neuroacanthocytosis

Hardie, R. J., Pullon, H. W. H., Harding, A. E., *et al.* (1991). Neuroacanthocytosis. A clinical, haematological and pathological study of 19 cases. *Brain* **114**, 13–50.

Tics

Lees, A. J. (1985). *Tics and related disorders*. Churchill Livingstone, Edinburgh.

Lees, A. J., Robertson, M., Trimble, M. R., and Murray, N. M. F. (1984). A clinical study of Gilles de la Tourette syndrome in the United Kingdom. *Journal of Neurology, Neurosurgery and Psychiatry* **47**, 1–8.

Pauls, D. L. and Leckman, J. F. (1986). The inheritance of Gilles de la Tourette's syndrome and associated behaviours. *New England Journal of Medicine* **315**, 993–7.

Stremmel, W., Meyerrose, K.-W., Niederau, C., Hefter, H., Kreuzpaintner, G. and Strohmeyer, G. (1991). Wilson's disease: clinical presentation, treatment and survival. *Annals of Internal Medicine*. **115**, 720–6.

Drug-induced movement disorders

Addonizio, G., Susman, V. L., and Roth, S. D. (1987). Neuroleptic malignant syndrome: review and analysis of 115 cases. *Biological Psychiatry* **22**, 1004–20.

Barnes, T. R. E. (1988). Tardive dyskinesia. *British Medical Journal* **296**, 150–1.

Editorial (1986). Akathisia and antipsychotic drugs. *Lancet* **2**, 1131–2.

Saltz, B. L., Woerner, M. G., Kane, J. M., *et al.* (1991). Prospective study of tardive dyskinesia incidence in the elderly. *Journal of the American Medical Association* **266**, 2402–6.

14 Multiple sclerosis

Multiple sclerosis is a relatively common neurological disorder in which episodes of demyelination of axons occur at intervals at different places in the central nervous system, and in those cranial nerves (olfactory, optic, and auditory) in which the axons are supported by oligodendroglial cells. Myelin is the compacted cell membrane of processes of oligodendroglial cells, which, during development, wrap themselves around axons in a way analogous to that of Schwann cells in the peripheral nervous system and other cranial nerves. The small areas of demyelination are known as plaques. The French name for the illness is *sclérose en plaques*, given by Charcot, who first described the clinical and pathological features of the illness at the Salpêtrière in 1868. Although the axons in small plaques survive, the interruption of saltatory nerve conduction and replacement by cable conduction,

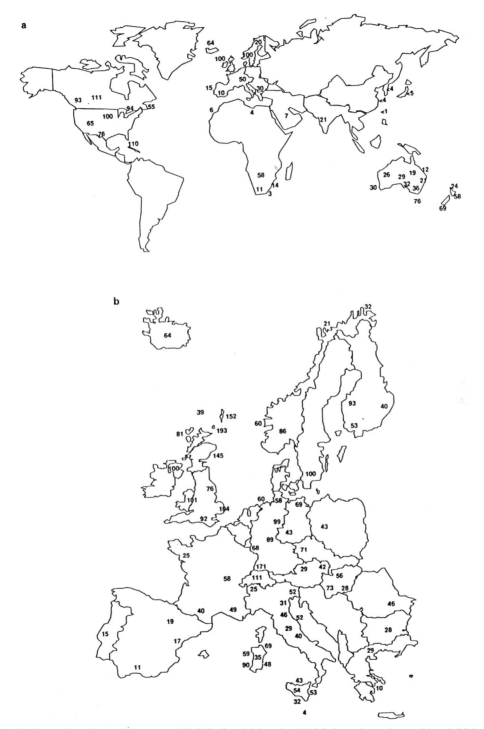

Fig. 14.1 Estimates for the prevalence per 100 000 of multiple sclerosis (a) throughout the world and (b) in Europe. (Reproduced with kind permission from Compston 1990.)

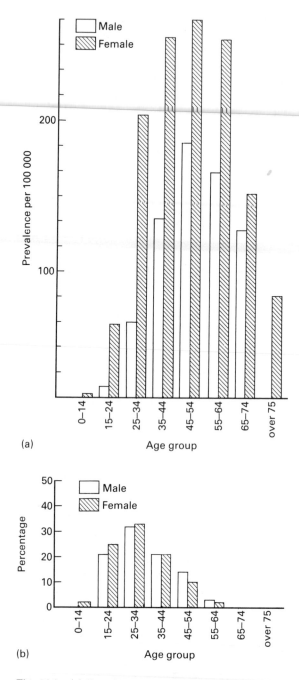

(a)

(b)

Fig. 14.2 (a) Prevalence per 100 000 of multiple sclerosis by age and sex in south-east Wales. (b) Age at onset of multiple sclerosis in prevalent patients in south-east Wales. Age at onset was not known for 8.9 per cent of males and 6.1 per cent of females. (Drawn from data in Tables 3 and 4 of Swingler and Compston 1988.)

or conduction block, results in symptoms if the plaque is in a functionally important part of the central nervous system, such as the brain stem, spinal cord, or optic nerve. Experience with MRI has shown that in areas of high signal, presumed plaques, often occur without symptoms.

14.1   Epidemiology and the cause of multiple sclerosis

The incidence and prevalence of multiple sclerosis varies markedly in different parts of the world, as shown in Fig. 14.1. Even within the high-risk areas, there are gradations of risk, such that the prevalence of the disease increases with increasing latitude in both northern and southern hemispheres. That is to say, the disease is more common in the northern states of the USA compared to the southern states, more common in Scotland, the Orkneys, and Iceland than in southern England, and more common in Tasmania and New Zealand than in the more northern parts of Australasia. As an example, the prevalence is 11.8 per 100 000 in Queensland (latitude 25.1° S) and 75 per 100 000 in Hobart (latitude 42.8° S). For the UK as a whole, the prevalence rate is about 100 per 100 000 population. As Fig. 14.2 shows, the age-specific prevalence in middle years of life is much higher. Figure 14.2b shows the age at onset. The incidence rate which, for the population as a whole in South Wales, reasonably representative of the UK, is about 5.4 per 100 000 per year. These figures indicate that the average family doctor in the UK will see one new case of multiple sclerosis about every 13–16 years, and have on his list at any time one or two patients who have the disease. The lifetime risk of developing multiple sclerosis for someone growing up in the UK is 1 in 800; this rises to 1:50 for the sibling of an affected person, and to 1:2 to 1:4 for the second identical twin if the first is affected.

Clues about the cause of multiple sclerosis come largely from epidemiological studies. The consensus view is that multiple sclerosis is probably caused by an infectious agent acquired in childhood and acting on genetically predisposed subjects. The evidence for this is based upon the occurrence of clusters of patients with multiple sclerosis, on the incidence of multiple sclerosis in migrants, and on studies on the familial incidence of multiple sclerosis and HLA antigens in those with the illness.

14.1.1 *Clustering of cases of multiple sclerosis in space and time*

In Scandinavian countries, where careful ascertainment of cases of multiple sclerosis is possible, there are geographical foci in which the prevalence of multiple sclerosis is up to six times the prevalence in other parts of the same country. Apart from such spatial clusters, there are instances of clustering in time. One notable example occurred in the Faroe Islands, in which multiple sclerosis appeared abruptly in 1943 and disappeared almost as abruptly in 1960. A large number of British troops were stationed in the Faroes in 1940. These temporal and spatial clusters suggest a disorder related to environment and time, and therefore that multiple sclerosis is probably a disorder acquired from the environment.

14.1.2 *Studies on migrating populations*

Further support for the idea that some factor in the environment is necessary for the development of multiple sclerosis comes from studies on people who have migrated at different ages from high- to low-risk areas and vice versa. Prevalence and morbidity rates for migrants, taking note also of the age at which migration occurred, show that those who migrate to low risk areas after the age of 15 from high-risk areas, such as northern Europe, retain much of the high risk of the place of origin. Those who migrate in early childhood to low-risk zones, such as South Africa, acquire the lower risk of their new home. However, other studies have shown that in high-risk areas, the illness can still be acquired in adult life.

14.1.3 *Studies on the familial incidence of multiple sclerosis and on HLA antigens in those with the illness*

The incidence of multiple sclerosis in the siblings or dizygotic twins of those with multiple sclerosis is about 6–8 times higher than would be expected by chance. This could, of course, indicate that the siblings are exposed to a common environmental factor. However, monozygotic twins have an even

higher chance than dizygotic twins of contracting the illness, giving clear evidence of some genetic predisposition to the illness. The concordance rate is about 25 per cent for monozygotic twins, but only 2 per cent for dizygotic twins and non-twin siblings. If human leucocyte antigen (HLA) typing is undertaken on northern Europeans with multiple sclerosis, an excess of those with A3, B7, Dw2, DR2, and DQw1 is found compared to the incidence of these antigens in the general population. It has been shown in a national study in the UK that multiple sclerosis is more common in areas of the country in which the population incidence of DR2 is higher. However, these antigens can in no way be considered a reliable marker for the illness. Twenty per cent of the healthy UK population are positive for DR2 or Dw2 and, although 70 per cent of those with multiple sclerosis are also positive for these antigens, 30 per cent are not. Furthermore, DR2 is common in some populations, such as the indigenous people of North America and in Zulus, in whom multiple sclerosis is rare.

14.2 Pathology

If the opportunity arises to see a recent plaque of demyelination at post-mortem, it is soft and pink. A plaque usually extends circumferentially around and along a small vein, with perivenular lymphocytic infiltrates and evidence of myelin degradation products, some of which—cholesterol esters—stain positively with the Marchi and Sudan stains. The axons are seen to remain intact. Similar lymphocytic infiltration is seen around the edge of a plaque. IgG can be demonstrated in a plaque. On occasion, a stereotactic biopsy of an active plaque has been undertaken. CD4+ and CD8+ lymphocytes and a remarkable degree of heterogeneity of surface markers can be seen in cells within a single lesion.

The 'vascular' component of the plaque—the peri-venular oedema and sheathing by lymphocytes—is reflected in evidence of vascular damage outside the nervous system. Sheathing of retinal vessels by oedema and cuffs of lymphocytes can be seen. There is no myelin in the retina, so some of the changes seen in both retina and brain probably reflect breakdown in the tight junctions of the capillary endothelium.

Chronic plaques feel firm to the touch post-mortem, hence the use of the word 'sclerosis' in naming the disease. Myelin degradation products have long been removed from chronic plaques, so the plaque will not stain with myelin stains, such as luxol fast blue. The edge of the plaque is sharply demarcated. Many axons are seen to survive amongst increased numbers of astrocytes and astrocytic fibres, often arranged in long parallel rows. Axons abruptly lose their sheaths as they enter the plaque. Plaques are particularly common in the cervical spinal cord, brain stem, and periventricular regions.

There is increasing evidence that suggests that multiple sclerosis is more diffuse than classically considered. Even in white matter that appears normal, MRI T_1 and T_2 relaxation times are significantly higher than in controls. Widespread gliosis with or without patchy small areas of demyelination is seen in areas of white matter that macroscopically look normal.

14.2.1 *The mechanisms of demyelination*

The observations listed in Section 14.1 suggest that multiple sclerosis is due to an environmental, possibly an infective agent, acquired by a genetically predisposed boy or girl near the time of puberty. Any proposed mechanism of demyelination has to take these epidemiological and pathological aspects into account, as well as a host of immunological and experimental observations. One function of the HLA antigens within the major histocompatibility complex, which lies on the short arm of chromosome 6, is participation in immune responsiveness. The population findings reviewed above, and the old observations of perivenular lymphocytic cuffing, have concentrated attention on the role of the immune system in multiple sclerosis.

A number of studies have shown a reduced number of suppressor T-cells in the blood of people with multiple sclerosis, and this number falls further during an acute episode, while the ratio of activated helper/inducer (CD4$^+$) to suppressor/cytotoxic (CD8$^+$) increases in the cerebrospinal fluid during an acute relapse. The role of T-cells in multiple sclerosis has been studied in an experimental model, experimental allergic encephalomyelitis, induced in susceptible animals by active sensitization with preparations of spinal cord or brain, compounded with suitable adjuvants. The specific component of cord or brain responsible for producing experimental allergic encephalomyelitis is known as myelin basic protein. It is also possible to induce experimental allergic encephalomyelitis by the injection of myelin basic protein-specific T-cell clones. This, and the electron microscopic evidence of mononuclear cells and macrophages actively stripping myelin, has formed the basis of much thinking about the immunological basis of multiple sclerosis.

A surprising finding is that whereas a very small number of myelin basic protein-specific T-cell clones will, if injected systemically, induce experimental allergic encephalomyelitis, injection directly into the brain does not. Other experiments have shown that oligodendrocytes are exquisitely sensitive to small concentrations of complement, and exposure to complement allows a sharp increase in intracellular calcium, which damages the oligodendrocyte, and hence myelin, its compacted cell membrane. It might be thought that any insult that damaged the blood–brain barrier by relaxation of endothelial tight junctions would, by allowing access of complement to the oligodendrocyte, result in demyelination. However, this does not happen after, for example, anoxic damage to endothelial tight junctions. Furthermore, there is no lymphocytic cuffing around venules damaged by anoxia.

It is not possible to induce experimental allergic neuritis in animals depleted of complement by pretreatment with cobra venom, nor, as noted above, can experimental allergic neuritis be induced by intracerebral injections of myelin basic protein-specific T-cell clones. It appears, therefore, that the presence of both activated T-cells and complement is necessary for demyelination. The inflammatory lesions of multiple sclerosis contain not only T-cells, but also B-lymphocytes and plasma cells, which synthesize the immunoglobulins that can be found in the spinal fluid. Experiments in tissue culture suggest an additive lytic effect of complement and circulating antibody.

Electron microscopic observations of experimental allergic encephalomyelitis, and limited observations on fresh human plaques, indicate that macrophages and mononuclear cells are actively engaged in stripping away and phagocytosing myelin lamellae. Presumably, these cells are activated by as yet unidentified lymphokines, released from the multiplying B-lymphocytes and by complement.

The mannose-binding protein known as cerebellar soluble lectin (CSL) may stabilize the structure of myelin by acting as a bridging molecule between glycoprotein glycans on the surface of oligodendrocytes. It is of considerable interest that CSL is not only found in these cells, but also on Schwann cells, and at endothelial tight junctions. Antibodies to CSL derange compacted myelin. Recently, antibodies to CSL have been found in the cerebrospinal fluid of patients with multiple sclerosis.

A general synthesis of these observations suggests that, in genetically susceptible individuals, activated T-cells, in response to some environmental trigger, interact with the tight junctions of the blood–brain barrier, to which the foot processes of astrocytes contribute. Alternatively, the initial damage to the tight junctions might be caused by circulating antibodies to CSL protein. Loosening of these junctions allows the passage of activated T-cells and complement into the brain; local proliferation of B-lymphocytes and plasma cells occurs. These produce antibodies, probably including anti-CSL, which, with complement, damage oligodendrocytes. Other lymphokines activate macrophages, which strip the damaged oligodendrocyte membrane (myelin) from the axon.

14.3 Clinical features

Figure 14.2b shows that the modal age of onset of multiple sclerosis lies in the mid-twenties for both men and women. Onset is rare before adolescence and after the mid-fifties. Women are rather more often affected than men, but the difference between sexes is not great.

Plaques of demyelination can occur virtually anywhere in the central nervous system, and in those cranial nerves which contain oligodendroglial cells (olfactory, optic, and acoustic/vestibular), so the range of possible symptoms is vast. However, three main groups of symptoms predominate, due to demyelination in the optic nerve, the brain stem, or the spinal cord (Table 14.1).

14.3.1 *Demyelination in the optic nerve*

This is called optic neuritis, or retrobulbar neuritis.

Table 14.1 Presenting symptoms and signs in 193 patients with multiple sclerosis (some patients have more than one at presentation) (data from Sanders *et al.* 1986)

	%
Posterior column	40
Pyramidal tract	37
Brain stem	30
Optic nerve	23
'Cerebellar'	17

The patient notices the sudden onset of blurring of vision. He or she may often remark upon the loss of intensity of colours, so that everything appears misty or grey. Although the visual acuity may be reduced to less than 6/60, it is unusual to lose vision completely. There may be a dull ache in or around the eye, which is exacerbated by movement, and pressure on the globe may be painful. Examination of the central visual field (Fig. 6.9) will show a central scotoma, with relative preservation of the peripheral field. Some patients can draw their own scotoma. If the impairment of central acuity is considerable, then the pupillary response to direct illumination will be impaired, though the pupil of the affected eye will still constrict briskly to illumination of the other eye. This is called an afferent pupillary defect. If the plaque of demyelination is far forwards in the optic nerve, the optic disc will be pink and swollen. If so, the associated impairment of acuity is useful in distinguishing between such a papillitis and papilloedema due to raised intracranial pressure, in which the acuity is near normal until the papilloedema is far advanced. If demyelination lies further back in the optic nerve, there will be nothing to see on fundoscopy in the acute stage, although, as the lesion settles, the optic disc becomes pale, most noticeably on the temporal side.

Magnetic resonance imaging shows a segment of high signal in the optic nerve in about 85 per cent of acute cases. The mean lesion length is about 10 mm. It has been calculated that about 12 million internodes are involved.

Demyelination may occur in the olfactory and auditory nerves, the only other cranial nerves in which oligodendroglial cells are present. Unilateral deafness is occasionally a symptom; audiometry and special tests of olfaction may show evidence of plaques in these nerves in some patients.

14.3.2 *Demyelination in the brain stem*

The hallmark of plaques in the brain stem is impairment of balance and, to a lesser extent, of coordination of the limbs and intention tremor due to demyelination of cerebellar connections. White matter pathways are so crowded together in the brain stem, however, that many other symptoms and signs may occur. Prominent among these are vertigo, clearly closely related to impairment of balance, and dysarthria due to impaired co-ordination of speech. Diplopia may be due to demyelination of the third, fourth, and sixth nerves before they leave the brain stem. Most commonly affected are axons of the sixth nerve, resulting in weakness of abduction of one eye. As these axons run in close proximity to axons of the fifth and seventh nerves, the palsy may be associated with ipsilateral numbness and facial weakness. Diplopia may also arise due to demyelination of the medial longitudinal bundle which links together the third and fourth and sixth nuclei. Characteristic of such a lesion is weakness of adduction of the eye on the side of the lesion on attempted lateral gaze, and prominent nystagmus of the other (abducting) eye. This combination is known as an internuclear ophthalmoplegia. If the demyelination occurs more anteriorly in the pons, then the pyramidal axons will be affected. A single brain-stem lesion can therefore account for both pyramidal and cerebellar connection signs. In advanced cases, bilateral demyelination of pyramidal neurons at various levels may result in a pseudobulbar palsy, with a spastic dysarthria and emotional lability (see Section 6.4.2).

14.3.3 *Spinal cord lesions*

Although both sensory and motor symptoms can arise from demyelination of afferent and efferent pathways in the brain stem, they often result from demyelination in the spinal cord. A common site for a plaque is high in the posterior columns and, as such plaques are often symmetrical, tingling may occur simultaneously in both upper limbs, commonly in the hands, and up the inner aspects of the forearms. The disturbance felt by patients is such that they may describe their fingers as swollen, or their hands as encased in boxing gloves. Depending on the site of the lesion in the posterior columns, sensory symptoms may also begin in the lower limbs, characteristically distally, and spread proximally up to the trunk, to the waist or mid-thorax. Demyelination of afferents from muscle spindles may result in marked incoordination and, from joint receptors, in loss of joint position sense. The two together, even if not associated with pyramidal signs, impair fine dexterous movements of the hands. The same defect in the lower limbs results in rombergism—instability of stance which worsens on closing the eyes.

A feature of active plaques in the cervical region is Lhermitte's sign (or, more properly, symptom). The patient notices that on bending the head forwards a shower of tingling spreads down the arms to the hands, and sometimes into the trunk and legs. This movement presumably stretches the plaque and stimulates impulse generation or ephaptic transmission (direct 'sideways' transmission of an action potential from one axon to a neighbour) in the demyelinated axons. Because this symptom occurs on flexion of the neck it is sometimes known as 'the barber's chair sign'. It can occur in diseases other than multiple sclerosis, most notably after trauma to the cervical spine, and in cervical spondylosis and subacute combined degeneration of the spinal cord (Section 23.2.4.4).

Demyelination of the pyramidal tracts in the spinal cord results in heaviness and dragging of one or both legs, which is notably worse after walking some distance. Demyelination may also be so extensive that an acute paraplegia occurs—a so-called transverse myelitis—but, more commonly, pyramidal weakness is less pronounced and the patient can continue walking with difficulty through an episode. Repeated pyramidal episodes, however, often in conjunction with demyelination of cerebellar connections, may eventually lead to a loss of ability to walk.

14.3.4 *Other clinical features of multiple sclerosis*

The cerebral control of the sphincters of the bladder reach the sacral cord by pathways immediately medial to the pyramidal tracts, and disorders of micturition are frequent in multiple sclerosis (Section 6.11.1.2). Complete retention of urine may occur, and is occasionally an early feature of the illness. More frequent is disinhibition of the detrusor muscle, so that reflex detrusor contractions occur as the bladder fills. The resulting rise in pressure produces a combination of urgency and incontinence—the involuntary passage of some urine after an urgent desire to void. Sometimes the physical disabilities associated with advanced disease prevent reaching the lavatory in time when the urgent desire to void is perceived. Usually such bladders empty reasonably well but, if not, the presence of residual urine after micturition encourages infection and the associated cystitis makes the urgency and incontinence even more troublesome.

In the earlier stages of the illness a transient worsening of symptoms may occur if the subject's body temperature is elevated by a hot bath or by exercise, the so-called Uhthoff's phenomenon. Studies on experimentally demyelinated nerve roots in animals have shown a remarkable sensitivity to temperature—a rise of only 0.5°C blocking conduction in some fibres.

Paroxysmal features occur in some patients with multiple sclerosis. There may, for example, be a transient dysarthria or ataxia. These phenomena may last only 20–30 minutes. It is inconceivable that demyelination and remyelination could occur in this short space of time. It is believed that such episodes are due to ephaptic ('short-circuit') conduction between adjacent demyelinated axons.

Epilepsy occurs in a small proportion of patients with multiple sclerosis. Some seizures are straightforward tonic–clonic or partial motor seizures, but others, tonic seizures, in which an abnormal posture may be maintained for a minute or two, may again be due to ephaptic conduction. Trigeminal neuralgia, indistinguishable from the spontaneous neuralgia of older people (Section 9.10.1), may have the same basis. Facial myokymia, an involuntary rippling of the muscles of one side of the face, may last for several weeks and is strongly suggestive of a diagnosis of multiple sclerosis, but the cause of this is not known.

In patients with advanced multiple sclerosis, mental changes often occur, of which the best known is euphoria—an elevated mood disproportionate to the disability of the illness. It is, however, important not to confuse conscious courage with euphoria. In other patients depression may occur. Social disinhibition, impaired memory, and frank dementia may afflict those with large zones of demyelination towards the end of their illness.

14.4   Laboratory studies in multiple sclerosis

14.4.1   *Examination of the cerebrospinal fluid*

Two-thirds of patients with multiple sclerosis have more than 5 white cells per microlitre of, the excess being accounted for by small and large lymphocytes. There is no particular correlation between the cell count and the duration of the disease, the degree of disability, or, rather surprisingly, whether the patient is in relapse or remission.

The protein in the CSF is largely albumin, identical with, and in equilibrium with, the plasma albumin. It diffuses into the spinal fluid through the walls of the capillaries in the choroid plexus. Relatively few endothelial tight junctions are affected in multiple sclerosis, and elevation of CSF fluid albumin does not occur to any significant extent. There is, however, good evidence of synthesis of immunoglobulin G (IgG) within the blood–brain barrier of patients with multiple sclerosis. The ratio between CSF IgG and albumin (or total protein) is therefore increased; in about two-thirds of patients with multiple sclerosis the proportion of IgG will exceed 15 per cent. A more sophisticated measure is the index described by Link and Tibbling, which incorporates the serum levels of IgG and albumin:

$$\frac{\text{IgG in CSF}}{\text{IgG in serum}} \div \frac{\text{Albumin in CSF}}{\text{Albumin in serum}}$$

In about 90 per cent of patients with clinically definite multiple sclerosis this index exceeds 0.7.

The greater part of the excess IgG synthesized within the nervous system of patients with multiple sclerosis is of restricted homogeneity, as judged by class and light-chain constitution, and by electrophoretic mobility. Electrophoresis of the CSF fluid of 90 per cent of patients with clinically definite multiple sclerosis shows several fractions that are not present in the blood of the same patients. The presence of these defined fractions, which form bands on the electrophoretic supporting medium, is known as oligoclonal banding. These bands are persistent and stable during the course of the illness, and their intensity does not correlate with the clinical progress of the disease. ACTH does, however, suppress the production of IgG in patients with multiple sclerosis.

It must be remembered that oligoclonal bands are found in conditions other than multiple sclerosis—conditions associated with immune reactions in the nervous system. These include neurosyphilis, sarcoidosis, systemic lupus erythematosus, Lyme disease, and other types of chronic meningitis. Oligoclonal bands are also found in HTLV-I myelopathy.

It is tempting to believe that the oligoclonal bands found in multiple sclerosis represent antibodies specifically directed towards the antigen (possible viral antigen) responsible for multiple sclerosis, but an alternative is equally likely, that oligoclonal IgG is synthesized in response to the presence of an antigen liberated by demyelination caused by some quite separate primary event.

Myelin basic protein is liberated into the spinal fluid at the time of a relapse. Higher levels are found in those whose disease is running a more aggressive course. Antibodies to cerebellar soluble lectin (CSL) we found in the spinal fluid of patients with multiple sclerosis. This protein stabilizes myelin structure by serving as a bridging molecule between glycoprotein glycans on the surface of oligodendroglia.

14.4.2 *Evoked responses*

The occipital cortical potential recorded about 100 ms after the reversal of a chequerboard pattern (Section 8.4) is the response most often used in the investigation of patients with possible multiple sclerosis. The response is usually distorted or absent in patients with clinically evident optic neuritis, but proponents of the investigation hope that, by detecting a clinically silent plaque in one optic nerve, the presence of a lesion elsewhere in the nervous system can be confidently supposed also to be demyelinating in nature. A common clinical problem is the investigation of someone with a mild paraparesis. This could be due to a spinal compressive lesion, or to a plaque of demyelination. Myelography or MRI can clearly distinguish these possibilities, and many neurologists do not feel that a delayed visual evoked response has sufficient status, bearing in mind the false positive and negative responses obtained, to allow avoidance of myelography or MRI in these circum-

stances, as missing a potentially remediable spinal compressive lesion could be disastrous.

Somatosensory and brain-stem evoked responses, and central motor conduction time after magnetic stimulation, may well also be abnormal in brain-stem and spinal lesions, but in many clinical circumstances such abnormalities cannot be reliably attributed to demyelination or, indeed, to a lesion of any type anatomically separate from that deduced on clinical grounds.

Many neurologists believe that the relative ease of recording evoked responses, using modern amplifying and computing equipment, has seduced clinical neurophysiologists into claiming more for their investigations than is justified. This is not to deny the fact that many patients with clinically definite multiple sclerosis have abnormal evoked responses, and that many patients with abnormal evoked responses progress to show clinically definite multiple sclerosis, but the diagnostic and predictive value in individual cases of possible multiple sclerosis is not high.

14.4.3 *Magnetic resonance imaging*

Figure 8.20 shows a scan from a patient with typical changes of multiple sclerosis, the T2 weighted axial images showing clearly areas of periventricular demyelination. Demyelination in this region is demonstrated in virtually all patients with clinically definite multiple sclerosis. In about two-thirds of patients with clinically 'isolated' optic neuritis, or brain-stem lesion, periventricular or other imaging abnormalities are seen. Plaques can also be demonstrated in optic nerves, the length of the abnormality correlating with the outcome for recovery of visual acuity. Serial studies on patients with multiple sclerosis have shown that appropriate high-signal lesions can become prominent within 2–3 days of the onset of symptoms. Conversely, new lesions can occur without clinical symptoms. The signal from new lesions is enhanced by the intravenous injection of gadolinium DTPA, which crosses the damaged blood–brain barrier. MRI has revolutionized the early diagnosis of multiple sclerosis, in countries in which the technology is available. However, in older patients with intermittent neurological symptoms due to vascular disease, the appearances and distribution of the zones of high signal, presumably associated with lacunes (see Section 10.1.2), may be indistinguishable from plaques of demyelination. A much rarer cause of periventricular areas of high signal is the adult-onset type of adrenoleucodystrophy (see Section 23.1.3.4).

14.5 Probable and definite multiple sclerosis

Epidemiological studies and clinical thinking have been clarified by the adoption of diagnostic criteria suggested by Poser and colleagues.

Clinically definite multiple sclerosis: Two attacks of neurological symptoms, each lasting at least 24 hours, separated by a period of 1 month, involving different parts of the nervous system. There must either be clinical evidence of two separate lesions on physical examination, or clinical evidence of one and paraclinical evidence (e.g. an abnormal evoked response) of another.

Laboratory-supported definite multiple sclerosis: Two attacks, clinical or paraclinical evidence of one lesion, and the presence of oligoclonal bands. One attack, clinical evidence of one lesion and paraclinical evidence of another separate lesion, and oligoclonal bands. Progressive course for 6 months, sequential discrete involvement clinically or paraclinically, and the presence of oligoclonal bands.

Clinically probable multiple sclerosis: Two attacks and clinical evidence of one lesion. One attack and clinical evidence of two lesions. One attack, clinical evidence of one lesion, and paraclinical evidence of another.

Laboratory-supported multiple sclerosis: Two attacks and the presence of oligoclonal bands.

14.6 Differential diagnosis of multiple sclerosis

Whenever a neurologist sees a patient who might have multiple sclerosis, he or she always tries to put that diagnosis to the back of his or her mind until other diagnostic possibilities have been excluded, as far as possible, on clinical grounds. The reason for this approach is that it is too facile a diagnosis. As demyelination can occur virtually anywhere in the central nervous system, it is possible to account for virtually any constellation of signs and symptoms by suggesting a multiplicity of

plaques. The approach outlined in Chapter 5 should be followed rigorously, so that a single anatomical lesion of an entirely different pathological type, treatable perhaps by surgical means, is not overlooked. The following points may help.

1. Lesions other than demyelinating plaques may have a relapsing and remitting course—notably, of course, vascular lesions. In younger patients, where atheromatous vascular disease is not very probable, the possibility of an angioma should be considered. Some tumours may also follow a fluctuating course, particularly pontine tumours. Other cerebral tumours may also fluctuate in size and in the symptoms they produce during pregnancy.

2. A progressive spastic paraparesis should never be considered to be demyelinating until a compressive spinal cord lesion has been rigorously excluded by myelography or MRI. Some patients with a progressive spastic paraparesis will prove to have an HTLV-I myelopathy or B_{12} deficiency.

3. Progressive failure of vision of one eye is seldom due to demyelinating disease but to local compression by, for example, a meningioma arising from a sphenoidal wing. Bilateral subacute visual loss may be due to Leber's atrophy (Section 23.1.4.1). An acute ischaemic optic neuropathy may mimic a retrobulbar neuritis, as may a toxic amblyopia (see Section 23.2.4.4). Friedreich's ataxia, neurosyphilis, and vitamin B_{12} deficiency may all be associated with clinical or electrophysiological evidence of optic nerve damage.

4. Significant muscular wasting does not occur in multiple sclerosis until the illness is far advanced. Focal wasting at an early stage should suggest some other type of lesion at that segmental level.

5. Focal lesions in the central nervous system that are clearly multiple or clinical on imaging grounds may be vascular, granulomatous, or neoplastic rather than demyelinating in nature. Areas of high signal on the MRI in the periventricular white matter are commonplace in older people.

6. A careful family history may allow distinction of a heredo-familial degenerative disorder with mixed pyramidal and cerebellar signs from multiple sclerosis (Section 20.3).

7. Occasional patients will have a monophasic

acute disseminated encephalomyelitis, with recovery over a few months (Section 14.13).

In general, MRI has been shown to be better in predicting a transition from laboratory-supported definite multiple sclerosis to the rank of clinically definite multiple sclerosis than the presence of abnormal evoked responses or oligoclonal bands.

14.7 Factors possibly precipitating the onset of, or a relapse of, multiple sclerosis

14.7.1 Trauma

Earlier authors reported an increased chance of relapse following trauma, including the trauma of surgery. However, case–control and prospective studies have failed to substantiate this. The belief arose possibly because patients with a disabling illness are more likely to recall trauma than the average healthy person going about his or her daily business. There remains one point for further research, however: if a new episode begins after trauma, symptoms appear more often in the traumatized limb than would be expected by chance.

14.7.2 Pregnancy and the puerperium

There is no increased chance of relapse during pregnancy, but during the first 3 months of the puerperium the risk of a relapse is tripled. Whether this is due to hormonal changes associated with the puerperium, or is in some way due to the effort of coping with a new baby is not known, but it would seem sensible to provide as much domestic help as practical to a woman with multiple sclerosis in the puerperium.

14.7.3 Immunization

Acute demyelinating encephalomyelitis did occur after smallpox vaccination. It was therefore considered unwise to vaccinate those with multiple sclerosis. Smallpox is now extinct, however, and there is no proven ill-effect of immunization against other infective agents such as tetanus or influenza, though many neurologists prefer to avoid immunization unless really necessary.

14.7.4 Other factors

Some patients attribute relapses to emotional stress, physical fatigue, or to getting cold or wet. It is impossible to be sure how seriously to take these suggestions, but recent observations on interactions between psychological states and immune responsiveness make such suggestions more credible than before.

There is no evidence that lumbar puncture induces exacerbations, but some neurologists feel that myelography may do so.

14.8 Treatment of acute episodes of multiple sclerosis

Most patients with acute exacerbations of multiple sclerosis, or episodes of demyelination which are probably the first evidence of multiple sclerosis, improve spontaneously over 4–6 weeks, so it is difficult to assess the additional benefit due to any medication. The problem is analogous to the management of facial palsy (Section 19.4.1.1), after which the vast majority of patients recover without any specific treatment.

There is no evidence that bed rest or time off work hastens the resolution of an exacerbation of multiple sclerosis, but the practicalities of the situation often determine these issues. As to pharmacological therapy during the acute episode, the principal intervention favoured by neurologists in the last 25–30 years has been adrenocorticotropic hormone (corticotropin, ACTH), intravenous methylprednisolone or oral corticosteroids such as prednisolone. The results have varied from trial to trial, probably because of the difficulties in scoring disability and progress and because of the relatively small numbers recruited into the trials. Furthermore, because of the clear-cut clinical effects of hypercorticolism, clinicians (and patients) in the trials often guess that a patient is on active treatment, so that 'blinding' is lost.

One recent trial (see Beck et al. Further Reading) has used optic neuritis as the study model. Impairment of function (visual acuity) is at least readily assessed in such demyelinating episodes. This study found that visual function recovered faster in patients receiving intravenous methylprednisolone 1 g per day for 3 days, followed by oral prednisone (1 mg/kg per day for 11 days) than in patients on placebo or oral steroids alone for 14 days. However, the 'life-table' curves to recovery of normal visual function were not widely separate in the three groups, and there was no significant difference in the numbers with poor visual outcome at six months. Unexpectedly, patients on oral steroids proved to be at unexpectedly higher risk of further episodes of optic neuritis in the next eighteen months, for reasons that are at present unexplained.

Methylprednisolone may cause facial flushing during the injection, and result in disturbed sleep and significant change in mood.

Faced with this data, it is difficult to recommend corticosteroid medication; probably even methylprednisolone should be reserved for those with acute devastating episodes of demyelination.

14.9   Long-term treatment of multiple sclerosis and prevention of relapses

Patients with multiple sclerosis are understandably keen to try anything that might prevent relapses or the slow progression of their disease. A vast number of different regimes have been proposed; the following require consideration at the present time.

14.9.1   *Modification of diet*

Exclusion of gluten from the diet has been associated with improvement in a few cases of multiple sclerosis, but there has never been evidence to suggest other than that this improvement was coincidental. A theoretical framework for this treatment is lacking, though that would not matter if it could be shown that the treatment worked. Another alternative—supplementation of the diet with polyunsaturated fatty acids—at least rests on some theoretical basis, as patients with multiple sclerosis have been found, in some studies, to have less linoleic acid in plasma-esterified cholesterol than normal subjects. Unsaturated fatty acids could influence the course of multiple sclerosis in a number of ways. They are constituents of oligodendroglial cell membrane (myelin); they are also precursors of prostaglandin, or they may themselves have a direct immunosuppressive effect.

Capsules of polyunsaturated fatty acids are available commercially, but there is no good evidence that supplementation of the diet by the ω-6 group of polyunsaturated fatty acids, as found in sunflower seed oil and oil of evening primrose, or the ω-3 fatty acids, as found in fish body oil, significantly influences the course of the disease. Diets low in animal fat, and supplementation of the normal diet by massive doses of vitamins important in other neurological illnesses (thiamine, cyanocobalamin) have not been shown to be of benefit.

14.9.2   *Hyperbaric oxygenation*

As plaques of demyelination tend to arise around small vessels, it has been suggested that capillary microthrombi might initiate demyelination, or that the plaques may arise in areas around veins occluded by fat emboli. The idea has arisen that the lesions could be helped by, as it were, forcing oxygen in. Unfortunately, controlled trials of hyperbaric oxygenation have failed to show any benefit. Furthermore, the pathological appearances of plaques and microembolism are quite distinct. Perivenous lymphocytic cuffing does not occur in anoxic tissue damage due to microembolism, although it is an obvious feature of plaques. Furthermore, if axons are damaged as a result of anoxia, myelin breaks down by Wallerian degeneration, not by demyelination, with sparing of axons.

14.9.3   *Manipulation of the immune system*

ACTH certainly inhibits the production of immunoglobulin G within the nervous system of those with acute episodes of multiple sclerosis, but there has been no evidence from trials that long-term administration of ACTH or steroids influences the course of the illness. Exceptionally, however, a neurologist encounters a patient who remains in remission on a small dose of steroids, and relapses as soon as this is withdrawn.

Trials of immunosuppressive treatment with azathioprine, cyclophosphamide, cyclosporin A, antilymphocytic serum, thoracic duct drainage, plasmapheresis, total body radiation, or thymectomy are unimpressive, and none of these has yet found international favour. Of these, the simplest to use is azathioprine. A meta-analysis of all trials shows no benefit at one year, but a slight difference in the Kurtzke disability score at two and three years, the difference favouring azathioprine. The chances of a new relapse in this time were also less. However, the trials reported a significant number of adverse effects, and there remains concern about azathioprine increasing the risk of the subsequent development of tumours.

Another method of modifying the immune system includes infusion of transfer factor—a dialysable extract of lymphocytes capable of transferring antigen-specific immunity. One trial of transfer factor did show a significant retardation in the progression of multiple sclerosis, but this has not been confirmed in another. The antiviral activity of interferons—glycoproteins released by cells infected with viruses—has also been studied. One trial of natural human fibroblast interferons reduced the rate of exacerbations of patients with a relapsing and remitting course by 57 per cent, but those on placebo treatment also showed a 25 per cent reduction in relapse rate. As interferon does not cross the blood–brain barrier, the drug has to be administered intrathecally. On the other hand, a trial of γ-interferon increased rates of relapse. Other trials have been carried out on Copolymer 1. This is a random polymer of certain amino acids simulating myelin basic protein, which probably acts through the production of antigen-specific suppressor T-cells. A reduction in relapse rate has again been reported. Both Copolymer 1 and the interferons probably act through their effects upon antigen-specific suppressor T-cells. Finally, on the grounds that a persistent viral infection may be involved, acyclovir and amantadine have been proposed as therapeutic agents. None of the treatments proposed is as yet in routine use.

14.10 Treatment of specific symptoms of multiple sclerosis

Troublesome symptoms of multiple sclerosis include spasticity, which is usually uncomfortable and sometimes painful. Treatments for this are similar to those used in the management of spinal cord lesions following trauma (Section 18.1.4.4). Urge incontinence is particularly troublesome, and the management of this is considered in Section

6.11.1.2. A sub-trigonal injection of phenol may produce remarkable relief. The unusual paroxysmal manifestations of multiple sclerosis (Section 14.3.4) respond well to carbamazepine, in doses similar to those used for the control of epilepsy (Section 12.8). Carbamazepine may sometimes help persistent troublesome sensory symptoms, but, all too often, these are unrelieved by any medication. Other symptoms for which medication is not beneficial include incoordination and impaired balance, and dysarthria. Physiotherapy may produce some improvement in stability and gait. The provision of aids should be considered as appropriate, and as outlined in Chapter 26.

14.11 Prognosis of multiple sclerosis

There is no illness in neurology, perhaps in the whole of medicine, about which a neurologist can be so aggravatingly uninformative to an individual, enquiring patient. Attempts to explain the varying course of the illness are often seen by the patient as prevarication, if not downright evasion. Yet the neurologist's task is very difficult when the following features are remembered.

1. Routine autopsies occasionally show advanced pathological evidence of multiple sclerosis, with no history of symptoms during life.

2. MRI of patients with multiple sclerosis may show many more plaques than clinically counted episodes. MRI of healthy young or middle-aged people occasionally may show areas of high signal in the periventricular region, indistinguishable from those seen in multiple sclerosis.

3. Some subjects have symptoms, signs, and a remission very suggestive of an initial episode of multiple sclerosis, yet never have any further problems; another subject with an identical history may remain free from symptoms for 20 years before the next undoubted episode, and yet another may be severely disabled from the effects of multiple sclerosis within 5 years.

4. Some subjects with multiple sclerosis never show the 'characteristic' relapses and remissions, but progress inexorably.

5. Some subjects have a number of episodes of diminishing severity, the illness burning itself out within a few years.

However, some definite statements can be made.

Patients with an older age of onset fare less well. Men do rather less well than women. Patients with sensory symptoms at onset have a better prognosis than those with motor symptoms at onset. Those with symptoms of incoordination at or near onset have the least favourable course. A long remission between the first and second episodes is a predictor of a favourable course. Those who have a progressive course from onset do less well. The persistence of sensory symptoms after an acute episode does not imply active demyelination any more than does the persistence of spasticity. There is no evidence that treatment of acute episodes influences the rate of overall progression of the illness.

Disability at 5 years after onset of multiple sclerosis correlates well with disability 10 and 15 years after onset; that is to say, the illness seldom suddenly accelerates its course. Another way of looking at this observation is that the disability of multiple sclerosis after the early episodes is due to the cumulative effects of randomly distributed plaques; the rate of accumulation is more or less constant for an individual patient.

The *average* duration of the illness to death is of the order of 25–30 years, and the majority of survivors to this time are still able to walk.

The average rate of clinical relapse is about one relapse every 2 years—0.5 relapses per patient per year. The relapse frequency lessens with time. Modification of this figure is at least a worthy target for any proposed new treatment. However, it can be calculated that, in order to show a reduction in the frequency of relapses by 25 per cent, more than 100 patients would need to be followed for more than 4 years. In future, moreover, the standing of this figure of 0.5 relapses per patient per year is likely to be diminished by more intensive noting of 'trivial' symptoms, recording of evoked potentials, and by MRI, as plaques causing little if anything in the way of symptoms are now known to be common. In prospective clinical studies, clinical exacerbations are more common than retrospective studies would suggest.

The probability of developing multiple sclerosis by 15 years after an episode of retrobulbar neuritis affecting one eye is of the order of 75 per cent for

women and 35 per cent for men. Female sex, an abnormal visual evoked response from the clinically unaffected eye, the presence of oligoclonal bands in the spinal fluid, the presence of high-signal lesions on MRI in the brain on presentation, and the possession of HLA DR2 (if with DR3) (Section 14.1.3), and winter onset all make the development of later multiple sclerosis more probable.

There is good evidence that simultaneous bilateral optic neuritis is a different disease. If this occurs in childhood, long follow-up shows that virtually no patient subsequently develops multiple sclerosis, and very few adults do so. Apart from the good prognosis, another important feature separates *bilateral* retrobulbar neuritis in childhood from multiple sclerosis—in many patients the visual evoked responses are normal after clinical recovery, whereas that is very seldom true for the affected eye of those with adult unilateral optic neuritis.

14.12   When and what to tell the patient

The paternalistic attitude of doctors protecting their patients against unpleasant information has largely passed, and most doctors appreciate that their patients want to know as much as possible about their illness. Not only is it right that they should have information that may allow them to plan their lives to the best advantage of themselves and their families, but there is also good evidence that patients tolerate disabilities much better once uncertainty has passed. Most patients now receive a balanced account of their illness when the diagnosis becomes clinically probable or definite.

The difficulties are, however, apparent when the diagnosis remains 'possible'. Even if, for example, 60 per cent of those with retrobulbar neuritis (men and women combined) do go on to develop clinically definite multiple sclerosis, 40 per cent do not, and is it right to cast a shadow over the lives of all? I adopt the following compromise, although others may have different views. I tell the patient who is suffering from an episode which I believe could prove to be the first episode of multiple sclerosis that he or she has a type of inflammation in the nervous system, possibly caused by a virus,

and that I expect the symptoms to settle spontaneously (or with methylprednisolone, if I decide
to use this). I go on to say that this type of
inflammation can, unfortunately, return, though I
hope it won't, and I shall be pleased to see the
patient again if there are further symptoms. If the
patient returns with a second episode, then I say
that one of the commoner causes of such recurrent
inflammation is multiple sclerosis, and that this is
a diagnosis that has to be considered. Over the
next consultations the word 'possible' shifts to
'probable', if appropriate. This technique has a
sound sociological pedigree, described by Goffman
as 'cooling the mark'—getting the 'mark' (the
patient) to come to terms gradually with a new and
unexpected situation. When the patient and I are
talking in terms of a diagnosis of 'probable' multiple sclerosis, then it is time to give a brief account
of the illness and prognosis, with a specific offer of
an appointment about 10 days ahead, the patient
bringing his or her partner if relevant, in order to
spend time answering the numerous questions that
will undoubtedly be generated in the interim.

14.13   Acute disseminated
encephalomyelitis

The relationship of this disorder to acute monophasic multiple sclerosis is unclear. Profound
neurological deficits, sometimes proceeding to
coma, are associated with a lymphocytic, and often
neutrophilic, pleocytosis in the cerebrospinal fluid.
Histological studies show marked perivenular clustering of T-lymphocytes and macrophages, with
surrounding demyelination. Areas of demyelination tend to be symmetrical on MRI. Oligoclonal
bands are present initially in the spinal fluid and
then disappear. The plaques of demyelination may
be so acute that they become haemorrhagic, and
so oedematous as to be seen as mass lesions on
imaging studies. Intravenous methylprednisolone
may reverse the fulminant process, but the disorder may prove fatal. The absence of subsequent
lesions appearing on MRI after six months is an
encouraging pointer that the illness should be
considered a monophasic episode of acute disseminated encephalomyelitis rather than multiple
sclerosis.

14.14   Further reading

General

Compston, D. A. S. (1990). The dissemination of multiple sclerosis. *Journal of the Royal College of Physicians
of London* **24**, 207–18.
Cook, S. D. (ed.) (1990). *Handbook of multiple sclerosis*. Marcel Dekker, New York.
Matthews, W. B. (ed.) (1990). *McAlpine's multiple sclerosis*. Churchill Livingstone, London.

Epidemiology and causation

Ebers, G. C., *et al.* (1986). A population based study of
multiple sclerosis in twins. *New England Journal of
Medicine* **315**, 1638–42.
Hughes, R. A. C. (1992). Pathogenesis of multiple sclero-
sis. *Journal of the Royal Society of Medicine* **85**, 373–5.
Larner, A. J. (1986). Aetiological role of viruses in
multiple sclerosis: a review. *Journal of the Royal
Society of Medicine* **79**, 412–17.
Roberts, M. H. W., Martin J. P., Mclellan, D. L.,
McIntosh-Michaelis, S. A., and Spackman, A. J.
(1991). The prevalence of multiple sclerosis in the
Southampton and South West Hampshire Health
Authority. *Journal of Neurology, Neurosurgery and
Psychiatry* **54**, 55–9.
Sibley, W. A., Bamford, C. R., Clark, K., Smith, M. S.,
and Laguna, J. F. (1991). A prospective study of
physical trauma and multiple sclerosis. *Journal of
Neurology, Neurosurgery and Psychiatry* **54**, 84–9.
Swingler, R. J. and Compston, D. A. (1988). The
prevalence of multiple sclerosis in South East Wales.
Journal of Neurology, Neurosurgery and Psychiatry
51, 1520–4.

Pathology

Estes, M. L., Rudick, R. A., Barnett, G. H., and
Ransohoff, R. M. (1990). Stereotactic biopsy of an
active multiple sclerosis lesion. *Archives of Neurology*
47, 1299–303.
Newcombe, J., Hawkins, C. P., Henderson C. L., *et al.*
(1991). Histopathology of multiple sclerosis lesions
detected by magnetic resonance imaging in unfixed
postmortem central nervous system tissue. *Brain.* **114**,
1013–24.

Clinical features and diagnosis

McDonald, W. I. (1989). Diagnosis of multiple sclerosis.
British Medical Journal **299**, 635–7.
Sanders, E. A. C. M., Bollen, E. L. E. M., and van der
Velde, E. A. (1986). Presenting signs and symptoms

in multiple sclerosis. *Acta Neurologica Scandinavica* **73**, 269–72.

Investigation

Jacobs, L., Munschauer, F. E., and Kaba, S. E. (1991). Clinical and magnetic resonance imaging in optic neuritis. *Neurology* **41**, 15–19.

Miller, D. H., Rudge, P., Johnson, G., *et al.* (1988). Serial gadolinium enhanced magnetic resonance imaging in multiple sclerosis. *Brain* **111**, 927–39.

Paty, D. W., McFarlin, D. E., and McDonald, W. I. (1991). Magnetic resonance imaging and laboratory aids in the diagnosis of multiple sclerosis. *Annals of Neurology* **29**, 3–5.

Zanetta, J. P., Waters, J. M., Kuchler, S., *et al.* (1990). Antibodies to cerebellar soluble lectin CSL in multiple sclerosis. *Lancet* **335**, 1482–4.

Treatment

Beck, R. W., Cleary, P. A., Anderson, M. M. Jr. *et al.* (1992). A randomized, controlled trial of corticosteroids in the treatment of acute optic neuritis. *New England Journal of Medicine* **326**, 581–8.

Editorial (1990). Lipids and multiple sclerosis. *Lancet* **336**, 25–6.

Goodin, D. S. (1991). The use of immunosuppressive agents in multiple sclerosis. *Neurology* **41**, 1072–6.

Hughes, R. A. C. (1991). Prospects for the treatment of multiple sclerosis. *Journal of the Royal Society of Medicine* **84**, 63–4.

The Canadian Cooperative Multiple Sclerosis Study Group (1991). The Canadian cooperative trial of cyclophosphamide and plasma exchange in progressive multiple sclerosis. *Lancet* **337**, 441–6.

Yudkin, P. L., Ellison, G. W., Ghezzi, A., *et al.* (1991). Overview of azathioprine treatment in multiple sclerosis. *Lancet* **338**, 1051–5.

Prognosis

Lee, K. H., Hashimoto, S. A., Hooge, J. P., Kastrukoff, L. f., Oger, J. J. F., Li, D. K. B., and Paty, D. W. (1991). Magnetic resonance imaging of the head in the diagnosis of multiple sclerosis: a prospective 2-year follow-up with comparison of clinical evaluation, evoked potentials, oligoclonal banding and CT. *Neurology* **41**, 657–60.

Miller, D. H., Ormerod, I.E.C., Rudge, P., *et al.* (1989). The early risk of multiple sclerosis following isolated acute syndromes of the brain and spinal cord. *Annals of Neurology* **26**, 635–9.

Phadke, J. G. (1990). Clinical aspects of multiple sclerosis in north-east Scotland with particular reference to its course and prognosis. *Brain* **113**, 1597–628.

Rizzo, J. F. and Lessell, S. (1988). Risk of developing multiple sclerosis after uncomplicated optic neuritis. A long term prospective study. *Neurology* **38**, 185–90.

Visscher, B. R., Liu, K.-S., and Clarke, V. A. (1984). Onset symptoms as predictors of mortality and disability in multiple sclerosis. *Acta Neurologica Scandinavica* **70**, 321–8.

Weinshenker, B. G., Bass, B., Rice, G. P. A., *et al.* (1989). The natural history of multiple sclerosis: a geographically based study. 1. Clinical course and disability. *Brain* **112**, 133–46.

Weinshenker, B. G. *et al.* (1989). The natural history of multiple sclerosis: a geographically based study. 2. Predictive value of the early course. *Brain* **112**, 1419–28.

Weishenker, B. G., Rice, G. P. A., Noseworthy, J. H., Carriere, W., Baskerville, J., and Ebers, G. C. (1991). The natural history of multiple sclerosis: a geographically based study. 3. Multivariate analysis of predictive factors and models of outcome. *Brain* **114**, 1045–56.

Coping with multiple sclerosis

Elian, M. and Dean, G. (1983). Need for and use of social and health services by multiple sclerosis patients living at home in England. *Lancet* **1**, 1091–3.

Gould, J. (1982). Multiple sclerosis. *Lancet* **2**, 1208–10.

Jee, M. (1990). *Living with MS*. King's Fund Centre, London.

Report of a Working Group. (1990). Standards of care for patients with neurological disease: a consensus. *Journal of the Royal College of Physicians of London* **24**, 90–7.

Acute disseminated encephalomyelitis

Case records of the Massachusetts General Hospital (1990). *New England Journal of Medicine* **323**, 1123–35.

Kesselring, J., Miller, D. H., and Robb, S. A. *et al.* (1990). Acute disseminated encephalomyelitis. MRI findings and the distinction from multiple sclerosis. *Brain* **113**, 291–302.

15 Head injury

The central nervous system lies protected within the hard axial skeleton, reflecting its central biological importance to the organism. The skull can protect the brain against penetrating injuries of low mass and velocity, but missiles of higher momentum will penetrate the bony vault, or result in a depressed fracture. Non-missile, closed, head injuries are of much greater importance in civilian life and, although the skull may often protect against penetration, it cannot protect the cranial contents against sudden decelerations on impact. Disruption of neuronal connections and small blood vessels by different angular accelerations on impact (Section 15.2) is the mechanism underlying all head injuries, except in the case of the very uncommon low velocity crush injuries of the skull.

15.1 Epidemiology of head injury

Head injuries range from a merely annoying knock on the head in a low doorway to an injury severe enough to cause immediate death. There is thus no epidemiological use in pooling data about injuries of such widely differing severity. The figures in Table 15.1 give some indication of the size of the problem.

Men are at greater risk from head injury than women, by virtue of their greater exposure to potentially dangerous physical occupations. They also drive vehicles for a greater number of miles, consume more alcohol, and participate to a greater extent in contact sports. Figure 15.1 shows the distribution of deaths due to head injuries at

Table 15.1   Epidemiology of head injury

	per 100 000	in UK
Annual incidence		
Attendances for head injury at Accident and Emergency Departments, both sexes (M:F ratio 2.5:1)	1800	1 000 000
Admissions for head injury	200–300	150 000
Deaths from head injury	9	5200
Severely disabled survivors	1.5	900
Prevalence		
Survivors of head injury with major persisting handicap	50–150	30 000–90 000

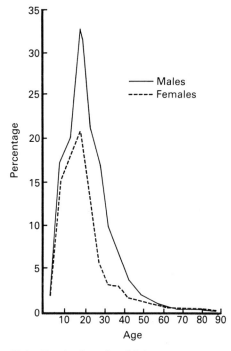

Fig. 15.1   Deaths from head injury as a percentage of all deaths in each age-range. (Reproduced by permission from Field 1976.)

Table 15.2   Causes of head injury (from Miller and Jones 1985)

	Severe (n = 93) (%)	All (n = 1919) (%)
Road traffic accident	70	29
Domestic or fall	21	41
Assault	3	20
Work	4	3
Sport	1	6

'Severe' indicates a Glasgow scale of 7 or less on admission.

different ages, and Table 15.2 the causes of head injuries attending Accident and Emergency Departments in a Scottish study.

Certain common-sense observations on prevention can be underlined by statistics. Motor cycles are dangerous machines. In the UK they account for only 2 per cent of all vehicle registrations but 22 per cent of all driver deaths. Crash helmets are effective against penetrating injuries, for example by the head hitting a car door handle. A deformable polystyrene liner within the shell provides only limited protection against deceleration injuries as the head hits the road.

The combination of high velocity and limited protection renders motor cyclists particularly vul-nerable to head injury, but increasing attention is being paid to protective headgear for pedal cycl-ists, who are often injured in low velocity accidents in towns.

Drivers of cars and trucks are afforded protection by the protective cage of their vehicles but, unless seat belts are worn, head and spinal injuries may occur as the occupants are thrown around the decelerating or overturning car. The compulsory use of seat belts in the UK has reduced serious injuries by about half. Unrestrained rear seat passengers do not seem to cause additional injuries to belted front seat occupants, but are themselves liable to cranial and spinal injuries, and legislation in the UK now makes the wearing of seat belts also compulsory for rear seat passengers. Fortunately, those working in the construction, mining, and quarrying industries now take the wearing of protective headgear more seriously than they did two decades ago, as do those who ride horses, a sport that places both head and spine at risk. Other physical sports resulting in head injury include rugby, football, skiing and rock-climbing. The special case of boxing, in which one of the principal criteria of success is to cause brain injury to an opponent, is considered in Section 15.8.2.

Alcohol plays a considerable part in domestic accidents and cases of assault, and greatly increases the risk of a road traffic accident—by a factor of three when the blood alcohol exceeds 80 mg/ 100 ml and by a factor of 10 when the blood alcohol exceeds 150 mg/100 ml.

15.2 Primary pathology of brain damage resulting from closed head injury

The principal cause of damage in cases of closed head injury is rotational acceleration of the brain within its rigid container—the skull. Different regions of the brain have a different resistance to movements induced by the accelerating force, and these differences result in shearing of fibres. A combination of physical distance from the centre of rotation and differences in compliance between grey and white matter results in shearing being maximal in the cortical and immediately subcortical zones. Shearing of fibres in the brain stem is seen only in more severe rotational head injuries. Small vessels bridging the subdural and subarachnoid space may be ruptured by such rotational movement, as may vessels within the substance of the brain. Severe head injuries may therefore show collections of subdural, subarachnoid, and intracerebral blood, in addition to damage to nerve fibres.

Direct linear impact without rotation will also accelerate the brain within its rigid container, divided into zones by the non-compliant falx and tentorium cerebelli. The sphenoid wing and petrous temporal bones are other non-yielding structures within the skull and, as the moving brain is decelerated by these bony or dural structures, local disruption and contusion occur at the non-compliant boundaries. This explains why a local injury (coup) in the parietal region may be accompanied by a contracoup contusion in the opposite temporal lobe. The effect of lesser injuries is shown by the presence of small surface contusions on the summits of the convexity of the gyri.

In most severe injuries there is, of course, a combination of rotational and linear accelerations, producing complex swirling movements within the brain. A good analogy is to take a blancmange or jelly within its mould and shake it vigorously. Cracks soon appear in the structure due to the shearing forces, though the mould itself is undamaged. In very much the same way, a patient can die from severe shearing damage within the brain without any fracture of the skull, or even a mark upon the scalp.

The changes seen on microscopical examination of the shear injuries depend on the time that has elapsed before death. Tearing of the axons results in retraction balls of axoplasm, seen with silver stains within the first 2 weeks. These balls then disappear, but evidence of Wallerian degeneration may be seen using the Marchi stain. Clusters of hypertrophied microglial cells are prominent. Some such clusters have been seen in patients who have died after recovering from minor head injuries, and this is one of the strands of evidence that suggests that the post-traumatic syndrome (Section 15.8) has, at least in part, a physical basis.

15.3 Secondary pathology of head injuries

15.3.1 Raised intracranial pressure

Widespread shearing of neurons and blood vessels results in elevation of intracranial volume in different areas of the brain. As the brain is divided by non-compliant septa—the falx and tentorium— these differences in volume are reflected in differences in pressure of sufficient degree to cause herniation of brain tissue between compartments. Usually the increased cerebral volume lies above the tentorium. The resulting increased pressure causes tissue necrosis and infarction in the parahippocampal gyri, as the medial parts of the temporal lobes are forced downwards against the edge of the tentorium. The posterior cerebral artery may be nipped and distorted by the edge of the tentorium and the descending temporal lobe. If severe, this will result in infarction in the medial occipital cortex. Other infarctions may be found in the 'watershed' areas of supply of the different major intracerebral arteries. A side-to-side shift may result in necrosis and infarction of the cingulate gyrus as it passes under the falx.

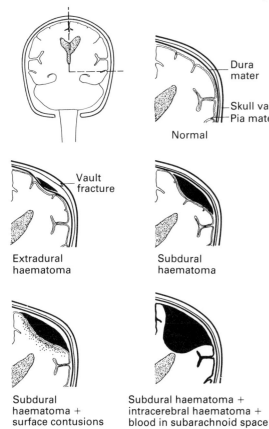

Normal

Dura mater

Skull vault

Pia mater

Vault fracture

Extradural haematoma

Subdural haematoma

Subdural haematoma + surface contusions

Subdural haematoma + intracerebral haematoma + blood in subarachnoid space

Fig. 15.2   Different types of intracranial haematoma.

15.3.2   *Intracranial haematoma*

Blood may collect at one or more of the sites illustrated in Fig. 15.2. An intracerebral haematoma arises if arteries or veins traversing brain tissue are sheared. Such haematomas are most common in the frontal regions. An acute subdural haematoma occurs most commonly in conjunction with surface contusions and lacerations of a temporal lobe. The volume of blood released contributes to the shifts described above. An extradural haematoma results from tears of branches of the middle meningeal arteries or veins in the temporo-parietal region. Less commonly, one may result from a torn venous sinus.

15.4   Management of head injuries

The part played by neurosurgeons in the manage-ment of head injury varies widely from country to country. In the USA a neurosurgery resident may well be available to give an opinion in the Accident and Emergency Room. In the UK the initial care rests in the hands of casualty officers and, if admission is considered necessary, this will usually be to a 'general surgical' bed.

Primary damage—disruption of neuron processes and of blood vessels—occurs at the time of impact. Surgical management is therefore confined to the detection and early treatment of features that lead to secondary brain damage. These include hypoxia and hypercapnia, elevation of intracranial pressure, the development of haematomas, the development of infection through open fractures, and the occurrence of seizures. The doctor on duty in the Accident and Emergency Department has the considerable task of sorting out, from the vast numbers of those attending with head injuries, who should be X-rayed, who should be admitted, and for whom he should seek urgent specialized neurosurgical help. The first priority is the establishment of an accurate medical record and of a chart on which serial observations at a stated interval can be made (Fig. 7.1), with a clear requirement of the nursing staff of the action that they should take (usually calling the medical staff) when observations change for the worse.

15.4.1   *Assessment of the severity of a head injury*

After ensuring an adequate airway and ventilation, the first necessity is to assess the level of consciousness on presentation to the examiner. This is best undertaken using the Glasgow coma scale, which is fully described in Section 7.1.1.1. The assessment should be compared immediately with what is known of the patient's conscious state immediately after the injury, so that a decision can be made about whether the patient is deteriorating or not. For example, a patient who has spoken a few words after a head injury, but who has then lapsed into deep coma, cannot have sustained severe diffuse white-matter injuries. The deterioration must be due to the presence of raised intracranial pressure, possibly from a haematoma, which will require urgent neurosurgical management (Section 15.5.1).

A patient may be apparently responsive, giving his or her name and address, and giving some account of the accident, yet subsequent examinations may show the patient to be amnesic for this conversation. The importance of the duration of post-traumatic amnesia in predicting the extent of recovery after a head injury is discussed in Section 15.7.2, but such assessment must by its nature be retrospective. Usually a careful assessment of the mental state of a patient who is still in his post-traumatic amnesia will show some degree of confusion when handling more complex ideas than just giving his or her name and address. Post-traumatic confusion may, of course, be much greater than this, displayed by irritability and aggression towards police and nursing staff.

Following an assessment of the level of consciousness and of the mental state, a full external examination of the skull by inspection and palpation should be undertaken. Depressed fractures can be felt easily with the fingers. An apparently simple laceration may overlie a fracture. Fractures of the anterior cranial fossa may be suspected from the development of bilateral periorbital haematomas, though a 'black eye' does not necessarily indicate a fracture. Fracture of the base of the skull may be suspected by the presence of blood in the auditory meati or behind the ear-drum. If cerebrospinal fluid is seen to be leaking from ear or nose, the diagnosis of a fractured base or anterior cranial fossa is certain. Some hours after a basal fracture, blood may track along the base of

Table 15.3 Need for skull X-rays after head injury (based upon guidelines of the Royal College of Radiologists 1989)

X-ray if one of these factors is present:
1. Suspected penetration of the skull
2. Loss of consciousness at any time, or altered consciousness at time of examination
3. Bleeding from the nose or ear, or haemotympanum (leakage of CSF makes fracture certain)
4. Focal neurological signs or symptoms
5. Patient lives alone
6. Patient is drunk—though poor co-operation may impair quality of X-rays
7. Patient has other neurological illness, such as stroke, that might confuse interpretation of physical signs
8. Circumstances of injury suggest particularly forceful impact

the skull and form dark bruising behind each ear—Battle's sign. Another sign of a basal fracture is a lower motor neuron facial palsy, which should not be confused with facial weakness resulting from damage to the contralateral hemisphere.

A full neurological examination should then follow, with particular reference to pupillary diameter and responses to light, posture, and movement of the limbs (Section 7.1.2). The focus of the examination should be to assess the degree of diffuse damage to white matter, and the presence of focal neurological signs indicating local cerebral damage, which might, for example, underlie a depressed fracture. Finally, it must never be forgotten that a patient who has sustained a head injury may have sustained spinal, limb, chest, or abdominal injuries as well, which all require evaluation.

15.4.2   Who should be X-rayed?

Until recently, about 80 per cent of the one million patients attending Accident and Emergency Departments in the UK with head injury were X-rayed, but serious attempts are now being made to cut down on the number of unnecessary films. Skull X-rays are clearly necessary to guide the management of those who are in any event going to be admitted, because of their level of consciousness or other injuries, but a number of patients who are alert at the time of examination have a closed linear fracture of the skull. If such a fracture is present, then the chances of the subsequent development of a haematoma is considerably increased (by a factor of 400 times in one study) so the detection of such fractures is of considerable importance. Studies have shown that if the criteria shown in Table 15.3 are adopted, the number of skull radiographs can be reduced by about half, and 94 per cent of patients with a fracture will still be detected.

15.4.3   Who should look at the X-ray?

Relatively inexperienced doctors have been shown to be nearly as good as radiologists at detecting skull fractures on X-rays, and their skills can be improved further by brief tuition. A knowledge of the normal sutures and meningeal vascular markings will save confusion of such linear shadows with a fracture of the vault. Diploic vessels draining to venous lakes may sometimes mimic star-shaped fractures. Air lying under the edges of a linear scalp laceration may give the false impression of a fracture. A fracture through the paranasal sinuses may be revealed by the presence of air within the cranial cavity. Depression of a fracture may be missed if the X-ray beam is parallel to the axis of the depression, and two sets of films at right-angles are required.

15.4.4   *Who should be admitted to hospital?*

There is no doubt about the need to admit patients who need treatment of obvious depressed fractures, or whose conscious level is depressed after head injury. The principal anxieties lie in deciding who should be admitted for observation, in case of subsequent deterioration due to the development of a haematoma. Table 15.4 lists the criteria suggested by a group of neurosurgeons in 1984. A brief amnesia after trauma with full recovery by the time of the examination is not sufficient indication for admission.

Table 15.4   Criteria for admission to hospital after head injury

1. Confusion or alteration of consciousness
2. Skull fracture
3. Neurological signs
4. Difficulty in assessing the patient due to co-existing medical condition or intoxication
5. Inadequate supervision available at home

Table 15.5   Criteria for consultation with a neurosurgeon after a head injury

1. Skull fracture in association with any of
   (a) confusion or worse impairment of consciousness
   (b) one or more seizures
   (c) neurological signs
2. Deterioration in level of consciousness
3. Coma persisting after resuscitation ⎫
4. Confusion or other   ⎬ even if no
   neurological disturbance   ⎪ fracture
   lasting more than 8 hours   ⎭
5. Depressed fracture of skull vault
6. Suspected fracture of skull base

15.4.5   *What advice should be given to those sent home?*

It is the custom in the UK to give patients sent home from hospital after a head injury written instructions that the patient should return in the event of undue sleepiness, headache, vomiting, or vertigo. Sometimes such instructions provoke undue anxiety, and they are generally unhelpful in the case of head injuries in young children, nearly all of whom are pale, sleepy, or irritable, and who often vomit, without grave significance.

15.4.6   *For whom is neurosurgical consultation or transfer required?*

Once immediate resuscitation and assessment has been undertaken, the next question is to decide whether specialized neurosurgical help is required, or whether the patient can safely be admitted under one of the 'general surgical' firms, a practice that may decline with increasing specialization in surgery. A group of British neurosurgeons has suggested that the criteria listed in Table 15.5 are suitable grounds for seeking consultation with a neurosurgeon. All neurosurgeons stress the need for early consultation and, if necessary, transfer. Initial resuscitation for extracranial injuries and simple immobilization for associated limb fractures should be arranged, and transfer supervised by adequately trained staff. All notes and X-rays must accompany the patient—a simple administrative procedure that is often neglected and, by alerting medical staff in the receiving hospital to a changing situation, may be life-saving.

15.5   Treatment of severe head injuries

The first priority is to ensure an adequate airway and oxygenation, if necessary by artificial ventilation, as hypoxia and hypercapnia considerably increase intracranial pressure and thereby exacerbate herniation and infarction. If, as is so often the case, an injury to the head is one of multiple injuries, assessment of these must continue and the volume of the circulation maintained. Following these initial measures, management must next be directed to the early detection and, if necessary, evacuation of intracranial haematomas, and the prevention of secondary cerebral damage due to raised intracranial pressure.

15.5.1 *Intracranial haematoma*

Haemorrhage may occur into the extradural, sub-dural or subarachnoid space, or into the substance of the brain (intracerebral haematoma) (Figs. 8.14, 8.15, 15.2). Cranial CT scanning and MRI have shown that small intracerebral haematomas are much commoner than previously realized. They may even be present in a patient who has not had a significant depression of consciousness at any time. They tend to be more common in the frontal regions, and are more superficial than the spontaneous intracerebral haemorrhage associated with hypertension. Their presence on a CT scan or MRI does not necessarily mean that evacuation is necessary, unless superficial and large, so that a local mass effect is occurring. The commonest situation in which this happens is a major contusion of one temporal lobe, in which disrupted brain is mingled with blood. In such cases blood must leak into the subarachnoid space, and some acute subdural collection is almost always present. Extradural haematomas are usually temporal or temporoparietal, resulting from damage to middle meningeal vessels, though sometimes from a torn venous sinus (Figs. 8.14 and 15.2). Their importance lies in the fact that very rapid deterioration in conscious level can occur due to brain shifts consequent upon the collection of blood, sometimes in patients who have been spared much in the way of diffuse neuronal injury.

Acute collections of blood causing shifts in the brain result in a classic sequence of events—deteriorating level of consciousness in association with ipsilateral dilatation of the pupil, as the shifted temporal lobe squeezes the third nerve against the tentorial opening, and contralateral hemiparesis. Yet if a doctor waits for the development of this classic picture, he or she will lose many patients through delay. Attention has shifted to a knowledge of those risk factors that make the development of a haematoma particularly likely, so that patients can be scanned at an early stage, and observed particularly closely. Table 15.6 outlines the findings of the Glasgow group of neurosurgeons. From this table, it is clear that all patients who are both disoriented and have a skull fracture should be immediately scanned and

Table 15.6 Risks of haematoma in adults attending Accident and Emergency Departments (based on data from Mendelow *et al.* 1983)

Skull fracture	absent	absent	present	present
Orientated	yes	no	yes	no
Absolute risk	1:6000	1:120	1:32	1:4
Relative risk	1	50	200	1400

observed closely, as they have a 1:4 chance of developing an intracranial haematoma of sufficient volume to require surgical decompression. If all patients who were only disoriented or who only had a skull fracture were scanned, the 'yield' of haematomata would be only 1–3 per cent.

The Glasgow neurosurgeons have calculated that if all disoriented patients with a skull fracture were scanned, this would result in slightly fewer than two scans a week in a neurosurgical unit serving a population of one million. Such a policy would yield one operable intracranial clot every 2 weeks.

The usual operation for a temporal extradural haematoma or the common temporal intracerebral haematoma, in association with an acute subdural haematoma, begins with a burr hole low in the temporal region, which may then be extended into a frontal flap if necessary. The results of surgery are best after early operation on purely extradural haematomata, but even for this most series show a 5–20 per cent mortality. In those cases with a severe temporal intracerebral and acute subdural clot, the mortality may reach 50 per cent.

The management of chronic subdural haematoma is considered in Section 15.6.

15.5.2 *Management of raised intracranial pressure*

Technical advances in electronics have made it comparatively simple to monitor intracranial pressure by means of subdural or extradural transducers, or through a catheter inserted directly into the frontal horn of a lateral ventricle. However, there is still considerable doubt as to how valuable numerical measures of pressure are, and many large centres manage well without their routine use, relying instead on conscientious clinical monitoring. There is no doubt that raised intracranial pressure may substantially increase morbidity by herniation and infarction. Intracranial pressure must therefore be kept as close as possible to the normal upper limit (<10 mmHg). A brief episode of airways obstruction will significantly increase intracranial pressure, as will, of course, an expanding haematoma. In the case of diffuse neuronal injury without haematoma, pressure may be temporarily reduced by elective hyperventilation; hypocapnia causes some cerebral vasoconstriction. Pressure may also be reduced by the use of intravenous osmotic diuretics, such as mannitol. This is usually given as a 25 per cent solution, in a dose of 0.5–1.0 g/kg, given over 15–20 minutes. Unfortunately, as mannitol equilibrates across the damaged blood–brain barrier fairly rapidly, the osmotic gradient gradually declines. Repeated doses may only elevate the plasma osmolality to dangerously high levels. On terminating treatment with mannitol there may be a rebound elevation of intracranial pressure. Other osmotic agents, such as 30 per cent urea or 10 per cent glycerol, have also been used, but the drawbacks are similar. Diuretics such as frusemide may also be temporarily effective, and high-dose corticosteroids have also been used, although most clinical trials have failed to show any benefit.

15.5.3 Management of open injuries and depressed fractures

A fracture is said to be depressed if the inner table is depressed by at least the thickness of the skull. The vast majority are associated with a scalp laceration, and are therefore said to be open, or compound. The local injury to the skull often does not result in the diffuse neuronal injury which results from deceleration injuries to the whole head, and many of the patients do not lose consciousness, and have only a brief post-traumatic amnesia.

After appropriate X-rays and imaging, the right policy is to debride carefully the wound of hair, necrotic scalp, dirt, and small bone fragments. Careful debridement is usually followed by local antibiotic spray. Many neurosurgeons do not use systemic prophylactic antibiotics for depressed fractures of the vault. However, basal fractures compound into the nasal sinuses or middle ear are so frequently followed by meningitis that prophylactic antibiotics must be used, penicillin being

most usually chosen. Depressed larger bone fragments may be elevated, though if the degree of depression is not great, and not cosmetically obvious, it may well be left unelevated, particularly if the depression lies over a major venous sinus.

During debridement and elevation of fracture, it will become clear whether the dura is torn. If so, the necrotic brain underneath should also be gently removed. Penetration of the dura, and therefore cortical damage, results in a substantially greater incidence of post-traumatic epilepsy (Section 15.7.1.4).

15.5.4 Other aspects of medical care of head injuries

15.5.4.1 Nutrition, nursing, and control of pain

The critical management discussed to this point should not deflect attention from less dramatic aspects of the clinical care. Nutrition should be continued, with due reference to any fasting required for surgical procedures, through a fine-bore nasogastric tube, aiming for between 2000 and 3000 kcal/day. Bed sores must be prevented by frequent turning, and the skin must be protected from abrasion against cot-sides or the foot of the bed, as abnormal tonic postures may bring the limbs into firm contact with these.

Damage to the cornea may be prevented by taping the eyelids shut, or by using hypromellose drops. Physiotherapists must show the nurses how to put all limbs through frequent passive movements to prevent the development of contractures. Tracheostomy care and suction may be necessary. Patients with head injuries are often restless because of cerebral damage, and may well be amnesic for pain experienced from the head or other bodily injuries. If pain appears to be contributing to restlessness, pethidine or morphine should be avoided, in part because of their potential of confusing pupillary responses. Injections of codeine phosphate, 60 mg, may help settle the patient.

15.5.4.2 Gastrointestinal bleeding

Gastrointestinal bleeding may follow severe head injury, as a result of so-called 'stress ulceration'.

Many neurosurgical units give H_2 antagonists such as cimetidine or ranitidine, but ulceration may still occur in spite of this, probably because the presence of gastric acidity is only one component of the mechanism of ulceration in these circumstances.

15.5.4.3   *Control of temperature*

Pyrexia may, of course, be due to infection, either intracranially, or at some other damaged site, or as a result of a chest or urinary infection. If such infection is eradicated, and high fever continues, then this is probably due to hypothalamic damage. Fans may be used to cool the patient, and sometimes chlorpromazine aids a reduction in temperature.

15.5.4.4   *Prevention of seizures*

About 5 per cent of patients admitted to a neurosurgical unit will have one or more seizures in the acute stages of their management. It has been shown that the occurrence of seizures in adults in the first week is a powerful predictor of the development of late post-traumatic epilepsy (Section 15.7.1.4). Seizures can usually be controlled by phenytoin, achieving rapid blood levels using the regime outlined in Section 12.10 on the management of status epilepticus. Prophylactic anticonvulsant medication is not much used as there is the possibility of confusing the clinical picture by the use of sufficient anticonvulsant medication to depress the level of consciousness. Furthermore, prophylactic anticonvulsant medication has not been shown to reduce the occurrence of late post-traumatic epilepsy.

15.6   Chronic subdural haematoma

The clinical problem presented by a chronic subdural haematoma is quite different from the acute lesion. About half those with chronic subdural haematomas cannot recall any significant head injury, and in the remainder the injury is often minor. Old age, male sex, cerebral atrophy, and excessive consumption of alcohol predisposing to falls and minor injuries are common relevant factors. A chronic subdural collection is unusual after severe head injuries, probably because

neurosurgical awareness leads to evacuation at an early stage.

Presenting features include fluctuating headache, apathy or confusion, and often a hemiparesis.

The cranial CT scan is usually diagnostic (Fig. 8.15). Fresh blood is radio-dense, but as it becomes autolysed, its density may match that of the underlying brain. Figure 8.15 shows that part of this subdural haematoma is isodense, and in this CT plane the only evidence is some shift of the midline structures. Sometimes the problem is more difficult than this, as about 15 per cent of those with a subdural have haematomas on each side, so that the ventricles remain more or less in their normal position. Carotid arteriography may show displacement of superficial vessels away from the vault of the skull. Most of the haematomas are over the parietal regions, but a few may be hidden under one temporal lobe. The evacuation of haematomas through burr holes is usually easy enough, but if the collection is small, and the patient frail and improving, conservative treatment may be justified.

15.7   Recovery from and after-effects of severe head injuries

Figure 15.3 shows that, as might intuitively have been expected, increasing age and deep coma are associated with an unfavourable outcome—death or survival in persistent vegetative state (Section 7.3.1). Attempts to devise a scoring system to predict death or such an unfavourable outcome that active treatment should be withheld have not met with success, although the Leeds prognostic score is a useful attempt along these lines.

With the exception of those so severely injured that they remain in a chronic vegetative state, without any behavioural evidence of cortical function, though with conjugate eye movements and reflex postural adjustments of the limbs, those survivors admitted in coma will, after a varying interval, begin to move their eyes and limbs and, after a further interval, utter some words. The global deficit may, of course, be modified by the effects of some prominent local cerebral contusion, so that aphasia or hemiparesis may be obvious. If not aphasic, meaningful communication gradually

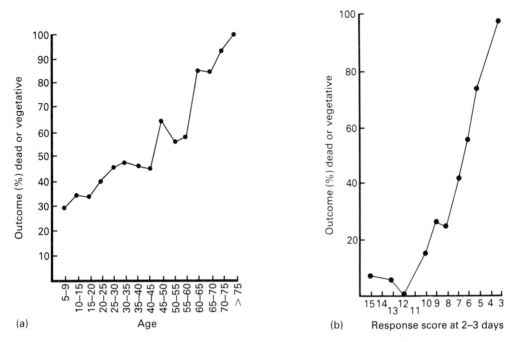

Fig. 15.3 (a) Effect of age upon outcome at 6 months after severe head injury. (b) Effect of Glasgow coma score (best in 2–3 day epoch) upon outcome at 6 months after severe head injury. (Redrawn with permission from Jennett and Teasdale 1981.)

returns, although the patient remains confused and restless. Sedation at this stage should be kept to the minimal necessary to prevent injury and disturbance of the whole ward. Thioridazine is an appropriate choice for this. Gradually, confusion lessens, and the patient becomes fully oriented and retains memory of day-to-day ward events—he or she has emerged from post-traumatic amnesia. There will, however, be residual after-effects, the prominence of which will depend upon the duration of coma and post-traumatic amnesia, in turn dependent upon the degree of cerebral damage sustained.

15.7.1   *Physical sequelae*

There are four principal groupings of *physical* handicap following cerebral injury, due to:

1   damage to the cerebral hemispheres;

2   damage to brain-stem connections;

3   damage to individual cranial nerves; and

4   epilepsy.

15.7.1.1   *Hemisphere syndromes*

Damage to the cerebral hemispheres may result in hemiplegia. As after stroke, the arm is almost always affected more severely than the leg. Spasticity in the hemiplegic arm may be painful. Nurses, and subsequently the patient, must learn how to minimize this by repeated passive movements. If the dominant hemisphere is affected, the hemiplegia may be complicated by aphasia. Non-dominant hemisphere lesions may result in disturbances of spatial orientation. Visual field defects may occur. A few patients have a dystonia, presumably due to damage to the deep basal ganglia.

15.7.1.2   *Brain-stem syndromes*

Damage to brain-stem connections may result in a troublesome limb tremor and unsteadiness of gait. Such patients may have little impairment of cognitive function.

15.7.1.3   *Cranial nerve syndromes*

Syndromes affecting the first eight cranial nerves

are commonly seen after head injuries. Anosmia is frequent after even minor injuries, presumably because the fine olfactory fibres passing through the cribriform plate are easily sheared by movements of the brain and olfactory bulb within the skull. As most of the enjoyment of food comes through smell rather than through taste receptors on the tongue, patients usually complain of loss of 'taste', saying, for example, that roast beef tastes like cardboard. The optic nerve may be damaged by a fracture passing through the orbit, or may atrophy secondary to a prolonged period of raised intracranial pressure. The third, fourth, and sixth cranial nerves may be damaged by an anterior or middle cranial fossa fracture, or the third as a result of tentorial herniation. Many patients therefore have double vision following head injury. This often settles in succeeding months, but if not, surgery on external ocular muscles may abolish diplopia for at least forward gaze. A seventh nerve palsy immediately following a head injury indicates a crack fracture across the axis of the petrous temporal, and is usually permanent. Delayed facial palsies usually recover. Petrous fractures also often cause sensorineural deafness and tinnitus due to cochlear damage. Vertigo is also frequent, due more to direct concussive injury of the membraneous labyrinth than to any damage to the eighth nerve. The last four cranial nerves are seldom damaged by injuries other than those caused by gunshot wounds.

15.7.1.4 *Epilepsy*

Epileptic seizures following some time after head injury occur in about 5 per cent of all patients admitted to hospital, and may prevent a return to previous employment for those who have otherwise made a good recovery. The careful studies of Jennett have clearly delineated those who are particularly at risk for developing seizures. The relevant factors are:

1 the occurrence of a seizure in the first week after injury;

2 the occurrence of a haematoma; and

3 the presence of a depressed fracture, particularly if the dura is torn.

These three factors all may perhaps be taken as evidence of focal cortical damage, and the first as an indicator of low seizure threshold (Section 12.6.1), and therefore an inbuilt propensity to seizures. In patients with depressed fracture, the risk of epilepsy varies according to these features, and to the duration of post-traumatic amnesia, as illustrated in Fig. 15.4.

Patients who have not had an early seizure, a haematoma, or a depressed fracture may be reassured that their chances of developing epilepsy are barely greater than that of the population as a whole. Of those who do develop post-traumatic seizures, about 70 per cent will have done so within 2 years of the injury. Electroencephalography gives little help in predicting who is likely to develop seizures. Early prophylactic treatment with phenytoin of those particularly at risk of developing epilepsy by the nature of their injuries does successfully reduce the incidence of seizures in the first week after the injury, but has no long-term effect in reducing the incidence of late post-traumatic epilepsy.

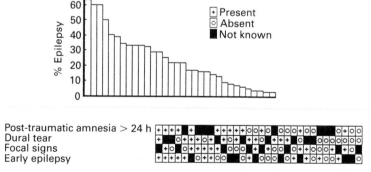

Fig. 15.4 Epilepsy after depressed fractures of the skull. (Redrawn with permission from Jennett 1975.)

15.7.1.5   *Other physical sequelae*

Other physical sequelae of head injury include chronic leakage of cerebrospinal fluid, usually from the nose. This may be relieved by the application of a dural patch across the fracture site in the anterior cranial fossa. The exact site of the leak is difficult to determine, but isotope studies may prove helpful. Bacterial invasion through such a fistula may result in meningitis. A severe head injury may be followed by communicating hydro-cephalus (Section 11.5.9), as blood and protein clog the absorptive mechanisms in the arachnoid villi. A severe injury is, in any event, often followed by some degree of cerebral atrophy with large ventricles, so the selection of those who truly have a significant obstructive component is difficult. Other rare physical complications include vascular occlusion, probably secondary to intimal tears in large vessels, and the development of carotico-cavernous fistulae.

15.7.2   *Neuro-psychological sequelae*

Most families find that coping with the later psychological effects of a severe head injury is far more exhausting and demoralizing than coping with the physical effects. Subtle or gross personality changes are the most troublesome feature for the family. A common complaint is that 'He's not the man he was'. The head-injured patient may be less interested in his spouse and family, and yet much more emotionally dependent upon them than before. Initiative for day-to-day household duties may be greatly decreased. Intolerance of the behaviour of others, especially children, is apparent, and small domestic upsets may result in aggression or despair. Intellect, memory, libido, and concentration are globally depressed, and there may also be focal deficits of cognitive function such as dysphasia. Patients have varying degrees of insight into these difficulties, the less severely injured often become significantly depressed as they are aware of how much less able they are than before the accident.

The extent of the neuro-psychological effects following a head injury can largely be predicted by the duration of post-traumatic amnesia. Broadly speaking, a person whose post-traumatic amnesia has extended for more than 28 days will have considerable difficulty in returning to paid employ-ment of any kind. Those whose post-traumatic amnesia has extended for more than one week are likely to have considerable difficulty in returning to tasks which involve considerable intellectual activity, such as the higher levels of business or the law. Those whose post-traumatic amnesia lasts for less than a day should be able to return to their original employment, although those with a post-traumatic amnesia of 12–24 hours may find significant difficulties for several months after first returning. These very broad statements are modified by the influence of the subject's age. Those in their 'teens and twenties recover very much better from severe head injuries than do those in their fifties.

The most important consequences of head injury on the social and vocational adjustment eventually achieved are not physical impairments, or even impairments of cognition, but changes in personality and behaviour. The most troublesome disorder of behaviour is increased irritability, or, in a more overt form, aggression, which may suddenly erupt after trivial stimulation. Such a brief outburst of abnormal and aggressive behaviour is sometimes known as the 'episodic dyscontrol syndrome'. This is often responsive, at least in part, to treatment with carbamazepine, in doses similar to those used for epilepsy (Section 12.8). Other drugs that have been used with limited success include the dopamine agonist methyl phenidate, or dopamine precursors such as L-dopa.

More prolonged disturbances of personality that follow cranial injury are not, in general, responsive to drug treatment, but abnormal behaviours can be improved, and sometimes quite markedly improved, by consistent behaviour modification in a controlled setting. The principle is that good behaviour is rewarded by a token, which can be used for subsequent small but, to the patient, important purchases. Bad behaviour is managed by periods of 'time out', in which the patient is removed briefly from social interaction with others.

Another common feature after cranial injuries is a general lack of drive, which is very difficult to treat, but drive may be somewhat improved by the use of a token economy as indicated above. There is little evidence that impairments of cognitive function or memory can be improved by specific programmes, although the patient can be taught useful strategies for his or her deficient memory, such as writing down shopping lists and keeping a diary.

Many of the deficits, such as impaired drive,

irritable and abrasive behaviour, impaired cognitive function and memory, interact so that a head-injured person may be grossly disabled socially, even in the absence of impairments of communication or motor performance. Social skills training short of formal behavioural modification may be useful in such patients. This extends not only from practising simple situations, such as shopping and role-playing with other patients, but more formal techniques encouraging appropriate eye contact, greeting and respect for the personal space and conversation of others. The benefits of cognitive rehabilitation, a systematic attempt to improve information processing and attention, are unproven.

15.8   Less severe head injuries and the post-traumatic syndrome

Fortunately, the vast majority of head injuries are not as grave as those discussed in the preceding paragraphs, but the persistence of symptoms thereafter gives rise to great distress for many patients. A typical story is of a man working in a factory who is struck by a falling metal bar. His head is cut, he is helped to the first-aid station and then to the local Accident and Emergency Department, conscious but 'dazed'. The head is X-rayed, the scalp sutured, and the patient sent home. Afterwards, it is clear that he has no recollection of the ambulance journey to the hospital—that is to say, his post-traumatic amnesia is about 30 minutes. When he arrives home he is tense and cross, has a splitting headache, and he may be sick. He goes to bed. The next day he gets up with a headache and is giddy. This persists for a few days. When he gets back to work after a week or two, he feels easily exhausted, and has difficulty in concentrating, so he stops work again. Headaches, dizziness, easy fatiguability, irritability, impaired memory and concentration and inability to work continue for what seems to be an inappropriate length of time for the apparent severity of the injury. This is the post-traumatic syndrome.

Many such injuries occur in the workplace, and are due to some fault in a machine or carelessness by a colleague. It is the employer's responsibility to provide a safe place of work and, if he fails, the injured man may claim compensation. Sometimes,

therefore, there is a feeling, often hinted at in reports prepared by doctors instructed by insurance companies, that the injured man is exaggerating his symptoms as a means of maximizing his claim. Although it seems probable that this sometimes happens, doctors have veered towards believing that some of the symptoms have an organic basis, particularly the post-traumatic vertigo, and probably the impaired concentration and memory. Other symptoms are an entirely understandable psychological reaction to the stress of and resentment about the accident, and to an inefficiently working brain. It used to be maintained that the syndrome was seldom seen if compensation was not an issue, and that symptoms disappeared when the claim was settled. Epidemiological studies have gone some way to disproving these statements. Neuropsychological examination after injuries with short periods of post-traumatic amnesia shows deficits, particularly on tests of reasoning, information processing, verbal learning, and the reproduction of a complex geometric design. All these abnormalities militate particularly against an early return to administrative or other office work.

Evidence for an organic basis to the syndrome comes from four other points. First, that there is often positional nystagmus in the early days after a concussive head injury. Secondly, neuropathological examination of the brains of those who have died from other causes after minor head injuries shows occasional clusters of hypertrophied microglial cells of the type seen after more severe head injuries. Thirdly, cumulative minor injuries in boxers and jockeys (see below) result in clear-cut organic syndromes. Finally, very long term follow-up shows persistently deficient memory amongst those who showed it early on.

15.8.1   Treatment of minor head injuries

It seems helpful to listen to patients, explain about their symptoms, disperse their resentment (identified as an unfavourable prognostic feature), and ensure a reasonable time off before attempting to return to work. When the patient does return to work, it should be at a lower level of activity or responsibility for a time. Depression may require specific pharmacological treatment.

15.8.2   *Cumulative head injuries in boxers and jockeys*

No neurologist now doubts that boxing damages brains, and virtually all would like to see the professional sport banned. To produce a cerebral acceleration sufficient to render an opponent unconscious is the principal purpose of the exercise. After suffering many knock-outs, boxers develop a characteristic syndrome of dysarthria, slowness of movement, tremor and unsteadiness, and intellectual impairment—the so-called 'punch-drunk' syndrome. Computed tomography or MRI shows cortical atrophy, ventricular dilatation, and a ruptured septum pellicidum. Less prominent evidence of brain damage is apparent in jockeys, who repeatedly fall on their heads.

15.9   Further reading

General

Jennett, B. and Teasdale G. (1981). *Management of head injuries*. F. A. Davis. Philadelphia.

Epidemiology

Field, J. H. (1976). *Epidemiology of head injuries in England and Wales*. HMSO, London.
Miller, J. D. and Jones, P. A. (1985). The work of a regional head injury service. *Lancet* 1, 1141–4.

Prevention

Bull, J. P. (1988). Cyclists need helmets. *British Medical Journal* 296, 1144.
Report of the Board of Science and Education working party on boxing (1984). *British Medical Journal* 288, 876–7.
Simson, J. N. L. (1989). Seat belts—six years on. *Journal of the Royal Society of Medicine* 82, 125–6.

Management

Bullock, R. and Teasdale, G. (1990). Head injuries I. *British Medical Journal* 300. 1515–18.
Bullock, R. and Teasdale, G. (1990). Head injuries II. *British Medical Journal* 300, 1576–9.
Feldman, Z., Contant, C. F., Robertson, C. S., Narayan, R. K., and Grossman, R. G. (1991). Evaluation of the Leeds prognostic score for severe head injury. *Lancet* 337, 1451–3.

Jennett, B. (1975). *Epilepsy after non-missile head injuries*. Heinemann, London.
Masters, S. J., McLean, P. M., Arcarese, J. S., *et al.* (1987). Skull X-ray examinations after head trauma. *New England Journal of Medicine* 316, 84–91.
Mendelow, A. D., Teasdale, G., Jennett, B. *et al.* (1983). Risk of intracranial haematoma in head injured adults. *British Medical Journal* 287, 1173–6.
Royal College of Radiologists (1989). *Making the best use of a Department of Radiology: guidelines for doctors*. London.
Suggestions from a group of neurosurgeons (1984). Guidelines for initial management after head injury in adults. *British Medical Journal* 288, 983–5.
Temkin, N. R., Dikmen, S. S., Wilensky, A. J., Keihm, J., Chabal, S., and Winn H. R. (1990). A randomized, double blind study of phenytoin for the prevention of post-traumatic seizures. *New England Journal of Medicine*. 322, 497–502.

Rehabilitation

Editorial (1990). Head trauma victims in the UK: undeservedly underserved. *Lancet*, 335, 886–7.
Medical Disability Society (1988). *The management of traumatic brain injury*. Royal College of Physicians of London Publications, London.
Tate, R. L., Lulham, J. M., Broe, G. A., *et al.* Psychological outcome for the survivors of severe blunt head injury: the results from a consecutive series of 100 patients. *Journal of Neurology, Neurosurgery and Psychiatry* 52, 1128–34.
Walsh, K. W. (1991). *Understanding brain damage: a primer of neuropsychological evaluation*. Churchill Livingstone, London.

Less severe injuries

Leininger, B. E., Gramling, S. E., Farrell, A. D., *et al.* (1990). Neuropsychological deficits in symptomatic minor head injury patients after concussion and mild concussion. *Journal of Neurology, Neurosurgery and Psychiatry* 53, 293–6.
Levin, H. S., Eisenberg, H. M., and Benton, A. L., (1989). ˙*Mild head injury*. Oxford University Press, Oxford.
Mittenberg, W., DiGiulio, D. V., Perrin, S., and Bass, A. E. (1992). Symptoms following mild head injury: expectation as aetiology. *Journal of Neurology, Neurosurgery and Psychiatry* 55, 200–4.
Wilson, B. (1992). Recovery and compensatory strategies in head injured memory impaired people several years after insult. *Journal of Neurology, Neurosurgery and Psychiatry* 55, 177–80.

16 Brain tumours

Virtually any of the multiplicity of cell types within the skull can give rise to tumours, although some, such as the glial series, do so more commonly than others. The bony confines of the base and vault mean that some tumours, which would be of comparatively little import if they arose from a similar tissue type elsewhere in the body, cause significant neurological symptoms by virtue of their displacement of normal neurological structures—hence the common, all-embracing phrase, *space-occupying lesion*. For example, a meningioma—a benign tumour derived from the meninges—can cause epilepsy, hemiparesis, dementia, or blindness, according to its site, simply by its distorting effect on neural and vascular structures, without invasion of neural tissue.

Other tumours, such as gliomas or metastatic tumours, do, however, invade and replace normal brain, and their total surgical eradication without leaving a grave neurological deficit is not possible.

16.1   Epidemiology and causation

Table 16.1 shows the incidence of brain tumours discovered during life in one large US national survey. Although published in 1985, the data was collected in 1973–74, before the era of modern imaging. A fuller population-based study, including autopsies, has shown that about one-third of brain tumours are not diagnosed during life. Most of these are small meningiomas or gliomas that

Table 16.1   Incidence of brain tumours (from Walker *et al.* 1985)

Primary intracranial neoplasms		Secondary intracranial neoplasms	
Incidence 8.2/100 000 per year		Incidence 8.3/100 000 per year	
Sex ratio M:F = 1.07:1		Sex ratio M:F = 1.5:1	
Distribution	%	Source	%
All gliomas	56	Bronchus	49
Meningioma	20	Breast	16
Neurinoma	7	Bowel	9
Medulloblastoma	2	Genito-urinary	8
Pituitary tumours	14	Other or unspecified	18*
Other	1		

* In some series melanoma is a frequent tumour of origin for cerebral metastases

gave rise to no symptoms in life, but some are unsuspected cerebral metastases in patients with known cancer. The increased interest in small pituitary tumours over the past 15 years, with neuroimaging techniques revealing microadenomas in many patients with hyperprolactinaemia, also makes these figures in Table 16.1 out of date in some ways, but the figures remain valuable in revealing the distribution of types of tumour that cause problems through space occupation or neural destruction.

Some tumours are much more frequent in, or virtually confined to, the years of childhood and adolescence. These include medulloblastomas, pilocytic cerebellar astrocytomas, teratomas, pinealomas, and craniopharyngiomas. Pontine gliomas and ependymomas also occur in adolescence, and are also seen in adult life. Gliomas of the hemispheres, meningiomas, neurinomas, pituitary adenomas, and metastatic tumours are seen in adult life through to old age.

A family doctor will see a new case of a primary cerebral tumour about once every 5–10 years. More people die of primary brain tumours than of multiple sclerosis, generally considered to be a common neurological disorder.

There is very little evidence about the cause of brain tumours other than the association with certain specific predisposing genetic disorders such as neurofibromatosis (see Section 16.8.1), tuberous sclerosis (see Section 16.8.2), and von Hippel–

Lindau disease (see Section 16.8.3). Meningiomas may have a familial occurrence, as may rare syndromes in which glioblastomas are associated with multiple tumours elsewhere. Oncogenes which potentiate or initiate cell mitosis may be expressed inappropriately in neoplastic cells, or neoplastic cells may have lost tumour-suppressor sequences, such as is known to occur in retinoblastoma. Restriction-fragment-length polymorphism analysis has been used to identify deletions on chromosome 22 in meningiomas, on chromosomes 17 and 22 in acoustic neuromas, on chromosome 3p in haemangioblastomas in families with von Hippel–Lindau disease, and on chromosomes 10 and 17 in astrocytomas. There is little evidence that any environmental factor causes the onset of brain tumours, but there is limited evidence that meningiomas may be precipitated by, or the course of their development accelerated by, cranial trauma.

16.2   Clinical features

The presenting symptoms of a brain tumour (other than a pituitary adenoma) are those of local neuronal damage or distortion. They include epilepsy, progressive hemiparesis or intellectual deterioration, or symptoms of raised intracranial pressure, such as headache. Pituitary adenomas may present with endocrine or visual effects (Section 6.8.3). A relatively small tumour, such as an ependymoma of the fourth ventricle, may present early in its development because of obstruction of CSF pathways, resulting in severe headache. Conversely, a slowly growing but very large oligodendroglioma may cause no more than occasional seizures for 10 years or more. Taking as an example all gliomas, the frequency of different initial symptoms of tumours are shown in Table 16.2.

Epilepsy is the most frequent initial symptom of a glioma or of a meningioma. Seizures may be tonic–clonic or partial. In a study of first epileptic seizures in adults, nearly all of whom had a CT scan, only 3.5 per cent turned out to have a tumour. From the perspective of a neurosurgeon, however, the facts are different, and more than half the patients with a glioma will have had one or more seizures by the time they come for neurosurgical assessment. Epilepsy is particularly likely to occur in frontal tumours. Such tumours may

Table 16.2 Symptoms of a glioma (from Thomas and McKeran 1990)

	Initial symptoms (%)	Symptoms by time of neurosurgical assessment* (%)
Epilepsy	38	54
Headache	35	71
Mental change	17	52
Focal neurological deficit		
hemiparesis	10	43
dysphasia	7	27
hemianaesthesia	3	14
hemianopia	2	8
Mental change	16	52
Vomiting	8	31
Impaired consciousness	5	25
Visual disturbance	4	18
Cranial nerve palsy	2	11

* More than one symptom may be present

present with status epilepticus. Tumours in the centro-parietal region, in the region of the Rolandic strip, are also particularly likely to cause epilepsy, whereas a parieto-occipital tumour may reach a considerable size without generating seizures.

Epilepsy occurs with roughly equal incidence in patients with gliomas and meningiomas. One of the sites at which the latter grow is the falx cerebri. Such a tumour may declare itself by a partial seizure beginning in one foot (see Fig. 12.3).

All patients whose epilepsy is of partial onset should have a CT scan or MRI, as a partial onset to a seizure indicates a structural lesion (see Section 12.4.1). The only exception is the benign Rolandic epilepsy of childhood (Section 12.5). Seizures of any type accompanied by physical signs, and seizures of any type accompanied by a post-ictal neurological deficit (Todd's paresis, Section 12.4.1) also require a CT scan, as these points again indicate a structural lesion.

Headache is an initial symptom of a hemisphere glioma in about 35 per cent of cases, but in tumours in the posterior fossa headaches occur early in practically all subjects. Headaches are not neces-

sarily due to an overall elevation of cranial pressure, but may be due to distortion of local structures containing afferent pain fibres, such as the meninges. For example, a small suprasellar extension of a pituitary adenoma may cause generalized headaches by distortion of the diaphragma sellae before the bulk of the tumour can significantly elevate intracranial pressure.

Characteristics of headaches that suggest that a patient should have a CT scan include headaches that are present on waking, or that are initiated by change in posture, or by coughing or straining. All these manoeuvres reflect some change in CSF dynamics and pressure. Other features to be taken seriously are if the headache is described as 'bursting', or some similar word, if the headache is predominantly occipital, and if headaches are a new symptom in someone never much previously prone to headaches. Headaches may or may not be lateralized to the side of the tumour.

A focal neurological deficit is the next most frequent initial symptom. A patient who presents with a progressive hemiparesis or dysphasia has a high probability of having a brain tumour. Ataxia is common in posterior fossa tumours. Sensory symptoms are uncommon. Progressive change in visual fields, although easily documented by a neurologist, are seldom presented as symptoms in hemisphere lesions.

Another group of symptoms comprise a change in personality, cognitive function, and memory. Apathy, depression, irritability, and declining performance at work are all suggestive features. Such symptoms are particularly likely in frontal tumours and tumours of the corpus callosum. It is not unknown for patients with frontal tumours to be 'rescued' by a visiting neurologist from a psychiatric hospital.

Vomiting occurs in a proportion of patients, particularly those with tumours in the posterior fossa. Patients with severe papilloedema may have sudden obscurations of vision. Finally, cranial nerve palsies may occur. There are two mechanisms for these. Either a nerve may be stretched by direct pressure from an expanding tumour, for example the facial nerve over an acoustic neurinoma (Section 16.8.1) or it may be stretched by displacement due to pressure effects from a distant lesion. A VIth nerve palsy is the most frequent of this second mechanism, which is commonly known as a 'false localizing sign'.

As a tumour within the skull expands, venous blood and CSF can be displaced without initially any elevation of total intracranial pressure. A point is reached, however, at which any further small increase in bulk results in a dramatic increase in intracranial pressure.

A tumour arising in one hemisphere will, as it expands, displace normal brain medially and downwards, producing a herniation through the tentorium. As the medial surface of the temporal lobe is squeezed through the tentorium, the IIIrd nerve is nipped between it and the tentorial edge, causing a IIIrd nerve palsy, often first manifest by pupillary dilatation. Haemorrhagic grooves on the medial surface of the temporal lobe can be seen at autopsy in such cases.

Lateral displacement of the brain under the falx also occurs, eventually being associated with altered consciousness. A displacement of 3 mm at the horizontal level of the pineal is usually tolerated, but a greater displacement is associated with drowsiness. If the displacement is greater than 8 mm, the subject is likely to be in coma.

An infratentorial (posterior fossa) mass will cause a similar 'plastic creep' of brain, the usual direction being towards the low pressure region below the foramen magnum, resulting in tonsillar herniation. Sometimes there is upwards herniation through the tentorium. However, it is a feature of posterior fossa tumours that they cause obstruction of the fourth ventricle inflow or outflow at an early stage, so that an obstructive hydrocephalus results, with dilated third and lateral ventricles containing CSF at high pressure. This probably limits the upward creep of the contents of the posterior fossa.

16.3   The natural history and management of different types of cerebral tumour

16.3.1   *Glioma*

Gliomas account for about 56 per cent of all primary brain tumours.

16.3.1.1   *Pathology*

A number of different pathological types are seen. Reasonably well-differentiated astrocytomas make up about 25 per cent of all gliomas. The common-est is the so-called fibrillary type, with spindle-shaped astrocytes filled with intracytoplasmic fibrils. Fluid-filled cysts may occur, and these may reach a considerable size, sometimes acting as space-occupying lesions in, as it were, their own right, so that evacuation of the cyst may result in considerable, albeit temporary, improvement. Fibrillary astrocytes invade and displace neurons, but many normal-looking neurons may survive, particularly near the edges of the tumour. There is no clear line of demarcation between the edge of the tumour and normal cells, and occasional malignant astrocytes may be found some distance from the apparent macroscopic limits of the tumour.

Although pathologists commonly grade the malignancy of the tumour, it must be remembered that the frequency of astrocytic mitoses and abnormal new vessel formation varies at different points within the same tumour. The better-differentiated tumours, or parts of tumours, are graded as I or II on the Kernohan scale. The less well-differentiated grade III is usually considered synonymous with an anaplastic astrocytoma. The least differentiated grade IV tumour is synonymous with a glioblastoma multiforme. This last group accounts for about 50 per cent of all gliomas. Glioblastoma multiforme is characterized by cellular pleomorphism, with astrocytes of different size and degrees of differentiation, frequent mitotic figures, occasional fused cells resulting in multinucleated giant cells, and marked proliferation of abnormal blood vessels, some of which rupture, resulting in haemorrhagic and necrotic cysts. Some glioblastomas appear to result from anaplastic changes in previously better-differentiated astrocytomas; some appear to arise primarily as poorly differentiated and rapidly expanding tumours. The advent of tissue culture techniques, and the development of monoclonal antibodies that allow the characterization of cell surface markers, have revealed marked heterogeneity in cell lines within gliomas. Histological characterization is at best a very crude assessment of a tumour's biological potential. A histopathological classification finding some favour is to consider simply an astrocytoma as one which is mildly hypercellular, with pleomorphism, but no vascular proliferation or necrosis; an anaplastic astrocytoma is one with these characteristics plus vascular proliferation (2 year survival, 50 per cent). A glioblastoma is one with the foregoing characteristics plus necrosis (2 year survival, only 5 per cent). Another simplified grading system included only four criteria—nuclear atypia, mitosis, endothelial proliferation, and necrosis.

There are characteristic chromosomal and cytogenetic abnormalities in most glioblastomas, which may gain chromatin on chromosome 7, and lose some of the material of 9 or 10. Oncogenes such as C-*sis* may be found. Loss of suppressor genes may also be important in facilitating the transfer of an astrocytoma to a glioblastoma, commonly involving losses of material from chromosome 10 or 17.

Other rare subtypes of astrocytoma occur. The cells within a protoplasmic astrocytoma contain few fibrils, and multiple microcysts are common. In a gemistocytic astrocytoma, the tumour cells are large and globoid, with abundant cytoplasm and few fibrils. The pilocytic astrocytomas are characterized by the tumour cells becoming elongated, in bundles parallel with accompanying axons. Eosinophilic rod-shaped structures (Rosenthal fibres) may be seen within them. These last tumours occur principally in the cerebellum of children, and have a good prognosis.

Oligodendrogliomas make up about 5 per cent of all gliomas. They are commonly seen to be calcified on the CT scan (see Fig. 8.17) or MRI, the calcification being related to blood vessels that divide up sheets of round cells with small nuclei and clear cytoplasm. Necrosis has a poor prognosis, but other pathological subdivisions have not proved helpful. Although, in general, slowly growing tumours, sudden acceleration of growth due to anaplastic change is not uncommon.

Ependymomas are derived from the specialized glial cells that line the ventricles and aqueduct. They account for about 6 per cent of all gliomas, being more frequent in childhood and adolescence. Histological examination in the better-differentiated examples shows the cells lined up in rosettes, forming little canals. Other cells orient themselves around blood vessels to give a characteristic halo. Ependymomas may project into the fourth ventricle or obstruct the foramen of Monro, causing hydrocephalus. Alternatively, they may multiply in subependymal regions.

Gangliogliomas are unusual tumours containing neoplastic neurons as well as neoplastic astrocytes. They are usually comparatively indolent tumours and may be cured by resection.

A papillary tumour may arise from the choroid plexus, usually in the fourth ventricle. Rarely,

tumours may also arise from the glial and other cell types in the region of the pineal gland.

16.3.1.2   *Diagnosis and management*

The clinical features of gliomas have been outlined in Section 16.2. The differential diagnosis includes other types of intracranial tumour, brain abscess (Section 17.2.1), fungal infections (Section 17.11), herpes simplex encephalitis (Section 17.12.3), tuberculoma (Section 17.5.2), a giant intracranial aneurysm producing local signs (Section 10.6.5), or a chronic subdural haematoma producing headache, confusion, and hemiparesis (Section 15.6). Vascular disease, such as internal carotid artery stenosis and subsequent occlusion, may cause a progressive hemiparesis that mimics that caused by a tumour.

The CT scan appearances of a glioblastoma are illustrated in Fig. 8.12, and of a cystic astrocytoma of a lower grade of malignancy in Fig. 8.13. The MRI of a glioma in the region of the craniocervical junction is shown in Fig. 8.19. Sometimes, particularly in the investigation of patients with epilepsy, the appearances are much less impressive, merely a small zone of low attenuation, often in this instance in the frontal region. Biopsy will show that these are almost invariably gliomas.

Most neurologists and neurosurgeons believe that all intracerebral mass lesions should be biopsied. In those with acute onset of symptoms, it is important to exclude an abscess. The CT appearances of a recent infarct with luxury perfusion may also mimic an astrocytoma with its peripheral enhancement after the injection of contrast.

If an astrocytoma or glioblastoma is strongly suspected on clinical grounds and on the appearances on the CT scan, the usual method of biopsy is through a burr hole. Most centres in developed countries now use coordinates derived from the scanner outputs to programme a stereotactic biopsy path, rather than a freehand biopsy. This increases the chances of obtaining relevant tissue, and provides the opportunity of avoiding important areas of cortex and deeper structures. The morbidity in such biopsies is now of the order of 2 per cent. Some increase in neurological deficit may occur if the lesion is in a clearly eloquent region of the brain.

Tissue obtained at needle biopsy is smeared on a glass slide. Tumour identification of this biopsy material correlates with paraffin-impregnated blocks of tissue taken at open biopsy or at autopsy reasonably well. However, the small amount of tissue removed leads to sampling errors and the higher grades of malignancy of primary tumours tend to be underestimated.

A formal craniotomy may be performed in some circumstances. This is indicated if it is planned to proceed after biopsy to a partial resection of the glioma. This is possible if the tumour lies in a frontal, temporal, or occipital pole. In other cases, partial debulking provides further room for new tumour growth without elevation of intracranial pressure. Another indication for craniotomy is if the initial CT appearances or histology are ambiguous. The surgeon may then decide that an open inspection of the part of the tumour that reaches the cortex is justifiable, possibly accompanied by multiple biopsies.

Removal of the maximal volume of abnormal tissue possible without leaving an intolerable neurological deficit should be the aim, as there is evidence that this increases survival. Adequate removal is aided by mechanical tissue fragmentation using the cavitron ultrasonic surgical aspirator (CUSA). Small, deeply seated gliomas may be tackled, though not eradicated, by a stereotactically directed CO_2 or Nd–YAg laser. This procedure is, as yet, available in few centres. Although it allows the precise removal of gliomatous tissue from parts of the brain which should be minimally disrupted to avoid morbidity, there is, as yet, no evidence that the long-term survival of these patients is improved.

If a biopsy confirms a glioma in an inaccessible part of the brain, such as the pons, hypothalamus, thalamus, or deep frontal regions, current practice is to advise radiotherapy. Radiotherapy is also given as an adjunctive treatment after partial excision of a glioma at a frontal, temporal, or occipital pole. The usual dose is 55 Gy fractionated over about 28–35 days. (1.8–2.0 Gy on 5 days a week). This is close to the maximal dose tolerated by normal brain. Attempts in the past decade at improving the results of radiotherapy have included the use of hyperbaric oxygen, misonidazole, and hyperfractionation—giving several fractions of the total dose in one day. This last may not greatly alter survival, but it does get the patient home more quickly.

The most promising advance in radiotherapy is the use of interstitial radiation, using radioactive seeds implanted either at open surgery or by stereotaxis; ^{125}I and ^{192}Ir have both been used. An alternative to the implantation of seeds is the use of removable catheters, which can be used to contain the source and placed in such a way as to maximize the tumour dose. An alternative way of delivery of finely focused local brain irradiation is by using megavoltage X-rays delivered from an isocentrically mounted linear accelerator, which rotates in a series of arcs. During treatment the beam always points at the lesion, which is positioned using a modified neurosurgical stereotactic frame. A further way of delivering finally focused radiation is by the use of charged heavy particles. As these slow in the tissues, ionization occurs at the end of their path length (the Bragg peak phenomenon). The calculation of where this will occur allows focused radiation damage at a defined point.

At various stages in management, corticosteroids are useful in reducing oedema in and around a tumour, which shifts cerebral structures. In general, if mid-line structures are shifted between 6 and 8 mm the patient is stuperose, and if more than 8 mm the patient is in coma. After the administration of corticosteroids, there may be remarkable recovery of lost functions or increase in alertness within 36–48 hours. In a situation where intracranial pressure is obviously high, the usual corticosteroid chosen is dexamethasone, 0.05 mg/kg four times a day (12–16 mg/day for an adult). Once as much recovery of function has occurred as can reasonably be expected, bearing in mind the destructive effects of the tumour, aside from oedema, then the dose should be reduced to the lowest level that maintains function. If a high dose of corticosteroids is used for more than a few days, it is usual to add an H_2 receptor antagonist, such as cimetidine, to minimize the risk of peptic ulceration although the evidence that this is effective is sparse.

Anticonvulsants are given in order to prevent seizures, or minimize the risk of further seizures. Carbamazepine or phenytoin are suitable drugs.

In view of the poor prognosis of most gliomas (Section 16.3.1.3), interest has naturally settled on the possibility of chemotherapy. The nitrosoureas have until recently found most favour, notably BCNU (1,3-*bis*(2 chlorethyl)-l-nitrosourea). However, interest is now focused on temozolomide, an

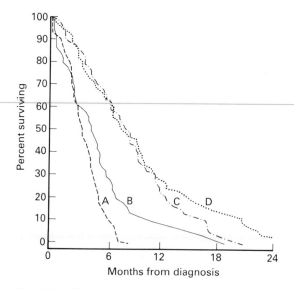

Fig. 16.1 The survival of patients with cerebral glioma who received: A. best conventional care, but no radiotherapy or chemotherapy; B. BCNU; C. radiotherapy; D. BCNU and radiotherapy. Data from Walker *et al.* 1978.

imidotetrazine derivative which can be given by mouth and crosses the blood–brain barrier. Dramatic resolution of CT scan changes have been reported in a few patients to date. Other groups are exploring the possibility of the infusion of antibodies targeted against glioma cells and lymphokines, but the studies are still at an early stage. Another novel experimental approach is to use mutants of herpes simplex virus deficient for the virus-encoded enzyme thymidine kinase. These mutants will kill dividing gliomatous cells in tissue culture and some experimental animals, leaving intact non-dividing neurons.

16.3.1.3 *Prognosis*

Unfortunately, many gliomas recur. Only occasionally is a second surgical procedure justified. As a near maximal dose of radiotherapy has been given, this, too, cannot be repeated. Headache and other unpleasant symptoms can usually be controlled by large doses of steroids, but these should be withdrawn when the quality of life is clearly unsupportable, and coma and death

due to raised intracranial pressure then soon ensue.

Studies have shown that repeated CT scanning or MRI is not an aid to follow-up after surgery, as on CT scanning post-operative areas of low attenuation and enhancement due to persistent tumour, response to anti-neoplastic therapy, necrosis and recurrent tumour cannot be distinguished. An increasing clinical deficit is all too obvious a warning of significant recurrence. PET scanning (Section 8.10.5) is of present research interest as increased glucose uptake appears to predict reliably the recurrence of tumour.

For patients with anaplastic astrocytomas or glioblastomas, in one study the median survival time after diagnosis was 14 weeks for conventional care, 18.5 weeks for those receiving BCNU, and 35 weeks for those receiving radiotherapy. The combination of BCNU and radiotherapy did not increase survival further, nor does the use of the sensitizing agent misonidazole. This study by the Brain Tumour Study Goup and the National Cancer Institute clearly shows a beneficial effect of radiotherapy. From this and other similar studies, it has emerged that age, degree of disability at diagnosis, and tumour type are all important variables in prognosis. Older patients, those who have significant disability at diagnosis, and those who have glioblastoma multiforme do less well.

Some neurologists and neurosurgeons make the point that the time occupied by surgery and radiotherapy in patients with such a short predicted survival is not 'worthwhile'. The short additional life span achieved may largely be spent in medical care, and the final stages of deterioration may well begin before convalescence from therapeutic procedures has been completed. The terminal stages of the illness are managed by continuing dexamethasone to relieve headaches, continuing control of seizures with anticonvulsants, control of vomiting by metoclopramide or domperidone, and, most importantly, the provision of adequate nursing and other support for the carer at home.

Astrocytomas of lesser grades (I and II) do have a better prognosis. Although no adequate controlled trial has been published, overall five-year survival rates are of the order of 10 per cent for partial tumour excision alone, improving to about 30 per cent if radiotherapy is added.

A recent population study has shown that oligodendrogliomas, generally considered to be the most favourable in outlook of the gliomas, in reality also have a poor prognosis, with a median postoperative survival time of 3 years, and a five-year survival rate of only 34 per cent.

Excision of a cerebellar pilocytic astrocytoma in childhood often results in a complete cure. Brain-stem gliomas in childhood often respond very well to radiotherapy, with good temporary remission of symptoms and signs. However, relapse soon occurs, and the five-year survival rate is of the order of 15 per cent. Gliomas also occur in the optic nerve or chiasma in childhood. These are compatible with long survival after radiotherapy, and useful vision is usually retained.

16.3.2   *Lymphoma and leukaemia*

Primary central nervous system lymphoma used to be called microglioma in the UK and reticulum cell sarcoma in the USA before it was recognized that the tumour was composed of B-lymphocytes, with a histological appearance similar to that of extranodal non-Hodgkin's lymphoma. The tumour may be multicentric. It is becoming a more frequent tumour, as it is prone to occur in AIDS or in patients immunocompromised after organ transplantation. However, it still only accounts for 1–2 per cent of all brain tumours. The CT scan or MRI appearances are rather different from those of a primary glioma, tending to enhance densely and diffusely with contrast. If the lesion is suspected, there are good grounds for not using dexamethasone as the histological changes may be so markedly altered that confirmation of the diagnosis then becomes difficult, due to tumour lysis. The tumour bulk can be considerably reduced by radiotherapy, but recurrence, or the origin of a further tumour at a new site, is common. The prognosis can be considerably improved by the adjunctive use of methotrexate and cytosine arabinoside.

Involvement of the central nervous system by leukaemia is very common. In acute lymphatic leukaemia of childhood (ALL), leukaemia cells invade the leptomeninges and the surface of the underlying brain. Leukaemic cells may be found in the CSF. The sensitivity of the search may be improved by staining the cells for the enzyme terminal transferase. The importance of meningeal relapse in the eradication of this condition is well known, and many trials have been undertaken to assess the best way of preventing this—by intrathe-cal methotrexate, cytosine arabinoside, or cranio-spinal irradiation.

Patients with ALL and acute myeloid leukaemia (AML) with very high white counts and thrombo-cytopenia are at considerable risk from intracereb-ral haemorrhage.

16.3.3   *Meningiomas*

Meningiomas can grow from any part of the meningeal covering of the brain. They constitute about 15–20 per cent of all primary brain tumours. They are particularly frequent over the convexity of the hemispheres, in relation to the falx or parasagittal region, and along the sphenoid wing (Fig. 8.22). Other sites include the subfrontal region, in relation to the olfactory groove, the parasellar region, the tentorium cerebelli, the neighbourhood of the trigeminal ganglion, and in the neighbourhood of the foramen magnum. The clinical presentation will, of course, depend on the site of origin of the tumour. Convexity, falx, and parasagittal meningiomas usually present with epilepsy. Subfrontal meningiomas present with change in personality and cognitive function. Meningiomas in the neighbourhood of the sphenoid wing often present with progressive unilateral visual failure, due to early compression of the optic nerve. Meningiomas in the region of the foramen magnum produce lower cranial nerve palsies, and may also compress the lower brain stem or the upper end of the spinal cord.

Various histological types of meningioma occur. The most benign is the syncytial type, in which fibroblasts are arranged in whorls. In other types vascular proliferation is prominent. The haem-angiopericytic type, a rare papillary type, and anaplastic meningiomas are all locally invasive, and often recur after what has been thought to be a total excision. Craniotomy is usually followed by radiotherapy in such cases.

Cytogenetic analysis has demonstrated multiple deletions on chromosome 22 in many meningiomas.

Meningiomas are well revealed by CT scanning and MRI, and enhance considerably after the injection of contrast. Being derived from meningeal cells, their vascular supply comes from the external carotid circulation. Carotid angiography with selective sequential catheterization of external and internal carotid arteries is therefore often used to identify a tumour as a meningioma before craniotomy.

Total removal of a syncytial meningioma usually results in a radical cure, but even if excision has been thought to be total, about 8 per cent do recur. The tumours have often reached a considerable size before diagnosis and, being highly vascular, operative morbidity is considerable. Sometimes, for example, a meningioma along the sphenoid wing becomes incorporated into bone, and only partial removal is possible. Such bony changes may be seen as areas of increased density on plain skull X-rays. Another variant is for tumour cells to grow in a sheet, for example along the floor of the middle fossa. It is not usually possible to remove totally such a meningioma-en-plaque.

Meningiomas usually occur in middle age, or later. Their slow rate of growth and the technical difficulties of surgery, and sometimes a relatively advanced age, are factors that justify a conservative approach without operation in some cases. They are notorious for enlarging rapidly during pregnancy.

16.3.4 Less common types of primary tumour in adults

16.3.4.1 Epidermoid and dermoid cysts

Epidermoid cysts are benign tumours which, on histological examination, prove to contain skin appendages such as sebaceous glands and hair. They may be located in the cerebellopontine angle, the parapituitary region, or the temporal lobe. The cysts are presumed to result from errors of infolding of the neural tube so that epithelial cells become misplaced between the surface ectoderm and developing nervous system. If epithelium and mesenchyme are misplaced, then a dermoid cyst develops. These are more frequently found in the mid-line, in the frontal region, in the vermis, and in the lumbosacral region of the spine, where they may be associated with other abnormalities such as spina bifida and diastematomyelia (see Section 22.1.4). Cystic teratomas contain elements from all germ layers, including mesodermal elements such as muscle and cartilage. Craniopharyngiomas, probably derived from ectodermal elements in Rathke's pouch, lie in the suprasellar region, and are lined with adamantinomatous epithelium, and

often contain whorls of squamous cells and cholesterol (see Section 16.6.5.1).

Epidermoid spinal cysts can very rarely be acquired after repeated lumbar punctures; presumably a plug of epidermal cells is carried towards the canal on the tip of the lumbar puncture needle, and there expands.

16.3.4.2 Tumours of the pineal region

Expansion of tumours in this region compresses or involves the upper part of the brain stem. This results in failure of upward gaze, a divergent squint, pupillary dilatation, and unresponsiveness to light or accommodation (Parinaud's syndrome). There is often pronounced hydrocephalus, as drainage from the third ventricle is obstructed.

Tumours in this region include germinomas and teratomas, which are radiosensitive. The CSF may contain elevated levels of α-feto protein and the plasma elevated levels of β-human chorionic gonadotrophin in these cases. Other tumours in this region include pinealblastomas or pinealcytomas. Gliomas may arise high in the brain stem and present in a very similar way.

16.3.4.3 Histiocytosis X

The nosology of this condition is obscure. It is characterized by abnormal proliferation of Langerhans cells, dendritic cells derived from the bone marrow, often containing inclusions known as Birbeck granules. The granulomatous proliferation may affect the orbit, the parapituitary region, and the skull vault. Although the lesions are not truly malignant, in the sense of not being monoclonal or with atypical cell structure, it may be necessary to control their growth with radiotherapy or chemotherapy. Lesions of histiocytosis X in the parapituitary region may result in diabetes insipidus.

16.4 Secondary intracranial tumours

The sources of cerebral metastases are shown in Table 16.1, and CT scans of two are illustrated in Figs. 8.10 and 8.11. More than half the patients have more than one metastasis imaged at diagnosis. Supratentorial metastases are commonly found

16.5 Brain tumours in children

in the watershed areas between the distributions of the main cerebral arteries, suggesting that most result from arterial tumour emboli. Metastases that are solitary are found rather more often in the posterior fossa, often arising from pelvic or gastrointestinal primary tumours.

Treatment for cerebral carcinomatous metastases is palliative. Dexamethasone may considerably relieve headache, and temporarily improve a neurological deficit. Radiotherapy with 3000 cGy delivered to the whole brain over 14–21 days may also be of benefit. The surgical excision of apparently solitary metastases is often worthwhile if a long period has elapsed after excision of the primary tumour; even if the operation is not curative, it produces better palliation than radiotherapy alone. More energetic treatment may be justifiable for non-Hodgkin's lymphoma, in which epidural deposits are common, resulting in cord compression or local spinal nerve root or cranial nerve signs.

16.4.1 *Malignant meningitis*

Multiple cranial nerve palsies can occur by direct extension of nasopharyngeal carcinomas, lymphomas or plasmacytomas, or by the local extension of a blood-borne metastasis from a carcinoma, commonly of the bronchus or breast. A melanoma is another common primary site. In such cases, malignant cells may be found in a cytocentrifuged specimen of CSF, but they are often infrequent. Clues to the diagnosis may emerge from the finding of a low CSF sugar.

Anaplastic gliomas or medulloblastomas may seed down the meninges in a similar way.

16.5 Brain tumours in children

The annual incidence of brain tumours in children is 2–3 per 100 000 per year. Although uncommon, primary brain tumours are the most common solid tumours of childhood. Of all childhood cancers, only leukaemia is more frequent.

About two-thirds of all childhood brain tumours are located below the tentorium cerebelli, whereas in adults three-quarters of all tumours lie above it. Although malignant supratentorial astrocytomas do occur, much more frequent are the tumours next described.

16.5.1 *Medulloblastoma*

This is the most common intracranial tumour of childhood, accounting for about 20 per cent. They arise in the cerebellum, most commonly in the vermis. They are believed to be of fetal external granular cell origin. Leptomeningeal seeding over the convexities and down the spinal canal is common. These tumours probably arise from primitive cells which may be capable of both neuronal and glial differentiation. Cytogenetic analysis often shows changes in chromosomes 1 and 17. Microscopy shows darkly staining tumour cells with little cytoplasm spread in uniform sheets. These tumours usually present with headaches, vomiting, and unsteadiness.

An initial ventriculo-peritoneal shunt is often necessary, followed by debulking surgery, and megavoltage cranio-spinal radiotherapy with enhancement of therapy at the local disease site. Spinal irradiation is necessary because of the frequency of leptomeningeal seeding. Adjuvant chemotherapy with lomastine and vincristine considerably improves survival in those aged less than 2 years, and in those with brain-stem involvement. Methotrexate and cisplatin are also effective, but their use is limited by the occurrence of a leucoencephalopathy and ototoxicity respectively. The overall five-year survival rate is of the order of 65 per cent, with 45 per cent surviving to 10 years. Unfortunately, the long-term follow-up shows substantial effects of radiotherapy upon endocrine and cognitive development, and chemotherapy is now the initial therapy of choice, particularly in children aged less than 2 years. Vincristine, cisplatin, procarbazine, and methotrexate are all useful.

16.5.2 *Ependymoma*

This is the second most common tumour in childhood, although ependymomas may be found in adult life as well. They arise from the cells lining the ventricles. In childhood, most tumours are infratentorial. Presentation, treatment strategies, and survival are similar to those outlined for medulloblastoma. Leptomeningeal seeding is particularly frequent.

16.5.3 *Brain-stem glioma*

Gliomas in the brain stem account for about 10–20

per cent of childhood brain tumours. Presentation is often with double vision, dysarthria, dysphagia, unsteadiness, and headache. Biopsy is not usually practical unless an exophytic protrusion of tumour occurs. Radiotherapy often results in a temporary remission. Chemotherapy is not effective.

16.5.4 Pilocytic cerebellar astrocytoma

The histology of these tumours is considered in Section 16.3.1.1. Radical excision is often possible, as the tumours lie laterally placed in one cerebellar hemisphere. Complete cure is then usually achieved.

16.5.5 Suprasellar gliomas

These are considered in Section 16.6.5.

16.6 Tumours of and near the pituitary gland

Striking advances in endocrinology in the past 20 years have led to a much closer relationship between endocrinologists and neurosurgeons.

Some functioning pituitary tumours are of such small size—microadenomas (<10 mm)—that they produce no local effect, but only humoral syndromes. An example is a small prolactinoma, resulting in amenorrhoea and galactorrhoea in women, and decreased libido and impotence in men. Clearly, there is no particular reason for a neurologist to become involved in such cases. In others, tumours are of such size that neurological syndromes occur.

16.6.1 Neurological symptoms and signs caused by a suprasellar lesion

Any adenoma growing within the pituitary fossa is for some time confined within it. There may be local ballooning or downwards deviation of the floor into the sphenoid sinus, but it is not until the tumour expands upwards or sideways that any neurological symptoms or signs occur.

Headaches are thought to arise from distortion of the diaphragma sellae, but have no characteristics distinguishing them from headaches of more banal origin. As the tumour balloons further

upwards, it begins to compress the inferior surface of the optic chiasma in which lie the crossing fibres from the upper temporal fields of each eye. A large expansion will result progressively in a bitemporal hemianopia (Fig. 6.1), and even, as the tumour spreads further upwards and forwards, loss of vision of one eye.

Expansion of pituitary tumours upwards from the pituitary fossa is well visualized by MRI, as are other tumours in the sellar and parasellar regions (Fig. 8.18). Lateral expansion of large pituitary tumours is also often seen on the CT or MR images but less often results in clinical signs. However, IIIrd, VIth, and IVth cranial nerve palsies can occur. The tumour may also invade the mesial temporal lobe and cause epilepsy. Larger tumours are prone to so-called pituitary apoplexy, in which a sudden haemorrhagic infarction of the tumour results in the onset of severe headache and ophthalmoplegia. The initial clinical syndrome may be suggestive of subarachnoid haemorrhage, the true state of affairs only being revealed by imaging studies.

16.6.2 Prolactinoma

Most prolactinomas are microadenomas, diagnosed initially by the finding in a subject with relevant clinical symptoms of a high serum prolactin (average of several random samples above 2000 mU/l). In practice, one sample taken in an unstressed patient after 11.00 hours with a serum level greater than 700 mU/l should raise a suspicion of a prolactinoma. However, it must be remembered that dopamine-receptor blocking agents, such as haloperidol, and dopamine-depleting agents, such as reserpine, can cause hyperprolactinaemia. Other causes of hyperprolactinaemia include pregnancy, oestrogens, and hypothyroidism. In this last case, elevated thyroid stimulating hormone (TSH) levels liberate prolactin.

So-called 'pseudoprolactinomas' occur when other tumours in the neighbourhood of the pituitary stalk, such as a craniopharyngioma, compress it and prevent delivery of dopamine from the hypothalamus. Normal pituitary lactotrophs then liberate an excessive quantity of prolactin. In large pituitary tumours, a serum prolactin of less than 2500 mU/l usually indicates a non-functioning tumour of this type; a true large prolactinoma is likely to have a serum prolactin of considerably more than this, usually 8000 mU/l or above. These observations only apply to large tumours.

In about a third of women with hyperprolactinaemia and a microadenoma, the serum prolactin will fall to within the normal range over a five-year period, and menstruation will return. Furthermore, microadenomas—or at least small areas of inhomogeneity—are seen on CT scans or MRI of about one-third of healthy women of childbearing age, and incidental microadenomas are found at autopsy in about a quarter of autopsies of subjects dying of endocrine disease. These figures suggest that functioning microprolactinomas are so common as to be virtually a normal variant. Clinical endocrine disorders may require treatment, but this may not be necessary for a high serum prolactin alone.

Symptoms associated with a high serum prolactin include delayed puberty or menstrual irregularities, galactorrhoea and infertility in women and, in men, impotence and also often galactorrhoea. These effects are due to the inhibition, in women, of positive feedback on the secretion of luteinizing hormone, and blockade of the effects of gonadotrophins at a gonadal level. In true prolactinomas, dopamine receptors are usually retained, and hyperprolactinaemia can be relieved by a dopamine-receptor agonist, such as bromocriptine. Nausea occurs with this drug, but this can usually be avoided by giving it in the middle of meals, with gradual increments to the usual maintenance dose of 2.5 mg two or three times a day. Pergolide is a longer-acting agent that allows once-daily treatment.

For those patients with small prolactinomas insensitive to dopamine agonists, or who cannot tolerate the drug, the tumour can be removed through a transethmoidal, transsphenoidal approach. In spite of their small size, it is usually practical to identify microadenomas by this route. Mild transient diabetes insipidus may follow in some patients, and others may develop a frontal sinus infection but, in spite of its apparent complexity, the operation is successful and safe. About 20 per cent of patients will be deficient in one or more of growth hormone, adrenocorticotrophic hormone (ACTH), thyroid stimulating hormone, or luteinizing hormone after the operation, and will require replacement therapy as appropriate.

Larger prolactinomas resulting in visual field defects are usually substantially reduced in size by dopamine agonists, with resultant improvement in the visual fields. It may then be possible to maintain the patient indefinitely on a smaller dose of dopamine agonist. Alternative strategies are to prevent re-expansion by external-beam megavoltage radiotherapy, or to remove the shrunken tumour by a transsphenoidal approach.

Prolactinomas may increase markedly in size during pregnancy. A dopamine agonist usually controls tumour bulk. If known about before conception, radiotherapy can be used to prevent further tumour expansion.

16.6.3   *Acromegaly and gigantism*

Growth-hormone-secreting adenomas result in these well-known syndromes with overgrowth of bone, soft tissues, and internal organs. The incidence is about 3–4 cases per million per year, and the prevalence about 60 per million. Endocrine diagnosis depends upon high fasting growth hormone levels (more than 10 μg/l) which are not suppressed to less than 2 μg/l by a 50 g oral glucose load. An insulin-like growth factor (IGF-1, also known as somatomedin C) is also elevated in acromegaly. About half the adenomas are less than 10 mm in diameter at diagnosis. Larger tumours produce similar neurological syndromes to large prolactinomas. Remote effects of the tumour include hypertension, a peripheral neuropathy, diabetes mellitus, and, very frequently, the carpal tunnel syndrome. Colonic polyps and cancer are being increasingly recognized. Growth-hormone-secreting adenomas are less responsive to dopamine agonists than prolactinomas. Normal growth hormone levels are achieved in only about 20 per cent of patients, often at the expense of unpleasant nausea and postural hypotension. Somatostatin, which normally exerts suppressive regulation of growth hormone secretion, will lower growth hormone levels to normal, but suppression lasts for only about 3 hours, and there is marked rebound hypersecretion. However, octreotide, a synthetic octapeptide analogue of somatostatin, has been developed with a longer duration of action, and this is now the drug of choice. It is given by injection every 8 hours. Gallstones may occur as an adverse effect of the drug.

Transsphenoidal hypophysectomy, and radiotherapy by an external conventional megavoltage beam or proton beam, or implanted ^{90}Y have also been used in the management of acromegaly, the choice depending upon the age of the patient, and the activity and size of the tumour. In general, tumours of less than 10 mm in diameter are well treated by transsphenoidal hypophysectomy, with rapid reduction in growth hormone levels. Adverse effects of the operation include hypopituitarism in about 15 per cent of the patients, with a need for subsequent replacement therapy, and sometimes the onset of diabetes insipidus or cerebrospinal fluid rhinorrhoea. External-beam radiotherapy can be used as an initial or adjuvant therapy, 40–50 Gy being usually administered over 4–6 weeks. The disadvantage of this type of treatment is the time taken for growth hormone levels to fall, and the late onset of hypopituitarism.

16.6.4   *Cushing's disease*

Cushing's *disease* is due to an adrenocorticotropin (ACTH)-secreting pituitary tumour, resulting in bilateral adrenocortical hyperplasia and excessive secretion of adrenal corticosteroids. Cushing's *syndrome* may be due to an adrenal tumour or to a cortisol-secreting ectopic source, such as a bronchial carcinoma. The diagnosis of Cushing's disease depends upon a failure of the pituitary source of ACTH to be suppressed by dexamethasone. Corticotropin-releasing hormone (CRH) given to those with a pituitary source of ACTH results in an exaggerated or normal corticotropin and cortisol response, but ectopic sources of ACTH or adrenal tumours do not respond. Treatment of Cushing's disease used to be by bilateral adrenalectomy, but in a large proportion of cases the pituitary adenoma enlarges subsequent to adrenalectomy and may become locally invasive. This is known as Nelson's syndrome. Transsphenoidal hypophysectomy is the treatment of choice, but external-beam radiation or intrasellar ^{90}Y is also effective. Initial medical therapy with metapyrone or ketoconazole may be useful to control the effects of hypercortisolism before surgery.

16.6.5   *Other tumours in the pituitary region*

Tumours secreting prolactin, growth hormone, adrenocorticotrophin, and (rarely) thyroid-stimulating hormone account for about two-thirds of all pituitary tumours in most surgical series, and apparently 'non-secreting' tumours make up the remainder. In recent years it has become clear that many of these non-secreting tumours are actually tumours of gonadotroph cells that produce gonadotropins or their subunits (luteinizing hormones or follicle-stimulating hormone). Hypersecretion of these hormones has little clinical effect, although hypogonadism may develop in both men and premenopausal women, and a small number of men have testicular enlargement secondary to the effects of follicle-stimulating hormone on the seminiferous tubules. Because of their relative clinical silence, many of these tumours previously thought to be non-secreting do present to neurologists and neurosurgeons with tumours of some size, with headaches and visual-field defects. Tumour size has not yet been shown to be reduced by any hormonal intervention, and surgery remains the treatment of choice.

There are also tumours not of pituitary origin that may result in syndromes of endocrine deficiency and visual-field defects—craniopharyngiomas and gliomas of the optic nerve, chiasma, or hypothalamus.

16.6.5.1   *Craniopharyngiomas*

These tumours are believed to arise from remnants of Rathke's pouch, a diverticulum of primitive ectoderm. They account for about 5 per cent of all childhood tumours. They usually present with endocrine or visual effects. The tumour is often calcified, especially peripherally. Surgical removal is not easy as the tumour tends to be adherent to neighbouring structures. Operation is followed by external-beam irradiation. Recurrences are frequent. Occasionally the tumour spreads vigorously into neighbouring structures, including the medial aspect of the temporal lobes, causing epilepsy.

16.6.5.2   *Suprasellar gliomas*

Gliomas of the optic nerve are common in children with neurofibromatosis 1 (Section 16.8.1.1). They present with visual loss or proptosis. The rate of progression is often slow. As the tumour often extends back into the chiasma, or has its origin there, there are obvious major difficulties in planning surgery. External-beam irradiation may be effective at slowing or halting tumour progression.

Gliomas can arise in the hypothalamus and

produce visual and endocrine problems as they extend downwards from the floor of the third ventricle.

16.7 Orbital tumours and other lesions

The orbit is a bony cone, and a mass lesion of any size will push the globe forwards. A unilateral proptosis therefore strongly suggests an orbital mass. In Graves' disease (see below), proptosis may be asymmetric, but there is usually bilateral proptosis.

Within the soft cone formed by the orbital muscles, a glioma or meningioma may affect the optic nerve, and metastatic tumours may arise, particularly from the bronchus. This is also a site at which deposits of malignant lymphoma occur, or a cavernous haemangioma arises.

16.7.1 *Non-malignant orbital lesions*

16.7.1.1 *Graves' ophthalmopathy*

Most patients with Graves' thyrotoxicosis have some eye signs when first seen, with lid retraction, proptosis, and a complaint of a gritty soreness affecting the eyes. More prominent symptoms lead to a diagnosis of Graves' ophthalmopathy, with immunologically mediated damage to the external ocular muscles. These become infiltrated by lymphocytes and oedematous, due to the hydrophilic properties of glycosaminoglycans which are released by proliferating fibroblasts. The swelling of the muscles leads to pronounced proptosis and exposure keratitis.

The pathogenesis of Graves' ophthalmopathy remains obscure, especially in its relationship to thyroid function. Ophthalmopathy occurs rarely in Hashimoto's thyroiditis and, occasionally, in the absence of any thyroid disease at all. It may get worse as thyrotoxicosis is brought under control by surgery or radio-iodine treatment. For these reasons, some believe that thyrotoxicosis and ophthalmopathy are two related but independent autoimmune disorders. The treatment of choice is immunosuppression with prednisolone, although cyclosporin may be combined with prednisolone in resistant cases. For thyrotoxic patients treated with radioactive iodine, concomitant treatment with prednisolone should be given to those already with considerable eye signs.

16.7.1.2 *Pseudotumour of the orbit*

This is another immunologically mediated orbital disorder, which also results in proptosis and ophthalmoplegia. It is characterized by a proliferation of T-lymphocytes in orbital fat and in external ocular muscles. It is responsive to prednisolone.

16.7.1.3 *The Tolosa–Hunt syndrome*

This is another type of painful ophthalmoplegia that is responsive to steroids, but in these cases there is a relative lack of proptosis. Granulomatous infiltration of nerves and muscles in the region of the superior lacrimal fissure has been reported in the few cases that have come to autopsy. Recurrent episodes of painful ophthalmoplegia may occur at intervals over years.

16.7.1.4 *Other orbital lesions*

Sarcoidosis is another type of orbital granuloma, causing a similar syndrome to those described above.

An orbital cellulitis may occur secondary to a frontal or ethmoidal cellulitis, sometimes in association with thrombosis of the cavernous sinus. Urgent intravenous antibiotic treatment is required.

The orbit may also be invaded by saprophytic fungi in diabetic patients (Section 17.11.6).

Lesions outside the cone of muscles that cause proptosis include a mucocele extending from the neighbouring sinuses, tumours of the lacrimal gland, and, again, a metastasis.

16.7.2 *Investigation of orbital lesions*

MRI usually gives reasonably clear evidence of the nature of the lesion causing proptosis. In vew of the frequency of cavernous haemangiomas, arteriography may be helpful. Orbital pseudotumour is remarkably responsive to steroids, and this may prove to be useful in supporting this diagnosis without biopsy.

16.8   Genetic disorders associated with tumours

16.8.1   *Tumours associated with neurofibromatoses 1 and 2*

These are two quite distinct disorders, the nature of which has been recently clarified by epidemiological studies and gene mapping. The diagnostic criteria are outlined in Table 16.3.

Table 16.3   Diagnostic criteria for neurofibromatoses (from Mulvihill *et al.* 1990)

Neurofibromatosis 1

The diagnostic criteria are met if a person has *two* or more of the following:

Six or more *café-au-lait* macules over 5 mm in greatest diameter in prepubertal persons and over 15 mm in greatest diameter in postpubertal persons

Two or more neurofibromas of any type or one plexiform neurofibroma

Freckling in the axillary or inguinal regions

Optic glioma

Two or more Lisch nodules (iris hamartomas)

A distinctive osseous lesion, such as sphenoid dysplasia or thinning of long bone cortex, with or without pseudoarthrosis

A first-degree relative (parent, sibling, or offspring) with neurofibromatosis 1 by the above criteria

Neurofibromatosis 2

The diagnostic criteria are met if a person has *either* of the following:

Bilateral eighth nerve masses seen with appropriate imaging techniques (for example, MRI or CT)

A first-degree relative with neurofibromatosis 2, and *either* unilateral eighth nerve mass or *two* of the following:

    neurofibroma
    meningioma
    glioma
    schwannoma
    juvenile posterior subcapsular lenticular opacity

16.8.1.1   *Neurofibromatosis 1 (von Recklinghausen's disease)*

This was first described in 1882 by von Recklinghausen. The diagnosis can be made if a person has two or more of the stigmata shown in Table

16.3, but there is considerable variability in phenotypic expression. The gene has been mapped to band 11.2 of the long arm of chromosome 17, and is inherited as a dominant disorder, which occurs about once in 3000 live births. However, about 30–50 per cent of all cases represent new mutations. It has recently been shown that a repetitive genetic element, the 282-base-pair Alu sequence, which is present on average every 5 kb of human genomic DNA has been found to be inserted, as a *de novo* mutation, into an intron on chromosome 17. Such inappropriate malplacements may be found in other genetic disorders. Apart from the *café-au-lait* patches and peripheral neurofibromata, central nervous system lesions are common, particularly gliomata of the optic nerve. MRI shows multiple areas of high signal on T2-weighted images in many symptomless children who may be presumed to be carrying the gene by their pedigree, and by the presence of *café-au-lait* patches. These areas of high signal represent hamartomatous areas of heterotopic or dysplastic tissues. Some may develop into low-grade gliomas. The spinal cord may be affected by intramedullary gliomas or, more commonly, be compressed by a intradural neurofibroma, which may extend out through the neural foramina as a 'dumb-bell tumour' (Section 18.4.2.1). Other cancers and multiple endocrine neoplasia, such as phaeochromocytoma and duodenal carcinoid tumours, occur more frequently than would be expected.

16.8.1.2   *Neurofibromatosis 2 (bilateral acoustic neurofibromatosis)*

Acoustic neuromas occur in two forms. Sporadic tumours are unilateral, there is no family history of tumour, and patients are usually aged over 40. Those who carry the gene for neurofibromatosis 2 often have a family history of affected relatives, the tumours occur at a younger age, and patients may develop other central nervous system tumours, such as meningiomas. Meningiomas commonly contain cells in which all or part of chromosome 22 is lost, and therefore, in view of the association, mapping of the gene for neurofibromatosis 2 initially concentrated on this chromosome. It has been found that both sporadic acoustic neuromas and bilateral acoustic neurofibromatosis have deletions of the middle of the short arm of chromosome 22 between bands 11.1 and 13.1. It is believed that this zone contains a tumour-suppressing gene on the normal allele. That is to say, although pedigrees of neurofibromatosis 2 show autosomal dominant inheritance, the mutant allele is, at the cellular level, recessive. It only becomes apparent after the loss of the tumour-suppressing gene on the normal allele.

The clinical features of acoustic neuromas

The usual initial feature is impairment of hearing, which on examination proves to be of sensorineural type. Further audiological examination will show poor speech discrimination, and an abnormal auditory evoked response, with, in particular, a reduction in amplitude of the V component of the response. The best available imaging is with MRI, with gadolinium enhancement, which will display tumours only a few millimetres in size. Plain films or tomograms of the internal auditory meati can play a useful screening role.

If the tumour expands beyond the meatus of the internal auditory canal, it may impinge upon and stretch neighbouring cranial nerves, including the Vth and VIIth. For this reason, the corneal reflex is often lost. Later still, a facial palsy occurs. The brain stem may become distorted by a large acoustic tumour, and nystagmus may result. Caloric testing will then show a mixture of canal paresis, due to the involvement of the vestibular component of the nerve, and a directional preponderance, due to distortion of the brain stem.

Many acoustic neuromas grow quite slowly in size, and the timing of surgery is always a matter for judgement. Partial removal alone may be appropriate, rather than the surgeon valiantly trying to remove all tumour and, in doing so, causing a severe and irrecoverable facial palsy. Often a combined transaural and posterior fossa surgical approach is undertaken.

16.8.2   *Tuberous sclerosis*

This is a disorder characterized by multiple intra-cerebral hamartomata, a proportion of which undergo malignant transformation and progress as gliomas. Tuberous sclerosis is transmitted as an autosomal dominant. Linkage analysis shows that in most families the gene is on chromosome 9q, but there is some evidence of non-allelic heterogeneity, with two other genes producing a similar phenotype on chromosomes 11 and ?12. About one-third of the cases appear to be new mutations.

Tuberous sclerosis is a cause of infantile spasms and other types of childhood epilepsy. The incidence is about 1 in 10 000 in early childhood. Mental retardation is frequent but not invariable. The diagnosis may be made clinically by the observation of characteristic skin lesions, adenoma sebaceum on face, rough patches of skin known as shagreen patches, and peri-ungual fibromas. Cardiac tumours occur.

The CT scan or MRI shows the hamartomata clearly, some of which are calcified (Fig. 8.16).

16.8.3   *Von Hippel–Lindau disease*

Von Hippel–Lindau disease is an autosomal dominant disorder characterized by a predisposition to a wide variety of tumours, particularly haemangioblastomas of the cerebellum, spinal cord, and retina, renal cell carcinoma, phaeochromocytoma, and renal, pancreatic, and epididymal cysts. About 60 per cent of people carrying the gene, which has been mapped to chromosome 3p, will develop a cerebellar haemangioblastoma, and about 40 per cent will present with cerebellar symptoms. About half of all patients will have presented their first tumour by their mid-twenties.

The cerebellar tumours can usually be excised, and spinal tumours often successfully debulked. Histologically the tumours show a network of endothelial-lined vascular channels and polygonal intervascular or stromal cells.

It is believed that the gene on 3p is a tumour-suppressor gene with dominant germ-line inheritance of a mutation in one copy, and tumour occurrence in somatic tissues when there is a second mutation in the normal allele. This mechanism is analogous to the gene for retinoblastoma.

16.9   Idiopathic intracranial hypertension
(synonyms: benign intracranial hypertension; pseudotumour cerebri)

A group of patients present with headaches, without focal neurological signs in the limbs, but with papilloedema, which may be so intense that obscurations of vision occur. The first thought—

that the patient must have a large supratentorial mass in a 'silent' part of the brain, or a posterior fossa tumour—fails to be substantiated by imaging studies, and all further investigations are unhelpful. This is the group of patients who have idiopathic or benign intracranial hypertension, also known as pseudotumour cerebri.

A similar picture is known to arise after extensive lateral and superior sagittal sinus thrombosis, commonly secondary to middle-ear infections. Such cases used to be known as 'otitic hydrocephalus', but are now rare in the developed world since the introduction of antibiotics. Sinus thrombosis does not often appear to underlie the mechanism of intracranial hypertension in the developed world, which can be found in a heterogenous group of patients listed in Table 16.4. The overall incidence is about 1 per 100 000 per year, or 20 per 100 000 obese women aged 20–45.

Table 16.4 Associations of benign intracranial hypertension

Venous sinus thrombosis
Endocrine disorders
   Obesity and menstrual irregularity
   Withdrawal from corticosteroid therapy
   Hypothyroidism
   Hypo- and hyperadrenalism
Pregnancy
Drug-induced
   Tetracycline
   Vitamin A
   Danazol
   Nitrofurantoin
   Lithium
Intoxication
   Chlordecone (a pesticide)
Acute infective polyneuropathy
Spinal cord tumours

Possible pathophysiological mechanisms include an increased rate of formation of cerebrospinal fluid, a decreased rate of absorption through the arachnoid villi, sustained increased venous pressure, and an overall increase in brain water. Despite intensive studies of the few cases that each unit has each year, no clearly defined mechanism has occurred. It used to be said, for example, that the high protein found in the cerebrospinal fluid in acute infective polyneuropathy (Section 19.3.9) or in spinal cord tumours 'clogged the arachnoid villi'. However, the syndrome may be found in patients with these conditions and with normal cerebrospinal fluid protein levels.

Imaging studies show rather small lateral ventricles, indicative of brain oedema. Lumbar puncture can be performed safely, after imaging to exclude mass lesions, as pressure is uniformly distributed throughout the cranio-spinal cavities. Although the pressure can be reduced briefly by lumbar puncture, it very rapidly increases to the previous levels. The mainstays of treatment are diuretics, such as frusemide, and corticosteroid drugs. In those with marked idiopathic intracranial hypertension, it is essential to monitor vision carefully. Central visual acuity is usually comparatively well preserved until late. More sensitive is constriction of the visual field, most particularly infero-nasally. If vision is declining rapidly, it may be necessary to undertake urgent surgical decompression in order to save vision. This can be performed by a subtemporal craniotomy, or the more local operation of fenestration of the optic nerve sheath.

A lumbar–peritoneal CSF shunt may be used for those who fail to respond to medical treatment.

16.10   Further reading

Gliomas—general

Thomas, D. G. T. and McKeran, R. O. (1990). In *Neuro-oncology: primary malignant brain tumours* (ed. D. G. T. Thomas), pp. 141–7. Edward Arnold, London.

Thomas, D. G. T. (ed.) (1990). *Neuro-oncology: primary malignant brain tumours*. Edward Arnold, London.

Walsh, A. R. W., Darling, J. L., and Thomas, D. G. T. (1990). Cerebral gliomas. In *Recent advances in clinical neurology*, (ed. C. Kennard), pp. 241–68. Churchill Livingstone, Edinburgh.

Epidemiology

Walker, A. E., Robins, M., and Weinfield, F. D. (1985). Epidemiology of brain tumours: the national survey of intracranial neoplasms. *Neurology* **35**, 219–26.

Pathology

Russell, D. S. and Rubinstein, L. J. (1989). *Pathology*

of tumours of the nervous system. Edward Arnold, London.

Treatment and prognosis

Black, P. McL. (1991). Brain tumours. *New England Journal of Medicine* **324**, 1471–6; 1555–64.

Cairncross, J. G. and Laperière, N. J. (1989). Low grade glioma: to treat or not to treat? *Archives of Neurology* **46**, 1238–9.

Committee on Health Care Issues (1989). Chemotherapy for malignant glioma. *Annals of Neurology* **25**, 88–9.

Garcia, D. M., Fulling, K. H., and Marks, J. E. (1985). The value of radiation therapy in addition to surgery for astrocytoma of the adult cerebrum. *Cancer* **55**, 919–27.

Mork, S. J., Lindegaard, K. F., Halvesson, T. B., *et al.* (1985). Oligodendroglioma: incidence and biological behaviour in a defined population. *Journal of Neurosurgery* **63**, 881–9.

Piepmeir, J. M. (1987). Observations on the current treatment of low grade astrocytic tumours of the cerebral hemispheres. *Journal of Neurosurgery* **67**, 177–81.

Plowman, P. N. (1990). Focal brain radiotherapy. *Journal of Neurology, Neurosurgery and Psychiatry* **53**, 541.

Walker, M. D., Alexander, E., Hunt, W. E., *et al.* (1978). The evaluation of BCNU and/or radiotherapy in the treatment of anaplastic gliomas—a cooperative clinical trial. *Journal of Neurosurgery* **49**, 333–43.

Wroe, S. J., Foy, P. M., Shaw, M. D. M., *et al.* (1986). Differences between neurological and neurosurgical approaches in the management of malignant brain tumours. *British Medical Journal* **293**, 1015–18.

Meningiomas

Schmidek, H. H. (1991). *Meningiomas and their surgical management.* W. B. Saunders, London and Philadelphia.

Lymphoma

De Angelis, L. M. (1991). Primary central nervous system lymphoma: a new clinical challenge. *Neurology* **41**, 619–21.

Malignant meningitis

Case records of the Massachusetts General Hospital (1988). *New England Journal of Medicine* **318**, 903–15.

Pituitary tumours

Editorial (1990). Management of prolactinoma. *Lancet* **336**, 661.

Jeffcoate, W. J. (1988). Treating Cushing's disease. *British Medical Journal* **296**, 227–8.

Klibanski, A. and Zervas, N. T. (1991). Diagnosis and management of hormone-secreting pituitary adenomas. *New England Journal of Medicine* **324**, 822–31.

Melmed, S. (1990). Acromegaly. *New England Journal of Medicine* **322**, 966–77.

Molitch, M. E. (1991). Gonadotroph-cell pituitary adenomas. *New England Journal of Medicine* **324**, 626–7.

Orth, D. N. (1991). Differential diagnosis of Cushing's syndrome. *New England Journal of Medicine* **325**, 957–9.

Orbital lesions

Fleck, B. W. and Toft, A. D. (1990). Graves' ophthalmopathy. *British Medical Journal* **300**, 1352–3.

Genetic disorders

Maher, E. R., Yates, Y. R. W., and Harries, R. (1990). Clinical features and natural history of von Hippel–Lindau disease. *Quarterly Journal of Medicine, New Series* **77**, 1151–63.

Mulvihill, J. J., *et al.* (1990). Neurofibromatosis 1 (Recklinghausen disease) and neurofibromatosis 2 (bilateral acoustic neurofibromatosis): an update. *Annals of Internal Medicine* **113**, 39–52.

Webb, D. W. and Osborne, J. P. (1992). New research in tuberous sclerosis. *British Medical Journal* **304**, 1647–8.

Idiopathic intracranial hypertension

Corbett, J. J. and Thompson, H. S. (1989). The rational management of idiopathic intracranial hypertension. *Archives of Neurology* **46**, 1049–51.

Wall, M. and George, D. (1991). Idiopathic intracranial hypertension. *Brain* **144**, 155–80.

17 Infections of the nervous system

17.1   Bacterial infections causing pyogenic meningitis

17.1.1   *Routes of bacterial invasion*

Bacteria may gain access to the nervous system through a break in the protective membranes. As an example, a fracture of the base of the skull may be associated with tears of the dura and arachnoid so that cerebrospinal fluid leaks from the ear or nose. Bacterial invasion may occur, and meningitis result. Therefore prophylactic antibiotics are usually given in these circumstances. Occasionally there are small developmental defects, usually in the mid-line, at the top or bottom of the spine, where infolding of the neuroectodermal plate and separation from the skin have been inadequate, leaving sinuses from the skin through to the epidural or subdural space, allowing recurrent infections. Infections may also spread from the paranasal sinuses or middle ear through into the epidural space, and thence into the subarachnoid space. Alternatively, paranasal sinus infection may result in infective thrombus in the cavernous sinus. This presents with proptosis, chemosis, and palsies of the IIIrd, IVth, Vth, and VIth cranial nerves. Infections may also enter the nervous system through infected implanted devices, such as shunts, used in the treatment of hydrocephalus.

Although all these routes of bacterial invasion of the nervous system occur, acute bacterial meningitis is most frequently due to haematogenous spread, although the initial portal of entry is often through the nasal or pharyngeal mucosa. Specialized components of the surface of virulent strains of meningococcus and other bacteria causing meningitis bind with cell surface receptors in the nasopharynx.

17.1.2   *Acute bacterial meningitis*

17.1.2.1   *Epidemiology and pathogenesis*

The incidence of acute bacterial meningitis is about 5–10 per 100 000 per year in developed countries, and far higher in countries still developing. Table 17.1 lists those organisms that are commonly found to cause acute bacterial meningitis. *Haemophilus influenzae*, the meningococcus (*Neisseria meningitidis*), and pneumococcus (*Streptococcus pneumoniae*) account for three-quarters of all cases. The organisms are commonly carried in the nasopharynx of the population. The carrier state is unrelated to the incidence of the disease, but the higher the carrier rate the greater the chance of a susceptible individual being infected.

These three genera of bacteria that commonly cause meningitis probably have similar mechanisms whereby they first gain adherence to the

Table 17.1   Bacteria causing acute meningitis in a developed country. Figures from the Public Health Laboratory Service, Colindale, UK.

	approx. % of cases
Haemophilus influenzae	28
Neisseria meningitidis (meningococcus)	35
Streptococcus pneumoniae (pneumococcus)	16
Mycobacterium tuberculosis	1
Other organisms (staphylococcus, other streptococci, *Escherichia coli*, *Listeria monocytogenes*)	20

nasopharyngeal mucosa, and secondarily penetrate the mucosa to enter the bloodstream. The poly-saccharides that make up their capsule go some way towards preventing phagocytosis, and allow their persistence in the circulation before entry through the blood–meningeal barrier.

Recent interest in meningococcal infections has centred on the increased incidence of the disease in adolescence, and on alterations in the subtypes found. The commonest antigenic groups in the UK are B, C, A, Y, and W135. Of group B, subtype B15 P1;16 sulphonamide-resistant organisms were until recently the most frequent, but now the majority of isolated organisms are non-typeable, which hinders the development of a vaccine.

17.1.2.2   *Clinical features*

In older children and adults, acute bacterial meningitis presents with fever, general malaise, headache, and vomiting. The patient is often drowsy and confused. If untreated, drowsiness progresses to stupor and unconsciousness. The characteristic clinical signs are those of meningeal irritation—a stiff neck and a positive Kernig's sign. This sign is elicited by first flexing the hip and knee, and then attempting to extend the knee. If meningitis is present, reflex spasm in the hamstrings can readily be felt.

Very young children may not show these symptoms and signs, presenting with poor feeding, lethargy, circulatory collapse, jaundice, and irregular breathing. Seizures may occur.

Patients with meningococcal fever may have a petechial rash, often first visible in the conjunctivae, but subsequently becoming widespread over the trunk and limbs. There may be profound hypotension in such patients, due to a combination of bacteraemia and release of endotoxins. Although meningococcal infection is the most common cause of such petechial rashes, petechiae may occur in pneumococcal, staphylococcal, and even some viral meningitides.

An acutely ill, stuporose febrile child or adult with bacterial meningitis may also have seizures in association with the meningitis and local venous infarcts. Papilloedema may be present due to diffuse cerebritis and generalized cerebral oedema.

17.1.2.3   *Investigation*

If there is considerable suspicion of the diagnosis of meningitis, particularly if other children are known to have recently been infected with *N. meningitidis*, then it may be wise to start parenteral benzyl penicillin before transfer to hospital.

In patients with evidence of raised intracranial pressure, a CT scan or MRI is mandatory before lumbar puncture, as the clinical features may be caused by a cerebral abscess (Section 17.2.1). Blood cultures should always be done as the infecting organism may more readily be identified in these than in the CSF.

The principal diagnostic investigation in meningitis is lumbar puncture. In bacterial meningitis the fluid will be turbid to the naked eye, and many hundreds or thousands of polymorphonuclear white cells per microlitre are readily seen on microscopy. A Gram stain will show pneumococci, meningococci, or *H. influenzae* in at least 80 per cent of those infected with these organisms. The concentration of glucose in the cerebrospinal fluid is reduced, not because bacteria metabolize the glucose and 'eat it up' but because meningeal inflammation interferes with the enzyme systems that transport glucose into the subarachnoid space. In addition to arranging an immediate Gram stain (and a Ziehl–Neelsen stain may also be necessary, Section 17.5.1.4), the fluid should be set up in culture for both aerobic and anaerobic organisms.

Sometimes a family doctor will have treated a febrile child with antibiotics before evidence of meningitis became apparent. The abnormalities in the spinal fluid may be modified by such partial treatment; there may be few polymorphs and no bacteria seen on Gram stain, although the glucose concentration often remains low. In order to distinguish such cases from those with viral meningitis, it may be helpful to estimate the concentration of CSF lactate. A level above 115 μmol/l indicates a bacterial infection. The amino-acid concentration may also be raised. It has also been shown that a serum level of C-reactive protein greater than 20 mg/l indicates a probable bacterial meningitis. More specific, however, is finding bacterial antigens that can be identified by counter-immunoelectrophoresis, radioimmunassay, or the ELISA technique (enzyme-linked immunosorbent assay).

17.1.2.4   *Treatment*

Antibiotics only influence the course of bacterial

meningitis if they gain access to the subarachnoid space. With the exception of chloramphenicol, which readily crosses the blood–CSF barrier, antibiotic penetration is dependent upon meningovascular inflammation. Bacteriocidal antibiotics must be chosen, as the encapsulated organisms that commonly cause meningitis resist phagocytosis.

The choice of antibiotic is dependent upon the age of the patient, and whether or not the infecting organism has been rapidly identified by Gram stain or other immediate techniques. It may, however, be some time before the organism is identified, and the gravity of the patient's illness brooks no delay. It is then necessary to begin antibiotic treatment based upon the most likely infecting organism. This is largely dependent upon age.

The neonate with meningitis is most likely to be infected with *Escherichia coli* or group B streptococci. Cefotaxime has replaced the aminoglycosides, which achieve poor levels in the CSF. Cefotaxime is highly effective against Gram-negative neonatal meningitis in a dose of 100 mg/kg/ day. It is only weakly effective against group B streptococcus. It is ineffective against *Listeria monocytogenes*, which accounts for about 7 per cent of cases of neonatal meningitis. It is therefore usual to combine cefotaxime with ampicillin, 150–200 mg/kg/day.

Children of pre-school age are most likely to be infected with *H. influenzae*. For many years ampicillin was the treatment of choice, but β-lactamase-producing strains are now common. Cefotaxime is now the preferred treatment, in a dose 50 mg/kg intravenously every six hours. Chloramphenicol is an alternative, and resistance to this drug is still rare. The dose is 75–100 mg/kg/day. Chloramphenicol penetrates the subarachnoid space very well. Good levels are achieved by oral dosage, so intravenous medication can be discontinued as soon as the child is well enough to swallow.

In older children and adults, infection with *Neisseria meningitidis* (meningococcus) and *Streptococcus pneumoniae* (pneumococcus) is frequent. The treatment of choice is benzyl penicillin. The dose for children is 150 mg/kg/day, given four-hourly, and for adults 1.2–2.4 g every four hours. Intrathecal penicillin should not be used. Chloramphenicol should not be given in conjunction with penicillin, as it antagonizes the latter's bacteriocidal action.

For the common specific organisms, the treatment is as described above. Other antibiotics may need to be used on occasions. Vancomycin is a useful drug for staphylococcal infections and penicillin-resistant *S. pneumoniae*. Cefotaxime is an effective alternative for meningococcal meningitis in those in whom penicillin cannot be used. Ceftazidime is the drug of choice for infections caused by *Pseudomonas aeruginosa*. It is also effective against *H. influenzae* and *N. meningitidis*. *Listeria* infections are best treated with ampicillin. Flucloxacillin (or, in the USA, nafcillin) is used for the treatment of meningitis due to *Staphylococcus aureus*. Vancomycin is an alternative.

Although the specific antimicrobial therapy has been considered first, there is much else to be done in the general supportive management of the patient acutely ill with meningitis. Septic shock may be resistant to volume replacement and sympathomimetic pressor agents. Although adrenal haemorrhages are found in some cases of meningococcal septicaemia (the Waterhouse–Friderichsen syndrome), the profound hypotension often seen probably is not related to this, and corticosteroids have not been shown to be of benefit in management. General nursing care, attention to urine drainage, to the integrity of the skin, and to fluid and electrolyte balance are important in reducing mortality. Although the bacteria are often relatively easily killed by an appropriately chosen antibiotic, the effects of circulating endotoxins are not at present reversible. However, trials are being made of the infusion of antibodies to endotoxins.

Trials have shown that dexamethasone, given early in acute bacterial meningitis in children, usually caused by *H. influenzae*, reduces the subsequent incidence of sensorineural hearing loss and other neurological abnormalities. Steroid treatment is not yet standard practice, but from the evidence it should be. A suitable dose is 0.15 mg/ kg given 20 minutes before the first dose of antibiotic, and continued four times a day for four days.

17.1.2.5   *Prognosis*

The mortality for acute bacterial meningitis remains high, particularly in the very young and in those over 60. The overall mortality in developed countries is about 5 per cent for infections with

H. influenzae, 10 per cent for *N. meningitidis*, and 20–30 per cent for *S. pneumoniae*. In the UK in 1989 there were 1142 notified cases of meningococcal meningitis, 228 of meningococcal septicaemia, and 203 deaths.

Survival with permanent neurological damage can occur. Children with high serum levels of C-reactive protein (>300 mg/l) during the acute illness are particularly likely to have neurological sequelae. Sensorineural deafness is common, and other cranial nerve palsies may occur. The cognitive development of younger children may be permanently retarded. Hydrocephalus may develop. Neonates may develop sterile collections of fluid over the brain—a subdural hygroma. Epilepsy may occur after an interval, due to focal areas of cortical damage. Those children who have no neurological signs after recovery of the acute illness are most unlikely to develop seizures.

17.1.2.6   *Prophylaxis*

Vaccines against some virulent subtypes of meningococcus (A, C, Y, W135, but not group B) have been raised, and are effective in localized communities. They are recommended to travellers to Mecca and the Sudan, where the disease is endemic. For those recently exposed to a case of meningococcal meningitis, rifampicin, 10 mg/kg twice daily for two days, will successfully clear the nasopharynx of the organism and prevent meningitis.

17.1.3   *Brucellosis*

Brucella abortus is usually acquired through the consumption of infected dairy products, but those who work in close association with cattle, such as dairy farmers and veterinarians, are particularly at risk. An acute or chronic meningoencephalitis may occur. Prolonged treatment with rifampicin and doxycycline is necessary to eradicate the infection.

17.2   Intracranial and spinal abscesses

17.2.1   *Brain abscess*

The routes of bacterial invasion resulting in a cerebral abscess are much the same as for bacterial meningitis. An abscess may arise through direct extension of infection in the middle ear or mastoid cavity, or in the paranasal sinuses. Haematogenous infection occurs as a result of metastatic infection from elsewhere in the body. Immunosuppression by drugs or by AIDS predisposes to brain abscesses, as does diabetes mellitus. Atrial or ventricular septal defects in congenital heart disease provide a direct path to the cerebral arterial circulation of venous blood potentially contaminated by minor infections of the hands or feet. An abscess may occur secondary to missile penetration of the skull.

The clinical features of a cerebral abscess are seizures, altered consciousness, and focal neurological signs, dependent upon its location. Systematic evidence of infection, such as a fever or peripheral leucocytosis, may not be obvious. Blood cultures should be performed, as the organism may be cultured.

Abscesses are readily visible on CT scans or MRI. The most characteristic appearance on CT is a zone of low attenuation surrounded by a ring of contrast enhancement, but a more irregular multilocular appearance may be seen, and enhancement may not be prominent. Imaging may also give evidence of the site of origin of the abscess, e.g. in the frontal sinus.

The treatment of cerebral abscesses includes surgical excision or aspiration, and antibiotic therapy. If the abscess is in the cerebellum or in the tip of a frontal or temporal lobe, then radical excision in the acute stage may be possible. Alternatively, repeated aspiration of pus through one or more burr holes is necessary, replacing the pus by instilled antibiotics. Shrinkage in the size of the abscess can be monitored by repeated CT scans or MRI.

Abscesses secondary to sinus infection are usually due to anaerobic streptococci. Penicillin, chloramphenicol, or metronidazole may be used. Abscesses of otitic origin usually yield mixed species, often including *Bacteroides* and *Proteus* species. A similar regime with the addition of ampicillin may be used. Traumatic abscesses often contain staphylococci, and fusidic acid, erythromycin, or clindamycin are all useful drugs in this instance.

In spite of early medical and surgical treatment, mortality from cerebral abscesses remains around 10–15 per cent. Epilepsy is a particularly frequent late complication. An abscess may recur many months after it has been thought to be eradicated.

17.2.2 *Extradural and subdural abscesses*

An extradural abscess (also known as an epidural abscess) is usually caused by extension of infection from the frontal sinuses, or from the mastoid cavity. There is intense local pain and oedema of the scalp. Extradural abscesses can also occur in the spinal column, usually secondary to an infection in a vertebral body. Surgical drainage and appropriate antibiotic therapy is urgently required. Pott's disease of the spine (Section 17.5.4) is one particular variety of spinal extradural abscess, in which the infecting organism is *Mycobacterium tuberculosis*.

A subdural abscess is often secondary to sinus or mastoid infection, the organisms spreading via the diploic veins without necessarily involving the vault. Once in the subdural space, the infection spreads rapidly, and results in thrombotic occlusion of many cortical veins. The prognosis is grave, as it may not be easy to eradicate the pus. Residual neurological deficits are common in survivors.

17.3 Bacterial infections associated with cerebrospinal fluid shunts

As does a catheter in the bladder, the presence of a shunt in the ventricles (see Section 22.2.2) is associated with a significant risk of infection. The shunt is usually colonized at the time of insertion, as retrograde haematogenous spread in the case of ventriculo-atrial shunts does not seem to occur. Most shunt colonizations are due to *Staphylococcus epidermidis*, but occasionally infection is due to *Corynebacterium* species, streptococci and yeasts. Serial monitoring of antibody levels to *S. epidermidis* against a pre-operative titre may be a useful way of detecting shunt infection. The measurement of C-reactive protein is also useful. There may be a secondary bacteraemia with symptoms of systemic infection, with positive blood cultures. The fact that the most frequent infecting organism is the organism that most frequently contaminates blood cultures during sampling compounds the difficulties in diagnosis.

Chronic infection of shunts may lead to so-called 'shunt nephritis' due to the deposition of antibody complexes in the glomeruli.

It is almost always necessary to remove the shunt in order to eradicate infection.

17.4 Spirochaetal infections

17.4.1 *Neurosyphilis*

Neurosyphilis has become uncommon since the Second World War, partly on account of a greater recognition of the risk of venereal disease from casual sexual encounters and a wider recognition of the early clinical manifestations of syphilis. A major factor in its decline, however, is the widespread use of bacteriocidal antibiotics in the treatment of incidental infections, which probably eradicate many cases of unsuspected asymptomatic neurosyphilis. The present epidemiology is confused. A greater incidence of protected intercourse since the advent of AIDS (Section 17.12.11) has probably led to a decline in infection rates. However, the immunosuppression of AIDS results in accelerated progress of neurosyphilis if there is co-incident infection with both HIV and *Treponema pallidum*.

Invasion of the nervous system by the spirochaete occurs early in the course of syphilis, the majority of patients having evidence of a lymphocytic meningitis during the secondary stage. This usually begins within 6 weeks of the healing of the primary chancre. In only a small proportion of patients is there clinical evidence of meningitic infection at this stage, but some will have headache and neck stiffness, cranial nerve palsies (particularly of the VIth, VIIth, and VIIIth cranial nerves), papilloedema, and seizures. This acute syphilitic meningitis, which may also occur up to 2 years after the primary infection, responds well to treatment with penicillin.

After the secondary stage, if untreated, a syphilitic infection of the nervous system will settle into a stage of asymptomatic neurosyphilis, in which the only evidence of infection lies in the spinal fluid (see Table 17.2). After this asymptomatic stage, neurosyphilis may develop as one or more of three clinical syndromes—meningovascular syphilis, general paresis, and tabes dorsalis.

Table 17.2   Stages of neurosyphilis, and the results of investigations

	Secondary syphilis	Acute syphilitic meningitis	Asymptomatic neurosyphilis	Meningovascular neurosyphilis	General paresis	Tabes dorsalis
Blood						
VDRL	+	+	usually+	+	+	maybe −
FTA-Abs	+	+	+	+	+	+
CSF						
cells/μl	moderate increase	many	moderate increase	many	moderate increase	normal or slight increase
protein	slight increase	increased	moderately raised	moderately increased	moderately increased	normal or slightly increased
VDRL	+	+	+ or −	+	+	often −
FTA-Abs	+	+	+	+	+	+

VDRL, Venereal Disease Reference Laboratory slide floculation test; FTA-Abs, fluorescent treponemal antibody-absorption test.

17.4.1.1   Meningovascular syphilis

Meningovascular syphilis usually occurs within 5–10 years of the primary infection. The pathology is that of a subacute meningitis, with infiltration of the thickened meninges with lymphocytes and plasma cells. Such a granulomatous infiltrate may reach some size, when it is called a gumma. These contain fibroblasts, histiocytes and giant cells, and may have a central necrotic region. Larger gummata may lie in the subcortical regions and act as a space-occupying lesion, and require surgical management.

In addition to the meningeal thickening, there is intimal proliferation in small arteries. A combination of meningeal and vasculitic lesions leads to cranial nerve palsies. Lesions of the VIIIth nerve are particularly common. Intimal proliferation in larger arteries is accompanied by perivascular infiltration with plasma cells and lymphocytes. This inflammatory arteritis (Heubner's arteritis) may lead to occlusion of a major artery, commonly the middle cerebral artery, and lead to a hemiplegia.

Meningovascular syphilis may also affect the spinal cord. The spinal roots are affected by the meningeal inflammatory response in a similar fashion to the cranial nerves (syphilitic cervical pachymeningitis). Combinations of multiple radicular lesions and long tract signs due to spinal cord infarction may occur (syphilitic meningomyelitis). The CSF is always abnormal in meningovascular

syphilis (see Table 17.2). Arteriography shows concentric narrowing and dilatation of smaller vessels. Arterial occlusions may be demonstrated. CT scanning may show multiple areas of infarction or gummata, which appear as avascular masses.

17.4.1.2   General paresis (synonym: general paresis of the insane, GPI)

Although this syndrome is associated with a chronic round-cell infiltration of the meninges and an arteritis of small vessels, the characteristic feature in this type of neurosyphilis is direct spirochaetal involvement of the brain. This results in loss of neurons and astrocytic proliferation, which is particularly marked in the frontal and temporal lobes. Spirochaetes are often readily visible microscopically.

General paresis affects about 40 per cent of those with neurosyphilis, beginning 10–20 years after the primary infection. Men are more often affected than women. The symptoms are similar to those seen in dementia of other types (Section 11.5.1.1), and are often accompanied by depression or agitation. The grandiose delusional picture—a man of humble means going out to order a Rolls Royce—is always remembered, but was always uncommon. Dementia is often accompanied by seizures, a tremulous dysarthria and ataxia, and dysphasia. The CSF is always abnormal (see Table 17.2).

17.4.1.3 *Tabes dorsalis*

This is about the most frequent form of neuro-syphilis. 'Tabes' means wasting. The name describes the typical wasting of the dorsal roots, which is the hallmark of the syndrome. The central processes of the dorsal root ganglion cells lie in the dorsal columns, and secondary degeneration in the dorsal columns is readily apparent at autopsy. Spirochaetes are not generally demonstrated in the dorsal roots or ganglion cells. Although there is mild leptomeningeal thickening over the roots and dorsal columns, the mechanism underlying the histological changes is uncertain.

Tabes begins about 10–20 years after the primary infection. A characteristic early feature is lightning pains. These are sudden stabbing paroxysmal pains, usually in the legs, which last a few seconds. Other types of painful paraesthesiae may occur. As the dorsal roots waste, symptoms due to deafferentation become prominent, with unsteadiness that is worse when the eyes are closed. This is the basis of Romberg's sign (See Section 6.3.1.3). As there is a loss of the sense of awareness of where the feet are in space, the patient adopts a high-stepping gait to reduce tripping. Deafferentation leads to a painless degenerative arthropathy, with much new bone formation (Charcot's joints). Deafferentation also affects the control of micturition, so a large bladder and painless overflow incontinence occur. Autonomic reflexes are impaired, so that impotence, constipation, and postural hypotension are common. Other poorly understood types of autonomic dysfunction result in acute abdominal pain—the so-called tabetic crisis—and laryngeal spasm with dyspnoea. Trophic changes in the skin cause painless ulcers on the soles of the feet.

On examination, the clinical findings are largely those indicated above, but other characteristics are loss of tendon reflexes in the lower limbs, loss of sense of passive movement in at least the distal joints, loss of perception of a vibrating tuning fork, and loss of perception of pain. The loss of pain perception classically first occurs over the nose, the inner aspect of the forearms, and the outer border of the legs and feet. The loss of myotatic reflexes due to deafferentation allows gross hypotonia, so straight leg-raising may reach 130° or more.

Tabes is often associated with optic atrophy, nerve deafness, and partial oculomotor palsies, often with ptosis. Of classical interest are the pupil abnormalities described by Argyll Robertson. The iris loses some pigmentation and appears atrophied. The pupil is small and irregular, and does not react to light, but does on accommodation. One explanation for this dissociation is that the afferent inputs to the Edinger–Westphal nucleus concerned with accommodation lie more anteriorly than those concerned in the light reflex, so that subependymal gliosis may differentially affect the afferent pathways. However, as dissociation between light and accommodation reflexes is seen in patients with hypertrophic neuropathy (Déjérine–Sottas disease, Section 19.3.8) and in some cases of diabetes, it may be that there is a more peripheral mechanism.

The diagnosis of tabes dorsalis often rests on clinical grounds, as the changes in the CSF are less prominent than in those of the other syndromes of neurosyphilis (Table 17.2).

17.4.1.4 *Congenital neurosyphilis*

The neurological syndromes are much as in acquired neurosyphilis, but brought forward to an earlier stage of life. Meningovascular syphilis is the commonest form, but general paresis can occur. A good portrayal of how the problem affected families is seen in Ibsen's play, *Ghosts*. We now have our similar plays about HIV infection.

17.4.1.5 *Coincident infection with human immunodeficiency virus (HIV)*

The alteration in the immune state induced by HIV may accelerate the progression of neurosyphilis. Difficulties in diagnosing neurosyphilis in association with HIV infection may arise. First, CSF pleocytosis is common to both conditions. Secondly, HIV can produce a clinical picture of dementia, strokes, and myelopathy similar to syphilis. Thirdly, the standard serological tests for syphilis may be non-reactive in the presence of HIV infection.

17.4.1.6 *Tests for syphilis*

Infection with *T. pallidum* results in two forms of antibodies—non-specific IgG and IgM antibodies against lipoidal antigens, and specific antibodies directed against components of the treponeme.

The first type of antibodies are assessed by the so-called reaginic tests—Rapid Plasma Reagin (RPR) or Venereal Disease Reference Laboratory (VDRL) slide floculation tests. The VDRL is not specific for treponemal infection, but its titre does reflect disease activity. The specific antibody test is known as the fluorescent treponemal antibody-absorption test (FTA-Abs). It is specific for treponemal infection, but cannot distinguish current or past-eradicated infection, nor infection with the yaws treponeme.

Table 17.2 shows the findings in blood and CSF in the different stages of syphilis affecting the nervous system.

17.4.1.7 Treatment

Treatment recommended by the World Health Organization is procaine penicillin, 600 mg/day for 20 days. Adequate CSF levels are not obtained with long-acting benzathine penicillin G. About 4 per cent of the population are allergic to penicillin. Tetracycline has been used for such patients.

A proportion of patients with neurosyphilis will demonstrate an exacerbation of symptoms and signs, with fever and tachycardia, within a few hours of the first injection of penicillin. The response, known as the Jarisch–Herxheimer reaction, is not related to the dose of penicillin, so there is no point in giving small doses initially. Corticosteroids are used for a day or two before penicillin by some physicians. This does not prevent the reaction, but may reduce its severity.

17.4.1.8 Prognosis

Fixed neurological deficits due to arterial occlusions or changes in the dorsal roots will clearly not be improved by eradicating infection, but progression appears to be prevented. There may be a modest improvement after treatment in the mental state in general paresis. Successful treatment is indicated by a return of the CSF pleocytosis and elevated protein concentration to normal. This may take several weeks. The serum RPR and VDRL titres fall and may become negative; the FTA-Abs rather more often remains positive.

17.4.2 Lyme disease

17.4.2.1 Epidemiology and pathogenesis

Lyme is a small town in Connecticut, near which this unusual and worrying disease was first clearly identified as being due to an infection caused by a spirochaete, *Borrelia burgdorferi*. However, the dermatological and neurological associations were previously recognized in Europe as the syndrome of Bannwarth, who described patients with a painful radiculopathy or facial palsies, and a pleocytosis in the spinal fluid. The organism is transmitted primarily by the bite of *Ixodes* ticks, the usual mammalian hosts of which are deer and raccoons. However, the spirochaete has also been isolated from the mouthparts of horseflies and mosquitoes.

17.4.2.2 Clinical features

The first stage of the disease is an expanding erythematous rash, usually centred on the tick bite. This is known as erythema chronicum migrans. However, secondary cutaneous eruptions may appear distant to the bite, and these are accompanied by malaise, fever, headache, and muscle aches and lymphadenopathy. These symptoms may settle without any treatment. However, about 15 per cent of patients go on to develop neurological problems. About 80 per cent of those neurologically affected have a meningitic illness, with a lymphocytic pleocytosis and elevated CSF protein. The CSF sugar is usually normal, but can be moderately reduced. The organism has been isolated from the fluid at this stage. Difficulties in diagnosis may arise as the patient may not have been aware of the original bite, and erythema chronicum migrans may not have occurred. Many of those with meningitis have an associated encephalopathy, ranging from drowsiness and depression to frank changes in cognitive function, ataxia, and seizures. Also prominent in the clinical picture are cranial neuropathies, commonly facial palsies, and a diffuse radiculoneuropathy. This may present as a mononeuritis multiplex or as a more diffuse but asymmetrical polyneuropathy. Root pains are frequent.

Cardiac involvement develops in about 8 per cent of patients. Features include either an atrioventricular block, or a diffuse myocarditis. Several months after infection, about 60 per cent of those infected develop a recurrent arthropathy affecting large joints, with effusions and subsequent chronic synovitis with erosion of joint cartilage.

Most of these pathological events are caused by direct borrelian invasion of tissues, but there is evidence that some late neurological events may be caused by immune-mediated processes.

17.4.2.3 *Diagnosis*

Specific IgM antibody to *Borrelia burgdorferi* antigen rises to a peak 3–6 weeks after infection, and specific IgG antibody rises later. In the acute stages of the illness, therefore, the diagnosis may rest upon clinical and epidemiological features.

17.4.2.4 *Treatment and prognosis*

Oral doxycycline 100 mg twice daily or amoxycillin 500 mg three times daily for 10–21 days will largely prevent the onset of neurological disease or arthropathy, but may be ineffective once neurological involvement has begun. High-dose intravenous penicillin (20 million units daily in divided doses for 10–21 days) may, however, still succeed in eradicating the disease. Ceftriaxone 2 g daily by single intravenous dose for 14–21 days is now appearing to be more effective than penicillin.

Some patients continue to experience chronic fatigue, poor memory, joint pains, and numbness of the extremities after treatment. This 'Post-Lyme disease' syndrome is probably due to persistent infection in the absence of detectable serum antibody, and may resolve after vigorous bacteriocidal therapy. A few patients develop a clear-cut chronic encephalomyelitis, with spasticity and sphincter disturbance.

17.4.3 *Leptospirosis*

Leptospira interrogans is excreted in the urine of wild and domestic animals, most often rodents, and may affect humans. Those particularly at risk are farmers, sewermen, and those who work in abattoirs. The organism usually enters through abraded skin. The illness commonly causes myalgia, fever, purpura, and jaundice (Weil's disease). However, *Leptospira* enters the nervous system within a day or two of infection. An aseptic meningitis may follow later, probably mediated by an immune response to leptospiral antigen, as the organism disappears from the CSF before active meningitis begins. Although polymorphonuclear cells may initially predominate, lymphocytes soon replace them, and may persist for several weeks after clinical resolution. Uveitis may occur with

meningitis. Occasionally an encephalopathy or an acute ascending polyneuropathy may occur. The treatment of choice is intravenous penicillin.

17.5 Tuberculosis

Tuberculosis of the nervous system is manifest either as a subacute meningitic illness or through the space-occupying effects of a tuberculoma, or of tuberculous pus.

17.5.1 *Tuberculous meningitis*

17.5.1.1 *Epidemiology*

This is still a common and often fatal illness in developing countries, and is still seen in the UK and USA, often in the socially and economically deprived. In the UK population, Asians are particularly likely to be affected. Children are most frequently affected, but the disease can occur at any age.

Tuberculous meningitis is increasing in those African countries in which HIV infection is widespread.

17.5.1.2 *Pathogenesis*

Mycobacterium tuberculosis does not gain widespread access to the nervous system at the stage of the primary infection. Tuberculous meningitis may not occur when other organs are widely affected by miliary tubercles. However, one or more meningeal tubercles may form at the time of the primary infection or soon after. The subsequent rupture of this tubercle, possibly in response to an immunological stimulus, allows free dissemination of bacilli into the subarachnoid space, and subsequent multiplication and the onset of clinical illness. This process was described by Rich in 1933. The meningeal tubercle is therefore called a Rich focus. Autopsy examination of those with the fully developed illness shows a number of tuberculous manifestations. These include disseminated meningeal tubercles, focal caseous meningeal plaques, and an acute inflammatory caseous meningitis, with a diffuse gelatinous exudate in the meshes of the pia arachnoid. This gelatinous meningitis is particularly prominent in the anterior basal cisterns, and, in life, this often results in cranial nerve palsies and a communicating hydro-cephalus. Less commonly, an obstructive hydro-cephalus occurs due to occlusion of the foramina of Luschka and Magendie. As the cranial arteries traverse the subarachnoid space, they too are affected, and an inflammatory arteritis may result in large areas of infarction. Similar changes affect the spinal meninges. Animal experiments suggest that the fully developed pathological picture depends, in part, upon a delayed hypersensitivity response to mycobacterial antigens.

17.5.1.3 *Clinical features*

The usual onset of tuberculous meningitis is insidi-ous. General malaise, headache, irritability, and other behavioural changes become increasingly apparent over 2–6 weeks. A low-grade fever and signs of meningeal irritation occur. If the diagnosis is not made at this stage, there is a rapid progres-sion with markedly increased headache, vomiting, neck stiffness, and drowsiness, and the develop-ment of cranial nerve palsies. Papilloedema often occurs, and fundoscopy may show the presence of choroidal tubercles. If untreated, stupor increases and death follows.

Occasionally, tuberculous meningitis may pres-ent much more abruptly, in a fashion similar to that of acute meningitis of other bacterial origin (Section 17.1.2).

17.5.1.4 *Investigations*

Although many patients with tuberculous menin-gitis have evidence of pulmonary or other tuber-culosis, this is not always the case, and a normal chest X-ray does not exclude the diagnosis. The Mantoux test is usually positive, but may be nega-tive in immunologically incompetent patients in whom tuberculosis may be an adventitious infection.

The crucial investigation is the examination of the spinal fluid. The total cell count is often between 40 and 400 per microlitre and, in the later stages, almost all of these are lymphocytes. Ini-tially, neutrophils may predominate. Of crucial importance in distinguishing a tubercular lympho-cytic meningitis from a viral lymphocytic meningi-tis is the finding of a low CSF sugar, often less than 2 mmol/l. The CSF protein is often considerably raised (>1 g/l). Mycobacteria can often be found

in the first specimen on microscopy of a Ziehl–Neelsen-stained sample. The chances of success are increased if the centrifuged deposit from a large (10–20 ml) sample is examined. Acridine orange and auramine-rhodamine stains are more sensitive, but these require a fluorescence micro-scope. However, bacilli are often not seen in subjects in whom clinical suspicion is high. Altern-ative diagnostic methods have been suggested, including the ratio of partition of bromide between blood and CSF, detection of adenosine deaminase activity in CSF, and various immunological meth-ods for the detection of mycobacterial antigens. These include the use of a murine monoclonal antibody to the 38 kDa antigen in a variant of the enzyme-linked immunosorbent assay, and the detection of cells in the spinal fluid which secrete antibodies to BCG. Another promising method is the use of the polymerase chain reaction to amplify the available quantity of bacterial DNA in the spinal fluid. Finally, specific chemical components of the bacterial wall, such as tuberculostearic acid, can be detected using gas chromatography/mass spectrometry.

17.5.1.5 *Differential diagnosis*

The differential diagnosis includes infection by fungi or parasites, e.g. *Cryptococcus neoformans* (Section 17.11.1) or *Toxoplasma gondii* (Sec-tion 17.10.1), partly treated bacterial meningitis (Sec-tion 17.1.2), sarcoid meningitis (Section 17.17.1), and diffuse meningeal involvement with malignant cells, including carcinoma, lymphoma, leukaemia, glioma, melanoma, and medulloblastoma (Section 16.4.1). Parameningeal abscesses (Section 17.2.2) may also cause a lymphocytic reaction in the spinal fluid.

Occasionally the CSF sugar may be significantly reduced in patients with herpes simplex encephali-tis, but not in any other viral infection.

17.5.1.6 *Treatment*

The outcome of tuberculous meningitis depends upon the stage at which treatment is commenced, morbidity and mortality considerably increasing with delay. It is always necessary to begin treat-ment with antituberculous therapy before the results of culture and sensitivity are known. It is also often necessary to begin treatment on suspicion alone, based upon a lymphocytic pleocytosis and a low CSF sugar, if clinical suspicion is strong and yet repeated Ziehl–Neelsen and other stains are negative.

The treatment of choice at present is isoniazid, 20 mg/kg/day for 1 month (maximum 600 mg/day), reducing to 10 mg/kg/day (maximum 300 mg), combined with rifampicin, 10 mg/kg/day (maximum 600 mg), and pyrazinamide, 30 mg/kg/day. All these drugs can be given in once-daily dosage. As isoniazid interferes with the metabolism of pyridoxine, increasing its excretion in the form of xanthenuric acid, it is essential to give pyridoxine supplements (10 mg twice a day for an adult). The necessary minimum duration of treatment is uncertain, but it is usual practice to stop pyrazinamide after 2 months and to continue rifampicin and isoniazid for 10 months.

In acutely ill patients, streptomycin can be added by intramuscular injection, in a dose of 20 mg/kg/day for the first 2 weeks or so, restraining the dose within the limits of ototoxicity. Some physicians add intrathecal streptomycin, 25–50 mg daily.

Rifampicin is expensive, and an alternative regime in developing countries is isoniazid, initial streptomycin, and thiacetazone or pyrazinamide. p-Aminosalicylic acid does not cross the blood–brain barrier and is of no use in the management of tuberculous meningitis. Corticosteroids have been used in the hope that the fibrous component of the meningeal reaction will be diminished, with a consequent reduction in the incidence of hydrocephalus, but there is no good evidence of their efficacy.

17.5.1.7 Prognosis

Although antibiotic therapy usually results in an early clinical improvement if given in the early stages of the illness, the pleocytosis and low sugar concentration in the spinal fluid take many weeks to resolve. Coexistent tuberculomas (Section 17.5.2) may show continued expansion on repeated CT scanning for many weeks, in spite of clinical improvement.

Mortality is directly related to conscious level and the extent of physical signs on beginning treatment. It is nowadays rare to lose a patient who is orientated at the time that treatment is started, but the disease continues to carry a high mortality in developing countries.

Even if the infection is eradicated from those severely affected, there may be residual neurological damage manifest by mental retardation, epilepsy, optic atrophy, and persistent cranial nerve palsies, resulting particularly in squints and deafness. Hydrocephalus may occur, and a shunt may be necessary.

17.5.2 Tuberculomas

Tuberculomas are granulomatous lesions with varying degrees of central necrosis within the brain or spinal cord, reaching sufficient size to produce epilepsy or focal neurological disability and signs. Although rare in developed countries, they are among the most frequent space-occupying lesions presenting to Asian neurosurgeons. They account for more than 40 per cent of all 'tumours' in Indian children aged less than 15 years. They are also particularly likely to develop in patients with AIDS (Section 17.12.12.3). It is not possible to distinguish reliably a tuberculoma from a glioma by the appearance on the CT scan, and biopsy is usually necessary, although a practical and economic method of management in developing countries is to try the effects of antituberculous treatment in the first instance. A tuberculoma less than 2 cm in size will often resolve on antibiotic treatment. Larger tuberculomas will require excision, presumably their greater radius preventing adequate diffusion of antibiotics to their centre.

As already noted, tuberculomas may coexist with tuberculous meningitis.

17.5.3 Tuberculous radiculomyelopathy

A gelatinous chronic tubercular exudate may ensheathe the spinal roots and cord over a varying length, the patient then presenting with paraplegia, disturbance of sphincter control, and root pain. This pathological picture can arise from a primary spinal tuberculous meningitis, or secondary to the more usual cranio-basal tuberculous meningitis.

17.5.4 Tuberculous disease of the spine (Pott's disease)

A patient may present with a sudden or rapidly

advancing paraplegia due to an extradural granuloma, or collection of extradural pus, extending from an infected vertebra. There may be an associated cold abscess. This is a fluctuant bag of pus, without the usual 'warmth' of pyogenic inflammation, which is found on the chest wall, in the groin, or upper thigh, depending upon the route by which the pus has tracked from the infected vertebra. Treatment is immediate surgical decompression combined with antituberculous therapy as described in Section 17.5.1.6.

17.6 Leprosy

Leprosy is the most common cause of peripheral nerve lesions world-wide. It is the only common cause of palpable thickening of peripheral nerves. The only other disorders that can cause enlargement of the peripheral nerves are some of the inherited hypertrophic neuropathies (e.g. Déjérine–Sottas disease, Section 19.3.8).

Leprosy is due to infection by *Mycobacterium leprae*. The clinical manifestations depend in part upon direct invasion of tissues by the organism, and in part due to the cell-mediated immune response. In those subjects who do not mount a good immune response, lepromatous leprosy is a generalized bacteraemic disease involving widely the skin, peripheral nerves, the upper respiratory tract, the eyes, and bone. It is probably through the nasal secretions of infected lepromatous patients that the disease is passed from person to person, the portal probably being the respiratory tract, although the epidemiological characteristics of the infectious process remain uncertain. The onset of clinical features following exposure is of the order of 5–10 years, as judged by the onset of symptoms in those who have visited briefly and then returned from endemic areas.

As already mentioned, the spectrum of clinical features is dependent upon the extent of the immune response mounted by the patient. In lepromatous (low resistance) leprosy, hypopigmented erythematous smooth macules with indeterminate edges are seen all over the body, with involvement of the nasal mucosa. Further invasion of the skin results in generalized thickening of the skin, particularly the skin of the face and the ear lobes. Dermal nerve fibres are gradually destroyed, and this results in progressive loss of sensation, usually most prominent distally, but eventually involving much of the skin of the body. Hairy areas of skin are relatively well preserved. Deeper involvement of dermal tissues and subdermal tissues results in bony infiltration and resorption of the phalanges and heads and shafts of the metatarsals. Many peripheral nerves may be enlarged. On histological examination, the dermis is diffusely infiltrated by large numbers of *M. leprae*, many lying within histiocytes. For lepromatous patients, formal biopsy is not necessary, a drop of tissue pulp being collected from the side wall of a deep incision, and stained for acid-fast bacilli.

If there is a high degree of cell-mediated immunity, infection by *M. leprae* leads to the development of only one, or a few, skin lesions, usually of larger size with a raised outer edge and a thin reddened rim. The destruction of dermal nerves results in loss of sensation in these lesions. Cutaneous nerve bundles are, however, involved to a comparatively limited extent, and only one or two thickened nerves may be found. On histological examination, acid-fast bacilli are rare, but biopsy of the active edge of the lesion shows a tuberculoid granuloma with epithelioid cells and lymphocytes.

Intermediate forms between tuberculous and lepromatous leprosy are also frequent.

From a neurologist's point of view, some cutaneous nerves and nerve trunks are particularly likely to be involved by leprosy. These include the superficial branch of the radial nerve as it passes near the radial styloid, the median nerve at the wrist, the ulnar nerve just above the medial epicondyle, and the greater auricular nerve as it runs towards the ear up the posterior border of the sternomastoid muscle. Lepromatous or tuberculoid infiltration of branches of peripheral nerves may result in areas of local anaesthesia conforming to the distribution of the nerve. Involvement of a nerve trunk, such as the ulnar nerve at the elbow, may result in a typical ulnar palsy (Section 19.4.2.5).

The detailed management of leprosy is beyond the scope of this book. The available drug regimens are, to some extent, dependent upon the financial and medical resources of those impoverished regions of the world in which leprosy is endemic. Rifampicin is a highly effective agent, but its expense precludes its global use. Where available, it can be effectively given in a single dose of 600 mg once monthly, under supervision in a field clinic, combined with two other drugs in order to prevent the emergence of bacillary resistance. The World Health Organization (WHO) regime adds to rifampicin (600 mg once a month), clofazimine—50 mg each day unsupervised, plus 300 mg as a supervised dose at a field clinic once a month. The third drug used is dapsone, 100 mg daily, unsupervised. Dapsone was the first drug to be introduced for the effective treatment of leprosy, and has the great advantage of being cheap. However, dapsone resistance commonly emerges, and a significant proportion of subjects are also allergic to this drug. Clofazimine is a fat-soluble dye, which is also bacillocidal. It is a successful drug for those with dark-brown or black skins. For those with light skins, a significant adverse effect is a prominent reddish-brown pigmentation of the skin, which becomes apparent within a few months.

The WHO regimen outlined above should be given for a minimum of 2 years, and continued until no bacilli are visible on a pulp smear. This may result in some patients receiving antileprous therapy for 10 years or so.

One type of reaction to antileprous chemotherapy is erythema nodosum leprosum, characterized by fever, general malaise, ulceration of the skin lesions, lymphadenitis, and the onset of pain in the infected nerves. Antileprous chemotherapy should be continued, the reaction being treated with prednisolone, 40 mg/day. This usually results in a brisk remission of symptoms. Another type of reaction is known as a reversal reaction, as treatment appears to initiate a change from the lepromatous end of the clinical spectrum towards the tuberculoid end. Painful neuritis is again a feature, the skin lesions may become swollen and oedematous, and new lesions may occur during the course of the reaction.

The prevention of leprosy is largely dependent upon the reduction of the numbers of those with active disease in endemic regions by appropriate chemotherapy. A vaccine consisting of killed *Mycobacterium leprae*, derived from armadillos (the only animal to which leprosy can readily be transmitted), combined with live BCG vaccine has been developed and is under test in various parts of the world.

17.7 Bacteria that produce neurological effects through toxins

17.7.1 *Tetanus*

The clinical syndrome of tetanus results from the effects of the neurotoxin produced by infection by *Clostridium tetani*. The spores of this anaerobic organism are widely distributed in soil and in street dust. Although *C. tetani* may be found in the bowel, virtually all clinical tetanus results from external contamination. In developed countries, the disease has largely been prevented by a policy of active immunization but, in those who are unprotected, a dirty penetrating wound, such as a dog bite or a compound limb fracture, can cause tetanus after a latent period. In developing countries, *C. tetani* infection of the umbilical stump (tetanus neonatorum) is a common cause of perinatal death.

17.7.1.1 *Pathophysiology*

The latent period after infection may be between 5 days and 2–3 months, probably depending upon the magnitude of the bacterial contamination. The multiplying *C. tetani* bacilli produce the toxin, known as tetanospasmin. This is coded for extrachromosomally by a plasmid. The toxin is bound to neuronal membranes. Toxin enters nerve endings near the site of the wound and travels centripetally in membrane-bound vesicles in axoplasm to spinal motor neurons. It then passes transsynaptically to the surrounding glycinergic inhibitory terminals, and prevents release of glycine and other inhibitory transmitters. The failure of presynaptic inhibition results in muscle spasms that may be induced by attempts to move, or occur spontaneously.

17.7.1.2 *Clinical features*

The local centripetal spread of toxin accounts for the rare phenomenon of local tetanus affecting only the wound-bearing limb. More frequently, the extent of toxin uptake is such that generalized tetanus occurs.

In generalized tetanus, the first features are trismus—'lockjaw'—and retraction of the angles of the mouth in the so-called 'risus sardonicus' (sardonic smile). Pain and stiffness in paraspinal and abdominal muscles follow. In some patients this muscular stiffness is the only feature, but in the more severely affected, spasms occur in which antagonists and agonist muscles are co-contracted, causing extreme pain and stiffness. Paraspinal muscle spasms may be so severe that dorsal vertebral fractures occur. There is, of course, no ventilation during spasms of respiratory muscles, and this is a major factor leading to death in the absence of effective treatment. Rhabdomyolysis may occur, resulting in myoglobinuria and renal failure.

Autonomic phenomena, including profuse sweating, excessive salivary and pharyngeal secretions, tachycardia, and hypotension occur, even in those who are electively paralysed for treatment (see Section 17.7.1.3). This indicates that the toxin also has a direct action upon the integration of autonomic outflow.

17.7.1.3   Treatment

There are three main objectives in treatment: to eradicate the infecting organism, to neutralize toxin before neural binding, and to overcome the physiological effects of toxin already bound within neurons.

The infecting organism is eradicated by wide wound excision, if the wound can be identified, and by the use of metronidazole 7.5 mg/kg every 6 hours orally, or intravenously if necessary. This drug has been shown to be superior to penicillin.

Circulating toxin is neutralized by passive immunization with 5000–10 000 units of human immune globulin intramuscularly.

Spasms may be prevented by intravenous diazepam; doses exceeding 5 mg/kg/day may be required. Dantrolene sodium, although acting peripherally on the sarcoplasmic reticulum, has also been shown to be beneficial. A suitable dose is 6 mg/kg/day. This drug can be given by nasogastric tube. Intrathecal baclofen has also been used on an experimental basis. In more severely affected cases, elective paralysis with neuromuscular blocking agents, positive pressure ventilation, and careful attention to fluid balance will be necessary. This approach has substantially diminished mortality in those severely affected.

17.7.1.4   Prognosis

As will be obvious from the foregoing, the mortality of tetanus in developing countries depends greatly upon the medical facilities available. Probably at least 50 per cent of infected children die. In developed countries, mortality remains high in those in whom frequent spasms are occurring before beginning treatment, and when the latent interval between the wound and the onset of tetanus is short, as this indicates a large infective inoculum.

Rather surprisingly, a dose of tetanus toxin that is potentially lethal is insufficient to cause active immunization. Recovered patients must therefore receive a full course of toxoid immunization. Tetanus is, of course, fully preventable with an adequate scheme of infant immunization, and proper care of the neonatal umbilical stump in developing countries.

17.7.2   Botulism

This paralytic illness is due to the toxin produced by *Clostridium botulinum*. As in the case of tetanus, the toxin is coded for extrachromosomally; however, several plasmids are involved, each producing a different subtype of toxin, known as A–G. In contrast to tetanus, however, toxin production by bacterial wound or bowel colonization is not common, and most cases result from the consumption of contaminated food, often canned, in which clostridial multiplication with toxin production has occurred (the word botulism comes from the Latin *botulus*, a sausage). Viable organisms may, however, be consumed along with the toxin, and further clostridial multiplication may occur in the gastrointestinal tract. In infants aged 2–6 months, botulism may arise from gut colonization with *C. botulinum*.

17.7.2.1   Pathophysiology

Clostridium botulinum toxin is probably the most potent biological agent known, the lethal dose being as little as 5 ng/kg in mice. It readily crosses the gut mucosa, is taken up by synaptosomes, and is then transmitted centripetally to neurons. The toxin prevents the quantal release of acetylcholine at neuromuscular junctions. Spontaneous non-quantal release can still occur. However, muscle fibres are effectively denervated and, as toxin-binding is irreversible, recovery has to wait until neural sprouting occurs—a process that may take several weeks.

17.7.2.2   *Clinical features and differential diagnosis*

Botulism in adults may present with nausea, vomiting, and abdominal discomfort, but neurological features soon predominate. The cranial nerves are particularly affected, with an external and internal ophthalmoplegia, followed by weakness of bulbar muscles, and then weakness of limb and trunk muscles, including respiratory muscles. The mental state remains normal, and there are no sensory signs. The differential diagnosis includes the Miller Fisher variant of acute infective polyneuropathy (Section 17.3.9.2) and diphtheria (Section 17.7.3). Myasthenia gravis (Section 21.12.2) is unlikely to be of such abrupt onset. In poliomyelitis, ocular muscles are not affected.

17.7.2.3   *Investigation*

Electrophysiological examination shows normal nerve conduction velocities. Repetitive stimulation of a motor nerve may cause a post-tetanic increase in amplitude of the evoked muscle response, but this is not as prominent as in the myasthenic syndrome (Section 21.12.3.1). It must always be remembered that a case of botulism raises the question that other members of a family or group may also have consumed the same toxin-contaminated food, and every attempt should be made to ascertain that they continue to be well.

17.7.2.4   *Treatment*

In infants, eradication of the organism is not recommended as there is concern that bacterial lysis may release large quantities of toxin. Furthermore, it has been shown that metronidazole can promote clostridial multiplication in animals.

Polyvalent antitoxin must be used as there are several different subtypes. Respiratory and circulatory support may be necessary for some weeks.

The prevention of botulism depends upon adequate sterilization of preserved foods prior to canning.

Bowel colonization by *C. botulinum* may be responsible for a few cases of the sudden infant death (cot death) syndrome.

Botulinum toxin is now used therapeutically for the control of blepharospasm and other facial dystonias (see Section 13.5.4).

17.7.3   *Diphtheria*

Corynebacterium diphtheriae produces a virulent neurotoxin through the intervention of a plasmid, which can pass to previously non-toxigenic strains. The principal early effects of upper respiratory tract diphtheria are due to the obstructive effects upon ventilation caused by a membrane that lies across the airway. This is formed from dead and dying epithelial cells, white cells, bacteria, and other constituents of the inflammatory exudate. Neurological effects occur about 3 weeks later.

17.7.3.1   *Pathophysiology and clinical features*

Diffusion of toxin from the site of infection leads to a local neuropathy affecting branches of nerves supplying the palate, pharynx, and larynx. Dangerous bulbar paralyses occur at a time when the child is often recovering from the primary effects of the infection. Occasionally a more generalized neuropathy results. In cutaneous diphtheritic lesions, the neuropathy may be manifest only as a zone of impaired sensation extending widely around the sore.

The effect of diphtheria toxin is exquisitely focused on Schwann cells, and for many years this toxin has been used as an agent for the production of an experimental demyelinating neuropathy in the laboratory. The toxin also damages the myocardium, and many infected children die with myocardial failure.

17.7.3.2   *Treatment*

The treatment of the toxic effects of diphtheria is with passive immunization with large doses of antitoxin, 50 000–100 000 units, of which half can be given intravenously. Antitoxin will only neutralize circulating toxin, and will have no effect upon toxin already bound to Schwann cells or to the myocardium. Ventilatory and circulatory support may be necessary until natural recovery from the paralysis occurs.

Diphtheria is eminently preventable with the usual schemes of infant immunization.

17.8   Rickettsial infections

Infections with the tick-borne *Rickettsia rickettsii* result in an encephalopathy in about 60 per cent of cases, with altered consciousness and focal signs. Seizures are rare. Examination of the CSF is usually uninformative. Pathological examination shows multiple cerebral vascular occlusions and microinfarcts, analogous to the purpuric cutaneous eruption, which gives the disease its name, Rocky Mountain spotted fever. Epidemic, or primary louse-borne typhus caused by *Rickettsia prowazekii*, is associated with delirium and agitation, progressing without treatment to coma in about 40 per cent of cases. Scrub typhus caused by *Rickettsia tsutsugamushi* also tends to affect severely the nervous system. Endemic or murine typhus caused by *Rickettsia typhii* tends to be a rather milder illness, although a meningoencephalitis can occur. Q fever, caused by *Coxiella burnetii*, rarely affects the nervous system. For all rickettsial infections, early treatment with tetracycline is essential. Chloramphenicol is also effective in many cases.

17.9   Mycoplasma infections

Infections with *Mycoplasma pneumoniae* are usually pulmonary, causing an atypical pneumonia. However, a number of neurological syndromes may occur in association—an acute infective polyneuropathy, an encephalopathy, an aseptic meningitis, or a transverse myelitis. Attempts to isolate the organism from the CSF or brain commonly fail. It is believed that most of the neurological manifestations have an immune basis.

17.10   Parasitic infections

17.10.1   *Toxoplasmosis*

Toxoplasma gondii is an intracellular protozoan parasite. The sexual stage of the parasitic cycle takes place only in cats. When oocysts are ingested by other hosts, including humans, they form trophozoites which persist for life. Infection in humans occurs through the ingestion of cysts from raw or undercooked meat, ingestion of sporulated cysts from cat faeces, and by the transplacental route. Congenital toxoplasmosis, caused by transplacental transmission of the organism if the mother acquires the infection in pregnancy, accounts for some cases of hydrocephalus. Hepatosplenomegaly, retinochoroiditis, and thrombocytopenia also occur.

Encysted cerebral trophozoites acquired through previous exposure can be reactivated in immunocompromised patients, such as those with AIDS. Clinical and other features are described in Section 17.12.12.2.

17.10.2   *Cysticercosis*

17.10.2.1   *Epidemiology and clinical features*

Cysticercosis occurs when a person becomes the host of the cyst stage of the pork tapeworm, *Taenia solium*. Usually humans host the worm stage, the only symptoms being nutritional, if diet is marginal, and the observation of the escaping proglottid. The cyst stage usually occurs in the muscle of pigs. In developing countries, food and drink may be contaminated by human faeces so that the eggs are ingested, and the cystic stage then occurs in humans. In endemic areas, such as rural Mexico, about 4 per cent of the population may be affected. The nervous system is frequently affected in such cases. The parasite cyst and the surrounding granulomatous infiltration may cause epilepsy. Damage to optic and oculomotor nerves results from granulomatous perineuritic meningal fibrosis.

17.10.2.2   *Investigation*

Early lesions are readily seen on the CT scan or MRI. Older lesions may become calcified, and may be seen on plain skull X-rays. If the disease is active, there will be an elevated concentration of protein and a number of mononuclear cells in the spinal fluid, even though clinical evidence of meningeal irritation is seldom present. The CSF sugar concentration may be reduced. The complement fixation test for cysticercosis (Nieto test) is positive in about 80 per cent of those with active disease, but only in about 20 per cent of those in whom the disease is no longer active. Enzyme-linked immunosorbent assay (ELISA) that measures specific IgM antibodies against Cysticercus antigens is more specific.

17.10.2.3   Treatment

Praziquantel 50 mg/kg/day for 15 days has been shown to be an effective treatment, but the eradication of the cysts is accompanied by severe headache, and in some patients by seizures and elevation of intracranial pressure. Dexamethasone may be used in the case of such reactions.

Freezing pork for 3 days has been shown to be sufficient to kill the cyst stage in pork, and is a useful public health precaution in endemic areas.

17.10.3   *Schistosomiasis*

Schistosomiasis (bilharziasis) is common in the developing world. Infective larvae, having escaped from the intermediate host, the freshwater snail, penetrate a person's skin, and then migrate via the lungs and the liver to the intestines and urinary bladder. All three species, *Schistosoma mansoni*, *S. haematobium*, and *S. japonicum* can affect the nervous system, but neurological involvement occurs in only about 2–4 per cent of those infected. The diagnosis is most easily made by searching the faeces for eggs, or by rectal biopsy.

Epilepsy is one neurological manifestation of *S. japonicum* infection, the CT scans showing enhancing lesions which have mass effect. Other neurological manifestations include a spastic paraparesis, resulting from infection with either of the two other species. The spinal cord may be compressed by granulomata around the roots and within the theca, or there may be ova within the cord, and an inflammatory response to their presence. A single day's treatment with praziquantel, 60 mg/kg in three divided doses, is sufficient to eradicate active infection, but residual symptoms usually continue.

17.10.4   *Paragonimiasis*

The larval stage of these flukes may occasionally migrate to the brain rather than their usual site in the lung, and there cause epilepsy, hemiparesis, or hydrocephalus. The cysts may readily be demonstrated by CT scanning. The treatment of choice is again praziquantel. Prevention depends upon proper cooking of the intermediate hosts, fresh-

water crabs and crayfish, common articles of diet on the eastern Asian littoral.

17.10.5   *Hydatid disease*

This is due to infection with the dog tapeworm *Echinococcus granulosus*. The usual life cycle is between dog and sheep, but in rural areas humans may ingest eggs from vegetables or water contaminated by dog faeces, or by handling dogs. The eggs hatch in the duodenum, and the embryo then migrates through the intestinal wall to liver, lungs, brain, and other organs, where the embryo further develops into cysts in which proto-scolices develop. Cerebral hydatid cysts present with epilepsy or from their effects as space-occupying lesions with hemiparesis. The CT scan appearances are of smooth-walled cysts filled with fluid of a Hounsfield number similar to cerebrospinal fluid. MRI shows analogous appearances. Surgical evacuation may be necessary if there is distortion of intracranial contents. Rupture and diagnostic aspiration must, as far as possible, be avoided in order to prevent the spread of daughter cysts. Medical treatment is disappointing, but benzimidazole derivatives are undergoing trial.

17.10.6   *Toxocariasis*

Infection with *Toxocara canis*, the common roundworm of the dog, is usually manifested as visceral larva migrans in young children with pica (perverted appetite). Occasionally an eosinophilic meningitis has been reported. Children with epilepsy have a higher incidence of anti-toxocara antibodies than a control population. The relationship is still debated—it is not clear whether cerebral toxocariasis is a significant cause of epilepsy, or whether the higher levels of antibodies reflect abnormal pica in young children with epilepsy who are exposed to dog-contaminated soil.

17.10.7   *Angiostrongyliasis*

Angiostrongylus cantonensis is a parasitic roundworm, the larvae of which develop in the giant land snail *Achatina*, prized as a gastronomic delicacy in South-East Asia. When the larvae are ingested they migrate to the central nervous system where they cause a radiculo-encephalomyelitis, characterized by the presence of eosinophils in the cerebrospinal fluid. No effective treatment has as yet been discovered, thiabendazole being ineffective. Adequate cooking destroys the larvae.

17.10.8   *Malaria*

Of the four *Plasmodium* species that infect humans, only *Plasmodium falciparum* produces cerebral malaria.

17.10.8.1   *Epidemiology*

The epidemiology of malaria is too vast a subject to review in a book of this type. *P. falciparum* is the predominant species in central Africa. Of particular concern to those working in developed countries is the possibility of a patient acquiring *P. falciparum* infection abroad, travelling home without symptoms during the stage of hepatic asexual multiplication, and becoming acutely ill with cerebral malaria some 2 weeks later in a country in which the diagnostic suspicion of malaria is not high.

17.10.8.2   *Clinical features*

The presenting features are fever for a few days, followed by altered consciousness and coma. The initial febrile stage may be very short in children. About half those with cerebral malaria have epileptic seizures, usually a tonic–clonic seizure, after which a deeper level of coma often ensues. Signs of meningism are rare. Papilloedema is virtually never seen, but retinal haemorrhages similar to the Roth's spots of infective endocarditis are common. The eyes of a comatose patient usually lie in the neutral position or are slightly divergent. Pupillary reflexes are retained. Tone in the limbs may be increased or decreased. The plantar responses are extensor in about half the cases.

17.10.8.3   *Pathophysiology*

A number of hypotheses have been advanced over the years, but none of these is entirely satifactory in explaining coma in cerebral malaria.

Although the brain is often swollen at autopsy, papilloedema during life is rare, and the spinal fluid is under normal pressure at lumbar puncture. There is no good evidence of severely raised intracranial pressure. Equally, there is no good evidence of a defect in permeability of the blood–brain barrier, and corticosteroids, so useful in treating other types of cerebral oedema, have been shown to increase rather than reduce mortality. There is no good evidence of a vasculitis or other immunological response to antigens derived from *P. falciparum*.

Red cells parasitized by *P. falciparum* are less deformable than healthy erythrocytes. This may contribute to the apparent obstruction of capillaries and venules, within which parasitized red cells are seen at autopsy to lie tightly packed. More important, however, are the changes in the red cell wall induced by the presence of mature trophozoites, which encourage the red cells to adhere to vascular endothelium. Parasitized red cells can be prevented from adhering in this way in primate experiments by the infusion of a strain-specific antibody. However, coma cannot be caused by focal or global ischaemia alone. The absence of focal physical signs in adults is one pointer against this, as is the complete physical recovery and recovery of cognitive function of those who survive malaria. However, focal neurological defects such as hemiplegia are common in surviving children.

Current views on the cause of coma in cerebral malaria are related to the observation that the concentration of lactate in the CSF is directly related to survival, high lactate being associated with an increased mortality. The adherent parasitized red cells in cerebral capillaries probably compete locally with the host cells for glucose, and the brain turns to anaerobic glycolysis. In overwhelming infections, systemic hypoglycaemia is a common pre-terminal event, lending some support to this hypothesis. In these terms, therefore, cerebral malaria can be considered as a metabolic coma. Residual deficits in children may be due to infarcts secondary to vascular occlusion.

17.10.8.4   *Diagnosis*

The diagnosis is confirmed by the observation of parasites in thick and thin films of peripheral blood stained by Field's and Wright's methods. Occasionally, parasitized erythrocytes may be sequestered in parts of the circulation through their cytoadherent properties, and it may be necessary to examine bone marrow to confirm their presence. The spinal fluid in cerebral malaria is virtually normal, although there may be a few white cells per microlitre.

The differential diagnosis of cerebral malaria extends to many of the causes of coma. The association of fever, convulsions, and coma is likely to focus attention particularly on bacterial meningitis (Section 17.1), septicaemia, and the acute viral encephalopathies (Section 17.12.2). It must be remembered that malarial parasitaemia is so frequent in adults in endemic areas that the finding of parasites does not necessarily exclude another cause of coma.

17.10.8.5   *Treatment and prognosis*

The drug of choice is chloroquine, 3.5 mg of base/kg diluted in 10 ml/kg isotonic fluid by intravenous infusion every 6 hours, to a total dose of 25 mg/kg. In areas where *P. falciparum* is resistant to chloroquine, quinine should be used. If the patient has not been receiving quinine, an initial loading dose of 20 mg/kg of the dihydrous salt (16.7 mg/kg of base) should be infused over 4 hours, followed by 10 mg/kg (8.3 mg/kg of base) over 4 hours, at intervals of 8 hours. When the patient can swallow tablets, a similar oral dose should continue for 7 days. An effective alternative, where available, is mefloquine 20 mg/kg orally in a single dose. This drug is probably teratogenic, and should not be given for prophylaxis or treatment to women who are not using a contraceptive method. The drug is not yet available intravenously for use in acutely ill patients. Attention to volume replacement, temperature, and to hypoglycaemia is necessary. Severe anaemia and renal failure may also occur.

At least 20 per cent of children and adults with cerebral malaria die. Mortality is related to the extent of parasitaemia, CSF lactate concentration, hypoglycaemia, and to the delay before initiating treatment.

17.10.9   *Trypanosomiasis*

Trypanosoma brucei gambiense and *T. brucei rhodesiense* cause West and East African sleeping sickness. The flagellated parasite is transmitted by a bite from an infected tsetse fly. Transmission is usually from human to human in the West African form, but game are involved in the life cycle in the East African form. Lymph nodes are infected early in the disease, but the parasite soon gains access to the nervous system. Changes in behaviour and a propensity to sleep during the day (hence 'sleeping sickness') are early evidence of the encephalopathy. Trypanosomes can be demonstrated in the CSF, which also shows a lymphocytic pleocytosis, and morular cells. These are plasma cells distended by large quantities of immune complexes.

Once the nervous system has been infected, the usual treatments of suramin and pentamidine are ineffective. Melarsoprol is effective in treating trypanosomal encephalopathy but relapses occur. A new agent, difluoromethyl ornithine, is at present showing great promise. This drug irreversibly inhibits ornithine decarboxylase, and blocks the synthesis of polyamines which play a prominent part in trypanosomal metabolism. The dose is 400 mg/kg/day intravenously for 14 days.

17.11   Fungal infections

Fungi, moulds, and yeasts are widely distributed in soil. Most probably gain access and cause disease through inhalation of spores. Subsequent involvement of the central nervous system occurs by haematogenous spread, but zygomycete fungi enter the cranium by direct spread from paranasal sinuses.

17.11.1   *Cryptococcosis (synonym: torulosis)*

Cryptococcus neoformans is usually widely distributed in avian faeces and soil. In developed countries, cryptococcal infections of the central nervous system usually occur in immunocompromised patients. Cryptococcal meningitis is now a frequent opportunistic infection in patients with AIDS (Section 17.12.12). However, in developing countries a subacute meningitis may occur in those previously fit. The presenting symptom is usually gradually increasing headache. Invasion of the subarachnoid space around the optic nerves often causes early papilloedema. The fungal masses may be sufficiently large to present as easily imaged space-occupying lesions. Granulomatous masses of fungi with little inflammatory response may be seen in the basal cisterns at autopsy.

The organism can usually be found in the spinal fluid, but repeated examinations may be necessary. The fungus is surrounded by a transparent capsule of large diameter, revealed by examining the centrifuged deposit in Indian ink. Mucicarmine will stain the capsule. This method, however, is less sensitive than detection of the polysaccharide capsular antigen. There is usually a moderate pleocytosis, and the CSF sugar is low. It is also possible to grow the organism in culture.

The treatment is amphotericin B intravenously, 0.3–0.5 mg/kg/day for a period of 6 weeks, i.e. a total dose of about 1 g in this period in adults. Oral 5-fluorocytosine, 150 mg/kg/day in four divided doses, should also be given. If given alone, resistance rapidly develops to 5-fluorocytosine. Another drug that appears to be more effective than amphotericin B is fluconazole, which, in a dose of 200 mg/day by mouth, has been shown to be effective in cryptococcal infection in AIDS patients. Previously fit patients have a good prognosis if treated early, but a poor prognosis if consciousness is altered before treatment. Immunocompromised patients fare much less well.

17.11.2 Aspergillosis

Aspergillus species (*fumigatus* and *flavus*) are widely distributed in soil. They occasionally invade the nervous system of immunocompromised hosts. With this fungus, meningitis is rare, the presentation being that of a space-occupying ball of fungus. Amphotericin B and 5-fluorocytosine should be used as described for cryptococcal meningitis (above), but the fungal burden should be initially lessened by surgical removal. The prognosis is poor.

17.11.3 Coccidioidomycosis

Coccidioides immitis is a mould widely distributed in hot, dry soils, and usually gains human access by inhalation. It may produce a chronic basal granulomatous meningitis similar in many clinical features to tuberculous meningitis (Section 17.5.1), with similar findings in the CSF—a pleocytosis, raised protein, and low sugar. Hydrocephalus may occur. Specific complement fixation tests are available, and mature and immature spherules may be seen in the CSF.

The treatment is high doses of amphotericin B, up to 1 mg/kg/day. 5-Fluorocytosine is not effective, as the mould lacks cytosine deaminase. The prognosis for eradication of meningeal infection is poor.

17.11.4 Histoplasmosis

Disseminated infection with *Histoplasma capsulatum* may occasionally affect the meninges, the clinical presentation being very similar to meningeal infection with *Coccidioides immitis*.

17.11.5 Candidiasis

Candida species are yeasts that are part of the normal skin and bowel flora. Budding is usually kept under control by competitive genera, but the use of antibiotics may alter the flora in such a way that candidiasis supervenes. Oral *Candida* infections are very common in intensive care units, for example. *Candida albicans*, however, may succeed in colonizing ventriculo-peritoneal or ventriculo-atrial shunts. Dissemination of the organism within the subarachnoid space results in a basal infiltrative meningitis with multiple cranial nerve palsies. The shunt may become blocked and hydrocephalus exaggerated. Successful treatment is usually dependent upon removal of any shunt and the use of amphotericin B and 5-fluorocytosine, as for cryptococcal meningitis (Section 17.11.1).

17.11.6 Zygomycosis (synonym: mucormycosis)

The clinical features of infection with this group of saprophytes (*Rhizopus*, *Rhizomucor*, *Absidia*) are quite different from the other fungal infections described above. The paranasal sinuses become stuffed with branching hyphae, which then extend into the orbit, and then posteriorly into the region of the cavernous sinus. The resultant proptosis and ophthalmoplegia are often mistaken for the signs of a cavernous sinus thrombosis. There may be vascular invasion by hyphae sufficient to cause arterial occlusion. Extensive bony necrosis occurs.

This 'rhinocerebral' form of zygomycosis is particularly likely to occur in poorly controlled diabetic patients. Facial pain and a black nasal discharge are often early features.

Mortality from zygomycosis is very high, successful treatment depending on extensive surgical debridement and early treatment with amphotericin B.

17.12   Viral infections of the nervous system

Research in this field is currently one of the most exciting in neurology. Some viruses cause clear-cut and relatively simple illnesses, for example the self-limiting meningitis of mumps (Section 17.12.1). Others can remain dormant in the nervous system for years, and then be reactivated to produce a new clinical illness, for example the occurrence of shingles (Section 17.12.7) many years after infection with chickenpox. Other viruses may induce post-infective demyelinating lesions through antibodies directed against both virus and myelin, for example measles encephalomyelopathy (Section 17.13.1). It is certainly a reasonable expectation that further research on virus–host interactions will lead to important increases in our understanding of other chronic neurological illnesses, such as multiple sclerosis.

Viruses may gain entry through the gut (e.g. enteroviruses), inhalation (e.g. measles and mumps), through inoculation through the placenta (e.g. cytomegalovirus), or by venereal contact (e.g. herpes simplex type 2 and HIV), or by transcutaneous inoculation, in drug abusers (HIV), and after bites (rabies).

Most neurological infections with viruses are acquired through the bloodstream, but some well-known viruses, such as rabies, are transported to the nervous system centripetally by axonal transport. Entry of virus into a cell requires interaction with a specific configuration on the cell surface. Matching of receptor and virus structure presumably accounts for the predilection of certain viruses for certain cell types (e.g. poliomyelitis virus for anterior horn cells).

For clinical purposes, viral illnesses of the nervous system are best considered by the clinical syndrome they produce.

17.12.1   *Acute viral meningitis*

A large number of viruses produce an acute viral meningitis, characterized by malaise, headache, moderate fever, drowsiness, and sometimes vomiting. Examination shows a moderately ill patient with some neck stiffness, but this is not usually as pronounced as with bacterial meningitis.

The most frequent viruses that cause viral meningitis in the UK are mumps and the enteroviruses echo and coxsackie B and A and the Epstein–Barr virus. Lymphocytic choriomeningitis virus is a cause in some countries of Europe and in North America. An acute self-limiting viral meningitis may occur after HIV infection (Section 17.12.11.2).

Examination of the spinal fluid shows a moderate pleocytosis. In the first few hours of the infection, polymorphs may predominate, but they are soon replaced by lymphocytes. The protein is only slightly elevated, and the CSF sugar is normal.

The most important differential diagnosis is tuberculous meningitis (Section 17.5.1). There is no specific treatment, but recovery after a few days' bed rest is the rule. However, patients may feel readily exhausted and have difficulty in concentrating for some weeks thereafter.

17.12.2   *Acute viral encephalitis*

The clinical distinction between an inflammatory response confined to the meninges—a viral meningitis (above)—and an encephalitis lies in the prominence of confusion and altered consciousness. The occurrence of seizures or of focal neurological signs certainly indicates cerebral involvement. Conversely, signs of meningism with clear consciousness indicate a predominantly meningeal involvement. Acute viral encephalitis may be defined as an illness of rapid onset and progression, with evidence of a diffuse or focal inflammatory disorder of the brain. The disorder must be distinguished from a post-viral encephalopathy mediated on an immune basis (Section 17.13.1).

Acute viral encephalitis can be due to infection with viruses that cause mumps, herpes simplex and zoster, and with Epstein–Barr virus, coxsackie and echoviruses. The Japanese B encephalitis virus is endemic in the northern part of India, and South-East Asia. This virus is transmitted by the bite of various species of *Culex* mosquitoes.

The differential diagnosis of a viral encephalitis includes bacterial meningitis (Section 17.1.2), tuberculous meningitis (Section 17.5.1), brain abscess (Section 17.2.1), cerebral infarction (Section 10.1.5), cerebral tumour (Section 16.2), diffuse vasculitides such as those accompanying systemic lupus (Section 10.2.5), and an acute metabolic encephalopathy.

The investigation of a case of suspected encephalitis will include CT scanning or MRI, electroencephalography, and examination of the CSF. CT scanning may show generalized oedema, or areas of focal low attenuation, often with surrounding enhancement by contrast. Electroencephalography may show diffuse, often symmetrical, slowing of background rhythms down to 3–4 c/s. There may be specific focal abnormalities; these are especially prominent with herpes simplex infections. Examination of the CSF usually shows an increased number of lymphocytes, but the CSF may be entirely normal. Evaluation of serum samples obtained during the acute illness and during convalescence for rising antibody titres is only helpful to the extent of clarifying in retrospect the nature of the illness.

Herpes simplex encephalitis is specifically considered, as there is an effective treatment available.

17.12.3. *Herpes simplex encephalitis*

17.12.3.1   *Epidemiology and pathophysiology*

Herpes simplex virus is a DNA virus, with two related antigenic subtypes, 1 and 2. The first usually affects non-genital areas, and is responsible for the common recurrent cold sore, which affects about 25 per cent of the population. Herpes simplex type 2 primarily affects the urogenital tract and skin below the waist.

Herpes simplex 1 is the commonest cause of acute encephalitis in adults, whereas type 2 is rather more frequent in neonates. The incidence is about 1 per 250 000–500 000 per year. Herpes simplex 2 occasionally causes encephalitis in neonates as part of a disseminated infection.

There is no obvious relationship between preexisting cold sores and herpes simplex 1 encephalitis. It is known that the virus remains in latent form in human sensory ganglia. It can be recovered from the trigeminal ganglion of about 50 per cent of individuals by co-cultivation of ganglion explants with monolayer cultures of susceptible cells. These show characteristic cytopathic changes in the presence of the virus. Although these are interesting observations, they fail to account for the sudden onset of viral replication in the temporal lobes, resulting in acute tissue necrosis and such local swelling that the area of encephalitis may mimic a space-occupying lesion.

In rabbits and mice, there is evidence that the virus gains access to the brain through the olfactory tracts.

17.12.3.2   *Clinical features*

Herpes simplex encephalitis can occur in patients of any age, at any time of the year. Headache, fever, and altered consciousness are the initial signs, but focal hemisphere signs such as a hemiparesis often follow. Seizures may occur.

17.12.3.3   *Investigation, treatment, and prognosis*

The CSF contains an increased number of lymphocytes, and in more than half the cases red cells may also be found. Occasionally the CSF sugar is low. Electroencephalography shows local slowing over one or both temporal lobes, and later the development of periodic complexes. CT scanning usually shows a swollen temporal lobe with areas of decreased and patchy increased attenuation and MRI shows patchy areas of high and low signal. Blood and CSF antibody titres to herpes simplex virus do not increase until the second or third week in the illness. This is too late to influence treatment, but samples should be obtained for subsequent analysis. Viral DNA in the CSF can be amplified by the polymerase chain reaction and identified by hybridization to a specific nucleotide probe by radioactive dot hybridization techniques at an earlier stage. Nevertheless, it is usually necessary to proceed to early treatment before the diagnosis is definitely established, as the mortality in untreated cases is about 70 per cent, and the outcome is clearly influenced by delay in treatment. Although some colleagues in the US advocate brain biopsy to establish the diagnosis, most physicians now begin treatment with acyclovir as soon as they suspect the diagnosis. Acyclovir should be given intravenously in a dose of 10 mg/kg delivered over 1 hour, every 8 hours for 10 days. Acyclovir is relatively non-toxic to normal cells. In the presence of herpes simplex viral thymidine kinase, acyclovir is monophosphorylated. Host cells then further phosphorylate the drug to its active triphosphate state which inhibits DNA synthesis and hence viral replication.

The prognosis of herpes simplex encephalitis is related to the conscious level at onset of treatment. All those who are only mildly obtunded will recover without significant cognitive or neurological deficit. Overall mortality has been reduced from 70 per cent to 20 per cent since the introduction of acyclovir. The prognosis for type 2 infection in neonates is worse than for type 1.

17.12.4   *Other viruses causing encephalitis*

Many arthropod-borne (arbo) viruses have been reported to cause encephalitis, the vectors being mosquitoes and ticks. Examples from different continents are St Louis encephalitis (USA), Murray Valley encephalitis (Australia), Japanese B encephalitis, and Central European encephalitis. This last is transmitted through drinking infected milk from goats carrying the virus, having been bitten by a tick. These viral encephalitides are of varying severity, but death and permanent neurological sequelae occur, particularly with Japanese B and Murray Valley infections. No specific treatment is as yet available. Protective vaccines are available for Japanese B encephalitis.

From 1915 to 1926, approximately, there was an epidemic of a form of encephalitis that has since disappeared. Von Economo's encephalitis was characterized by fever and stupor—hence the popular term 'sleeping sickness'. Perivascular mononuclear cell infiltrates were present in the mid-brain. Considerable interest remains in this condition on account of the late neurological effects—post-encephalitic parkinsonism, characterized by rigidity, akinesia, and oculogyric crises (Section 13.1.4).

17.12.5   *Rabies*

17.12.5.1   *Epidemiology and pathophysiology*

The word rabies comes from the Sanskrit 'rabhas', which means madness or rage. The bullet-shaped rabies virus is distributed throughout the world, with the exception of western Europe, Japan, Australasia, and many of the islands of the western Pacific and Indonesia. In North America, northern Europe, and northern Asia the virus is confined to wild species such as foxes, badgers, and bats. In South America, Africa, and southern Asia there is a significant risk to people as the virus is endemic in urban dogs and is present in their saliva. Transmission occurs through dog bites. Transmission occasionally occurs from bats to those exploring their cave habitats, possibly by inhalation of the virus.

Cases occur from time to time in the UK, but the virus has always been acquired abroad, as have most of the cases in the USA. The latent period before the onset of neurological symptoms is usually 1–2 months, but may be shorter or longer. The incubation period is shorter in children and in bites around the head and neck. Virus gains access to the central nervous system by centripetal spread within the axoplasm of peripheral nerves. Intense multiplication of virus occurs centrally, most prominently in the mid-brain and medulla. The most characteristic pathological change is the presence of Negri bodies, which represent masses of viral ribonucleoprotein.

17.12.5.2   *Clinical features*

The initial symptom of neurological involvement is often paraesthesiae and itching or pain in the bitten limb. This is followed by a prodromal stage of headache, fever, malaise, and lethargy. Most patients then develop intensely painful spasms of the larynx, pharynx, and inspiratory muscles, often precipitated by attempts to drink—hence 'hydrophobia'. As the disease progresses, spasms become more and more widespread, and may be associated with generalized convulsions. In between the spasms there may be few physical signs. This, and the rarity of the disease in developed countries, often leads to a delay in diagnosis. In about 20 per cent of cases rabies is manifest by an ascending paralysis rather than hydrophobia, although mixed forms are common.

The diagnosis of rabies can most easily be confirmed by examining the brain of the suspect dog for Negri bodies. If the dog is not available, virus in small nerves obtained at skin biopsy may be demonstrated by fluorescent specific antibody techniques.

17.12.5.3   *Treatment and prognosis*

With the very rarest of exceptions, rabies is rapidly

fatal once neurological symptoms have developed, and care is limited to sedation to minimize muscle spasms and terror. There are three reports of survivors after skilled intensive care.

With such a terrible prognosis, every effort must be made to prevent the acquisition of rabies to areas in which it is not at present endemic. Hence the rigour of the UK quarantine laws, under which any imported dog is kept caged under observation for 6 months. For those bitten, the wound must be vigorously cleaned with detergent and water, and flooded with iodine. Crushed tissue should be debrided surgically and the wound left open. Active and passive immunization should commence at once. Human rabies immune globulin, if available, or horse antirabies serum should be used, half the calculated dose being infiltrated around the wound, and half in the deltoid muscle. Active immunization is obtained by using vaccine grown in human diploid cells and injected into the deltoid muscle on days 0, 3, 7, 14, and 28 days after exposure. This vaccine is safer than that derived from phenol-treated virus grown in animal nervous tissue. This last method, a variant of the original Pasteur method, is followed by neuroparalytic events in about 2 per 1000 subjects, with about a 20 per cent mortality. Pathological study of these neuroparalytic events shows a multifocal inflammatory perivenular demyelinating process. This results from an immunological reaction to myelin basic protein.

17.12.6   *Poliomyelitis*

Rabies is a very neurotropic virus, and poliomyelitis is even more specifically targeted, in this case to anterior horn cells.

Poliomyelitis virus is, like echo and coxsackie viruses, an enterovirus. These RNA viruses spread through faecal contamination of food and water. Some of them cause neurological disease. Poliomyelitis damages anterior horn cells. Occasionally, other enteroviruses cause an acute ataxic syndrome or other evidence of an encephalitis.

17.12.6.1   *Epidemiology*

The introduction of polio vaccine has vastly altered the epidemiology of poliomyelitis, but where rates of immunity in the population fall to less than

50–60 per cent, the disease may break out again. The World Health Organization estimates that there are 400 000 cases of persisting paralytic poliomyelitis in developing countries.

One particular risk is immunization of only some members of a family. It is then possible for other members of the family who are not immune to acquire a paralytic illness as the immunized members excrete virus. This occurs because some strains of virus increase in neurovirulence on passage through the human bowel. It is therefore essential to ensure that programmes of community immunization are as widespread as possible, although even immunization of 60 per cent of a population will substantially reduce episodes of paralytic illness.

17.12.6.2   *Clinical features*

Polio virus may induce a febrile illness, without any neurological feature, or may induce an aseptic meningitis without paralysis. Some patients with an aseptic meningitis progress to a paralytic illness, often preceded by considerable muscle pain. Acute necrosis of anterior horn cells and/or cranial nerve motor nuclei occur. Bulbar palsy, respiratory insufficiency, and various patterns of lower motor neuron paralysis occurs. The spinal fluid contains 10–500 lymphocytes/μl. The protein is slightly elevated initially, more so later. The CSF sugar is normal.

17.12.6.3   *Treatment and progress*

Apart from relief of muscle pain and ventilatory support, and appropriate nutrition in those with a bulbar palsy, there is no effective treatment in the acute stage. Those who survive this stage may be left with a variable amount of permanent lower motor neuron paralysis. If the illness has occurred in early childhood, there may be asymmetries of skeletal growth, the bones of the paralysed limb(s) failing to develop their usual mass and length. Orthopaedic corrections may therefore be required in later life. Some patients with ventilatory insufficiency may require intermittent or continuous ventilatory support in a tank respirator, the so-called 'iron lung'. There are other methods of ventilatory support, such as the cuirasse ventilator, or the rocking bed.

17.12.6.4   *The post-poliomyelitis syndrome*

A small proportion of patients previously afflicted by acute poliomyelitis develop some 25–30 years later further weakness in the affected muscles. For many years this was dismissed as being no more than due to the additional handicapping effects of ageing, or to the normal age-related loss of anterior spinal neurons that occur at age 55 and beyond. However, there now seems no reasonable doubt that new active denervation can occur 30 years after an initial episode of polio in those people infected young, and long before age-related loss of neurons might reasonably be expected to begin. It is not certain whether delayed post-polio loss of anterior spinal (and bulbar) motor neurons is due to an immunologic process, or to very delayed effects of the virus upon neuronal metabolism.

17.12.7   **Herpes zoster**

The varicella–zoster virus is a DNA herpes virus that causes both chickenpox (varicella) in children, and zoster (shingles) in adults.

17.12.7.1   *Epidemiology*

Shingles is a common disorder in primary care practice, occurring in about 3–4 cases per 1 000 per year. The word shingles comes from the Latin 'cingulum' meaning belt, reflecting the dermatomal distribution of the vesicular eruption.

It is believed that shingles is a result of reactivation of varicella–zoster virus that has lain dormant in trigeminal and other sensory root ganglia since the primary childhood chickenpox infection. Viral DNA can be demonstrated (by amplification, using the polymerase chain reaction, and binding to a specific oligonucleotide probe) in the neurons of the trigeminal ganglia at autopsy of subjects without recent zoster, confirming the potential long-term dormancy of the virus. Susceptible children can acquire chickenpox from an adult with zoster, but exposure of an immune adult to a child with chickenpox or to another adult with zoster does not usually result in his own virus reactivation, although exceptions have been reported. However, changes in immunity in adult life, resulting from radiotherapy or the onset of a lymphoma, may activate zoster. More often there is no obvious predisposing cause. Older people are more commonly affected, possibly because cell-mediated immunity declines with age.

Other rare neurological manifestations of varicella–zoster virus occur, and are described in Sections 17.12.7.4 and 5.

17.12.7.2   *Clinical features*

The cardinal feature of zoster is the dermatomal eruption of vesicles. However, pain and paraesthesiae may precede the eruption by several days. The first warning of the eruption is a maculopapular rash, but vesicles soon appear. After 2–3 days, the vesicles may become pustular. After a few more days they dry up and crust over. The crusts separate after about 3 weeks and leave an area of skin that may remain depigmented. These areas are often locally hypoalgesic thereafter. The thoracic dermatomes are most often affected, but the skin of the face supplied by the trigeminal nerve is affected in about 15 per cent of all cases. Unfortunately, it is usually the ophthalmic division that is involved, so that there is a risk of ocular complications such as scleritis, iritis, and subsequent glaucoma and keratitis. Isolated vesicles elsewhere on the body reflect the viraemia that occurs in about 30 per cent of subjects with shingles.

17.12.7.3   *Treatment and prognosis*

Acyclovir is now the drug of choice. Its method of action is described in Section 17.12.3.3. An oral dose of 800 mg five times daily for 7 days has been shown in a controlled trial to reduce the formation of new lesions in those patients treated within 48 hours of the onset of the rash. Pain is also markedly relieved. However, treatment with acyclovir has no influence upon the incidence or severity of post-herpetic neuralgia.

An episode of zoster does not confer immunity, and about 5 per cent of patients can expect to have a further attack. Immunologically incompetent patients may develop life-threatening disseminated varicella on exposure to the virus. Hence the rigorous exclusion of children with chickenpox from the wards in which children with leukaemia and other childhood malignancies are being treated.

Post-herpetic neuralgia

Apart from the complications of ophthalmic zoster already mentioned, zoster has only one important late complication, and that is post-herpetic neuralgia. All pain settles within 1 month of onset in about half the patients with zoster, but about 20 per cent will continue to have some pain 6 months after onset. In some, the pain is severe and burning and accompanied by hyperaesthesiae in the affected dermatome. Pain is exacerbated by the lightest touch of the affected area. The incidence of neuralgia after zoster is much greater in older people. Women are more likely to be affected than men.

The pathophysiology of post-herpetic neuralgia is related to a selective loss of large diameter dorsal root afferents following the acute infection. It has been suggested that these normally exert a modulating effect on spontaneous and evoked discharges in unmyelinated (C) fibres in the root-entry zone of the spinal cord. It also appears that second-order neurons in the cord, which would normally transmit impulses concerned with nociception, become accessed by large-fibre mechanoreceptor afferents. That is to say, some form of central sensory reorganization may play a part in post-herpetic neuralgia.

The pain of post-herpetic neuralgia does not respond to conventional analgesia. The affective component of the pain may be prominent, particularly in an elderly person living alone, so anti-depressants have some part to play. Even without overt depression, tricyclic antidepressants may significantly relieve pain. Some patients are helped by carbamazepine, but the relief is not nearly so striking as in trigeminal neuralgia (Section 9.10.1). Local treatments have a major role. Stimulation of surviving large-diameter afferents by brisk manual kneading (which causes much less pain than a light stroke), or by a vibrator, may be useful. Acupuncture has its adherents, but the results are unconvincing. Transcutaneous electrical stimulation helps about one-third of patients to some extent. Local injections of long-acting anaesthetics such as bupivicaine may provide longer relief than would be expected from their known anaesthetic effect. Unfortunately, all treatments fail in a substantial minority of patients, although there is often a gradual spontaneous improvement over a period of 2–3 years. Treatment of zoster in the acute stage with prednisolone or acyclovir does not alter the incidence or severity of post-herpetic neuralgia.

17.12.7.4   *Variants of herpes zoster*

Zoster virus may affect more than one adjacent dermatome, but rarely is bilateral. Zoster affecting the dorsal roots of the cervical and lumbar regions may be associated with the development of a lower motor neuron weakness in the same segment. Almost certainly this happens in thoracic zoster as well, but it is difficult to note if one intercostal muscle is weak, whereas the changes of wasting and weakness in one hand in a T1 lesion, for example, are obvious. Presumably the virus spreads out of the dorsal root into the anterior root or anterior horn cells but, as the prognosis is good, there are no adequate pathological reports. Occasionally weakness affects a motor segment distant from the dermatome affected, which cannot be explained on the hypothesis of direct spread. Zoster in sacral segments may be accompanied by retention of urine, or disturbance of anal sphincter control.

Zoster may affect cranial nerves other than the trigeminal (Section 17.12.7.2). The best known example is the Ramsay Hunt syndrome, or 'geniculate herpes', the name given to zoster infection with vesicles in or around the auditory meatus, and associated with a facial palsy. Vesicles may also appear on the palate. The syndrome probably reflects simultaneous activation of virus in the neurons of more than one afferent cranial nerve. The facial palsy in some cases is due to the necrotic swelling of those afferent fibres travelling in company with the facial nerve. However, the cause of the facial palsy may sometimes be direct local involvement of the facial nucleus in the brain stem, analogous to the segmental motor weakness described above.

Occasionally pain apparently similar to that caused by zoster may occur in a dermatomal distribution. If accompanied by a rise in antibody titre, this can fairly be called 'zoster sine herpete'.

17.12.7.5   *Other complications of varicella–zoster infection*

There are more substantial and serious neurological diseases associated with the varicella–zoster virus, following a clinical episode of either zoster or chickenpox.

Encephalomyelitis may occur after either type of clinical expression of the virus. The clinical features are not very different from other types of encephalitis, with the exception that an acute cerebellar syndrome is frequent in children exposed to varicella. Direct viral invasion of the brain may occur in association with zoster infection, although immune-mediated mechanisms may contribute in some cases. The pathological evidence is that the encephalitis after varicella is similar to that after measles (Section 17.13.1), in being of a demyelinating type. The prognosis after either type of encephalitis is not good, there being a significant morbidity and a mortality of 5–10 per cent. The elderly and the immunocompromised are particularly at risk, a quarter of the survivors having some neurological deficit.

A few cases of a late onset encephalopathy have been reported, cognitive impairment and focal motor signs and seizures beginning slowly some months after zoster. The clinical picture, imaging and pathological appearances are similar to progressive multifocal leucoencephalopathy (Section 17.14.3.2). This syndrome presumably reflects the effects of chronic intracerebral viral replication.

Varicella is one of the most frequent viruses incriminated in the encephalopathy of Reye's syndrome (Section 17.13.2.1).

An acute infective polyneuropathy, indistinguishable, apart from the rash, from other cases of the Guillain–Barré syndrome may occur after either zoster or varicella. The prognosis is much worse in the former group, but this may reflect no more than the known inferior prognosis of older patients requiring ventilatory support.

In a rare, but interesting, group of patients, trigeminal zoster is followed by a contralateral hemiplegia. Pathological studies have shown a necrotizing granulomatous angiitis of meningeal and cerebral arteries. Herpes zoster virus particles have been detected in the outer layers of the arterial wall.

17.12.8   *Epstein–Barr virus infections*

A variety of neurological syndromes have been associated with infection with the Epstein–Barr virus, including aseptic meningitis, an acute infectious polyneuropathy, transverse myelitis, acute psychosis, facial palsy, and an acute cerebellar ataxia. Most of the recorded cases have been young people. It is not clear whether the syn-

dromes are due to a direct viral or post-infectious immune effect.

17.12.9   *Cytomegalovirus infections*

Cytomegalovirus (CMV) is a common opportunistic infection in AIDS (see Section 17.12.12.4). The virus is also implicated in the cause of epilepsy in a proportion of children with infantile spasms (see Section 12.5). Genomic material of CMV has also been found in Rasmussen's encephalitis, a disorder of young people in which intractable partial epilepsy and focal neurological deficits occur. Some patients with such seizures come for surgical control of their epilepsy, and histological examination shows microglial nodules, perivascular lymphocytic cuffing, neuronal loss, astrocytosis, and leptomeningeal inflammation.

17.12.10   *Human T-cell lymphotrophic virus type I infection (HTLV-I)*

One of the original names for HIV virus was human T-lymphotrophic virus type III (HTLV-III). Antibodies to another retrovirus, HTLV-I, have been identified in the sera of those suffering from tropical spastic paraparesis (Jamaican or West Indian myelopathy), or a similar myelopathy in Japan. This syndrome is clinically similar to the progressive spastic paraparesis that occurs in some cases of multiple sclerosis in Europids, without brain-stem or optic nerve demyelination. MRI shows some evidence of intracerebral demyelination, in so far as areas of high signal are seen on T2 weighted images in a proportion of cases. Visual and somatosensory evoked responses may be abnormal.

There is strong evidence that HTLV-I is the cause of tropical spastic paraparesis, as intrathecal synthesis of antibodies directed against the virus can be demonstrated, and nucleic acid sequences found in the virus can be demonstrated in blood and cerebrospinal fluid lymphocytes. However, the disease is comparatively rare considering the extensive seroprevalence of HTLV-I, and it may be that genetically determined or acquired host factors determine the extent of neurological involvement. Indeed, as the HTLV-I virus is the aetiological agent of adult T-cell leukaemia and lymphoma, it is probably host factors that determine whether there is a non-clonal expansion of peripheral blood lymphocytes and the development of a spastic paraparesis, or a clonal expansion leading to adult T-cell leukaemia.

The route of transmission of HTLV-I is not well defined, but probably includes sexual and parenteral transmission. In Japan, there is evidence of transmission by breast milk.

The related virus HTLV-II has also recently been associated with a degenerative disorder similar to the olivopontocerebellar variant of multiple system atrophy (Section 12.2.3.1).

17.12.10.1   Treatment

Some patients, particularly those with the Japanese variant of the illness, benefit from corticosteroid therapy.

17.12.11   Human immunodeficiency virus (HIV) and associated neurological syndromes

17.12.11.1   Epidemiology

Human immunodeficiency virus (HIV) has emerged as one of the most important causes of rapidly progressive neurological disease in younger adults. Some of the neurological syndromes are caused by direct invasion of the nervous system. These can occur soon after acquisition of the virus, and even before seroconversion. The virus can be recovered from the spinal fluid in those without neurological symptoms, and intrathecal synthesis of antibodies to HIV can be demonstrated at around the time of seroconversion. Other neurological syndromes result from opportunistic infections in patients who go on to develop the acquired immunodeficiency syndrome (AIDS). The Centers for Disease Control in the USA report that about 10 per cent of AIDS patients will present with a neurological problem, and about 40 per cent will have a neurological problem at some stage, most commonly AIDS dementia. Autopsy studies of patients dying with AIDS show that fewer than 5 per cent of the brains are normal. Multiple neurological syndromes in one subject are common.

17.12.11.2   Neurological syndromes occurring near the time of seroconversion

An acute self-limiting lymphocytic meningitis has been shown to be due to HIV infection. Features atypical of other viral meningitides, such as recurrence or chronicity, or associated cranial nerve palsies (V, VII, VIII) are common. Other peripheral syndromes include an acute polyneuropathy, similar to the Guillain–Barré syndrome (Section 19.3.9), facial palsy, and an acute ataxic neuropathy due to dorsal root ganglionitis. The acute polyneuropathies may respond to plasmapheresis. Later in the course of HIV infection, a distal symmetrical sensori-motor neuropathy occurs frequently, and is probably often overlooked in a setting of weight loss associated with multiple opportunistic infections or malignancies.

Acute myelopathy resulting in a paraparesis with an increased number of white cells in the CSF has been described, and also an acute encephalopathy, with fever, general malaise, confusion, or depression of consciousness and fits. Both syndromes occur around the time of seroconversion. It is not yet known whether these early neurological manifestations indicate an increased risk of the subsequent chronic neurological syndromes, or the earlier development of AIDS.

17.12.11.3   Chronic neurological syndromes

Some of the chronic syndromes are due to the results of infection with the HIV virus itself; others are associated with opportunistic infections consequent on the immunodepression of AIDS.

Neurological syndromes due to the direct effects of HIV itself affect the peripheral nerves, spinal cord, and brain. A subacute or chronic sensorimotor neuropathy, similar to that described in Section 19.3.1, can occur. Although painful dysaesthesiae are frequent, sensory signs are usually mild. Less frequent is a subacute mononeuritis multiplex (Section 19.6). Many patients develop a chronic myelopathy with sensory dysaesthesiae, a spastic paraparesis, and disturbance of urinary control. The lateral and posterior columns are affected. The characteristic pathological finding is vacuolation and intramyelinic oedema.

HIV (AIDS) dementia

The most frequent neurological syndrome of HIV infection is the AIDS dementia complex, characterized by impairment of cognitive function and memory, and later motor disturbance. Although a similar clinical syndrome can result from opportunistic infections with other viruses and organisms, there seems no doubt that HIV alone is responsible in most cases. The dementia is produced by primary neuronal loss, and, in many cases an inflammatory encephalopathy.

The earliest symptoms of HIV dementia are impairment of concentration, loss of interest in pastimes, and impairment of memory. It is often difficult to distinguish these early symptoms from the psychological symptoms associated with anxiety and depression about being aware of HIV seropositivity. Mild slowing of background rhythms on the electroencephalogram and slightly delayed somatosensory evoked responses have been reported as early evidence of neurological abnormality in seropositive subjects. Occasionally, more dramatic psychiatric manifestations of HIV cerebral infection may occur—agitation, inappropriate behaviour, and hallucinations. The dementia in most patients progresses rapidly, with marked apathy and prominent impairment of cognitive function. Depression of consciousness and seizures are uncommon. Towards the end, many patients develop ataxic spastic para- or tetraparesis, and become mute and incontinent. Some of the signs may well be accounted for by a coexistent vacuolar myelopathy.

Lumbar puncture in HIV encephalopathy usually shows a moderate pleocytosis. Electroencephalography shows a moderate degree of generalized slowing, but no specific features. CT scanning shows cortical atrophy, ventricular enlargement, and sometimes diffuse attenuation of white matter. MRI shows areas of increased signal in the central white matter in T2 weighted images. At post-mortem the principal findings are multifocal perivascular rarefaction and focal vacuolation of white matter, reactive astrocytosis, and collections of macrophages and multinucleated giant cells. There are also perivascular lymphocytic infiltrates. In many cases without obvious inflammatory change, quantitative neuronal counts show substantial losses of neurons in the frontal cortex.

17.12.11.4 Treatment of HIV infections

Some of the neurological syndromes of HIV infection and survival can be improved by zidovudine, 3.5 mg/kg orally every 4 hours. An essential step in the replication of HIV is the formation of a viral DNA transcript which can become integrated into the host-cell DNA. This process is mediated by the enzyme reverse transcriptase, and requires the presence of thymidine for incorporation into the DNA chain. Zidovudine (azidothymidine), after metabolism to its triphosphate, is recognized by reverse transcriptase as true thymidine, and is inappropriately bound into the DNA transcript, resulting in premature chain termination of the viral DNA. Unfortunately, bone marrow toxicity is a serious drawback with this drug. If the dose is reduced because of myelotoxicity, an acute meningoencephalitis may occur. The drug may also cause a necrotizing inflammatory myopathy (Section 21.3.4.3). However, there is no doubt that zidovudine, in a dose of 500 mg/day in asymptomatic HIV-seropositive subjects, will slow the rate of CD4+ lymphocyte depletion and progression to AIDS. Symptomatic patients require larger doses: 1200–1500 mg per day. As yet, it is not certain that zidovudine slows the rate of HIV dementia (Section 17.12.11.3). Acyclovir in combination with zidovudine has been shown to be more effective than zidovudine alone in one trial.

17.12.12 Associated infections and neoplasms in immunodeficient subjects

Infection with HIV causes chronic, progressive depletion of CD4+ helper/inducer T-lymphocytes. Together with infection of macrophages, this depletion results in an immune deficiency that allows opportunistic infection.

17.12.12.1 Fungal infections

Cryptococcus neoformans commonly causes a meningitis in patients with AIDS, and may be the first evidence of the development of AIDS. Although headache is frequent, frank clinical evidence of meningitis in the form of neck stiffness may not be apparent. There is some evidence that co-infection with *Cryptococcus* enhances HIV infection. Treatment is with fluconazole (Section 17.11.1). *Aspergillus*, *Candida*, *Histoplasma*, and *Mucor* infections also occur.

17.12.12.2 Parasitic infections

Toxoplasma gondii is the most frequent CNS parasitic infection in AIDS patients. The trophozoite invades and kills glial cells and neurons, producing a necrotic area surrounded by an intense mono-nuclear cell reaction. Perivascular mononuclear inflammation may result in the extension of the areas of necrosis by infarction. AIDS patients with *Toxoplasma* infections present with headache, con-fusion, focal neurological signs (these in contrast to patients with HIV dementia), and seizures. CT scanning usually shows one or more areas of focal necrosis surrounded by ring enhancement, but occasionally the infection is diffuse throughout the brain. *Toxoplasma* IgG antibody is found in the serum of most patients. The diagnosis may be confirmed by brain biopsy, but the imaging appear-ances in AIDS patients are usually sufficiently typical to warrant a therapeutic trial with pyrimeth-amine and sulphadiazine or clindamycin. How-ever, the mortality from *Toxoplasma* in AIDS patients approaches 70 per cent.

17.12.12.3   *Bacterial infections*

Bacterial CNS infections other than syphilis or tuberculosis in AIDS patients are unusual. The occurrence of neurosyphilis may represent no more than coincident infection, although immunodefi-ciency allows much more rapid progress of the spirochaetal disease. CNS tuberculosis complicates AIDS, and is an increasing cause of deaths from AIDS in Africa, but more often in the West, if a mycobacterium is found, it is an atypical organism (e.g. *M. avium intracellulare*). Two specific organ-isms, however, affect other immunocompromised patients.

Listeria monocytogenes

Although not particularly frequent in patients with AIDS, this is the commonest cause of bacterial meningitis in patients with other causes of immuno-suppression, for example after renal transplan-tation, or in those receiving chemotherapy for lymphomas. Headache, fever, and confusion pre-dominate in *Listeria* infections, and clinical evi-dence of meningeal inflammation may be slight. A local brain-stem encephalitis may occur. It is diffi-cult to demonstrate the Gram-staining rod on microscopy, but the organism can be readily cul-tured. Ampicillin, intravenously in a dose of 12 g/day (for an adult), is the treatment of choice.

Nocardia asteroides

This Gram-positive branching rod is related to the mycobacteria and actinomycetes. It affects the same type of immunosuppressed patient as does *Listeria*. As the organism commonly forms an abscess, rather than meningitis, focal signs are common. The organism is sensitive to sulphadiazine.

17.12.12.4   *Viral infections*

Cytomegalovirus (CMV) inclusions and microglial nodules occur in nearly 25 per cent of the brains of AIDS patients at autopsy. The clinical effects of superadded CMV to HIV infection are uncertain. CMV infection of the choroid and retina is more clinically important in AIDS. Vascular occlusion and perivascular exudates and haemorrhages are seen on fundoscopy. CMV can probably cause an encephalopathy independent of HIV infection, as confusion and lethargy in association with this virus occur in renal transplant patients. Ganciclovir may be used at a dose of 5 mg/kg intravenously over 1 hour every 12 hours, for 14–21 days. Significant neutropenia and a variety of other side-effects prevent widespread use of the drug.

Herpes simplex encephalitis and progressive multifocal leucoencephalopathy due to infection with the JC papovavirus (Section 17.14.3.2) have also been reported. Herpes simplex produces the usual acute encephalitic picture described in Sec-tion 17.12.3. The progression of JC infection is difficult to distinguish from HIV dementia.

Neoplasms

Primary CNS B-cell lymphomas have been reported in a number of patients with AIDS, some possibly related to Epstein–Barr virus-induced transformation of B-cells. Ante-mortem distinction from the much more common HIV dementia is again difficult. Initial symptoms are commonly changes in cognitive function, headache, focal motor deficits, and ataxia. Focal seizures and cran-ial nerve palsies may occur. Imaging may show solitary or multiple lesions, with some degree of enhancement on CT scanning.

17.13   Post-viral syndromes

A number of different neurological syndromes can follow viral infections. Their clinical features and pathogenesis are heterogeneous.

17.13.1   *Post-infectious encephalomyelitis*

After measles, varicella, and rubella, and previously after smallpox, a post-viral demyelinating or allergic encephalopathy can occur. The incidence after measles is about 1 in 1000. A similar encephalomyelitis can occur after measles vaccine.

17.13.1.1   *Pathophysiology*

The histology of post-infectious encephalomyelitis is indistinguishable from that described in Section 17.12.5.3 for neuroparalytic events after neural rabies vaccine. If measles is taken as an example, demyelination could theoretically result through direct infection of oligodendroglia, death of which would result in breakdown of the myelin membrane, as in progressive multifocal leucoencephalopathy (Section 17.14.3.2). However, measles virus is not identified in the brain at this stage, nor is there evidence of intrathecal production of anti-measles antibody. Interest centres on the observation that antibodies to myelin basic protein are present. There is some homology in sequence between the measles nucleocapsid protein and myelin basic protein, so antibodies directed against measles protein could possibly be directed against myelin as well. It has been suggested that the presence of a complementary antigen, analogous to adjuvant, is necessary for the fully developed syndrome, accounting for its relative rarity. There are certainly alterations in general immune responsiveness at this stage. For many years it has been known that positive Mantoux tests may revert to negative for some weeks after measles infection, and epidemics of measles have been noted to be followed by epidemics of tuberculosis.

17.13.1.2   *Clinical features*

The onset of measles encephalomyelitis begins 2–7 days after the onset of the rash, often at a time when the child's general state is otherwise improving. Alterations in conscious level, seizures, hemiparesis, ataxia, and involuntary movements are all frequent features. The clinical features of other types of post-viral encephalomyelitis are similar.

17.13.1.3   *Treatment and prognosis*

Neither hyperimmune γ-globulin nor cortico-steroids significantly alter the course of post-viral encephalomyelitis. There may, however, be a surprising degree of recovery, even after periods of profound coma, so supportive therapy should be energetic. Unfortunately, however, mental retardation and late epilepsy are frequent residual features.

Programmes of immunization against measles and rubella and the abandonment of smallpox vaccination have led to a gratifying reduction in the frequency of post-viral encephalomyelitis.

17.13.2   *Other post-viral syndromes*

Infectious mononucleosis may be complicated by a meningoencephalitis, or by a peripheral neuropathy. An acute cerebellar syndrome may also occur, the pathophysiology of which is poorly understood.

17.13.2.1   *Reye's syndrome*

This poorly understood syndrome is characterized by the sudden development of profuse vomiting, an encephalopathy with stupor, and acute fatty degeneration of the liver. It affects a child or young adult who has recently been infected with a common virus, such as influenza B or, less commonly, influenza A, varicella, or the Epstein–Barr virus. The median age of affected children is about 14 months in the UK, but as high as 8 years in the USA.

Pathophysiology

The cause of Reye's syndrome is unknown but is probably multifactorial. That is to say, there is an abnormal reaction to a viral infection occurring in a genetically susceptible host. This reaction is in some way influenced by the concurrent consumption of aspirin, as case control studies show that aspirin has been given for the viral infection in a high proportion of instances. These factors interact to disrupt mitochondrial structure and function, particularly in the liver. Blood ammonia accumulates, as do hepatic enzymes such as transaminase. Salicylic acid has been shown to uncouple oxidative phosphorylation, inhibit mitochondrial dehydrogenases, and alter membrane permeability in hepatic cells. There is electron microscopic evidence of mitochondrial damage. Aspirin also inhibits lymphocyte transformation and interferon production in response to viral infection. Aspirin seems to play a less important part in adult cases. The CSF is usually normal.

The differential diagnosis includes other causes of fulminant hepatic failure, including viral hepatitis, overdosage with paracetamol, halothane anaesthesia, and urea cycle diseases such as ornithine transcarbamylase deficiency and systemic carnitine deficiency.

Cerebral oedema rather than hepatic failure is the principal cause of death. If this can be controlled by ventilation and reduction of $P_{a\,CO_2}$ and mannitol, and if there is careful attention to fluid and electrolyte balance, and if arterial perfusion pressure is maintained, then the outcome is generally satisfactory. Dietary protein restriction is probably also useful.

17.13.2.2 Chronic fatigue syndrome (synonyms: myalgic encephalomyelitis, post-viral fatigue syndrome, Royal Free disease)

This poorly understood condition occurs principally in epidemics in partly closed communities, such as hospitals or schools. Vague malaise, muscle aches, and fever are then followed for many months or even years by easy fatiguability and mild depression. Some advocate a psychological explanation for these symptoms, others incline to the view that they represent the late results of viral infection. The syndrome is further discussed in Section 25.2.4.

17.13.2.3 Exacerbation of pre-existing neurological illness

It has been recognized for many years that intercurrent viral infections may precipitate an exacerbation of multiple sclerosis. Some of the inherited ataxias (Section 20.3) may also be made worse.

17.14 Persistent viral infections

17.14.1 Chronic virus infections

Examples of chronic virus infections are congenital rubella and congenital cytomegalovirus infection, in which the virus can be isolated from infected

infants for years after birth. Host defences are insufficient to eliminate the virus.

17.14.2 Latent virus infections

Herpes zoster (Section 17.12.7) and herpes simplex (Section 17.12.3) are examples of infections in which the virus can lie latent for many years, being reactivated by unknown mechanisms to cause a new acute clinical illness.

17.14.3 'Slow' virus infections

The term 'slow virus infection' is used to describe persistent infections with a long latency before the clinical onset of disease. Both conventional viruses and unconventional agents may cause such syndromes. Measles virus is associated with subacute sclerosing panencephalitis, and the JC papovavirus with progressive multifocal leucoencephalopathy. Unconventional agents are associated with Creutzfeldt–Jakob disease and kuru (Section 17.15).

17.14.3.1 Subacute sclerosing panencephalitis

This is a serious virus-mediated encephalopathy of children and young adults. The annual incidence is about 1 per million. Males are more commonly affected, as are those living in rural areas. Mortality is very high. Those who survive do so with considerable intellectual impairment and physical disability.

At post-mortem, there is perivascular cuffing, with lymphocytes and plasma cells. Gliosis is prominent. Eosinophilic intranuclear inclusion bodies are characteristic, most often being found in oligodendrocytes. Fluorescent antibody techniques demonstrate the presence of measles virus, but the virus can only be recovered by co-cultivation.

Although an unusual illness, subacute sclerosing panencephalitis (SSPE) is of great biological interest. How is it that measles virus is eradicated from the vast majority of children, and yet in a few can persist in the brain and cause devastating neurological illness, although there are high levels of measles antibody in the blood and CSF? The mechanism is not fully understood, but some facts are known. Genetic factors are not important, as identical twins are usually discordant for SSPE. Those who develop SSPE are likely to have had measles at an unusually early age, often before 1 year of age. Cases follow immunization with measles vaccine, but at a lesser frequency than after natural measles. Children with SSPE appear to be of normal immunological competence in other ways. Many peripheral lymphocytes also contain measles virus in patients with SSPE.

The measles virus associated with SSPE appears to be different from the usual measles virus. The virus assembled within the nervous system is defective in the matrix (M) protein of measles virus, and serum antibodies against this protein are deficient in patients with SSPE.

One hypothesis is that SSPE is due to a mutant measles virus which has an abnormality in the gene coding for M protein. Alternatively, the defect of M protein production could lie within the host brain cells. In either event, measles nucleocapsids then accumulate within the brain and spread from cell to cell by directly traversing cell membranes. When sufficient accumulation of unassembled virus has occurred, the clinical illness begins.

Clinical features

The initial features are behavioural disturbances or a decline in school performance. The child is subsequently affected by myoclonic jerks, seizures, dysarthria, and spastic weakness of the limbs, becoming mute and rigid before death.

Measles antibodies are present in high titre in the blood and CSF. The CSF contains a high concentration of IgG, which can be shown to be anti-measles IgG. The EEG shows characteristic stereotyped triphasic high-voltage discharges occurring on a relatively featureless background.

Treatment

The most widely followed treatment is isoprinosine, but unfortunately this has not been shown to influence the course of the illness significantly.

17.14.3.2   *Progressive multifocal leucoencephalopathy*

This disorder was first described in 1958 in patients with lymphomas, but is now recognized to occur in patients who are immunologically incompetent for any reason. The cause is infection with a papovavirus, a group of DNA viruses, many of which are potentially oncogenic. Virtually all the virus isolates have been JC virus, the initials of a patient in

Wisconsin. (Note there is potential confusion with the initials of the Creutzfeldt–Jakob agent, which is quite different.) Another papovavirus, 'SV40', has occasionally been isolated. The virus infects and destroys oligodendrocytes, and hence demyelination occurs. Multinucleated enlarged astrocytes are found in these areas of focal demyelination. It is not known whether immunological incompetence allows a previously latent virus to replicate, or whether the illness occurs as a new infection in an immunologically incompetent subject. However, as nearly 80 per cent of individuals over the age of 20 are serologically positive for JC virus, the former suggestion is more likely.

Clinical features

The initial symptoms and signs reflect the foci of myelin destruction. Personality change, cognitive impairment, hemiparesis, dysarthria, and ataxia are all found. Severe dementia follows. Headaches and seizures are unusual.

CT scanning shows focal zones of decreased attenuation which enlarge gradually as the disease progresses. They do not enhance after the injection of contrast. The low attenuation zones often follow the border between grey and white matter. MRI also demonstrates the lesions well.

Treatment

Cytosine arabinoside has been used, with some possible effect upon the progress of the disease, but unfortunately the illness is usually rapidly progressive, death following within 2–4 months of the onset of symptoms.

17.15   The prion diseases

Prion protein is the normal product of a gene found in many organisms. Little is known of its function, but it is bound to membranes. An abnormal form of prion protein is found in human brains and in those of animals with a variety of diseases, collectively known as the spongiform encephalopathies. Examples are Creutzfeldt–Jakob disease, Gerstmann–Sträussler–Scheinker disease and kuru in humans, and scrapie, a degenerative disease of sheep, transmissible mink encephalopathy, and bovine spongiform encephalopathy in animals (see below). Histological examination of the brains of affected humans or animals shows varying degrees of neuronal loss, vacuolation of the cytoplasm and dendrites of surviving neurons (hence the term 'spongiform'), marked astrocytosis (gliosis), and deposition of amyloid in fibrils. These fibrils are the abnormal form of the prion protein. As they were first identified in scrapie, they are known as scrapie-associated fibrils (SAF). They are 6 nm in length and often lie in pairs. They appear to be associated with infectivity, and contain a specific proteinase-resistant host-encoded glycoprotein, the modified prion protein.

The history of the prion-protein-associated spongiform encephalopathies is of great interest. A number of rapidly advancing dementing illnesses associated with ataxia and myoclonic jerks were described by Heidenhain, Creutzfeldt, Jakob, and Nevin, and the typical spongiform changes recognized by Creutzfeldt in the 1920s. Similar histological changes were recognized in the brains of members of the Fore highlanders in Papua New Guinea afflicted by kuru, an ataxic, paralysing, and dementing illness. This tribe practised ritual cannibalism, and epidemiological evidence suggested that this was associated with kuru. The realization that kuru might be transmissible, and the similarity of the spongiform changes of kuru to Creutzfeldt–Jakob disease eventually led Gadjusek to demonstrate the transmissibility of Creutzfeldt–Jakob disease to chimpanzees, but only by intracerebral injection. It is now recognized that person-to-person transmission of Creutzfeldt–Jakob disease can occur through corneal grafting, the use of pituitary-derived human growth hormone, the use of dural grafts, or by the implantation of contaminated electrodes. The incubation period after such exposure is variable, between 18 months or 10 years or more. Furthermore, there is strong circumstantial evidence that the current epidemic in the UK of bovine spongiform encephalopathy resulted from feeding meal containing sheep offal to normally herbivorous cows. The scrapie agent from sheep brains can be transmitted by intracerebral or intraperitoneal injection to mice or hamsters.

All this implies an infective agent, but, if so, the agent is, unlike a virus, highly resistant to heat, irradiation, and glutaraldehyde. It can be inactivated by 2 per cent hypochlorite or by autoclaving at 134–138 °C in a porous load system. The agent cannot be cultured, and cannot be detected by tests for any known antigen, nor has any systemic antibody response been detected. However, modified prion protein can be localized in the brain by specific antibodies (immunocytochemistry and Western blotting), and the modified prion protein found in these diseases is thought to be the major if not the only component of the agent responsible for transmission.

Then there is the problem that 15 per cent of patients with Creutzfeldt–Jakob disease are familial, and, in the histologically identical Gerstmann–Sträussler–Scheinker disease, transmission appears to be by an autosomal dominant gene. Molecular studies of the prion protein gene have shown three gene variants that occur only in families with familial Creutzfeldt–Jakob disease (a codon 117 valine substitution and insertions of six tandem repeat sequences of codon 53, or a codon 200 lysine substitution) or the Gerstmann–Sträussler–Scheinker syndrome (codon 102 leucine substitution). A case has been described of a demented patient whose brain after death showed *no* spongiform change, but who had one of these gene variants. A recent further prion disease has been described—familial fatal insomnia, characterized also by dysautonomia and motor signs, with a gene variant at codon 178.

A synthesis of this evidence suggests that a small proportion of the population carries a prion protein gene variant that places them at particular risk of developing a dementing illness, usually but not invariably characterized by the production of amyloid fibrils and spongiform change. In non-genetic cases, the presence of abnormal prion protein (e.g. by intracerebral injection) triggers conversion of the normal form into more of the variant associated with the disease.

17.15.1   *Creutzfeldt–Jakob disease*

Creutzfeldt–Jakob disease is a rare disorder, the annual incidence being about 1–2/million, but fifty times more common in Libyan Jews in whom the codon 200 lysine substitution described above is common. Older people are usually affected. After a vague prodromal illness of change of mood and general malaise, focal neurological deficits, such as dysphasia, ataxia, or visual hallucinations, occur. Myoclonic jerks are frequent. At a later stage, cortical blindness, rigidity, muscle wasting and mutism occur. Survival may be for only a few weeks, and most patients are dead within 10 months.

Investigations short of brain biopsy are of little help. This procedure has naturally become unpopular since it has become clear that neuro-surgical instruments sterilized in the usual way can transmit the disease. However, with suitable pre-cautions, biopsy can be done, and specific im-munostaining of amyloid plaques and the presence of protease-resistant prion protein will confirm the diagnosis. Examination of the CSF is unhelpful. The EEG may show stereotyped generalized tri-phasic complexes occurring once or twice a second, but these only occur late in the disease. No treat-ment has as yet been found to modify the course of the illness.

The differential diagnosis includes rapidly advancing Alzheimer's disease, in which myoclonus may be prominent. Other diagnoses to be considered include Parkinson's disease with dementia, normal pressure hydrocephalus, and limbic encephalitis. The pathology is described above.

17.16   The problem of vaccine-induced brain damage

Herd immunization against polio, diphtheria, per-tussis, tetanus, measles, mumps, and rubella has been achieved in developed countries, and serious morbidity and mortality have been enormously reduced. There have been particular problems with ascertaining whether pertussis vaccine, in particu-lar, causes brain damage. The vaccine certainly causes fever in a significant number of children, and some of these children have febrile convul-sions. At the time the vaccine was introduced, it was recognized that other vaccines, such as small-pox, rabies, and tetanus toxin, could cause immu-nological events and, in the case of the first two at least, an encephalopathy. The scene was therefore set for considering that pertussis may do the same. The National Childhood Encephalopathy Study in the UK suggested a risk of permanent brain damage arising from pertussis vaccination of 1 per 330 000 doses and of encephalopathy 1 per 140 000. Further calculations by others suggest that these risks are an artefact of the data; the increased relative risk of febrile convulsions in the first 7 days being offset by a decreased risk over the next 21 days. In a large study of more than 100 000 vaccine doses given to children enrolled in Medi-caid in Tennessee, no child who was previously neurologically normal had a seizure within 3 days of immunization with diphtheria–tetanus–pertussis vaccine that heralded the onset of either epilepsy or developmental abnormality. However, earlier studies have led to encephalopathy following vac-cine damage as being the object of compensation in the UK, and of litigation in the USA.

17.17   Inflammatory disorders of the nervous system which may or may not have an infectious origin

17.17.1   *Sarcoidosis of the nervous system*

Sarcoidosis is a multisystem granulomatous dis-order of unknown origin, characterized by the presence in affected organs of epithelioid-cell gran-ulomas, without caseation. Mycobacterial DNA can be identified in some lesions, but other infectious causes may occur. The most common clinical pres-entations include bilateral hilar adenopathy, uveitis, peripheral adenopathy, and erythema nodosum and other skin lesions. The nervous system is affected in about 5 per cent of cases. The most frequent neurological manifestation is cranial neu-ropathy affecting one or more cranial nerves. The facial nerve is most commonly affected, but ophthalmoplegia and nerve deafness also occur. Cranial neuropathies may be accompanied by evi-dence of a lymphocytic meningitis, with an ele-vated CSF protein and reduced CSF sugar. Granulomatous meningeal and juxta-ependymal involvement may result in hydrocephalus.

Granulomas may affect the parenchyma of the brain. They show a predilection for the hypothala-mus. Diabetes insipidus, hypersomnolence, and impaired temperature control may reflect lesions in this area. Such a granuloma may invade the optic chiasma and result in visual defects. Other cerebral granulomas may cause epileptic seizures. A combination of spinal meningeal involvement and intramedullary granulomas may cause a spastic paraparesis. The local effects of these parenchy-matous granulomas is compounded by the pres-ence of a vasculitis. A similar vasculitis in the peripheral nervous system can cause a mononeuritis multiplex, but a symmetrical chronic sensory neuropathy is also seen. Rarely, acute or chronic myopathies occur, but muscle biopsy shows granulomas in about half the patients with widespread sarcoidosis, even if the muscles are not clinically affected.

17.17.1.1 Diagnosis and treatment

The diagnosis of neurosarcoidosis often depends upon evidence of the disease elsewhere, such as hilar adenopathy and uveitis, in association with one of the syndromes just described. Examination of the CSF, imaging, biopsy of an enlarged gland or skin lesion, muscle or nerve all play a part in the diagnosis. The serum angiotensin-converting enzyme may be elevated, and the Kweim test may prove useful.

Corticosteroids prove useful in many cases of sarcoidosis, resulting in a shrinkage of parenchymatous granulomata and often a recession of meningitis. However, disabilities due to neurosarcoidosis often advance in spite of treatment.

17.17.2 Vogt–Koyanagi–Harada syndrome

This rare but interesting disorder is characterized by a meningoencephalitis, uveitis, oculomotor palsies, and vitiligo. It is thought that the cause may be an abnormal immune response to a viral infection.

17.18 Further reading

General

Lambert, H. P. (ed.) (1991). *Infections of the central nervous system*. Edward Arnold, Sevenoaks.

Bacterial meningitis

Editorial (1989). Meningococcal meningitis. *Lancet* 1, 647–8.

Odio, C. M., Faingezicht, I., Paris, M., *et al.* (1991). The beneficial effects of early dexamethasone administration in infants and children with bacterial meningitis. *New England Journal of Medicine* 324, 1525–31.

Pomeroy, S. L., Holmes, S. J., Dodge, P. R., and Feigin, R. D. (1990). Seizures and other neurological sequelae of bacterial meningitis in children. *New England Journal of Medicine* 323, 1651–7.

Spanos, A., Harrell, F. E., and Durack, D. T. (1989). Differential diagnosis of acute meningitis. An analysis of the predictive value of initial observations. *Journal of the American Medical Association* 262, 2700–7.

Tunkel, A. R., Wispelwey, B., and Scheld, W. M. (1990). Bacterial meningitis: recent advances in pathophysiology and treatment. *Annals of Internal Medicine* 112, 610–23.

Welsby, P. D. and Golledge, C. L. (1990). Meningococcal meningitis. *British Medical Journal* 300, 1150–1.

Brain abscess

Editorial (1988). Treatment of brain abscess. *Lancet* 1, 219–20.

Sparrow, O. C. (1991). The importance of early detection of intracranial suppuration. *Journal of the Royal Society of Medicine* 84, 187–8.

Neurosyphilis

Davis, L. E. (1990). Neurosyphilis in the patient infected with human immuno-deficiency virus. *Annals of Neurology* 27, 211–12.

Davis, L. E. and Schmitt, J. W. (1989). Clinical significance of cerebrospinal fluid tests for neurosyphilis. *Annals of Neurology* 25, 50–5.

Hook, E. W. and Marra, C. M. (1992). Acquired syphilis in adults. *New England Journal of Medicine* 326, 1060–9.

Lyme disease

Kaslow, R. A. (1992). Current perspective on Lyme Borreliosis. *Journal of the American Medical Association* 267, 1381–3.

Logigian, E. L., Kaplan, R. F., and Steere, A. C. (1990). Chronic neurologic manifestations of Lyme disease. *New England Journal of Medicine* 323, 1438–44.

Rahn, D. W. and Malawista, S. E. (1991). Lyme disease: recommendations for diagnosis and treatment. *Annals of Internal Medicine* 114, 472–81.

Leptospirosis

Reik, L. (1987). Spirochaetal infections of the nervous system. In *Infections of the nervous system*, (ed. P. G. E. Kennedy and R. T. Johnson), pp. 43–75. Butterworths, London.

Tuberculous meningitis

Bateman, D. E., Newman, P. K., and Foster, J. B. (1983). A retrospective survey of proven cases of tuberculous meningitis in the Northern Region

1970–1980. *Journal of the Royal College of Physicians of London* **17**, 106–10.

Lu, C.-Z., Qiao, J., Shen, T., and Link, H. (1990). Early diagnosis of tuberculous meningitis by detection of anti-BCG secreting cells in cerebrospinal fluid. *Lancet* **336**, 10–13.

Shankar, P., *et al.* (1991). Rapid diagnosis of tuberculous meningitis by polymerase chain reaction. *Lancet* **337**, 5–7.

Tuberculomas

Loizou, A. and Anderson, M. (1982). Intracranial tuberculomas: correlation of computerised tomography with clinicopathological findings. *Quarterly Journal of Medicine* **202**, 104–14.

Tuberculous radiculomyelopathy

Freilich, D. and Swash, M. (1979). Diagnosis and management of tuberculous paraplegia with special reference to tuberculous radiculomyelitis. *Journal of Neurology, Neurosurgery and Psychiatry* **42**, 12–18.

Tuberculous (Pott's) disease of the spine

Gorse, G. J., Pais, M. J., Kusske, J. A., and Cesario, T. C. (1983). Tuberculous spondylitis. *Medicine* **62**, 178–93.

Leprosy

Bryceson, A. and Pfaltzgraff, R. E. (1990). *Leprosy* (3rd edn). Churchill Livingstone, Edinburgh.

Tetanus

Ahmadsyah, I. and Salim, A. (1985). Treatment of tetanus: an open study to compare the efficacy of procaine penicillin and metronidazole. *British Medical Journal* **291**, 647–50.

Botulism

Lund, B. M. (1990). Foodborne disease due to *Bacillus* and *Clostridium* species. *Lancet* **336**, 982–6.

Rickettsial infections

Shaked, Y. (1991). Rickettsial infections of the central nervous system: the role of prompt antibiotic therapy. *Quarterly Journal of Medicine, New Series* **79**, 301–6.

Toxoplasmosis

McCabe, R. and Remington, J. S. (1988). Toxoplasmosis: the time has come. *New England Journal of Medicine* **318**, 313–15.

Cysticercosis and paragonimiasis

Case records of the Massachusetts General Hospital (1990). *New England Journal of Medicine* **322**, 1446–58.

Schistosomiasis

Scrimgeour, E. M. and Gajdusek, D. C. (1985). Involvement of the central nervous system in *Schistosoma mansoni* and *S. haemotobium* infection: a review. *Brain* **108**, 1023–38.

Toxocariasis and echinococcosis

Arpino, C. and Curatolo, P. (1988). Toxocariasis in children. *Lancet* **1**, 1172.

Elliot, D. L., Tolle, S. W., Goldberg, L., and Miller, J.B. (1985). Pet associated illness. *New England Journal of Medicine* **313**, 985–95.

Malaria

Phillips, R. E. and Solomon, T. (1990). Cerebral malaria in children. *Lancet* **336**, 1355–60.

Trypanosomiasis

Pepin, J., Guern, C., Milford, F., and Schechter, P. J. (1987). Difluoromethylornithine for arseno-resistant *Trypanosoma brucei gambiense* sleeping sickness. *Lancet* **2**, 1431–3.

Fungal infections

Galgiani, J. N. (1990). Fluconazole, a new antifungal agent. *Annals of Internal Medicine* **113**, 177–9.

Tjia, T. L., Yeow, Y. K., and Tan, C. B. (1985). Cryptococcal meningitis. *Journal of Neurology, Neurosurgery and Psychiatry* **48**, 853–8.

Walsh, T. J., *et al.* (1985). Aspergillosis of the nervous system: clinicopathological analysis of 17 patients. *Annals of Neurology* **18**, 574–82.

Wiles, C. M. and Mackenzie, D. W. R. (1987). Fungal diseases of the central nervous system. In *Infections of the nervous system*, (ed. P. G. E. Kennedy and R. T. Johnson), pp. 93–117. Butterworths, London.

Encephalitis

Aurelius, E., Johannsson, B., Sköldenberg, B., Staland, A., and Forsgren, M. (1991). Rapid diagnosis of herpes simplex encephalitis by nested polymerase chain reaction assay of cerebrospinal fluid. *Lancet* **337**, 189–92.

Hoke, C. H., *et al.* (1988). Protection against Japanese encephalitis by inactivated vaccine. *New England Journal of Medicine* **319**, 608–14.

Whitley, R. J. (1990). Viral encephalitis. *New England Journal of Medicine* **323**, 242–50.

Rabies

Baer, G. M. and Fishbein, D. B. (1987). Rabies post-exposure prophylaxis. *New England Journal of Medicine* **316**, 1270–2.

Poliomyelitis

Bateman, D. E., Elrington, G., Kennedy, P., and Saunders, M. (1987). Vaccine related poliomyelitis in non-immunised relatives and household contacts. *British Medical Journal* **294**, 170–1.

Munsat, T. L. (1991). Poliomyelitis—new problems with an old disease. *New England Journal of Medicine* **324**, 1206–7.

Herpes zoster

Editorial (1990). Post herpetic neuralgia. *Lancet* **336**, 537–8.

Kennedy, P. G. E. (1987). Neurological complications of varicella-zoster virus. In *Infections of the nervous system*, (ed. P. G. E. Kennedy and R. T. Johnson), pp. 117–208. Butterworths, London.

Epstein–Barr virus infections

Erzurum, S., Kalavsky, S., and Watanakunakorn, C. (1983). Acute cerebellar ataxia and hearing loss as initial symptoms of infectious mononucleosis. *Archives of Neurology* **40**, 760–2.

Human T-cell lymphotrophic virus type I infections

Bhagavati, S., Ehrlich, G., Kula, R. W. *et al.* (1988). Detection of human T-cell lymphoma/leukaemia virus type I DNA and antigen in spinal fluid and blood of patients with chronic progressive myelopathy. *New England Journal of Medicine* **318**, 1141–7.

Brew, B. J. and Price, R. W. (1988). Another retroviral disease of the nervous system. Chronic progressive myelopathy due to HTLV-I. *New England Journal of Medicine* **318**, 1195–6.

Editorial (1988). HTLV-I comes of age. *Lancet* **1**, 217–19.

Morgan, O., St. C., Montgomery, R. D., and Rodgers-Johnson, P. (1988). The myeloneuropathies of Jamaica: an unfolding story. *Quarterly Journal of Medicine, New Series* **67**, 273–81.

Post-infectious encephalomyelitis

Arnason, B. G. W. (1987). Neuroimmunology. *New England Journal of Medicine* **316**, 406–8.

Johnson, R.T. and Griffin, D.E. (1987). Postinfectious encephalomyelitis. In *Infections of the nervous system*, (ed. P. G. E. Kennedy and R. T. Johnson). Butterworths, London.

Chronic fatigue syndrome

See references to chronic fatigue syndrome at the end of Chapter 25.

Reye's syndrome

Editorial (1987). Reye's syndrome and aspirin: epidemiological associations and inborn errors of metabolism. *Lancet* **2**, 429–31.

Jenkins, J. G., Glasgow, J. F. T., Vlack, G. W. *et al.* (1987). Reye's syndrome: assessment of intracranial monitoring. *British Medical Journal* **294**, 337–8.

HIV infection

Brew, B. J., Sidtis, J. J., Rosenblum, M., and Price, R. W. (1988). AIDS dementia complex. *Journal of the Royal College of Physicians of London* **22**, 140–4.

Case records of the Massachusetts General Hospital (1990). *New England Journal of Medicine* **323**, 1823–33. (This contains a useful review and source of references for opportunistic infections in AIDS.)

Dalakas, M. G. and Pezeshkpour, G. H. (1988). Neuromuscular diseases associated with human immunodeficiency virus infection. *Annals of Neurology* **23** (suppl.), S38–S48.

Denning, D. W., Anderson, J., Rudge, P., and Smith, H. (1987). Acute myelopathy associated with primary infection with human immunodeficiency virus. *British Medical Journal* **194**, 143–4.

Everall, I. P., Luthert, P. J., and Lantos, P. L. (1991). Neuronal loss in the frontal cortex in HIV infection. *Lancet* **337**, 1119–21.

Fischl, M. A., Parker, C. B., Pettinelli, C., *et al.* (1990). A randomized controlled trial of a reduced daily dose

of zidovudine in patients with the acquired immunodeficiency syndrome. *New England Journal of Medicine* **323**, 1009–14.

Friedland, G. H. (1990). Early treatment for HIV–the
time has come. *New England Journal of Medicine* **322**,
1000–2.

Hammersmith Staff Rounds (1990). Cerebral mass
lesions in patients with AIDS. *British Medical Journal*
301, 226–8.

Lantos, P. L., McLaughlin, J. E., Scholtz, C. L. *et al.*
(1989). Neuropathology of the brain in HIV infection.
Lancet **1**, 309–10.

Petito, C. K., Navia, B. A., Cho, E.-S., *et al.* (1987).
Vacuolar myelopathy pathologically resembling subacute combined degeneration in patients with the
acquired immunodeficiency syndrome. *New England
Journal of Medicine* **312**, 874–9.

Pinching, A. J. (1988). Neurological aspects of the
acquired immune deficiency syndrome. *Journal of the
Royal College of Physicians of London* **22**, 136–9.

Quinn, T. C., Zacarias, F. R. K., and St. John, R. K.
(1989). AIDS in the Americas—an emerging public
health crisis. *New England Journal of Medicine* **320**,
1005–7.

Rosenblum, M. L., Levy, R. M., and Bredesen, D. E.
(ed.) (1987). *AIDS and the nervous system*. Raven
Press, New York.

Progressive multifocal leucoencephalopathy

Lipton, H. L. (1991). Is JC virus latent in brain? *Annals
of Neurology* **29**, 433–4.

Richardson, E. P. (1988). Progressive multifocal leucoencephalopathy 30 years later. *New England Journal
of Medicine* **318**, 315–16.

Subacute sclerosing panencephalitis

Case records of the Massachusetts General Hospital
(1986). *New England Journal of Medicine* **314**,
1689–1700.

Creutzfeldt–Jakob disease and other prion diseases

Collee, J. G. (1990). Bovine spongiform encephalopathy. *Lancet* **336**, 1300–3.

Collinge, J., *et al.* (1990). Prion dementia without characteristic pathology. *Lancet* **336**, 7–9.

Harrison, P. J. and Roberts, G. W. (1992). How now
mad cow? (bovine spongiform encephalopathy). *British Medical Journal* **304**, 929–30.

Hsiao, K., Meiner, Z., Kahana, E., *et al.* (1991). Mutation of the prion protein in Libyan Jews with Creutzfeldt–Jakob disease. *New England Journal of Medicine*
324, 1091–7.

Johnson, R. T. (1992). Prion disease. *New England
Journal of Medicine* **326**, 486–7.

Will, R. G. and Matthews, W. B. (1984). A retrospective
study of Creutzfeldt–Jakob disease in England and
Wales. *Journal of Neurology, Neurosurgery and Psychiatry* **47**, 134–40.

Will, R. G., Matthews, W. B., Smith, P. G., and
Hudson, C. (1986). A retrospective study of Creutzfeldt–Jakob disease in England and Wales 1970–79.
II: Epidemiology. *Journal of Neurology, Neurosurgery
and Psychiatry* **315**, 279–83.

The problem of vaccine-induced brain damage

Ad hoc Committee for the Child Neurology Society
Consensus statement on pertussis immunization and
the central nervous system (1991). *World Neurology*
9–10.

Editorial (1990). 'Pertussis vaccine encephalopathy': it is
time to recognise it as the myth that it is. *Journal of
the American Medical Association* **262**, 1679–80.

Sarcoidosis

Saboor, S. A., Johnson, N. McJ., and McFadden, J.
(1992). Detection of mycobacterial DNA in sarcoidosis and tuberculosis with polymerase chain reaction.
Lancet **339**, 1012–15.

Stern, B. J., *et al.* (1985). Sarcoidosis and its neurological
manifestations. *Archives of Neurology* **42**, 909–17.

18 Diseases of the spinal cord and nerve roots

Many neurological diseases affecting the brain affect the spinal cord as well. Multiple sclerosis, for example, is commonly disseminated in both regions. On the other hand, vascular disorders of the spinal cord are surprisingly rare, considering the frequency of transient ischaemic attacks and stroke.

The mobility of the spinal column is associated with articular degenerative changes (spondylosis), which are important causes of radicular syndromes (Section 18.2.2) and myelopathy (Section 18.2.3). The vertebrae are common foci for metastatic tumours or pus, which may invade the extradural space, so that compressive lesions of the spinal cord are comparatively common. These are known as extramedullary lesions, as opposed to intramedullary lesions within the cord, such as an astrocytoma of the cord (Section 18.5.3). The spinal cord terminates at the lower border of the second lumbar vertebra. The spinal canal below that level is filled with a leash of nerve roots—the cauda equina. The physical signs of spinal cord and cauda equina syndromes are described in Sections 6.9 and 6.10.

Table 18.1 provides a framework for considering disorders of the spinal cord and nerve roots. As traumatic lesions of the spinal cord provide a convenient model for severe cord lesions of any aetiology, this is considered first.

18.1   Traumatic injuries of the spinal cord

Spinal trauma often occurs in the prime of life. The necessary emotional and physical adjustments to a life of disability usually take 2–3 years, the first part of which is usually spent in a special unit devoted to the care of those with spinal injuries. The avoidance of the late complications begins in the earliest stages of management, and such early care, and advice about rehabilitation is best given in such units. There is usually about one unit per 5 million people. Amongst the best known of these is at Stoke Mandeville in the UK, where Guttmann and colleagues introduced many of the principles and techniques now widely employed throughout the world.

18.1.1   *Epidemiology of spinal trauma*

The annual incidence of spinal cord injury is about 20 per million per year. The commonest cause is motor cycle and car accidents, but falls at home down stairs or at work are also a frequent cause. Injury sustained in sporting and recreational activities, particularly falls from horses, rugby football, swimming, and gymnastics are also unfortunately common. Rugby injuries are usually due to hyperflexion of the neck during a collapsing ruck, and attempts have been made to minimize this risk by modifying the rules of the game. Injuries during swimming usually occur by diving into water that is unexpectedly shallow, so that the head is hyperextended and the neck compressed on striking the bottom. It should be the law that the depth of water should be marked at intervals around all swimming pools, domestic or private, and all young swimmers must be instructed to check the depth before diving from river banks or from rocks into the sea. In crowded swimming pools, impacts may occur between a diver and a swimmer already in the pool, either party then sustaining a spinal injury. Motor cycle accidents, sporting accidents,

Table 18.1   Classification of neurological disorders of the spinal cord

Extramedullary compression by
   trauma (vertebral misalignment and haemorrhage)
   vertebral destruction (e.g. by metastasis)
   spondylotic bars
   soft disc extrusion
   benign tumours (e.g. meningioma)
   pus (e.g. tuberculous pus)
   Paget's disease
Intramedullary disorders
   inflammatory disorders, unknown cause
      acute transverse myelopathy
      multiple sclerosis
   inflammatory disorders, known cause
      HTLV-I infection (tropical myelopathy)
      HIV infection
      Epstein–Barr infection
      syphilis
   vascular disorders
      atheroma
      angiomatous malformations
      inflammatory arteritis
      haemorrhage (e.g. in haemophilia)
   tumours
      astrocytoma
      ependymoma
   congenital anomalies
      syringomyelia
      cord tethering
   toxic disorders
      cyanide
      triorthocresyl phosphate
   deficiency disorders
      vitamin B_{12} deficiency

Also, a number of degenerative disorders and motor neuron disease, considered in Chapter 20, cause prominent histological changes in the spinal cord, but are not usually considered under the heading of spinal cord diseases.

and accidents at work (often on construction sites) are particularly likely to occur in young men.

18.1.2   *Mechanism of injury and pathology*

Hyperflexion of the spine occurs when the head and body are in forward motion, and then suddenly decelerated, the blow tilting the head forwards. Head-on collisions in cars may result in such injuries, particularly if safety belts are not worn. Falling down stairs may result in a hyperflexion injury as the back of the head strikes a wall on the turn of the staircase. The interspinous ligament, the capsule of the articular facetal joints, and the posterior fibres of the intervertebral disc are all torn, and there may be a forward dislocation of the upper vertebra on the lower, often C5 on C6.

Hyperextension injuries occur as a result of a forward fall on to the face. The anterior longitudinal ligament and anterior fibres of the disc rupture. The ligamentum flavum buckles and compresses the cord from behind, and the spinal cord itself is hyperextended. In older people, who already have some degree of cervical spondylosis (Section 18.2), there is an increased risk of cord damage due to the reduced cross-sectional area of the spinal canal. A rear-end motor vehicle impact may cause a sufficient hyperextension (whiplash) injury to damage the spinal cord, without direct impact to the head. All cars should be provided with head restraints.

Combinations of compression and flexion forces may result in cervical compressive fractures, with extension of the crushed vertebral body, and haematoma, into the spinal canal. Crush fractures also occur in the dorsal and lumbar spine, and may result in paraplegia. For example, the first lumbar vertebra may be crushed as a result of the impact forces arising from a fall from a height on to the heels. This will result in paraplegia due to damage to the lower spinal cord. A crush fracture of L3–5 will, however, cause paraplegia through injury to the cauda equina.

Atlanto-axial dislocation resulting in spinal cord damage may occur as a result of relatively minor trauma in subjects with Down syndrome (Section 23.1.2.1), or in rheumatoid arthritis. In both these instances, the transverse ligament of the atlas is insufficient to restrain the odontoid peg, which can move backwards to impinge on the high cervical cord (Section 18.4.2.2).

18.1.3 Clinical features and immediate management

Conscious patients are usually immediately aware of lack of feeling and paralysis below the level of the lesion. Bystanders and ambulance crew should only move the patient when there are sufficient numbers of people to transfer him or her without further significant movement of the spine. Unconscious patients should be assumed to have a spinal injury in addition to a cranial injury until X-ray of the spine has disproved this.

In conscious patients, the level of the injury to the spinal cord can readily be ascertained by brief clinical examination of the sensory and motor 'level', as outlined in Section 6.9. The spine is then X-rayed. The lower cervical vertebrae may be obscured by the shadow cast by the shoulders, which need to be pulled down. Oblique views may be necessary to reveal cervical facetal dislocation. Special views through the mouth may be necessary to reveal a fractured odontoid process. Other evidence of a cervical spine injury may come from an increased pre-vertebral soft tissue shadow. It must not be forgotten that acute cervical spinal cord injuries due to hyperextension may not be associated with any evidence of bony injury, the cord being damaged by the mechanism outlined above. Severe compressive forces are usually necessary to damage the thoracic and lumbar vertebrae, and lateral and anterior–posterior films are usually sufficient to identify injuries in these regions, although tomography may be necessary to reveal details of the upper thoracic vertebrae. Further details of bony extensions and haemorrhage into the spinal cord can be obtained, as necessary, by CT and MRI, and there is now no indication for myelography in developed countries.

There is some evidence that the long-term outcome is favourably influenced by very high doses of methylprednisolone (30 mg/kg) given by bolus intravenous injection. A randomized controlled trial showed benefit in both those initially evaluated to have complete lesions as well as those having incomplete lesions, but only if the steroid was given within 8 hours of the trauma. There is considerable interest in the use of GM-1 ganglioside in the acute stage of spinal cord injury. Gangliosides are complex acidic glycolipids which form a major component of the cell membrane. There is experimental evidence that they augment neurite outgrowth in tissue culture, and induce regeneration and sprouting of neurons. A recently published trial has shown that 100 ml infused intravenously for 18 to 32 doses, with the first dose within 72 hours of the injury, produced a marked improvement in long term functional outcome compared to a group given a placebo infusion. However, to date the results of only one study have been published, and further observations are clearly essential.

After initial evaluation, immediate transfer to a spinal injuries unit is recommended. Consideration should be given to the use of helicopter transport. According to the facilities available, the level of the fracture, and the complicating problems of other injuries, the spine should be immobilized during transport. In the case of cervical injuries, transfer is best accomplished on a Stryker frame, on which traction can be maintained and the patient rotated to alter points of weight-bearing. Catheterization (see below) must be performed before transfer. Traction is best performed by Crutchfield tongs—large calipers, the points of which are inserted into small holes drilled under local anaesthesia into the outer table of the skull.

18.1.4   *Further management*

Consideration must be given to the possibility of surgical intervention in the acute stage. Experience has shown that there is usually little to be gained by early surgical reduction of a dislocation and evacuation of extradural debris and haematoma. However, some centres suggest that an early Cloward-type operation (see Section 18.2.3.2) in the case of cervical injuries, or Harrington rod fixation in the case of dorso-lumbar injuries, improves the overall result. Most centres, however, believe that maintenance of reduction of dislocations by continued traction, in the case of cervical injuries, or by immobilization in an appropriate posture, in the case of dorsal or lumbar injuries, affords the best prospect of at least a partial recovery of function.

Leaving aside the question of surgery, there are problems of immediate and subsequent management, detailed attention to which has revolutionized the survival and abilities of patients with spinal injury.

18.1.4.1   *Pressure sores*

Pressure sores are caused by tissue hypoxia, exacerbated by shearing forces to the skin. Ischaemia occurs in skin and subcutaneous tissues if the local tissue pressure exceeds capillary perfusion pressure. Obviously, in healthy people this happens frequently during the day, for example over the ischial tuberosities when sitting, but frequent

minor shifts in position ensure that, in health, no area is hypoxic for a sufficient time to cause tissue necrosis. Para- and tetraplegic patients cannot make such changes in position, and tissue necrosis can begin within the first few hours of the spinal cord injury. The commonest sites are over the ischial tuberosities, the sacrum, the greater trochanters, the heels, and, less commonly and in tetraplegics, over the shoulder blades and elbows. The only way to prevent sores is to disperse pressure as evenly as possible over the body surface, either by repeated turning, or by the use of a low air loss or other similar type of bed. A low air loss bed consists of a number of sacs of fabric through which large volumes of warmed air are pumped at low pressure. The sacs leak the air continuously. The patient effectively 'floats' on the low pressure sacs. The leaking warm air also effectively dries the skin, as skin macerated by sweat or urine is particularly likely to break down. During the stages of wheelchair rehabilitation, the sacrum and ischial tuberosities must be protected by a special cushion, such as a Roho cushion, which distributes weight evenly.

Established sores should be treated by debridement of necrotic tissue, often aided by using a desloughing agent such as Eusol. Avoidance of further pressure will rapidly heal smaller sores, but operative management is indicated if there is infected bone at the base of the sore (which is excised before closure), or if there is a discharging sinus with an underlying infected cavity. All sores are, of course, infected with a multiplicity of organisms, but systemic antibiotics are not indicated. Occasionally topical antibiotics, in the form of gentamycin beads, may be used in order to eradicate infection following closure. The size of the sore alone may be sufficient indication for surgical closure, as the rate of spontaneous healing may be so slow that rehabilitation is unduly delayed. In such cases, it may be necessary to turn a skin flap with a vascular pedicle.

18.1.4.2   *Bladder management*

In the early stages after a cord injury, some spinal units use intermittent catheterization every 6 hours, using a strict aseptic technique. Others recognize that the chances of maintaining the urine sterile with repeated catheterization are limited, and employ continuous urinary draining using an indwelling catheter. A 12 or 14 French Gauge 5 ml Foley catheter is recommended. If made of latex, the catheter should be changed weekly, if of silicone it may be left for about 6 weeks. A further alternative is suprapubic catheterization, which avoids the urethral trauma of repeated or chronic catheterization, with the associated risk of urethral fistula or diverticulum.

Tetraplegics, and paraplegics whose disabilities are due to cord lesions (rather than lesions of the cauda equina), develop involuntary detrusor activity after about 6 weeks. This activity occurs reflexly in response to elevated bladder pressure. The aim of further management is to encourage this reflex activity by avoiding overdistension of the bladder in the early stages, and by tapping in the suprapubic region as reflex responsiveness begins, followed by firm suprapubic pressure in an effort to minimize residual volume. As spontaneous detrusor contractions also occur, most men will require urinary collection through what is known as a Texas condom—a condom to which is fused a collecting tube leading to a urinary bag. Unfortunately, no satisfactory system of collecting urine externally from women has as yet been devised, and absorbent pads and plastic pants are often needed. For those who fail to establish an automatic bladder, usually because their paraplegia is due to a conus or cauda equina lesion, continued intermittent self-catheterization is often necessary, although manual expression combined with a sphincterotomy to reduce outflow resistance may be effective. Indwelling catheters may be necessary in tetraplegics who have insufficient hand function for self-catheterization, or in the elderly.

The immobility following spinal cord injury results in considerable calcuria due to mobilization of skeletal minerals. A catheter may become blocked by calcium deposits, and bladder stones may form. A bi-weekly bladder wash-out with Suby-G solution may reduce this tendency. Bladder stones may require crushing by urethral instrumentation.

Urinary infection is an ever present hazard, and until the advent of newer methods of management in the Second World War, accounted for most deaths. In the early stages, urine is cultured weekly, and an appropriate antibiotic used if there is systemic evidence of sepsis or if there are more than 10^5 organisms/ml or more than 50 leucocytes/ml. Sometimes local urinary antiseptics

such as mandelic acid may be useful. Avoidance of urinary infection long term is helped by maintenance of a high fluid intake, and by maintaining a low residual urine volume. Residual urine volume may be monitored by catheterization after manual expression, or by an ultrasound scan. In those who have well-established automatic bladder activity, a sphincterotomy may sufficiently reduce outflow resistance to allow better emptying.

Some help with bladder emptying may be obtained from the judicious use of drugs. Carbachol and bethanechol increase detrusor activity, and increase the responsiveness to suprapubic tapping. Sometimes, however, spontaneous detrusor activity may be excessive, and repeated small quantities of urine are passed between larger evacuations, causing problems, particularly to women. Detrusor activity may then be reduced by propantheline or oxybutynin. Phenoxybenzamine reduces outflow resistance.

From what has been written above, it is clear that urodynamic studies are a useful aid to understanding any one individual's problems with bladder emptying. Intravenous urography is also advisable about 3 months after the spinal injury, and follow-up urography is necessary at intervals of 2–3 years, so that painless stones or hydronephrosis can be noted at a relatively early stage.

Modern techniques that are likely to come into more widespread use include the use of an artificial sphincter—an inflatable and deflatable cuff placed around the bladder neck, with a pump placed in the scrotum or one labium. This is useful for those with no detrusor activity, as may occur in a conus or cauda equina lesion. For those with higher lesions, bladder emptying may be achieved by the use of implanted electrodes used to stimulate the second, third, and fourth sacral anterior roots.

18.1.4.3   Bowel management

There is a transient ileus for 2–3 days after a spinal injury. As spontaneous bowel movements return, there will be spontaneous evacuation of faeces. In the early stages, these can be made of easy consistency by the careful use of aperients such as bisacodyl or docusate sodium. As rehabilitation proceeds, many patients can achieve a spontaneous evacuation at a convenient time by adjustment of the diet, with special regard to fruit and bran, and the reflex stimulation afforded by the insertion of a suppository. Sometimes digital evacuation is required, with aid from a carer if the subject is tetraplegic.

18.1.4.4   Control of spasticity and contractures

Paralysed limbs must be moved daily through a complete range of movement at each joint, so that contractures do not have a chance to occur. Contractures are fibrotic changes in muscles, joint capsules, and tendons secondary to a joint remaining in a fixed position. They are common at the hip and knee. It is particularly important not to neglect extension of the hip, which means turning the patient prone for part of each day, in itself a useful adjunct for avoiding sores and spasticity.

As spinal reflexes return in the early weeks after the stage of spinal shock, flexor withdrawal reflex responses ('flexor spasms') result from slight stimuli to the lower limbs, and are exacerbated by pressure sores, or by a distended or infected bladder. If neglected, the patient spends more and more time with his hips and knees flexed in spasm. This in turn means that he spends more and more time on his side, and this is a sure precursor of trochanteric and ischial sores. Daily passive movements and periods of lying prone will do much to reduce this, but antispastic drugs may be useful. Of these baclofen is most useful. A suitable starting dose is 10 mg twice a day. Doses of up to 120 mg/day may be required, but drowsiness becomes common with higher doses. Drowsiness also often prevents the use of high doses of diazepam, otherwise a very useful antispastic agent. Dantrolene sodium is also useful, but occasional cases of hepatotoxicity have been reported. In patients with partial lesions, spasticity may interfere with recovering gait, and baclofen is particularly useful.

Occasionally, surgical treatment to relieve contractures is necessary. Partial tenotomies and incision of joint capsules may bring a patient into a posture that more comfortably fits a bed or a wheelchair. Spasticity may be helped by multiple motor point injections of phenol, which interrupts the reflex arc. Occasionally intrathecal phenol is used; the induced damage to the anterior roots converts an upper motor neuron lesion into a lower motor neuron lesion. As any automatic bladder control will be lost following this procedure, and

as pressure sores are more likely after it, the procedure is not often performed.

18.1.4.5   Other complications of spinal injury

The incidence of deep vein thrombosis and pulmonary embolism has been greatly reduced by the routine use of heparin in the early days, followed by warfarin. A suitable dose of heparin is 5000 units subcutaneously every 12 hours, followed by warfarin in a dose titrated by estimation of the prothrombin time.

Autonomic dysreflexia is a well-recognized complication of spinal injury. Acute attacks of hypertension and sweating occur. The blood pressure may reach levels of the order of 300/160. The reason is that the efferent limb of the baroreceptor arc, that should reduce pressure from these heights by diffuse vasodilatation particularly in the trunk and lower limbs, is disconnected by a high spinal injury. The initial stimulus to an elevated blood pressure often comes from a distended or infected bladder, or a peripheral infection. In the stage of active rehabilitation the reverse problem can occur, as severe postural hypotension cannot be controlled by baroreceptor-mediated peripheral vasoconstriction. Other autonomic phenomena in those with spinal cord injuries include unwanted erections (priapism), and episodes of profuse sweating.

18.1.5   Longer-term management and rehabilitation

After the initial stages of management, the patient's hope is followed by disbelief, and then by anger as the patient recognizes the permanence of his disability. Nurses, therapists, and doctors must accept that some of this anger will be directed at them. Eventually resentment usually fades to depression, followed by acceptance, and keen enthusiasm for learning techniques of coping with everyday life.

In contrast to those who receive rehabilitative therapy after, for example, a stroke, patients with spinal injuries have, of course, a normal brain. This, and their relative youth, means that the target for paraplegics is a return to work, and for tetraplegics to a level at which they can, as far as possible, care for themselves. Active physical rehabilitation cannot really begin until the bony injury is stable. If pain is a continuing feature due to bony instability, then the spine may be stabilized across the fracture site by the use of Harrington rods. These may also be used to prevent or correct deformity arising at the fracture site. The patient is then gradually sat up more and more in bed, so reducing the chances of postural hypotension. He can then learn basic wheelchair skills and, if paraplegic, strengthen the muscles of the upper part of his body, which will enable him to transfer more easily from chair to bed, or from chair to lavatory, to car, etc. Sports such as archery are of value.

With lesions below the cervical spine, erect mobility can be achieved with various devices. Patients with high dorsal lesions can support the body on crutches, and swing the legs braced by calipers forwards to the crutches. However, most patients will require assistance to 'get up' to this position, and only a few swings can usually be accomplished before fatigue and pelvic imbalance stops progress. With dorso-lumbar lesions (D10–L2), pelvic control through latissimus dorsi is sufficient to allow a four-point gait, in which a crutch and the ipsilateral leg are moved in sequence, followed by the contralateral crutch, and then the contralateral leg. Lesions below L2 allow normal hip flexion, and gait is relatively easy with below-knee calipers and crutches or sticks.

Considerable efforts have been made in bio-electronic research, so that some paraplegics can stand and 'walk' by programmed sequential stimulation of anti-gravity and propulsive muscles. There are enormous emotional gains for those few who are in successful research programmes, but early 'fatigue' is at present a limiting factor, as a high level of expenditure of energy in upper limb and trunk muscles is required, and the stimulated muscles also fatigue. Probably the best compromise is an orthotic device which largely supports the trunk, accompanied by functional electrical stimulation to drive the legs forward.

Tetraplegic patients are not, of course, capable of the same degree of self-care as the paraplegic, and mobility comes only through an electric wheelchair. Attention is primarily devoted towards maximizing the function of the hands. A common lesion is between segments of C6 and C7, so that the patient retains elbow flexion and wrist extension (see Table 6.3), but not elbow extension (C7), finger extension (C7), or finger flexion (C8) or opposition (T1). Elbow extension can be partly restored by transferring the posterior part of the deltoid into the triceps tendon. Finger flexion can be partly restored by transferring extensor carpi radialis longus into flexor digitorum profundus. Thumb flexion can be achieved by transferring brachioradialis tendon to flexor pollicis longus. A useful 'pinch-grip' can be obtained by fixing the tendon of flexor pollicis longus to the lower end of the radius, and fusing the interphalangeal joint. As the wrist is extended, the thumb will then 'oppose' the radial side of the index.

Apart from the physical aspects of rehabilitation, attention must also be given to modifications to the home and, if appropriate, at work, to allow subjects to achieve the fullest possible physical independence and satisfaction in life. Some of these aspects are considered in Chapter 26.

18.1.5.1   Later complications

A number of late complications, such as renal failure due to recurrent infections, and inaction associated with multiple pressure sores, have already been touched upon, but there is one additional, poorly understood, late effect of spinal injury. This is post-traumatic cystic myelopathy (often called post-traumatic syringomyelia). In this condition, which affects about 2 per cent of all patients with spinal injuries, cavitation in the spinal cord ascends several or many segments above the level of the traumatic lesion, resulting in pain,

Table 18.2   Survival of patients with spinal injury (information from Geisler *et al.* 1983; as modified by Swain *et al.* 1986)

Age at injury (years)	Type of lesion	Life expectancy (years)
20	Incomplete paraplegia	46
40	Incomplete paraplegia	28
20	Complete paraplegia	40
40	Complete paraplegia	23
20	Incomplete tetraplegia	44
40	Incomplete tetraplegia	27
20	Complete tetraplegia	30
40	Complete tetraplegia	15

dissociated sensory loss, and advance of muscle weakness to a higher level. Drainage of the cavity may relieve pain but has little effect on motor disability.

18.1.6   *Survival*

As Table 18.2 shows, survival is influenced both by the level of the lesion and by the age at which the injury is sustained.

I have first considered in this chapter the effects of acute spinal trauma, as damage to the spinal cord so produced is a model, albeit an exaggerated one, for most disorders of the spinal cord. Table 18.1 lists a classification of disorders of the spine, spinal cord, and nerve roots. In view of the frequency with which patients present with symptoms due to cervical and lumbar spondylosis and disc prolapse, (Table 3.3), these disorders are next considered.

18.2   Cervical spinal and radicular syndromes

There are few of us who reach middle age without some episodes of cervical muscle spasm—waking with a stiff neck, or a sudden unguarded movement producing pain accompanied by spasm and tenderness in the cervical spinal muscles. Assessment of the mechanism of cervical pain by conventional clinical examination is notoriously difficult, and we probably have much to learn from those who practise osteopathic medicine. Radiological studies of patients suffering from chronic cervical pain are also notoriously unsatisfactory, as some degree of spondylotic change—narrowing of intervertebral disc spaces, irregular osteophytic degeneration of the intervertebral and apophyseal joints—is invariable by middle age. It is therefore very difficult to say more than that as the degree of spondylotic changes increases, so does the propensity to cervical pain and radicular syndromes.

18.2.1   *Whiplash injury*

Rear-end collisions account for about 20 per cent of all vehicle accidents. As the trunk is moved forwards, the inertial mass of the head results in a forced hyperextension strain of ligaments and muscles. This type of injury has increased since the requirement that seat belts be worn. Head restraints seem insufficiently well designed to prevent all but the most severe degree of hyperextension injury. Although rear-end collisions are most likely to result in whiplash injuries, a collision from any direction may cause a cervical strain. Women are much more troubled than men, possibly because of the lighter mechanical structure of their necks. Cervical pain may be of immediate onset, but there is often a latency of several hours before cervical pain, exacerbated by movement, and occipital headache and giddiness occur. Patients with more extensive injuries, and older patients with pre-existing spondylotic change may have radicular symptoms as well (see Section 18.2.2).

Cervical pain and limitation of cervical movements may persist for weeks or months, or intermittently even longer, after the injury. Assessment of the situation is bedevilled by the fact that the injured person is often an innocent victim of someone else's careless driving, and is making a claim on the other driver's insurance policy. However, it must be said that one careful prospective study showed that affect, personality traits, psychosocial stress and other somatic complaints were not associated with outcome, whereas initial neck pain intensity and injury-related cognitive impairment clearly were. No good radiographic or other evidence exists to confirm or refute the extent of symptoms, and clinical examination is not very helpful, as pain and apparent limitation of movement are usually the only findings.

It has been traditional to advise a supporting soft collar in the early weeks, with gradual subsequent mobilization. However, a recent controlled trial from Ireland showed that ice packs for the first 24 hours, to relieve muscle spasm, followed by exercises designed to move the spine within the patient's tolerance, were more effective in relieving pain and increasing the range of movement than a supporting collar.

18.2.2   *Cervical radicular syndromes*

Spondylotic degenerative changes in the intervertebral and apophyseal joints may allow incursion of degenerate disc material and osteophytes into the foramina through which the spinal roots exit from the canal. The sixth and seventh cervical roots are by far the most commonly affected. The syndrome of the sixth root is of a deep boring pain referred to the shoulder and upper arm, which is often worse on neck movement, or in some particular position of the neck. The pain may be accompanied by tingling and numbness in the index finger and thumb, the distribution of the sensory fibres in the root. The biceps and brachioradialis tendon reflexes are usually depressed, and in severe lesions these muscles are weak. The syndrome of the seventh root is similar, except that the pain is referred to the arm, forearm, and sometimes the chest wall, the sensory disturbance is in the middle finger, and it is the triceps reflex that is depressed. In severe lesions, this muscle is weak.

18.2.2.1 Pathology

It is unclear why symptoms should suddenly arise from a root that has been chronically compressed by bony spondylotic changes that have clearly been present for a long time. Equally, it is not clear what causes the symptoms to settle spontaneously, as they usually do. Presumably an unguarded movement causes some minor injury in the periradicular structures, and the resulting oedema and inflammation of the root cause pain. A younger subject with cervical radicular syndrome may have a 'soft' cervical disc prolapse, the pathology then being a partial rupture of the annular ligament.

18.2.2.2 Treatment

Most patients are more comfortable in a collar, but care must be taken to support the neck in the position in which pain is least, and for this reason individually moulded, lightweight plastic collars are more successful than the commercially available 'off the peg' variety. Traction may sometimes be useful. The pain is often very severe, and disturbs sleep. Adequate analgesia is necessary.

Whether a collar actually makes any difference to the time taken for the radicular syndrome to settle is uncertain, but fortunately most patients become pain-free within a few months, although recurrent episodes are frequent. Occasionally continuing pain and weakness necessitate surgical decompression of the root in the exit canal.

18.2.3 Cervical spondylotic myelopathy

In contrast to what might intuitively be thought, patients with cervical radicular symptoms are not particularly disposed to spondylotic myelopathy. This usually presents with spastic weakness of the legs, but as the usual level of the myelopathy is at C5/6 or C6/7, there may be clumsiness of one or both hands due to a mixed afferent and pyramidal deficit, the former usually predominating.

18.2.3.1 Pathology

The principal cause of the myelopathy is probably compression of the spinal cord from in front by degenerate disc material becoming converted to spondylotic bars, and from behind by thickening of the ligamentum flavum. It is noteworthy that there is an association between the anterior–posterior diameter of the spinal canal and severity at presentation, suggesting that the congenitally determined capacity of the canal is an important factor in determining whether or not spondylotic myelopathy develops. Post-mortem studies show loss of myelin around the circumference of the cord, and it may be that compression results in secondary ischaemic effects. Apparent fluctuations in the severity of the disability suggest that secondary vascular events may occur.

18.2.3.2 Natural history, investigation, and treatment

The disability may insidiously progress, fluctuate with occasional improvements, or there may be no or little change for many years. There is no clear benefit from cervical immobilization in a collar, but this is commonly used.

As stated in Section 8.13, a necessary investigation of an advancing spastic paraparesis is MRI or myelography, to demonstrate the site(s) and degree of spinal compression, if the diagnosis is spondylotic myelopathy, and to exclude other causes of spinal compression, as listed in Table 18.1. In practice, investigation with a view to decompressive surgery will be reserved for those who are young and fit enough for surgery, whose history is relatively short (months or years rather than decades), and who are deteriorating to a level of significant disability.

If these criteria are fulfilled, and if significant

compression is imaged at one intervertebral level, then the operation of choice is the Cloward operation. In this procedure, the spine is approached from in front through a horizontal incision over and in front of sternomastoid, which is then retracted. A cleavage plane between the carotid artery and the oesophagus is found, and the oesophagus retracted laterally to expose the pre-spinal tissues. After detaching the pre-vertebral muscles, the intervertebral disc is drilled out using a guarded drill, the guard being set by reference to X-rays so that the drill cannot penetrate too far. The disc fragments are then removed, and the two adjacent vertebrae fused with a peg of bone taken from the iliac crest.

The natural history of cervical spondylotic myelopathy does appear to be influenced favourably by such an approach if patients are well selected. However, the different 'thresholds' at which different neurological and neurosurgical units advise decompression makes it difficult to record reliable figures for outcome. In one recent series, 52 per cent of the patients operated upon returned to full employment, and a further 39 per cent to light employment. The risk of spinal cord injury or infarction occurring at the time of operation is of the order of 2 per cent in good hands, but of course a disaster if it occurs, as the patient becomes tetraplegic.

18.3   Lumbar spinal and radicular syndromes

Low back pain of mechanical origin is considered in Section 25.2.1. Here I first consider the specific syndrome of sciatica due to compression of a lumbar or the first sacral nerve root.

18.3.1   *Degenerative lumbar spondylosis, and prolapsed intervertebral discs*

18.3.1.1   *Pathology*

Although these descriptive terms are used by some almost interchangeably for those with radicular symptoms, the pathology is different. A prolapsed intervertebral disc may occur in a young person, maybe aged even less than 20, following an awkward lift or other strain. It is due to rupture of the annular ligament, and extrusion of soft disc material from the nucleus pulposus. In middle-aged and older people, the water content and thickness of the intervertebral disc decreases, and herniation of soft disc material is much less frequent. Lateral radiculograms or MRI of symptomless middle-aged people usually show smooth backward displacements of the posterior longitudinal ligament over the disc spaces. These 'bulges' are a combination of thickened fibrotic annulus and hard bony ridges extending across the full width of vertebral body. They do not, in themselves, have sufficient volume to compress roots unless the anterior–posterior diameter of the canal is reduced, as in lumbar canal stenosis (see Section 18.3.3).

Radicular lesions in middle-aged people are largely due to hypertrophic degenerative changes in the facetal joints, with subsequent compression of the nerve root as it leaves the spinal canal through the intervertebral canal. Awkward lifts and strains may pull the nerve root through a tight canal, resulting in subsequent inflammation in the periradicular tissues, as described for cervical radicular symptoms; or there may be a true herniation of a small amount of disc material into a canal, the diameter of which is already compromised by facetal hypertrophy. As in the case of the cervical canal, the smaller the cross-sectional area of the spinal canal and radicular exit canals, the less room there is for the encroachment of disc material or osteophytic new bone formation without the precipitation of symptoms.

18.3.1.2   *Clinical features*

About 70 per cent of disc protrusions arise at the L5/S1 level, compressing the first sacral root, and 25 per cent at the L4/5 level compressing the fifth lumbar root. Both radicular syndromes are characterized by 'sciatica', i.e. pain in the buttock, and down the back of the thigh and leg. Back pain is often less intense than the sciatic pain. First sacral (S1) radicular lesions are characterized by tingling along the outer aspect of the foot. Examination shows impairment of sensation in this area—the dermatomal distribution of the first sacral root. The ankle tendon reflex is depressed, or absent. In severe lesions the gastrocnemius/soleus muscles in the calf may waste, but plantarflexion usually remains fairly strong as there is S2 supply to these muscles. Fifth lumbar (L5) lesions are characterized by some degree of foot drop, and more particularly by weakness of extensor hallucis longus. There may be a vague area of sensory impairment down the outer aspect of the leg and on the dorsum of the foot. There is no convenient tendon reflex as in the case of an S1 radicular lesion.

Patients over age 60 have a higher chance of having a radicular lesion affecting the fourth, third, and second lumbar roots. In L4 lesions, foot drop is prominent due to weakness of tibialis anterior; in L2 and L3 lesions, pain radiates down the front of the thigh. Quadriceps may be weak, and the knee jerk depressed.

Although limitation of straight leg raising is by no means pathognomonic of a disc or other compressive radicular lesion, as opposed to back pain due to mechanical causes (see Section 25.2.1), the probability of a disc lesion increases as the angle necessary to reproduce sciatica by raising a straight leg decreases. If sciatica is reproduced by raising the contralateral straight leg, then a radicular lesion is probable.

18.3.1.3 *Investigation, treatment, and prognosis*

The diagnosis of most disc lesions is clear from the history and physical examination. As many patients with sciatica settle with simple rest, it is not usual to investigate such patients unless surgery is being entertained. Plain X-rays or MRI will show degenerate discs, increasing proportionately to age in patients without sciatica; as in cervical spondylosis (Section 18.2.2), there is little correlation between symptoms and imaging changes. If surgery is being considered, then radiculography, CT scanning, or MRI will image the region of nerve root compression. Electromyographic evidence of denervation (Section 8.7.1.2) in the muscles supplied by the affected roots is often found, but this is a test of low specificity.

No more than 5–10 per cent of patients with sciatica require operation, as the pain usually settles with a short period of bed rest. Pain can usually be relieved by non-steroidal anti-inflammatory agents or indomethacin. Epidural analgesic or steroid injections have been shown by controlled trial not to be of benefit. Traction may also diminish pain, but probably does not alter the time to become free of pain. Injection of chymopapain

into the disc may relieve symptoms after an initial exacerbation, but many surgeons find that the results are no better than rest alone can achieve. There are, furthermore, occasional anaphylactic reactions to chymopapain.

For those few patients who continue with severe pain for more than 2 weeks, or for those who have foot drop, imaging procedures with a view to surgical decompression should follow sooner rather than later. Operation is now best performed using an operating microscope and a lateral incision, through which the extruded disc material can readily be seen and removed. The short-term success rate is of the order of 90 per cent, and the risks are, of course, substantially less than those of operation on the cervical spine.

Neurologists, neurosurgeons, and orthopaedic surgeons all acknowledge that success rates of this order can only be achieved by careful selection of cases. There is absolutely no case for operation unless clinical and imaging assessments clearly indicate significant nerve root compression. If these guidelines are followed, then the surgeon will be less troubled by patients with 'failed back surgery' who return with continual back pain and unconvincing signs, who may, because of the persistence of their symptoms, be again submitted to inappropriate exploratory surgery.

The problem of low back pain of mechanical origin, and of back pain due to other diseases such as ankylosing spondylitis, is considered briefly in Section 25.2.1.

18.3.2 *Lumbar disc protrusion and the cauda equina syndrome*

In most cases of prolapse of a lumbar intervertebral disc, the annular ligament ruptures laterally, and the nerve root is compressed, producing a syndrome of sciatica, as described above. Occasionally a large volume of nucleus pulposus is extruded more or less in the mid-line, resulting in a cauda equina syndrome, as described in Section 6.10. Immediate operative decompression is required.

18.3.3 *Lumbar canal stenosis*

Both the anterior–posterior and transverse diameters of the spinal canal vary considerably from person to person, the latter being particularly dependent upon the position and shape of the posterior intervertebral joints. The available cross-sectional area in those with massive pedicles may be only just sufficient for the passage of the cauda equina. A relatively minor postero-lateral disc protrusion or central bulge of the annular ligament or hypertrophy of the posterior ligaments will then compromise the roots (Fig. 18.1). This is the condition known as lumbar canal stenosis. The patient may present with recurrent low back ache and sciatica. Other patients present with reversible neurological deficits on exercise, such as tingling in the feet, or foot drop, relieved by rest. Erections on walking have also been described. The similarity of the time-course of these symptoms to those induced by peripheral vascular disease resulting in ischaemic painful claudication has led to the neurological syndrome being named 'intermittent claudication of the cauda equina'. Once considered, the limits of the spinal canal can be imaged readily by CT scanning or MRI. Radiculography may prove to be difficult as the roots are so tightly packed that there is insufficient cerebrospinal fluid to allow identification of the subarachnoid space on lumbar puncture. Usually, it is necessary to remove laminae at several levels in order to obtain adequate decompression, following which the patients are often markedly improved.

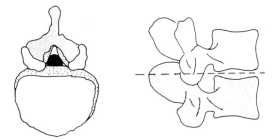

Fig. 18.1   Spinal stenosis. Plain X-ray films or CT scans may significantly underestimate the available space in the spinal cord. The addition of intrathecal contrast will outline the true extent of the available space for the cauda equina.

18.4   Extramedullary compression of the spinal cord and cauda equina

Ancient physicians considered the spinal cord to be the vertebral 'marrow' or medulla—hence 'intramedullary' nails for fixing a fractured shaft of femur, 'intramedullary' tumours, for tumours arising within the substance of the spinal cord (see Section 18.5.3), and 'extramedullary' tumours for those lying outside the cord (Section 18.4.2.1).

Just as the brain is enclosed in its protective cranial vault, with finite capacity, so is the spinal cord within the confines of the spinal canal. Both brain and spinal cord can therefore be compressed by disorders of the bony and membranous coverings. However, the cranial vault is a static box and, with the exception of expanding lesions such as subdural and extradural haematomas secondary to

trauma, and meningiomas, extracerebral disorders affecting the brain by direct invasion or displacement are not common. However, the mobility of the spinal canal is associated with degenerative changes (spondylosis) involving the central (disc) and apophyseal intervertebral joints. If the subject has, by chance, a spinal canal of rather narrow dimensions (spinal stenosis) then the hypertrophied degenerative intervertebral and apophyseal joints may intrude significantly on the spinal canal, again causing compression (Sections 18.2.3.1 and 18.3.3). However, spondylosis is probably not a very good example of a compressive lesion as there is some evidence that secondary vascular factors also play a part. The 'purest' example of spinal compression arises from expansion of an extramedullary tumour, such as a neurofibroma or meningioma. More frequently, spinal compression is caused by a metastatic deposit in a vertebra eroding through into, and occupying, the extradural space. Compression can also be caused by pus extending into the extradural space from an osteomyelitic vertebra.

When considering *any* extramedullary or intramedullary lesion it is helpful to think both in terms of vertebral level (Table 18.3) and segmental level (Section 6.2.2.4 and Table 6.3).

18.4.1   *Compression due to disease within the vertebrae, but outside the dura*

18.4.1.1   *Tumours*

The vertebrae are common sites for secondary

Table 18.3 Vertebral and spinal cord segmental levels

Vertebral level		Spinal cord segmental level
Body	Spinous process	
C7	C7	C8
T2–3	T3	T5
T10	T9	T12
T11	T10	L1–2
T12	T11	L3–4
L1	T12	L5
L2	L1	S1–5

The cord terminates at the lower border of the body of L2. In the lower thoracic/upper lumbar region the spinous process overlies the body of the vertebra below, owing to the obliquity of the spinous processes.

deposits of carcinoma. The most frequent sites of primary origin are breast, bronchus, and prostate. Primary tumours such as plasmocytomas also occur within vertebrae. The centre of the vertebral body may collapse, allowing soft tumour tissue and softened bone to be extruded into the extradural space, with compression of the cord or cauda equina and consequent paralysis. Vertebral malignant disease does not always readily show on plain X-ray films until collapse is gross. Tumour does not readily cross the intervertebral disc space, in contrast to tuberculous infiltration. Prostatic deposits are often readily visualized as many are sclerotic. Isotope scans may show the extent and number of vertebra involved. The compromised spinal canal can be imaged by metrizamide radiculography or MRI. Local palliative radiotherapy usually relieves pain and may be successful in causing a temporary partial remission of weakness. There is evidence that this is at least as effective in metastatic disease as urgent surgical decompression.

18.4.1.2   Infection

Tuberculous infection of one or more vertebrae is known as Pott's disease of the spine. Tuberculous granulation tissue readily crosses the intervertebral disc spaces. Granulation tissue and pus may spread into the paravertebral tissue planes, and be visualized on X-rays as a fusiform paravertebral shadow. Back pain is an early symptom. Evidence of systemic tuberculous disease is not always present.

Tuberculous pus may track from the paravertebral region anteriorly in the fascial planes, to present as a cold abscess on the chest wall, or in the groin. Tuberculous granulation tissue and pus may also track into the extradural space, compressing the spinal cord. The treatment is immediate decompression, usually by approaching the vertebra and abscess from behind, by removing the head of a rib if the abscess is in the dorsal region. If bony instability due to vertebral destruction is considerable, then vertebral fusion may be performed using an anterior bone graft. Antibiotic therapy is also, of course, essential (see Section 17.5.1.6).

Staphylococcal septicaemia may occasionally result in acute vertebral osteitis and subsequent vertebral collapse, with an associated extradural abscess.

18.4.1.3   Paget's disease of the spine

Paget's disease is characterized by a massive osteoclastic proliferation, with marked bone resorption, and little osteoblastic activity. There is considerable evidence that osteoclastic proliferation is precipitated by an RNA virus of the syncytial paramyxovirus family, perhaps a respiratory syncytial virus. Paget originally described the polyostotic form of the disease, with enlargement of the skull vault, bowing of the tibia, and shortening of stature due to vertebral involvement. However, monostotic forms are common, particularly in the spine. The proliferating mass of diseased bone may compress the spinal cord or, less commonly, the cauda equina. Surgical decompression may be performed, but adequate decompression is often rapidly achieved by the use of disodium etidronate.

18.4.2   Compression due to disease within the vertebral canal, but outside the dura

18.4.2.1   Extramedullary tumours

Meningiomas and neurofibromas are about equally frequent, and about three times as common as intramedullary tumours. Meningiomas usually arise in the dorsal region, and result in a slowly advancing spastic paraparesis, often with few sensory signs. A neurofibroma (Section 16.8.1) may arise at any level. In addition to the spastic para-paresis, there may be a unilateral band of pain and distorted sensation at the level at which the tumour is arising. A neurofibroma may extend out of the canal through the exit foramen of the root on which it lies, and continue to grow in the para-vertebral space. Such a 'dumb-bell' tumour, if in the dorsal region, may then be seen on the chest X-ray. Extramedullary tumours are readily dem-onstrated by myelography or MRI (Fig 8.21).

18.4.2.2 *Other causes of medullary compression*

Metastatic tumours may cause extradural com-pression without vertebral involvement. Hodgkin's and non-Hodgkin's lymphoma may also be found in this tissue plane. An extradural abscess may arise as part of a staphylococcus septicaemia. An extradural haematoma may compress the cord or cauda equina; the bleeding is most often associated with anticoagulant therapy. There is a significant risk of inducing an extradural haematoma if lumbar puncture is performed while a subject is anticoagulated.

The high cervical cord may be compressed by the odontoid peg of the axis if the usual ligament that restrains it—the transverse ligament of the atlas—is disordered. This occurs in rheumatoid arthritis. About 12–20 per cent of those with Down syndrome (Section 23.1.2.1) also have congenital anomalies at the same level. These include undue laxity of the transverse ligament, or an abnormally thin and small atlas vertebra. Both those with Down syndrome and those affected with rheuma-toid arthritis are at risk from a sudden tetraparesis due to atlanto-axial subluxation. X-rays of the cervical spine in flexion readily show the degree of separation between atlas and odontoid.

18.4.3 *Chronic arachnoiditis*

An adhesive granulomatous arachnoiditis, with secondary damage to the spinal cord and nerve roots, can occur as a result of a tuberculous, syphilitic, or parasitic infection (such as schisto-somiasis). A non-specific sterile arachnoiditis may result from myelography using oil-based contrast (now obsolete) or from previous spinal surgery. In general, further operations 'to free the roots' are not successful.

18.5 Intramedullary disorders

18.5.1 *Inflammatory disorders*

18.5.1.1 *Acute transverse myelopathy*

In this condition, a flaccid paralysis and sensory loss ascend from the feet to the mid-thoracic region or higher. These neurological symptoms are usu-ally associated with spinal pain. Acute transverse myelopathy can occur as a remote (non-metastatic) manifestation of carcinoma of the bronchus, and has also been described in association with herpes zoster, herpes simplex, HIV, and Epstein–Barr virus infections. Although the clinical picture is identical to that of a large plaque of demyelination in a patient with multiple sclerosis, long-term follow-up indicates that in at least half those who present with an acute transverse myelopathy, the patient has suffered an acute monophasic illness, and does not develop other lesions indicating multiple sclerosis. Many are left with permanent residual deficits.

MRI or myelography must be performed to exclude an acute compressive lesion. The cord may appear slightly swollen but often appears normal on imaging. The cerebrospinal fluid usually con-tains an excess of lymphocytes, but may also be normal. Treatment with steroids seems to have little effect.

18.5.1.2 *Other inflammatory disorders*

The spinal lesions of multiple sclerosis are described in Section 14.3.3. Tropical spastic para-paresis due to HTLV-I infection is described in Section 17.12.10, and HIV myelopathy in Sections 17.12.11.2 and 3. Parasitic infections such as schis-tosomiasis can also cause paraplegia (see Section 17.10.3).

18.5.2 *Vascular disorders*

Vascular disorders of the spinal cord are surpris-ingly rare, considering the frequency of athero-embolic brain infarction. The anterior spinal artery is formed in the cervical region by the fusion of a branch derived from each vertebral artery within the cranial cavity, and in the thoracic region by branches from intercostal segmental arteries, which are occasionally damaged during the surgical repair of coarctation of the aorta. The lower thoracic and lumbo-sacral cord is supplied by a large segmental arterial branch of the aorta known as the artery of Adamkiewicz. The cord is particularly liable to infarction in the watershed territories at the limits of supply of each of these contributors to the anterior spinal system. This supplies the anterior two-thirds of the cord, so that the lateral corticospinal (pyramidal) tracts, the spinothalamic tracts, and anterior horn cells are all damaged if the artery is occluded. The posterior columns are supplied by posterior spinal arteries and are spared if the anterior spinal artery is occluded. The clinical presentation of an acute anterior spinal artery occlusion is of a flaccid paralysis with areflexia, and dissociated sensory loss—impairment of pain and thermal sensation, but preservation of vibration sense and sense of passive movement. As anterior horn cells are involved, wasting becomes prominent after a few weeks. The diagnosis is essentially a clinical one. Spinal cord infarction is usually a diagnosis of exclusion, after MRI or myelography has excluded a compressive lesion, in an age-group in which transverse myelopathy seems unlikely. It is inappropriate to attempt to visualize the occluded artery by angiography.

The cord may suffer anoxic infarction, paraplegia then resulting from a period of profound hypotension, such as may occur during the course of an operation. Rather surprisingly, anoxic infarction of the cord may occur in the absence of any evidence of cerebral damage. Infarction may also occur as a result of atheromatous disease, sickle-cell disease, arteritis, or as the result of a dissecting aortic aneurysm occluding the origin of the intercostal segmental arteries which supply the spinal cord. Gas embolization in deep-sea divers may also occur and result in paraplegia if decompression has been too rapid.

18.5.2.1 Arteritis

Arteritis used to be a well-recognized cause of paraplegia of sudden onset in those with meningo-vascular syphilis.

18.5.2.2 Spinal vascular malformations

Malformations of the longitudinal arteries and veins on the anterior and posterior aspects of the cord may occasionally rupture, causing a spinal subarachnoid haemorrhage. More commonly, however, there are recurrent small infarctions in the territories supplied by, or drained by, the abnormal vessels. The relapsing spinal cord syndromes may mimic the recurrent episodes of multiple sclerosis. The abnormal vessels can be demonstrated by angiography by selective catheterization of the big segmental feeding arteries, a procedure not without risk. Operative control of the angioma is difficult, as it is usually not possible to occlude abnormal vessels without the risk of further infarction, but sometimes this can be accomplished successfully either at open operation or by interventional radiology by selective embolization.

18.5.3 Intramedullary tumours

Malignant intramedullary tumours may arise from the ependymal lining of the central canal (ependymoma) or from cells of the glial series, the most frequent being an astrocytoma. Secondary deposits from carcinomas occur occasionally, most often from a bronchial primary tumour. Malignant intracranial tumours, such as glioblastomas or medulloblastomas, may seed cells into the subarachnoid space, resulting in secondary tumours ensheathing and invading the cord. Intramedullary tumours are most frequent in the thoracic and cervical cord. The clinical presentation is usually of a spastic paraparesis with sensory signs reminiscent of syringomyelia (Section 18.5.4.1).

The investigation of choice is MRI. A biopsy may exacerbate the neurological deficit, but sometimes cystic cavities within tumours can be drained with some temporary advantage. Radiotherapy may slow tumour progression.

18.5.4 Congenital anomalies

18.5.4.1 Syringomyelia

This disorder figures more prominently in some neurological text books than its rarity justifies—the incidence is about 1 per million per year. This is probably because thinking about the pathology and effects of the disorder is a nice anatomical exercise. A central cavity forms in the cord, disrupting the spinothalamic pathways, which carry impulses ultimately perceived to be concerned with pain and temperature, as they cross in front of the cord and then ascend as the spinothalamic tracts. As the dorsal columns are usually spared, sensory examination reveals what is termed a dissociated sensory loss, with impairment of painful and thermal sensations, but preserved sense of passive movement and vibration sense.

Pathology

Most cases of syringomyelia are of the 'communicating' type, communicating with the central canal. Many patients with communicating syringomyelia have a malformation at the cranio-cervical junction, usually an Arnold–Chiari type I abnormality (see Section 22.1.4). This may be due to a congenital dysplasia of growth of the posterior fossa bones, so that the contents are crowded out into the spinal canal. Patients with syringomyelia are found to have been born in a difficult labour more often than control subjects. It is suggested therefore that the pressure gradients that may arise during a difficult birth alter the normal dynamics that exist between the fourth ventricle and the central canal of the cervical spinal cord, possibly rupturing the ependymal lining. In subsequent life, the cystic dilatation of the central canal is further enlarged by a persistent communication of the central canal into the ventricular system, and by the effects of physiological pressure waves associated with coughing and straining. It has also been suggested that the difference in pressure between the head and spinal canal during cardiac systole could gradually enlarge the cyst. Rupture of the ependymal lining may lead to secondary cysts that track up and down the cord adjacent to the central canal.

Some cases of syringomyelia are not associated with anomalies at the cranio-cervical junction. Some of these are associated with basal arachnoiditis following an episode of meningitis in early childhood. Other cases of syringomyelia are of a 'non-communicating' type. These are due to cystic degeneration in intramedullary tumours, or occur as a late effect of spinal cord trauma (Section 18.1.5.1).

Clinical features

True 'communicating' syringomyelia of the type described above affects the cervical and upper thoracic spinal cord. Cysts seldom track lower than this, but a secondary cyst after rupture of the ependyma may track upwards into the brain stem,

producing syringobulbia. The cyst is usually more prominent on one side, at least initially. Therefore, early symptoms are impairment of painful and thermal sensations in one hand. The subject may notice this, or he may first notice burns from cooking or from cigarettes that he has not felt. A deep boring pain is also often felt in the affected limb and forequarter. This may begin abruptly after a bout of coughing, an occurrence which supports the hydrodynamic mechanisms of origin of the cyst, as described above. The cavity usually extends forwards and laterally, disrupting anterior horn cells, so that there is often wasting and weakness of the small muscles of one hand. The tendon reflexes in the affected limb are lost at an early stage of the disease; the terminal part of the IA afferent fibres from the spindles are damaged as they sweep through close to the centre of the cord to synapse on the anterior horn cells. As spinothalamic pathways from the lower trunk and lower limbs are placed most laterally in the spinothalamic tracts, they are least affected by a centrifugal expansion of a centrally placed cyst, so the loss of painful and thermal sensations, even when advanced, may be suspended like a cape over the shoulders, with normal sensation below about the middle of the chest. Because the descending tract of the trigeminal nerve descends into the cervical cord, there may be dissociated sensory loss over the face. The lamination of fibres in these tracts is such that the impairment of sensation begins posteriorly on the face, advancing forwards but sparing the tip of the nose.

As the cystic cavity enlarges, wasting and weakness affects other muscles supplied by cervical segments. There is often also compression and destruction of the descending pyramidal pathways, so that a spastic paraparesis results.

Increasing deafferentation from painful sensations results in trophic lesions affecting skin and nails. There may also be hypertrophic destruction of joints, most often of the shoulder, similar to Charcot's joints, seen in tabes dorsalis (Section 17.4.1.3).

If the cavity extends into the brain stem (syringobulbia), then there may be wasting of the tongue, a vocal cord palsy, palatal paralysis, and nystagmus.

Investigation

The investigation of choice is now undoubtedly

MRI, which will display well in sagittal section both any cranio-cervical congenital anomaly, and the cyst.

Cranial CT scanning is much less effective at analysing the anatomy of this region, not only because of its incapacity to form sagittal views, without reconstruction (Section 8.13.2), but also because of the high Hounsfield number of bone and the amount of bone in the region of the foramen magnum. MRI will also distinguish the cystic cavity in the thoracic spinal cord from a cervical tumour (Section 18.5.3). Cavities in the brain stem are only rarely demonstrated.

In centres without MRI, the investigation of choice is to outline the dilated cord, and Chiari malformation if present, with myelography. Sometimes the contrast will enter the cyst some hours later.

Treatment

A number of different surgical procedures have been proposed. Most include decompression of any Chiari malformation by removal of part of the posterior rim of the foramen magnum and by a high cervical laminectomy, associated with decompression of the cyst. This is achieved by drainage through a catheter brought out from the cyst to lie subcutaneously in the flank and then pass to the peritoneum. The operation is most successful in relieving pain. It may apparently slow the progression of the disease, but it has little influence on established neurological signs. There appears to be no advantage in operating on patients with prominent physical disability unless pain is a feature. Short lived improvements after surgery are unfortunately often not maintained.

18.5.4.2   *Tethering of the spinal cord*

In some subjects, the conus medullaris is placed abnormally low, tethered down by a short and thickened filum terminale, or by abnormal structures such as an intraspinal lipoma or cyst. Diastematomyelia or hydromyelia also occur. These defects may occur in spina bifida occulta, and are readily revealed by MRI or myelography immediately followed by CT scanning. About 30 per cent of such children have a cutaneous abnormality of the lower back, such as a hairy patch or an area of atrophic skin. A sacral subcutaneous lipoma may also be present.

Neurological abnormalities associated with a tethered cord include asymmetrical muscle weakness in the legs, trophic ulceration of the feet, and the development of a neurogenic bladder (Section 22.1.4).

18.5.5   *Traumatic syringomyelia*

In about 2 per cent of cases of severe lumbar or thoracic spinal cord injury, a secondary cavity (syrinx) may form above the level of the lesion, and gradually ascend proximally in the cord. Fortunately, this only very rarely reaches the cervical region.

18.5.5.1   *Myelopathy following electrical shock*

In industrial electrical accidents, the current pathway is often from one hand to the other, necessarily passing through the cervical cord. If the current density is high, there may subsequently develop a syndrome reminiscent of motor neuron disease (Section 20.1), with wasted hands and a spastic paraparesis.

18.5.6   *Toxic disorders affecting the spinal cord*

Lathyrism is the name given to a paraplegia of almost a pure upper motor neuron type that occurs in parts of Central India, particularly after a poor monsoon, when poorer members of the population eat large quantities of the chickling pea, *Lathyrus sativus*. Lathyrism is also seen in Africa. Disturbance of sphincter function and parasthesiae also occur, but sensory signs are not prominent. Experimental studies on primates indicate that a potent agonist of the excitatory neurotransmitter, glutamate, named β-N-oxalylamino-L-alanine (BOAA), a known constituent of the chickling pea, may induce upper motor neuron signs. Glutamate agonists can kill neurons by enhancing the entry of calcium. It is of great interest that a closely related compound β-N-methylamino-L-alanine (BMAA) has been found in the seeds of the false sago palm, *Cycas circinalis*, which is a traditional food of the Chamorros of Guam, an area in which a disease with some similarities to motor neuron disease is endemic (Section 20.1.3.2).

For many years it has been suggested that cyanogenic glycosides present in cassava, a tuber which is a source of carbohydrate in the diet of deprived people in tropical Africa, are responsible for outbreaks of spastic paraplegia.

Other known toxins affecting the spinal cord are tri-orthocresyl phosphate (Section 19.3.7) and clioquinol; the latter, when used to treat infective diarrhoea, occasionally resulted in an illness that came to be known as subacute myelo-optic-neuropathy (SMON).

18.5.7   Deficiency disorders

The syndrome of subacute combined degeneration of the cord (combined degeneration of pyramidal pathways and the posterior columns) results from deficiency of vitamin B_{12}. This, and the effects of a deficiency of vitamin E are described in Sections 23.2.4.3 and 23.2.4.2.

18.6   Further reading

Spinal cord injury

Epidemiology

Kurtzke, J. F. (1975). Epidemiology of spinal cord injury. *Experimental Neurology* **48**, 163–236.

Management

Bliss, M. R. (1992). Acute pressure care: Sir James Paget's legacy. *Lancet* **339**, 221–3.

Bracken, M. B., Shepard, M. J., and Collins, W. F. (1990). A randomised, controlled trial of methylprednisolone or naloxone in the treatment of acute spinal cord injury. *New England Journal of Medicine* **322**, 1405–11.

Geister, F. H., Dorsey, F. G., and Coleman, W. P. (1991). Recovery of motor function after spinal cord injury—a randomized, placebo-controlled trial with GM-1 ganglioside. *New England Journal of Medicine* **324**, 1829–38.

Swain, A., Grundy, D., and Russell, J. (1986). *ABC of spinal cord injury*. British Medical Journal Publications, London.

Rehabilitation

Bedbrook, G. M. (ed.) (1985). *Lifetime care of the paraplegic patient*. Churchill Livingstone, Edinburgh.

Woolsey, R. M. (1985). Rehabilitation outcome following spinal cord injury. *Archives of Neurology* **42**, 116–19.

Prognosis

Geisler, W. O., Jousse, A. T., and Wynne-Jones, M. (1983). Survival in traumatic spinal injury. *Paraplegia* **21**, 264–373.

Whiplash injury

Editorial (1991). Neck injury and the mind. *Lancet* **338**, 728–9.

Mealy, K., Brennan, H., and Fenelon, G. C. C. (1986). Early mobilisation of acute whiplash injuries. *British Medical Journal* **292**, 656–8.

Newman, P. K. (1990). Whiplash injury. *British Medical Journal* **301**, 395.

Pearce, J. M. S. (1989). Whiplash injury: a reappraisal. *Journal of Neurology, Neurosurgery and Psychiatry* **52**, 1329–31.

Radanov, B. P., di Stefano, G., Schnidrig, A., and Ballinari P. (1991). Role of psychosocial stress in recovery from common whiplash. *Lancet* **338**, 712–5.

Cervical spondylosis

Heller, C. A., Stanley, P., Lewis-Jones, B., and Heller, R. F. (1983). Value of X ray examinations of the cervical spine. *British Medical Journal* **287**, 1276–8.

Jeffreys, R. V. (1986). The surgical treatment of cervical myelopathy due to spondylosis and disc degeneration. *Journal of Neurology, Neurosurgery and Psychiatry* **49**, 346–52.

Atlanto-axial instability

Collacott, R. A. (1987). Atlanto-axial instability in Down's syndrome. *British Medical Journal* **296**, 988–9.

Prolapsed intervertebral disc

Deyo, R. A., Loeser, J. D., and Bigos S. J. (1990). Herniated lumbar intervertebral disk. *Annals of Internal Medicine* **112**, 598–603.

Editorial (1988). Microsurgical lumbar discectomy – another surgical gimmick? *Lancet* **1**, 394–5.

Frymoyer, J. W. (1988). Back pain and sciatica. *New England Journal of Medicine* **318**, 291–300.

Kerr, R. S. C., Cadoux-Hudson, T. A., and Adams, C. B. T. (1988). The value of accurate clinical assessment in the surgical management of the lumbar disc protrusion. *Journal of Neurology, Neurosurgery and Psychiatry* **51**, 169–73.

Lumbar canal stenosis

Editorial (1985). Neurospinous claudication. *Lancet* **2**, 704.

Chronic arachnoiditis

Bourne, I. H. J. (1990). Lumbo-sacral adhesive arachnoiditis: a review. *Journal of the Royal Society of Medicine* **83**, 262–5.

Paget's disease of the spine

Case records of the Massachusetts General Hospital (1986). *New England Journal of Medicine* **314**, 105–13.

Syringomyelia

Mariani, C., Cislaghi, M. G., Barbieri, S. *et al.* (1991).

The natural history and results of surgery in 50 cases of syringomyelia. *Journal of Neurology* **238**, 433–8.

Acute transverse myelopathy

Editorial (1986). *Lancet* **1**, 20–1.

Tethered spinal cord

Editorial (1986). *Lancet* **2**, 549–50.

Toxic disorders

Martyn, C. N. (1987). Neurological clues from environmental neurotoxins. *British Medical Journal* **295**, 346–7.

19 Peripheral neuropathy

The wide range of clinical disorders and the different types of pathological processes that affect peripheral nerves do not make this an easy subject for analysis. Virtually the whole of the rest of this book is devoted to diseases of the central nervous system; it is not surprising that the peripheral nervous system has its fair share of diseases.

19.1 Nomenclature

Primary disorders of the anterior horn cells, such as poliomyelitis or motor neuron disease, are by convention not referred to as neuropathies. However, the effect upon these cells of various toxins which induce changes in their axons is so considered. Conversely, disorders of the analogous primary sensory neuron in the dorsal root ganglion *are* usually considered in discussions on neuropathy, sometimes under the name of sensory neuronopathy.

A peripheral lesion of a single nerve, such as of the ulnar nerve at the elbow, is sometimes known as a mononeuropathy. A mononeuritis multiplex indicates damage to more than one named nerve, for example a median nerve lesion in one arm, an ulnar nerve lesion in the other, and a common peroneal nerve lesion in one leg.

The word polyneuropathy implies a diffuse symmetrical disturbance of all peripheral nerves, although symptoms and signs are usually most prominent in the extremities—the feet and hands. Sometimes motor and sometimes sensory fibres are more prominently affected. The term 'neuritis' has, with the exception of its occurrence in the term mononeuritis multiplex, largely been superseded by the term neuropathy. Although the term could be taken to apply to a pathological process affecting any neuron, by convention it is taken to indicate a peripheral neuropathy.

A root or radicular lesion (a radiculopathy) implies a pathological process affecting one root, very often a prolapsed intervertebral disc. These are considered in Sections 18.2 and 18.3. On the other hand, polyradiculopathies have much in common with peripheral neuropathies, and are considered in this chapter.

Finally, the term autonomic neuropathy indicates that symptoms and signs are due to disordered afferent fibres subserving vegetative functions, such as the control of blood pressure, or to a disordered efferent sympathetic system.

19.2 The principal pathological processes affecting peripheral nerves

These are listed in Table 19.1 and illustrated in Fig. 19.1. In Fig. 19.1a the axon is seen in longitudinal section, surrounded by the compacted Schwann cell membrane, which is myelin. Each Schwann cell is separated from its neighbour by a node of Ranvier. At the far right is the nerve ending, containing vesicles of transmitter, and the motor end-plate. Disorders of this end-plate complex result in myasthenia gravis, and myasthenic syndromes (Sections 21.12.2 and 3). Disorders of the nerve fibre itself may be located in the axon, or in the Schwann cell. If Schwann cells are primarily affected, the axon may become demyelinated, but itself continue intact. In Fig. 19.1b the myelin of two adjacent Schwann cells has disintegrated. This process is known as segmental demyelination. The purest example of this is the neuropathy due to diphtheria toxin (Section 17.7.3.1), which has a potent but selective effect upon Schwann cells. Diffusion of toxin away from the site of infection causes a localized demyelinating neuropathy. In this type of neuropathy, the axon and its effector apparatus remain intact. However, the demyelinated node has an increased capacitance, so that the current available for distal depolarization is reduced. If sufficient lengths of axon are demyelinated, conduction in that particular axon may be blocked. If demyelination is less extensive, conduction alternates between fast saltatory conduction in the myelinated lengths and cable conduction in the demyelinated segments, the net velocity over a long length of fibre being considerably slowed. The hallmark of this type of neuropathy, therefore, is slow conduction velocity

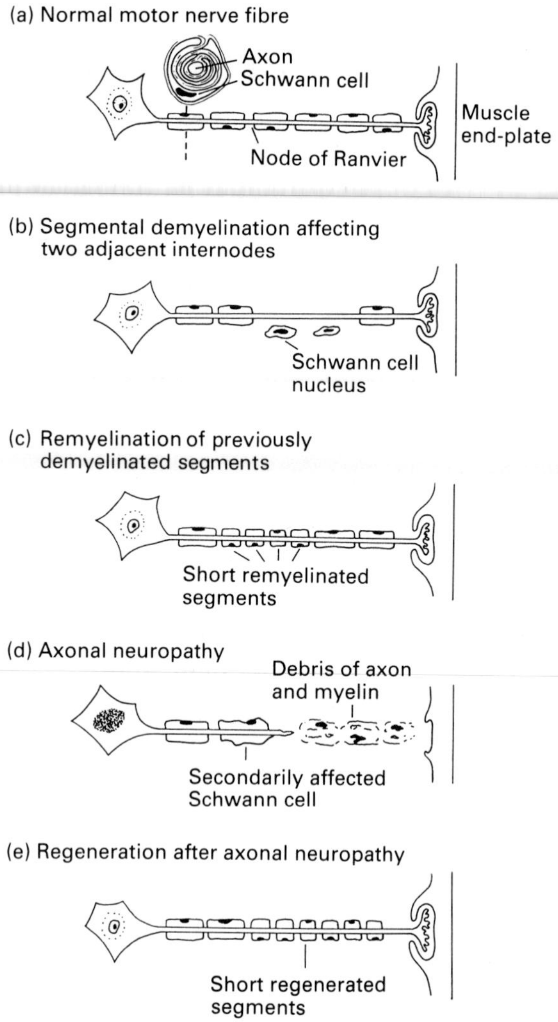

Fig. 19.1 Different types of pathological process affecting peripheral nerves. (a) Normal. Myelin is compacted Schwann cell membrane, which is laid down as a spiral around the axon. (b) Segmental demyelination. Seen in its purest form in diphtheritic neuropathy, the axon and motor end-plate region remain intact. (c) Remyelination after segmental demyelination. The new internodes are of shorter length. (d) Axonal neuropathy. Often due to defects in axonal transport. Longest fibres are first affected. The axon dies back from the periphery. Schwann cells are secondarily affected. The motor end-plate region becomes disorganized. (e) Regeneration after axonal neuropathy (or after neural transection and distal Wallerian degeneration). The axon sprouts and is associated with new, short Schwann cell internodes.

Table 19.1   Pathological changes in peripheral nerves

Pathological process	Typical disease process
Wallerian degeneration break-up of axon and myelin from site of injury	Nerve transection
Segmental demyelination loss of internodes, preservation of axon	Diphtheria
Axonal degeneration 'dying back' from periphery; some Schwann cell changes, but these are secondary	Many industrial toxins and drugs
Acute compression invagination of axoplasm and nodes of Ranvier away from site of pressure	'Saturday night' radial palsy
Chronic compression detachment and retraction of loops of myelin from nodes of Ranvier; thinning of axon	Carpal tunnel syndrome
Microvascular infarction Wallerian-like degeneration	Polyarteritis nodosa
Local infiltrations and inflammation; multiplication of abnormal cells within epineurium	Leprosy

on electrophysiological examination (Section 8.8). A demyelinating neuropathy recovers as Schwann cell nuclei divide and spin new myelin lamellae around the axon. Such remyelinated internodes are short, although their diameter approximates to the original thickness. Remyelination can therefore always be recognized by the presence of internodes which are inappropriately short for that diameter fibre. Conduction velocity through such fully remyelinated segments is again saltatory, and therefore recovers to virtually normal values.

The other principal type of neuropathy is an axonal neuropathy. In these circumstances the primary lesion affects the axon, or the metabolic processes located in the cell body responsible for maintenance of the axon and transport of organelles and metabolic products down it. Axons so affected die back from the periphery, so these are sometimes called 'dying-back neuropathies' (Fig. 19.1d). As an affected motor axon becomes disconnected from its muscle end-plate at an early stage, it follows that velocity of conduction in only surviving fibres can be measured by the normal techniques (Section 8.8). However, as dying back usually begins in the most rapidly conducting fibres of largest diameter, the rather slower velocity of surviving smaller fibres is measured. Any reduction in velocity is less than in the demyelinating neuropathies.

As the axon shrinks prior to dying back, the Schwann cells may become disorganized at the nodes of Ranvier. There may be some widening of these nodes, and even some loss of whole internodes proximal to a level at which the axon and its associated myelin disintegrates; but these changes appear to be secondary to the primary axonal changes. An axonal neuropathy, if it recovers, does so by regeneration. The axon sprouts are of smaller diameter than the parent, and are myelinated, as they grow back towards the effector organ, by a continuous chain of short internodes. Regeneration may be aberrant as the sprouts do not necessarily connect with their original end-plates. The best example of this is recovery after a facial palsy, when regenerating fibres from cells of the facial nucleus in the pons, originally destined for muscles of the lip, may regenerate and supply periocular muscles. Consequently, when the subject smiles he or she may also wink.

There are four other types of peripheral nerve

lesion to be considered. The first is simple transec-tion, such as may occur after a wound by a sliver of glass at the wrist (Section 19.4.2.1). Below the level of transection the changes of Wallerian degeneration occur, and recovery is by regenera-tion. The diagrams for this would be broadly similar to Figs 19.1d and 19.1e.

Another type of lesion, very common in clinical practice, is a peripheral nerve lesion caused by pressure (Section 19.4.2.3). For example, a radial nerve palsy may be caused by going to sleep after a Saturday night party with an arm draped over the back of a chair. The radial nerve is then compressed between the chair and the spiral groove in the humerus. Electron-microscopic stud-ies of an analogous experimental situation in ani-mals show that the myelin at the point of pressure is intussuscepted proximally and distally away from the site of pressure rather like a tube of toothpaste squeezed in the middle. The paralysis resulting from such a lesion is called a neuropraxia. Figure 19.2 shows this process. Not all compressive neuropathies are of this acute type, however. Chronic entrapment neuropathies can occur at sites of constriction, such as within the carpal tunnel at the wrist. The pressures here are prob-ably insufficient to cause invagination of axons and nodes of Ranvier, but it appears that terminal loops of myelin at a node shear away from their attachment to the axon and are displaced away from the site of pressure. The displacement of myelin leads to a 'tadpole'-like appearance of teased single fibres—the heads of the 'tadpoles' facing away from the site of pressure.

Another type of lesion of peripheral nerves is a microinfarct. Nerves are very resistant to general-ized ischaemia, hence neuropathy is not a feature of atheromatous peripheral arterial disease. How-ever, connective tissue disorders such as polyarter-itis nodosa may be associated with microinfarcts of a number of different peripheral nerves (mononeu-ritis multiplex) due to an obliterative inflammatory arteritis. The resulting focal areas of ischaemia result in Wallerian degeneration.

The final type of peripheral nerve lesion is caused by infiltration of inflammatory, malignant, or lymphomatous cells. By far the commonest cause is lepromatous neuropathy. The *Mycobac-terium leprae* bacillus enters and multiplies within Schwann cells, and this, and the associated immune response in the tuberculoid form, results in extensive demyelination and axonal degenera-tion (Section 17.6).

19.3   The polyneuropathies

19.3.1   *Clinical aspects of a typical subacute sensorimotor polyneuropathy*

Patients usually first notice unpleasant sensations in the tips of the toes or balls or soles of the feet. The sensations (paraesthesiae) may be described as pricking, or burning, or the feet may just be described as sore. As symptoms become more prominent, abnormal sensations spread to the dorsum of the feet and involve the fingertips. Patients sometimes say that textured objects feel rougher than they should. Muscular weakness in many patients with neuropathies of slow onset is not very prominent but, if present, usually involves dorsiflexion of the toes and feet, so that the feet trip on kerbs and stairs. Distal muscles may waste. The tendon reflexes become depressed or absent, the ankle jerks being first affected. Sensory exam-ination shows impairment of perception of passive movements of the toes, and later of the fingers. Perception of vibration is usually lost at an earlier stage than light touch. Discrimination between two points on the fingertips is impaired. A pinprick may be felt as less or more painful, the latter because the stimulus of the pin may precipitate painful dysaesthesiae (hyperpathia). The impair-ment of sense of joint position and impaired affer-ent information from muscle spindles may cause prominent ataxia, and a positive Romberg's sign (Section 6.3.1.3). Although the distal onset of sensory and motor symptoms can easily be under-

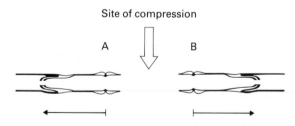

Site of compression

A   B

Fig. 19.2   Intussusception of myelin at the site of pres-sure. (Reproduced with permission from Gilliatt and Harrison 1984.)

stood in the case of an axonal neuropathy with dying back from the periphery, it is not so easy to understand the distal onset of symptoms in a segmental demyelinating neuropathy. In some cases the reason is probably just that a longer fibre stands a statistically greater chance of being 'hit' somewhere along its length. However, this cannot be the only reason, as in some acute polyradiculo-pathies, in which pathological changes are virtually confined to the spinal roots, symptoms and signs are also first prominent distally. The reasons for root fibres destined for the periphery being selec-tively damaged in such cases are not clear.

19.3.1.1   *Differential diagnosis*

A lesion of the cervical spinal cord can mimic the symptoms of a peripheral neuropathy. The sensory phenomena associated with demyelination due to multiple sclerosis must always be considered. If such plaques are confined to the posterior columns, there will be no helpful pyramidal signs (Section 6.2.3) such as brisk tendon reflexes or an extensor plantar response. Conversely, if there is sym-metrical distal weakness, without sensory disturb-ance, the cause may be a disorder of the anterior horn cells, such as motor neuron disease (Section 20.1), or a primary muscle disorder (Section 21.2).

19.3.2   *Causes of a subacute polyneuropathy*

Table 19.2 lists some of the very many causes of a typical subacute mixed motor and sensory poly-neuropathy of this type. From this extensive list some of the commoner syndromes are now con-sidered in more detail.

19.3.3   *Metabolic neuropathies*

19.3.3.1   *Diabetic neuropathy*

This is the most common cause of neuropathy in developed countries, and may take several forms.

Table 19.2   Causes of subacute or chronic symmetrical mixed motor and sensory polyneuropathy

Metabolic	Drugs
Diabetes mellitus	Antineoplastic
Chronic renal failure	vincristine, procarbazine, nitrofurazone, etoposide,
Hypothyroidism	chlorambucil
Acromegaly	Antimicrobials
Inherited metabolic abnormalities (see Table 19.3)	isoniazid, ethionamide, nitrofurantoin,
Deficiency states	metronidazole, clioquinol, dapsone
Thiamine (B_1)	Cardiovascular drugs
Pantothenic acid (B_2)	perhexilene, amiodarone
Pyridoxine (B_3)	Antirheumatic agents
Hydroxocobalamin (B_{12})	gold, penicillamine
Starvation	Anti-convulsants
Malabsorption	phenytoin
Hyperemesis	Miscellaneous drugs
Toxins	disulfiram
Alcohol	Neuropathy associated with carcinoma
Thallium, arsenic, lead	Neuropathy in association with disordered immune states
n-hexane	In association with lymphomas and paraproteinaemias
Acrylamide	Subacute infective polyneuropathy
Tri-orthocresyl phosphate	Infections with HIV, Epstein–Barr, cytomegalovirus,
Carbon disulphide	and herpes zoster virus
	Injections with horse serum—anti-tetanus toxin
	Inherited neuropathies, see Table 19.3

Males are more usually affected. There is a relation between the incidence of neuropathy, the degree of hyperglycaemic control, and the duration of diabetes. The most frequent type is a largely sensory distal neuropathy, with a painful burning sensation in the feet and toes. Motor features are usually slight or absent. Assessment of the frequency of occurrence of this type of neuropathy in those with diabetes depends upon the diagnostic criteria. For example, it is not uncommon to lose ankle jerks and vibration sense in the legs, and yet have no symptoms. The principal pathological change is axonal degeneration, possibly secondary to microvascular changes, with secondary Schwann cell changes, although some authors have described prominent segmental demyelination. Loss of sensation carried in large fibres may be so prominent that the patient is markedly unsteady. If such a patient is asked to hold out his outstretched hands, the lack of sense of position results in slow, wavering fingers, sometimes known as 'pseudo-athetosis' (Section 6.3.1.3). Other patients with diabetic neuropathy may be tortured by persistent painful, burning dysaesthesiae, although they are, paradoxically, relatively insensitive to painful stimuli. The loss of sensation from skin may result in injuries that would normally be painful being overlooked, resulting in painless, deep, penetrating, indolent ulcers on the sole or plantar aspects of the toes. Sometimes such 'trophic' ulcers appear to arise spontaneously, without pre-existing injury. Patients should be advised to inspect their feet daily. Repeated minor painless trauma to the joints may result in gross hypertrophic osteoarthropathy, the deformities of the joints becoming visible without radiography. These are analogous to Charcot's joints of tabes dorsalis (Section 17.4.1.3).

The treatment of diabetic neuropathy is not easy. Although strict control of hyperglycaemia does not guarantee resolution of the neuropathy, it is clearly the first step, and probably allows a greater chance of fibre regeneration. However, some patients develop a severe sensory neuropathy at a time when their good diabetic control seems no different from preceding years. Pain is usually the most troublesome feature, and may be relieved, in part, by analgesics, and by hypnotics at night. Antidepressants are sometimes useful. On the grounds that there are similarities between the dysaesthesiae of trigeminal neuralgia (Section

9.10.1) and diabetic neuropathy, carbamazepine or phenytoin have also been used. Recent interest has centred on increased polyol pathway activity associated with hyperglycaemia. Although aldose reductase inhibitors, which block the rate-limiting enzyme in the polyol pathway have no effect on ouabain sensitive ATP ase activity, a multicentre trial has shown some evidence of benefit even in patients with long established neuropathy, and there is evidence of worsening of nerve function on withdrawal of these experimental drugs, such as Tolrestat. In experimental animals, these compounds prevent the accumulation of myoinositol in nerves, improve nerve conduction and albumin leakage from nerves.

It is helpful to reassure patients with diabetic neuropathy that pain usually disappears spontaneously after about 12 months or so.

Apart from a symmetrical sensory or sensorimotor polyneuropathy, diabetic patients may develop diabetic amyotrophy (Section 19.5.3.1), entrapment neuropathy (Section 19.4.2.5), cranial mononeuropathies (Section, 19.4.1), and autonomic neuropathy (Section 19.7).

19.3.3.2   *The neuropathy of chronic renal failure*

Uraemic neuropathy was not recognized until the advent of dialysis in the early 1960s, although with more effective dialysis and transplantation the incidence has again declined. Neither urea nor creatinine appear to be implicated directly in the causation of the neuropathy. The presumably dialysable substance involved has not been clearly identified.

19.3.3.3   *The neuropathy associated with hypothyroidism and acromegaly*

Although each of these endocrine disorders may cause a generalized sensory neuropathy, a physician is far more likely to see these patients present with compression of the median nerve due to the laying down of abnormal connective tissue within the carpal tunnel (Section 19.4.2.5).

19.3.4   *The neuropathy of deficiency states*

Deficiencies of thiamine alone virtually never occur in clinical practice. Nutritional neuropathies are due to mixed deficiencies of a number of vitamins—thiamine, pyridoxine, pantothenic acid, and biotin all playing a part. Some species, such as pigeons, are exquisitely sensitive to deficiency of thiamine alone and rapidly develop a neuropathy. A thiaminase in pet food has led to an outbreak of feline neuropathy.

Although deficiency of vitamin B_{12} is usually considered under the heading of subacute combined degeneration of the cord (Section 23.2.4.4), the earliest pathological change is in the peripheral nerves. The combination of absent ankle jerks, due to the neuropathy, and extensor plantar responses, due to degeneration of the lateral columns, should always bring to mind a deficiency of vitamin B_{12} as a possible diagnosis.

Patients with malabsorption may develop a neuropathy that may persist and advance even if all recognized nutritional factors are replaced systemically.

19.3.5   *Neuropathy associated with carcinoma*

A neuropathy, often with particularly marked sensory involvement, may occur in carcinoma. The lung is most commonly the site of the primary tumour, but neuropathy has also been reported in patients with carcinoma of the breast or ovary, or gastrointestinal tract. The severity of the neuropathy bears no relation to the bulk of the tumour—indeed, the neuropathy may precede the appearance of a carcinoma of the lung by up to 3 years.

19.3.6   *Neuropathy in association with disordered immune states*

Neuropathy can occur in association with multiple myeloma, monoclonal gammopathy, cryoglobulinaemia, and macroglobulinaemia. Plasma exchange has been shown to be of benefit in monoclonal gammopathies, particularly of the IgG of IgA type. Lymphomas may also be associated with a neuropathy. Certain virus infections, particularly herpes zoster, mumps, and glandular fever may all be associated with a syndrome very similar to acute infective polyneuropathy (Section 19.3.9).

19.3.6.1   *Chronic inflammatory demyelinating polyneuropathy*

This condition develops slowly over months or years, and is usually characterized by a relapsing and remitting course, although occasionally a steady monophasic course is seen. There is no family history of neuropathy. As in acute infective polyneuropathy (see Section 19.3.9), the protein in the CSF is greatly raised, but there are few or no lymphocytes. Segmental demyelination and remyelination occur, the latter sometimes being so prominent that the nerves become thickened and palpable. Nerve condition velocities are extremely slow. Histological examination shows Schwann cells arranged in lamellae, like 'onion bulbs', indicating the repeated episodes of de- and remyelination. The 'onion bulbs' are infiltrated by lymphocytes, suggesting a delayed-type tissue hypersensitivity. However, as plasmapheresis is effective, circulating antibodies are probably also important. Steroids are also of benefit.

19.3.7   *Toxic and drug-induced neuropathies*

Alcohol is a common cause of neuropathy in rich societies and is particularly considered in Section 23.4.2.7.

Table 19.2 lists some industrial toxins particularly likely to cause neuropathy. Solvents of adhesives, such as *n*-hexane have produced outbreaks of neuropathy in leather-workers. Acrylamide is the monomer of polyacrylamide used as a waterproofing agent in tunnels and for foundations. Tri-orthocresyl phosphate is a constituent of high-temperature lubricating oils. This looks like high-quality cooking oil, so it has been purloined and sold as such in developing countries, with disastrous results. Subtle alterations of chemical structure may vastly alter neurotoxicity. For example, the change from methyl iso-butyl ketone to methyl butyl ketone in a factory manufacturing photographic products resulted in a major outbreak of neuropathy.

The list of chemicals known to cause a neuropathy grows almost monthly. It is justifiable to be suspicious of any chemical to which a patient is exposed in the course of his or her work, or any drug being taken by a patient who develops a neuropathy. Table 19.2 lists only some of the commoner possibilities. The mechanism of neurotoxic action of few of the drugs is known, but usually factors that lead to a high blood level of the drug are important. For example, those who, for genetic reasons, acetylate isoniazid slowly, or who oxidize perhexilene slowly, are particularly likely to develop neuropathy. Similarly, those who excrete nitrofurantoin slowly because of renal impairment are also at risk.

The case of disulfiram is worthy of special comment. It can sometimes be difficult to decide whether a neuropathy arising in an alcoholic is due to the toxic effects of alcohol and malnutrition, or to his or her treatment with disulfiram.

19.3.8 *Inherited neuropathies*

Table 19.3 lists some of the many inherited disorders of peripheral nerves. Discussion of virtually all these is beyond the scope of this work, they are listed solely for future recognition of their names, and as an acknowledgement of the fact that research is, in some instances, revealing their basic genetic and metabolic defect. The commonest of the inherited neuropathies is Charcot–Marie–Tooth disease. There are two principal phenotypes, both inherited as an autosomal dominant. In both types, slowly progressive distal wasting of the lower limbs and later wasting of the hands occur. The toes become hyperextended (clawed) and the foot may become highly arched. The disorder is sometimes known as peroneal muscular atrophy, as these muscles are characteristically predominantly involved. Sensory symptoms are uncommon, but there may be minor distal sensory loss. The onset of significant symptoms is usually in the second decade of life. In type 1, conduction velocity is very slow due to repeated demyelination and remyelination, which may lead to some hypertrophy of nerves. This type is genetically heterogeneous. One gene has been located to chromosome 17p11.2, with a duplication in this region being associated with apparent sporadic cases. A similar phenotype is associated with a gene on chromosome 1. A very similar clinical picture occurs in type 2 Charcot–Marie–Tooth neuropathy, although in this case the primary disorder is neuronal, with axonal degeneration. This type tends to begin rather later in life than

type 1. The gene for this type has not yet been mapped. Both types are entirely compatible with a normal life span. Although dominantly inherited, the severity of clinical expression may vary widely within the same families so that one affected member may have only clawed toes and high-arched feet, and another marked distal wasting and weakness.

A more profound neuropathy, with marked hypo- and demyelination, and slowing of conduction, with easily palpable nerves, is inherited through an autosomal recessive gene (Déjérine–Sottas neuropathy).

A dominantly inherited axonal neuropathy affecting sensory cells in the dorsal root ganglion is associated with such severe trophic changes in the feet that digits may be lost, and the sole largely destroyed by giant trophic ulcers. The names of Thévenard and Denny-Brown are often attached to this type of neuropathy. A similar condition arising in infancy, or present at birth, is the recessively inherited (congenital) sensory neuropathy of Ohta and Dyck. Also inherited in this way is the Riley–Day syndrome, in which not only large sensory fibres but also unmyelinated axons are severely affected, resulting in marked insensitivity to pain, and disordered autonomic function, with episodes of vomiting and disturbed control of blood pressure.

Amyloid neuropathy results when a single amino-acid residue change in the plasma pre-albumin molecule, determined by a single base change in the genomic DNA, makes the abnormal pre-albumin amyloidogenic, so that amyloid fibrils are laid down in peripheral nerves. A number of different kindreds have been described from different parts of the world, with a variety of pre-albuminic changes. The same variant occurs in Portugal and Ireland, possibly reflecting spread of the gene through trading routes, or through survivors of the Armada. Changes in painful and thermal sensation and in autonomic function are particular features of this type of neuropathy.

Of the other inherited neuropathies with a known metabolic defect, only porphyria is sufficiently common to warrant discussion in this chapter. In acute intermittent porphyria (Section 23.1.4.8) there may occur a fulminant neuropathy, principally affecting motor nerves, often accompanied by abdominal pain and psychiatric symptoms. Episodes may be precipitated by barbiturates, sulphonamides, and other drugs which induce δ-aminolevulinic acid synthetase activity. In an acute episode porphobilinogen accumulates in the urine and causes this to darken after a few hours' exposure to light. Clues to the diagnosis may emerge from a history of recent exposure to the relevant drugs, and the fact that the neuropathy often affects proximal rather more than distal muscles. The ankle jerks may be preserved. Any sensory loss may be in a 'bathing-trunk' distribution. Another feature is the rapidity with which wasting occurs, but the recovery of function, even of severely wasted muscles, is surprisingly good.

19.3.9   *Acute infective polyneuropathy (synonym: the Guillain–Barré syndrome)*

This uncommon fulminating neurological illness may occur at any age. It may lead to death from progressive paralysis of the ventilatory muscles within 48 hours. However, adequate ventilatory support should tide most patients over to complete or nearly complete recovery. The disorder was first described by Guillain, Barré, and Strohl towards the end of the First World War. It is now considered identical with 'Landry's ascending paralysis'. The incidence is about 2 per 100 000 per year.

About two-thirds of patients mention that the symptoms of a flu-like illness had preceded the onset of the polyneuropathy by about 2 weeks. As a virtually identical disorder can follow infections with HIV, herpes zoster, mumps and Epstein–Barr (infectious mononucleosis) viruses, and with cytomegalovirus it is tempting to consider that 'idiopathic' examples of the illness occur in response to an infective agent. Other cases follow elective surgery, trauma, myocardial infarction, or even, it seems, as a general response to management in an intensive care unit, suggesting that the illness arises as part of a deranged immune response. Some workers have reported that the serum of patients with acute infective polyneuropathy contains a factor capable of demyelinating axons in tissue culture.

19.3.9.1   *Pathology*

Histological examination of the nerve roots and peripheral nerves of those dying from acute infective polyneuropathy shows extensive perivenular inflammation, with invasion of lymphocytes, and some macrophages. This cellular infiltrate is associated with segmental demyelination. If this is very extensive, there is Wallerian-type degeneration as well. Sometimes the pathological process appears to be virtually confined to the spinal roots, on other occasions to the nerves. Most commonly, both are involved.

19.3.9.2   *Clinical features*

After their prodromal illness, patients say that their legs begin to feel weak and rubbery, and are often painful. The pace of the illness is such that weakness may advance to a quadriparesis and ventilatory insufficiency within 48 hours (10–20 per cent of patients), or evolve slowly to a level insufficient to cause great alarm over 3 weeks. Eighty-five per cent of patients have reached their maximum deficit within 3 weeks, and it is most unlikely that artificial ventilation will be required if it has not been needed by this time. Sensory disturbances include numbness and tingling, but sensory findings on examination are often relatively slight, although ataxia may be prominent due to deafferentation of muscle spindles. The tendon reflexes may not be depressed for the first day or two, even when weakness is quite prominent. The cranial nerves, particularly those supplying the bulbar musculature, and the seventh pair are often affected. In one variant of the illness— the Miller Fisher syndrome—there is a marked external ophthalmoplegia, in association with ataxia, due to the neuropathy affecting spindle afferents. Selective involvement of some nerve fibres is particularly striking in this disorder, as horizontal movements of the eyes can be much more affected than vertical gaze.

The autonomic nervous system is also affected, with urinary retention occurring in about one-third of patients. More important, perhaps, are irregularities of cardiac rhythm: both paroxysmal tachycardias and bradycardias have been reported. Occasionally patients require pacing in addition to artificial ventilation, and this should be undertaken prophylactically if there is profound bradycardia. Paroxysmal arrhythmias are particularly likely to occur if suxamethonium is used to facilitate intubation. Other features of autonomic involvement include ileus, hypotension, and blurring of vision. About 5 per cent of patients develop papilloedema. The mechanism of this is not clear, but it may be related, in some way, to the high protein content of the cerebrospinal fluid.

It is clear that all patients with such a devastating, though potentially recoverable, illness must be nursed in an intensive therapy unit. It is easy for the inexperienced to overlook the early signs of ventilatory insufficiency. To wait for cyanosis is to wait until the patient is nearly dead! Although the increased work of the surviving ventilatory motor units may be detected by tachypnoea, tachycardia, and sweating, such signs can, of course, occur in someone who is simply frightened. A poor cough and utterances interrupted by inspiration may give some warning, but there is no substitute for the hourly recording of vital capacity. Once vital capacity drops below 15 ml/kg (1.05 litres for a 70 kg subject) intubation and artificial ventilation is mandatory. It is usual to set the machine to give a high tidal volume to prevent atelectasis, with about 5–10 cm H_2O of positive end-expiratory pressure.

19.3.9.3 *Differential diagnosis*

The differential diagnoses of acute infective polyneuropathy are few. In countries in which anterior poliomyelitis is still endemic, this is probably the more likely diagnosis. Of the neuropathies listed in Tables 19.2 and 19.3, infection with the human immunodeficiency or other viruses, porphyria, and acute (and possibly malicious) heavy metal poisoning are likely to mimic acute infective polyneuropathy. It is sometimes more difficult to distinguish this acute polyneuropathy from other quite different causes of a flaccid quadriparesis. An acute transverse myelopathy, or a compressive lesion of the spinal cord, may result in a flaccid and temporarily areflexic paraplegia (Section 18.5.1.1). A brain-stem infarction may result in a bulbar palsy and weakness of all four limbs (Section 10.1.5). Myasthenia gravis (Section 21.12.2), periodic paralysis (Section 21.8.3) and acute polymyositis (Sec-

Table 19.3　Examples of inherited neuropathies

	Inheritance	Nerve pathology
Unknown metabolic defect		
Charcot–Marie–Tooth disease, types 1 and 2	D	Type 1 Demyelinating
		Type 2 Axonal
Déjérine–Sottas disease	R	Demyelinating
Hereditary sensory neuropathy (Thévenard, Denny-Brown)	R	Axonal (DRG)
'Congenital'—(very early onset sensory neuropathy (Ohta, Dyck)	R	Axonal (DRG)
Familial dysautonomia (Riley–Day)	R	Axonal (DRG)
Amyloidoses	D	Axonal
Inherited liability to pressure palsies	D	Demyelinating
Known metabolic defect*		
Uroporphyrinogen 1 synthetase deficiency—acute intermittent porphyria	D	Axonal
Arylsulphatase A deficiency—metachromatic leucodystrophy	R	Demyelinating
Galactosyl ceramide β-galactosidase deficiency—globoid cell dystrophy	R	Axonal
High-density lipoprotein deficiency—Tangier disease	R	Axonal
Abetalipoproteinaemia—Bassen–Kornzweig disease	R	Axonal (DRG)
Phytanic acid storage disease—Refsum disease	R	Demyelinating
α-galactosidase A deficiency—Anderson–Fabry disease	X-linked R	Axonal (DRG)

Abbreviations: D, dominant; R, recessive; DRG, dorsal root ganglion.
* See Chapter 23

tion 21.3) can also mimic acute infective polyneuritis. Acute botulism (Section 17.7.2) is also a worrying possibility because of the possibility of contaminated food having affected many others. In this illness the ocular accommodation reflex is affected early, and bradycardia is usual. Finally, a few unfortunates are dismissed at an early stage as 'hysterics'.

The diagnostic tests to consider these other various possibilities are listed in the Sections cited. Investigation of acute infective polyneuropathy in the early stages may often be surprisingly unhelpful. The cerebrospinal fluid (CSF) may be normal at first, or contain an excess of lymphocytes. Within a day or two, however, the number of lymphocytes, if previously elevated, falls to normal, but the level of protein rises, and may later reach very high levels—5 g/l or more. The normal cell count and high protein were stressed by Guillain and Barré ('dissociation albuminocytologique') as a diagnostic point to distinguish their syndrome from poliomyelitis in which the cell count is raised. However, it is often not possible to make this distinction on the CSF alone at an early stage of the illness.

Nerve conduction velocity may also be normal at an early stage of the illness. However, the method of measuring this uses only a length of nerve trunk in forearm or leg. More sophisticated examinations, such as measurement of the latency of the H reflex, which traverses both anterior and posterior roots, or the F response, which traverses the anterior root first antidromically and then orthodromically, are often abnormal (Section 8.8). Although electromyography may be unhelpful at an early stage of the illness, it may be useful as a guide to prognosis after about 3 weeks. If there is then extensive fibrillation, then there is much Wallerian-type degeneration, and recovery will be slower and less complete than if the pathological process is largely confined to segmental demyelination.

19.3.9.4   Treatment

In an illness with a mortality of between 7 and 22 per cent, according to different series, treatment other than general supportive measures has often been proposed. The use of corticosteroids seemed appropriate with a view to suppressing an abnor-

mal immune response, but controlled trials have failed to show any benefit over the expected natural resolution of the disease. No benefit has been shown even with high-dose intravenous methylprednis alone. It is, however, possible that the trials were not powerful enough to identify a subgroup that might benefit from steroid therapy. As it has been shown that the serum contains a circulating factor that demyelinates cells in tissue culture, plasmapharesis was tried. From controlled trials, there is no doubt that this is beneficial. In the North American study, the time spent on a ventilator was halved from 48 to 24 days, and the time prior to ambulation in ventilator patients was nearly halved, from 169 to 97 days. The benefits seem greatest in those started on plasmapharesis within 7 days. Unfortunately, plasmapharesis is not easy to arrange, even in some developed countries.

Apart from plasmapharesis, ventilatory support, and energetic treatment of pulmonary infections as they arise, general supportive measures include avoidance of pressure sores by careful positioning. Drainage of the bladder by catheter is necessary in the early days in about 20 per cent of patients. Aching pain in the buttocks, thighs, and legs is often troublesome, requiring appropriate analgesic treatment. Some units give twice-daily injections of heparin in an attempt to minimize venous thrombosis and pulmonary embolism.

19.3.9.5   Prognosis

Patients with acute infective polyneuropathy require continuing psychological support, and reassurance that total recovery can reasonably be expected. There is a significant mortality due principally to cardiac dysrhythmias, pulmonary infections, and thromboembolism. Of the survivors, about 15 per cent will have a residual neurological deficit, usually a bilateral foot-drop. Prognostic features have been identified: muscle weakness sufficient to require ventilatory support, and failure to begin to improve within 3 weeks of reaching peak neurological deficit. If both features are present, then there is an 85 per cent probability of a persistent deficit. There is also a significant association between a poor outcome and a small amplitude of the compound muscle action potential from abductor pollicis brevis, indicating prominent axonal loss. Age over 40 is also a less favourable prognostic feature. Fortunately, most patients make a good recovery, with no residual functional deficit. Physiotherapy from the early stages is essential in order to prevent contractures at joints.

19.4 Mononeuropathies

19.4.1 *Cranial mononeuropathies*

19.4.1.1 *Facial palsy (synonym: Bell's palsy)*

Bell's palsy is one of the commonest neurological conditions seen by general practitioners, the annual incidence being at least 25 per 100 000 per year. Although doctors know that the ultimate prognosis in most cases is good, the distress that sudden facial disfigurement causes should not be underestimated.

Pathology and aetiology
Remarkably little is known about the causes and pathological changes of Bell's palsy. Facial palsies also occur in association with mumps and infectious mononucleosis, and occasionally other viral infections, but the vast majority of patients do not show any evidence of preceding or concurrent viral infection. In some patients, careful clinical examination and study of the spinal fluid suggests that a facial palsy is the most visible evidence of a mild acute infective polyneuropathy (Section 19.3.9). It is believed that many viral infections or a mild subclinical generalized neuropathy may cause a minor degree of oedema of nerves. In the particular case of the facial nerve, any significant swelling at all renders it liable to compressive and ischaemic injury as it lies within its long and tortuous canal within the petrous temporal bone. Depending upon the extent of the oedematous compression, there will either be a conduction block, with segmental demyelination (the axons remaining in continuity), or infarction of the nerve with distal Wallerian degeneration. One particular variety of facial palsy is due to a herpes zoster infection of the geniculate ganglion. This can be identified by the presence of vesicles containing virus on the drum, or in the territory of the posterior auricular branch. This combination of signs is known as the Ramsay Hunt syndrome (Section 17.12.7.4).

Facial palsy may occur as a complication of accelerated hypertension, particularly in children. Some studies suggest that it is more likely in pregnancy and in patients with diabetes.

Clinical features
The facial palsy usually becomes complete or nearly complete within a few hours of the onset of symptoms. It is often accompanied by, or preceded by, pain in or behind the ear. Patients often describe the face as being 'twisted' to the side opposite to the palsy, although all that they are observing are the normal facial movements, which seem unduly prominent when matched against the weak side. An early symptom is lacrimation, as the lower eyelid everts away from the globe; tears then spill down the cheek rather than following the gutter of the lower eyelid to the nasolacrimal duct. The failure of conduction in one branch of the facial nerve (the nerve to stapedius) results in distorted hearing or hyperacusis, and in another (the chorda tympani) in a perception of unpleasant taste on the anterior part of the tongue on the same side.

In Bell's palsy, weakness usually affects the upper and lower parts of the face equally, in contrast to an upper motor neuron facial weakness. In this latter case, there is relative sparing of the frontalis and periocular muscles, as each side of the upper part of the face receives a dual innervation from each cerebral hemisphere.

Relaxation of levator palpebrae is insufficient to cause tight eye closure by itself, and patients with Bell's palsy are unable to close the eye on the affected side at night. Attempted eye closure is accompanied by reflex upward rotation of the globe, so that the sclera is seen under the partly closed lid (Bell's sign).

Investigation
Electromyography has not proved as useful as might be thought. Fibrillation potentials indicating Wallerian degeneration do not appear until about 17 days after axonal section, so their absence before this time does not necessarily imply the good prognosis that is associated with conduction

block. There seems little virtue in extensive needle sampling of facial muscles to search for some units under voluntary control. This is quite painful, and flickers of contraction can readily be seen through the skin.

Differential diagnosis

Many patients with facial palsy believe that they have suffered a stroke, but an analysis of the facial movements, as described above, will usually readily show that the palsy is of lower motor neuron type.

Although only the facial nerve is affected in a true Bell's palsy, patients often say that the skin feels different over the two sides of the face. This probably reflects only a distortion of trigeminal receptive fields as the face sags. If there is clear-cut evidence of trigeminal or other neighbouring nerve or nuclear involvement, then further investigation is clearly required. The facial nerve may be compressed by tumours in the cerebello-pontine angle. A lateral brain-stem infarction (Section 10.1.5) may affect the nucleus of the facial nerve.

Treatment and prognosis

Without any treatment at all, nearly 85 per cent of all patients with facial palsy will make a complete recovery. About 10–13 per cent will have a mild degree of residual weakness, and 2–5 per cent a moderate or severe residual palsy. Recovery usually begins with a few days of onset. Unfavourable features include advanced age, the presence of initial pain, a complete palsy, and a disturbance of taste and/or hyperacusis.

As such a large proportion of subjects recover spontaneously, it is difficult to show any benefit from therapy. None the less, a number of controlled trials have shown that corticosteroids do reduce the numbers of those with residual facial weakness. Medication probably has to be commenced within 24 hours of onset if there is to be benefit. Steroids certainly relieve retro-aural and facial pain. A suitable course for an adult is prednisolone, 60 mg/day for one day, reducing by 10 mg/day at daily intervals. Methylcellulose eye drops should be used to protect the exposed eye. Occasionally, antibiotic eye drops (e.g. sulphacetamide, 10 per cent) are required. There is no evidence that vitamin therapy, electrical stimulation of the muscles, or operative decompression of

the nerve within the facial canal make any difference to outcome.

In patients with Wallerian degeneration distal to the site of the lesion, recovery is by regeneration, which may be aberrant. For example, a neuron programmed centrally to close the eye may regenerate and reach lower facial muscles around the lips. Consequently, when the patient closes his eye, there may be a twitching movement of the mouth. These are known as synkinetic movements. Aberrant regeneration can also affect autonomic fibres. For example, a secretomotor fibre originally destined for a salivary gland may be diverted, as it regenerates, down the greater superficial petrosal nerve to the sphenopalatine ganglion, where it synapses with fibres going to the lacrimal gland. The end result is that stimuli resulting in salivation may also result in lacrimation—the so-called crocodile tears, as it is alleged (probably untruthfully) that a crocodile weeps as it eats its victim.

The occasional patient left with a severe residual facial palsy may sometimes be helped by surgery. For example, a sling of fascia lata can be passed subcutaneously from the zygoma to the drooping angle of the mouth. The operation of hypoglossal nerve–facial nerve anastomosis is now seldom performed, as synkinetic movements are a major problem.

19.4.1.2 *Other cranial mononeuropathies*

Other isolated cranial mononeuropathies (with the exception of optic nerve lesions, not usually so considered) are much less common than a facial palsy, and the pathogenetic mechanisms are clearly different. For example, a IIIrd nerve lesion may be caused by a diabetic microinfarct, or by lateral extension of a pituitary tumour. Unexplained isolated trigeminal neuropathies always give concern in case there is a lesion invading the skull base, for example a nasopharyngeal carcinoma. Isolated VIth nerve lesions are common after cranial injury and as a manifestation of the distortions caused by raised intracranial pressure (Section 16.2). An isolated VIIIth nerve lesion may be due to an ischaemic lesion or to an acoustic neuroma.

Multiple cranial mononeuropathies may occur as a result of a diffuse infiltrating lesion at the base of the skull. One common cause is a nasopharyngeal carcinoma that erodes through the skull base. An extradural secondary deposit of, for example, bronchial carcinoma may have the same effect. Inflammatory lesions causing multiple cranial mononeuropathies include sarcoidosis (Section 17.17.1), 'malignant' otitis due to *Pseudomonas* infection, and basal tuberculous meningitis (Section 17.5.1.2).

19.4.2 Peripheral nerve injuries and entrapment

19.4.2.1 Complete division of nerves (neurotmesis)

Such injuries are commonly caused by knife or glass wounds, the median and ulnar at the wrist being particularly exposed to such trauma. Unfortunately, injuries to nerves may be initially overlooked and the skin alone sutured. Immediate repair is best, using an operating microscope in an attempt to rotate the nerve so that the perineum of appropriate fascicles can be sutured together. However, the presence of infection, or the initial absence of a surgeon with suitable skills may make it advisable to suture the nerve at a later stage, but the delay should not be such that muscle atrophy becomes far advanced. If there is a significant gap between the two ends of the nerve, then this may be bridged by a short sural graft, although of course this itself undergoes Wallerian degeneration; only the epineurium survives, as a skeletal tube down which regenerating fibres grow.

Axon sprouts regenerate from the severed central stump of a cut nerve within a few hours, advance to meet proliferating Schwann cells in the distal stump, and gain new myelin. However careful the repair, some cross-innervation to the 'wrong' muscle or sensory receptor is inevitable. The new axons grow at a rate of about 1 mm/day, but the longer the distance required to re-innervate a muscle fibre or sensory receptor, the less likely is it that functional reunion will occur. That is to say, the results of suturing a divided ulnar nerve at the wrist will be better than if the injury has arisen in the upper arm.

19.4.2.2 Incomplete division of nerves: causalgia and post-traumatic dystrophy of the extremities

An incomplete lesion of a peripheral nerve obviously results in less weakness and sensory disturbance than a complete division. However, some of those who have suffered an incomplete division subsequently develop causalgia—the name given to a constant dull ache, with throbbing pain on activity, and episodes of sharp pain superimposed. Initially the pain lies in the distribution of the affected nerve, but later may spread well outside it. The hand or foot becomes stiff and cold, and there are often trophic changes in the nails and in the skin, which becomes sweaty, blue, and shiny. Similar changes may follow comparatively minor soft-tissue and bony injuries to limbs, when the condition is known as post-traumatic dystrophy or Sudeck's atrophy. X-rays of the disabled limb show a considerable degree of bone resorption. The pathophysiology of post-traumatic dystrophy secondary to partial nerve damage is uncertain. It is thought that there may be 'short circuits' (ephaptic transmission) between damaged nerve fibres. There is also alteration in the afferent drive from the periphery to the autonomic nervous system. The character of the pain, however, is so similar to that which follows avulsion injuries of the brachial plexus (see Section 19.5.1) that the central effects of deafferentation are certainly also important. It has also been suggested that there is a secondary failure of opioid peptide modulation in regional sympathetic ganglia. The first treatment of this distressing condition is to encourage the fullest use of the disabled hand, in order to restore as far as possible the pattern of central afferent stimulation. However, sympathetic blockade by intra-arterial guanethidine or transcutaneous nerve stimulation may be useful.

19.4.2.3 Acute compression injuries of peripheral nerves

These occur when a nerve is acutely compressed between some hard object and underlying bone. A good example is the so-called 'Saturday night' palsy—a radial palsy, caused by hanging the upper arm over the back of a chair, then dropping off to sleep, often while intoxicated. The patient notes a wrist drop that is usually painless. Examination shows normal triceps contraction, but weakness of brachioradialis, the extensors of the wrist, fingers, and thumb, and the long abductor of the thumb. Supinator is also weak, but as supination is effected by biceps this is not obvious. There may be some tingling or slight sensory impairment in the anatomical snuff box.

The function of the hand can be improved considerably, while nerve repair is under way, by the provision of a volar splint that holds the wrist cocked up in a functional position so that the fingers can be used for most day-to-day tasks.

Another common lesion is a foot drop due to acute compression of the common peroneal nerve at the head of the fibula. Sometimes the compression is due to some external force, such as trapping the nerve between the fibula and the side of a knee-hole in a desk. Sometimes the injury associated with a fracture of tibia or fibula is responsible, or even the top edge of a below-knee plaster of Paris splint used for treating such a fracture. Sometimes no external object can be blamed. For example, in the prolonged squat necessary to weed a flower bed, or pick strawberries, the common peroneal nerve may be squeezed at the knee, with resulting foot drop.

Examination shows weakness of the tibialis anterior and extensor hallucis muscles, and, usually, of the muscles which evert the foot, the peroneus longus and brevis. If the compression lies above the origin of the cutaneous superficial branch, there will be impairment of sensation over the whole of the outer aspect of the lower part of the leg, and most of the dorsum of the foot. If below the origin of this branch, then sensory loss is confined to the area of supply of the terminal branch of the anterior tibial nerve, a small zone on the dorsum of the foot extending to the cleft between the great and second toes.

There are, of course, other causes of foot drop, and one which sometimes gives rise to difficulty in differential diagnosis is an L 4 or 5 radicular lesion due to a prolapsed intervertebral disc. Back and sciatic pain does not always occur with such disc protrusions, but there will, in such cases, be weakness of *inversion* of the foot due to weakness of the tibialis posterior. Sensory loss also extends rather higher up the outer aspect of the leg in L5 lesions than it does in peroneal nerve palsies.

Other common acute compressive nerve palsies are ulnar nerve compression or sciatic nerve compression arising during prolonged periods of recumbency during anaesthesia or unconsciousness. A tourniquet left on too long will also damage nerves in the limb to which it has been applied.

The primary lesion of acute compressive nerve injuries is, as described in Section 19.2, Table 19.4, and illustrated in Fig. 19.2, invagination of axoplasm and nodes of Ranvier away from the site of compression, with subsequent demyelination and block in conduction (neuropraxia). If the changes are more pronounced, then some axons degenerate (axonotmesis), with consequent fibrillation and wasting of denervated muscles. As the epi- and perineurium remain intact, however, regeneration is much more effective than that following a division of the whole nerve by, for example, a glass injury.

Complete conduction block and axonotmesis both result in paralysis and sensory loss distal to the lesion. A neurologist can, however, decide the type of underlying pathology, and prognosis, by certain clinical and electrophysiological points. Immediately after an axonotmesis, the length of nerve distal to the lesion is still capable of conducting, if stimulated distally, for about 3 days before Wallerian degeneration develops fully. Stimulation below the lesion will then evoke no muscle response. In conduction block, however, the axons remain intact and stimulation below the lesion continues to evoke a normal muscle response, whereas stimulation above the blocked zone evokes no response or, if a partial lesion, a delayed dispersed response of low amplitude. After axonotmesis, the denervated muscles waste, but this is much less pronounced in a conduction block due to a demyelinated compressive lesion. Finally, electromyography shows that denervated muscles fibrillate, though this does not begin for 17 days. These changes are summarized in Table 19.4. Of course, intermediate lesions are often seen, and probably are the rule. It may be 2 or 3 months before conduction can be detected following a severe neuropraxic lesion, with marked changes in a number of nodes of Ranvier, so there may not be that much difference in the time-course of clinical recovery following severe neuropraxia or axonotmesis, though clearly the former is more favourable.

19.4.2.4 *Chronic compressive lesions*

Certain occupations or pastimes may cause chronic focal neuropathies. Examples include compression of the deep ulnar branch of the ulnar nerve by bicycle handlebars, and compression of the termi-

Table 19.4 Summary of changes in acute nerve lesions

	Conduction block (neuropraxia)	Axonotmesis
Pathological changes	Invagination of nodes of Ranvier and subsequent demyelination	Wallerian degeneration
Voluntary effort	No muscle response	No muscle response
Stimulation of nerve		
above lesion	No muscle response	No muscle response
below lesion		
first 3 days	Normal muscle response	Declining muscle response as fibres degenerate over 3–4 days
after 3 days	Normal muscle response	No response until much later regeneration (perhaps >300 days)
Wasting	Not marked	Becomes marked
Electromyography	No fibrillation	Fibrillation begins after 17 days

nal part of the anterior tibial nerve by tight ski-boots. The pathological changes are similar to the spontaneously occurring chronic compressive lesions known as entrapment neuropathies. Avoidance of the precipitating cause usually results in spontaneous resolution.

19.4.2.5 *Entrapment neuropathies*

This is the term used to describe focal disturbances of peripheral nerve function due to entrapment in fibro-osseous tunnels such as the carpal tunnel. Very similar lesions result from recurrent stretch and angulation, such as that which affects the ulnar nerve at the elbow. The pathological changes are described in Section 19.2. Table 19.5 lists the common, and some of the less common, varieties. Only the common varieties are further discussed.

The carpal tunnel syndrome
The classic symptom of this common condition is nocturnal awakening by painful paraesthesia in the affected hand. Although it might be expected that patients would localize the tingling to the lateral three and a half digits (the distribution of the median nerve), about two-thirds of patients say that all digits tingle and that pain and tingling often extend well up the arm. The patient attempts to get relief by shaking his hand or by hanging it down out of the bed. Women are affected three times as often as men. Many patients have bilateral

symptoms, though the dominant hand is usually first affected. It has been shown that affected women tend to have carpal tunnels of smaller cross-sectional area than controls matched for age. Any encroachment upon the tunnel may precipitate symptoms, so that those who have thickening of the synovial sheaths of tendons traversing the tunnel may well develop the syndrome. Such thickening is seen in occupational or rheumatoid tenosynovitis, or following a fracture of the lower end of the radius, or of one of the carpal bones. Pregnancy is particularly likely to precipitate symptoms, usually from the end of the second trimester. Other patients develop symptoms following a gain in weight, or consequent upon the enlargement of distal soft tissues in acromegaly, or as a result of hypothyroidism.

Clinical examination of patients presenting with this story is often unremarkable, and no convincing sensory changes may be found. If there is sensory loss, it is most often found in the middle finger. Some patients may prove to have wasting and weakness of the thenar muscles innervated by the median nerve, particularly abductor pollicis brevis. Percussion over the affected median nerve in the carpal tunnel may produce tingling in the lateral three digits (Tinel's sign). In many patients, unforced but full flexion of the wrist for 60 seconds may reproduce the symptoms (Phalen's sign).

The clinical story is so suggestive that often no confirmation is required, but electrodiagnostic

Table 19.5   Entrapment neuropathies

Nerve	Site of entrapment	Predisposing factors	Clinical features
Common			
Median	In carpal tunnel	Female sex Small carpal tunnel Pregnancy Recent gain in weight Tenosynovitis Rheumatoid disease Previous fracture Hypothyroidism Acromegaly	Nocturnal paraesthesiae Weakness of thenar muscles
Ulnar	At elbow	Male sex Heavy manual occupation Increased carrying angle Previous fracture Osteoarthritis of elbow	Paraesthesiae in and clawing of fourth and fifth digits, weakness of muscles innervated by this nerve, particularly interossei
Lower trunk of brachial plexus	Cervical rib or band	Anatomical variation	Pain in arm and hand Wasting and weakness of *all* hand muscles, and medial forearm muscles
Lateral cutaneous nerve of thigh ('meralgia paraesthetica')	In inguinal ligament	Male sex Prolonged exercise Recent gain in weight Tight pants	Paraesthesiae on front and outer aspect of thigh
Less common			
Median or anterior interosseous	Below elbow by tendinous bands within pronator teres or flexor digitorum superficialis	Anatomical variation	Pain and tenderness in forearm Weakness of flexor pollicis longus and indicis
Ulnar	At wrist in ulnar canal bounded by pisiform and hook of hamate bones	Ganglion at wrist Manual occupation Previous fracture	Pain in wrist, weakness of small hand muscles innervated by deep ulnar branch
Posterior interosseous	On interosseous membrane, by tendinous band within supinator muscle	Anatomical variation Lipoma or ganglion at this site	Weakness of extensor carpi ulnaris, extensor digitorum communis and indicis, abductor and extensor pollicis longus
Peroneal	Between fibula and head of peroneous longus	Anatomical variation Previous fracture	Weakness of tibialis anterior, extensor hallucis longus, sometimes of peroneal muscles
Posterior tibial	Tarsal tunnel below and behind lateral malleolus	Anatomical variation	Burning pain in sole of foot, sometimes sensory loss, particularly in medial plantar area

Diabetes mellitus or a mild generalized underlying neuropathy predispose to the development of an entrapment neuropathy. These should be considered in all cases of entrapment neuropathy.

studies may be useful in some patients. The cardinal findings are:

(1) a prolonged latency and/or diminution in amplitude of sensory action potentials derived from the lateral three digits. These observations can be reinforced by the observation of normal sensory action potentials from the little finger (Fig. 8.6);

(2) a prolongation of the latency of the muscle response of the thenar muscles evoked by stimulation at the wrist.

The principal differential diagnosis of carpal tunnel syndrome is a radicular lesion affecting the sixth cervical dermatome, with pain and tingling also in the lateral part of the hand. Those with C6 root lesions may have pain in the neck, are not usually awakened at night by paraesthesia, and may have other evidence of dysfunction of the C6 root, such as a weak biceps muscle, or a depressed biceps reflex. Electrodiagnostic studies are particularly useful in distinguishing radicular lesions from compression of the median nerve within the carpal tunnel.

Patients with severe symptoms, definite sensory loss, and weakness of the thenar muscles will require operative decompression of the carpal tunnel. The flexor retinaculum is divided by a curvilinear incision extending distally from the wrist crease. Patients with minor symptoms, or those who have transient exacerbations during pregnancy, may be helped by the provision of a volar splint which holds the hand slightly dorsiflexed, or by the injection of methylprednisolone (20 mg) just proximal to the carpal tunnel. Operative decompression is, however, so straightforward and successful that there should be no hesitation in recommending it if symptoms are not readily relieved by conservative treatment. If both hands are affected, it will be sensible to operate upon the more severely affected hand first, as the necessary post-operative firm bandaging will incapacitate the patient for a few days if both hands are done together.

Ulnar nerve compression at the elbow

All of us are familiar with the shower of pins and needles running down the ulnar aspect of the forearm into the ring and little finger after unwittingly striking the 'funny bone'—the ulnar nerve as it lies in its fibro-osseous tunnel behind the medial epicondyle of the humerus. Recurrent minor trauma during life, and probably recurrent stretch and damage caused by friction as the nerve slides back and forth during flexion and extension of the elbow are responsible for the development of a chronic focal ulnar neuropathy. Predisposing factors include a previous fracture of the elbow joint, or an increased carrying angle at the elbow. Other patients may develop a pressure palsy following a prolonged period of unconsciousness or nursing in the intensive therapy unit as the nerve lies posteriorly when the patient is supine. Most frequent symptoms are paraesthesia in the fourth and fifth digits, but some patients present with weakness. A common presenting motor symptom is an inability to use a Yale key, due to weakness of the adductor pollicis, which is used in pinching the head of the key between thumb and index finger. Other patients notice wasting of the web between thumb and index finger, formed by the first dorsal interosseous muscle.

Examination usually shows wasting of this muscle, of abductor digiti minimi, and of the other dorsal interossei, as revealed by the appearance of gutters lying between the extensor tendons on the dorsum of the hand. In severe cases, there may be noticeable thinning on the medial aspect of the forearm. The wasting and contractures of the interosseous and lumbrical muscles and weakness of the long flexors of the fourth and fifth fingers result in a characteristic posture of the hand, in which these fingers are held slightly hyperextended at the metacarpo-phalangeal joint, and slightly flexed at the interphalangeal joints.

Testing each muscle in a patient with ulnar palsy at the elbow will show weakness of all muscles innervated by the ulnar nerve (flexor carpi ulnaris, flexor digitorum profundus 4 and 5, all interosseous muscles, abductor digiti minimi, and adductor pollicis). In early cases, weakness of finger abduction and adduction is most easily detected, the latter movement being tested by the ability of the adducted fingers to squeeze a thin card, and prevent the examiner from withdrawing it. Impairment of sensation in an ulnar lesion at the elbow may be found affecting the medial 2 cm of both palmar and dorsal aspects of the hand (not extending onto the medial aspect of the forearm), all the fifth finger, and ulnar half of the ring finger. Occasionally the sensory impairment splits the middle finger instead.

Electrophysiological examination will support the diagnosis of an ulnar lesion at the elbow by:

(1) showing normal conduction velocity in the length of ulnar nerve below the elbow;

(2) reduced velocity across the elbow segment;

(3) evidence of a conduction block across the elbow segment;

(4) evidence of denervation in muscles innervated by the ulnar nerve, with normal findings in thenar muscles; and

(5) reduced or absent ulnar sensory action potential derived from the little finger, with normal sensory potential from the index finger.

The differential diagnosis of an ulnar nerve lesion at the elbow includes a lesion affecting the deep branch of the ulnar nerve in the palm. This may arise in certain occupations (for example, in woodworkers, the head of a screwdriver is repeatedly pushed into the palm). In deep-branch palsies, there is no sensory impairment, as the superficial branch is given off above the wrist. This superficial branch also supplies abductor digiti minimi, which is usually, therefore, preserved, as is flexor digitorum profundus of the fourth and fifth digits.

The differential diagnosis of ulnar nerve lesions includes those that cause wasting of all the small muscles of the hand—thenar and interosseous—notably motor neuron disease, a cervical rib, or a spinal tumour or syrinx at the first thoracic segmental level. Cervical radiculopathy, as a result of spondylosis, must also be considered.

Patients with minor symptoms due to compression of the ulnar nerve at the elbow should be advised to protect the nerve against minor damage in everyday life, for example by avoiding chairs with wooden or metal arms, and by avoiding leaning on the elbow when writing or telephoning. More substantial lesions should be relieved by transposition of the nerve to the front of the elbow. Although the nerve may be left lying superficially on the front of the forearm, it is better placed beneath the common flexor muscle mass. Unfortunately, patients who present with a great deal of wasting, weakness, and sensory involvement may not be greatly helped by transposition.

Compression by a cervical rib

Although a lesion of the brachial plexus, and not

nearly as common as the next syndrome discussed, this syndrome is best considered here on account of the diagnostic distinction from the median and ulnar lesions just described. The eighth cervical and first thoracic roots unite to form the lower trunk of the brachial plexus, which normally lies on the first rib. The lower trunk may be stretched over an extra rib articulating with the seventh cervical vertebra, or by a fibrous band running from the tip of the transverse process of this vertebra to the scalene tubercle on the first rib.

Patients complain of pain in the forearm and hand, and weakness of the hand. Examination usually shows wasting of all the small muscles of the hand, although sometimes the thenar pad seems more prominently affected. Wasting extends up the medial aspect of the forearm, as these muscles are supplied by C8. Electrophysiological studies show denervation in the wasted muscles, a normal sensory action potential from the index finger, and a reduced or absent sensory action potential from the little finger. Operative decompression usually relieves pain, but if the patient presents with prominent wasting of the hand, there may be little recovery of function.

The distinction between the various symptoms affecting the hand and forearm is not easy, but a clear record and analysis of which muscles are weak, their nerve and segmental supply, and the distribution of any sensory loss usually allows a firm diagnosis to be reached, confirmed by electrodiagnostic studies. Table 19.6 summarizes these findings.

Entrapment of the lateral cutaneous nerve of the thigh

This condition is known as *meralgia parasthetica* (Greek, *meras* = thigh). The lateral cutaneous nerve of the thigh passes deep to or through the inguinal ligament. The nerve may be compressed by repeated exercise; for example it is common in young soldiers, with exacerbations after route marches. It is also common in middle-aged men, who have put on weight. It sometimes appears that the thigh holes of underpants or jeans may be too tight. The symptoms are of an unpleasant burning sensation and numbness in the distribution of the nerve. The borders of impaired sensation are fairly sharply defined. As the nerve is purely cutaneous, there is no muscle wasting or weakness, nor any

Table 19.6 Evaluation of some common lower motor neuron lesions affecting one hand

	Carpal tunnel syndrome	Ulnar lesion at elbow	Ulnar lesion (deep palmar branch)	Cervical rib	Cervical spondylotic radiculopathy C8/T1	Motor neuron disease
Wasting and weakness						
thenar muscles	+	0	0	+	±	+
interosseous muscles	0	+	+	+	+	+
abductor digiti minimi	0	+	0	+	+	+
flexor digitorum profundus 4+5	0	+	0	+	±	+
Sensory impairment						
Thumb, index, and middle	+	0	0	0	0	0
Ring finger	split	split	0	±	0	0
Little finger	0	+	0	+	±	0
Medial forearm	0	0	0	+	±	0
Sensory action potential						
From index	impaired	normal	normal	normal	normal	normal
From little finger	normal	impaired	normal	impaired	normal	normal

Note: The contents of this table imply that the lesion is fully developed and, in the case of cervical spondylotic radiculopathy and motor neuron disease, that the hand is wasted, which is, of course, by no means always the case.

change in the knee jerk—points that distinguish this condition from a more proximal lesion affecting lumbar roots or plexus. Surgical decompression of the nerve is disappointing; patients should be encouraged to lose weight, if appropriate, and put up with their symptoms, confident in the knowlege that the sensory impairment will spread no further.

Before leaving compression and entrapment neuropathies, three additional points should be stressed. First, patients with diabetes mellitus are particularly predisposed to such focal neuropathies, and an estimation of a fasting blood sugar often proves worthwhile. The usual decompressive procedures should be undertaken, but recovery may not be so good as in the non-diabetic. Secondly, minor degrees of generalized neuropathy, apart from diabetic neuropathy, predispose to entrapment neuropathies. This may be discovered at routine electrophysiological examination for what was thought to be a straightforward carpal tunnel syndrome; it is then found that there is diminution in amplitude of all sensory action potentials. Thirdly, there are rare families in which a tendency to pressure palsy and entrapment neuropathy is inherited through an autosomal dominant gene (Table 19.3).

19.5 Plexus lesions

Table 19.7 lists some of the disorders of the brachial and of the lumbar plexus.

19.5.1 *Acute injuries of the brachial plexus*

The majority of brachial plexus injuries are due to sudden excessive traction occurring as a result of road traffic accidents, particularly those involving motor cycles. A high velocity impact of the tip of the shoulder with the road, or a distraction between head and shoulders will tear the upper part of the plexus. The lower part may be torn by a forceable abduction of the arm. Unfortunately, components of the plexus tear at their weakest point, where they are unsupported by perineurium, which is within the spinal canal. The roots are often avulsed from the cord. The tear therefore lies proximal to the dorsal root ganglion and there is no possibility of regeneration of the central axon of the primary sensory neuron into the spinal cord, nor of surgical repair.

Clinical assessment of brachial plexus lesions depends, therefore, on judging whether the lesion affects the upper or lower part of the plexus,

Table 19.7 Disorders of the brachial and of the lumbar plexus

Brachial plexus
  Acute traction injury
    motor accidents
    birth injury
  Compressive lesions
    cervical rib
    rucksack palsy
  Invasion by carcinoma
    lung or breast
  'Immunological' causes
    neuralgic amyotrophy
    injection of serum
    abuse of heroin
Lumbar plexus
  Diabetic amyotrophy
  Bleeding after excessive anticoagulation
  Invasion by tumour
    retroperitoneal sarcoma
  'Immunological' causes
    neuralgic amyotrophy
    injection of serum
    abuse of heroin

whether the lesion is proximal or distal, and, if proximal, whether pre- or post-ganglionic.

Upper plexus injuries involve the muscles innervated by the fifth and sixth cervical roots, particularly the supraspinatus and deltoid. The nerve to rhomboids and the long thoracic nerve to serratus anterior arise proximally in the plexus, and involvement of these muscles is, therefore, a poor prognostic sign. In severe upper brachial plexus injuries, the supraclavicular nerves from the cervical plexus may also be involved, and analgesia in their territory, over the neck, is also a very unfavourable sign.

Lower plexus injuries are characterized by involvement of the finger flexors and small muscles of the hand, innervated by C8 and T1. A proximal lesion will damage sympathetic fibres passing to the stellate ganglion, resulting in unilateral ptosis and meiosis—a Horner's syndrome (Section 19.7.2.4).

In pre-ganglionic injuries, the peripheral sensory axon still has its cell body intact, although the affected dermatome is anaesthetic. Integrity of the pre-ganglionic axon can be deduced unequivocally if sensory nerve action potentials (Section 8.8) are of normal amplitude from an anaesthetic digit. A helpful bedside test is the response of anaesthetic skin to a scratch, or more reliably, the intradermal injection of 1 per cent histamine. If the axons are in continuity into intact cell bodies, then a flare and wheal occur. If the injury is post-ganglionic, then there is only a wheal, and limited local vasodilation.

Early surgical exploration of the plexus is indicated if the damage is caused by a knife or glass wound, as suturing damaged upper components of the plexus under the operating microscope may lead to worthwhile regeneration, and recovery of shoulder movement and elbow flexion. Attempts to repair the lower part of the plexus do not, in general, result in worthwhile recovery of function of the hand. Another indication for early surgical exploration is if there is associated damage to the subclavian or axillary artery or vein. Intra-operative stimulation and recording of evoked potentials may help to analyse whether identified structures are in continuity. If it is certain that the lower roots are avulsed from the cord, then the ulnar nerve with its intact sensory root ganglia, may be used as a vascularized nerve graft to repair post-ganglionic upper plexus damage.

Fortunately, not all brachial plexus injuries result in rupture of roots or trunks, and about two-thirds of patients with initially clinically complete C5, C6 lesions recover shoulder abduction and elbow flexion by regeneration. The more roots initially involved, the worse the prognosis. If the arm remains flail, then a three-component splint should be provided, supported by a harness over the opposite shoulder. One component prevents subluxation of the shoulder, another locks the elbow at five different angles of flexion, and the third supports the wrist. On the flexor aspect of the wrist support can be slotted appropriate appliances, such as a split hook or tool holder. Amputation used to be offered for useless flail arms, but carefully designed splinting avoids amputation and gives some worthwhile function.

Most of those with pre-ganglionic lesions suffer severe burning pain in the paralysed limb, with paroxysms of shooting pain on a background of severe burning pain. The management of this very difficult problem is considered with other painful peripheral nerve symptoms in Section 19.4.2.2.

High-velocity traction is not the only type of trauma to the brachial plexus. Low-velocity traction injuries to the plexus may occur during birth. If the head, during delivery, is forcibly pulled away from the shoulder, then the upper part of the plexus may be torn, with transient or lifelong weakness of the shoulder abductors. The lower plexus may also be injured during birth by traction on an extended arm, in which case the finger flexors and small hand muscles are affected—Klumpke's paralysis.

The commonest compressive lesion of the brachial plexus—by a cervical rib—was considered in Section 19.4.2.5. In addition, heavy rucksacks were found, during the Vietnam war, to produce compressive injuries of the plexus as the webbing support compressed the plexus between the clavicle and first rib.

19.5.2   Brachial plexopathies

19.5.2.1   Neuralgic amyotrophy

Although obscure in origin, this is a clearly defined clinical syndrome. The first symptom is usually a deep, aching pain in the shoulder and upper arm, which increases rapidly in severity. Because of the pain, the patient may avoid moving his arm, but when he does so, he finds it weak. The muscles most prominently affected are the serratus anterior, deltoid, and periscapular muscles, although more distal muscles may also, or independently, be affected. Sensory loss is usually slight, but, if present, is most often over the territory of the axillary nerve, i.e. over the lateral part of the arm. The pain usually fades after a week or so but muscle wasting (myoatrophy or amyotrophy) then begins. Electrodiagnostic studies show denervation in the affected muscles, but normal conduction in surviving fibres. Recovery is often incomplete, and slow, taking up to a year. The cause of this condition is not known, nor is there any information about the histopathology from autopsy studies. Biopsy of distal affected nerves has shown only uninformative axonal degeneration. Occasionally neuralgic amyotrophy is recurrent. There are also families reported with several affected members.

The differential diagnosis of neuralgic amyotrophy is principally from painful brachial weakness caused by a prolapsed cervical intervertebral disc. Serratus anterior is seldom, if ever, affected by a disc protrusion, but is commonly affected in neuralgic amyotrophy. Treatment is with analgesics. It may be helpful to rest the arm in a sling, or collar and cuff. Steroids have not been found to be useful.

19.5.2.2   Other brachial plexopathies

One possible explanation of neuralgic amyotrophy is that it is related to some immunological process, as a very similar condition follows injections of horse-serum, frequently given before tetanus toxoid replaced antitetanus serum as routine prophylaxis. Other cases follow heroin abuse, particularly if contaminated heroin has been used. Similar spontaneous serum- or heroin-induced lesions can, less commonly, affect the lumbar plexus.

The brachial plexus may also be invaded directly by malignant disease. The lower trunk, or medial cord, may be destroyed by the upward spread of an apical carcinoma of the lung (Pancoast's syndrome). Secondary glands in the neck, common with carcinoma of the breast, may form a diffuse mat of solid tissue palpable above the clavicle, and affecting virtually any part of the plexus. Local radiotherapy may give some worthwhile partial recovery of function, and relieve pain. Very occasionally, radiotherapy itself induces a brachial plexitis and the distinction between this and local recurrence of carcinoma may be very difficult.

19.5.3   Lumbar plexopathies

19.5.3.1   Diabetic amyotrophy

The most frequent lumbar plexopathy is diabetic amyotrophy. Occasionally patients with this condition present to the neurologist, who makes the diagnosis of diabetes mellitus for the first time. Other patients with established diabetes may present during a time of poor control. Conversely, it sometimes appears that amyotrophy is precipitated at a time when insulin therapy is initiated or diabetic control improved. In general, however, the disorder is more common in non-insulin-dependent diabetics, and in older people.

The clinical symptoms are of severe constant pain in one thigh, then accompanied by wasting and weakness of the quadriceps muscle. However, clinical examination and electromyography show that more muscles than this are denervated, fibrillation and fasciculation potentials being found in the paraspinal muscles innervated by the posterior primary rami, and clinical weakness often being apparent in adductor magnus and iliopsoas. There are no sensory findings. The number of autopsy examinations is limited, but it seems likely that the lumbar plexus is affected by multiple microvascular infarcts. Most patients recover following improved diabetic control, in spite of the anomalies mentioned above, but they may have a miserable few months before the pain settles. Whether or not it is the better control which speeds recovery, or whether recovery would occur anyway, even if control was lax, is not clear. This condition is still not as widely recognized as it ought to be, and a number of patients are submitted to radiculography and even spinal surgery as the symptoms are mistakenly attributed to a prolapsed intervertebral disc, which only rarely occurs at these high lumbar levels.

19.5.3.2   *Other lumbar plexopathies*

These may be spontaneous, as in neuralgic amyotrophy of the brachial plexus, or induced by heroin abuse. Local tumours on the posterior abdominal wall, for example retroperitoneal sarcoma, may also affect the plexus. Neurofibromas may arise from different parts of the plexus and lie buried in iliopsoas muscle. Excessive anticoagulation may cause bleeding into the posterior abdominal wall and plexus. The symptoms and clinical signs of all these plexopathies depend upon the roots or nerves affected, but common symptoms include pain in the thigh, and the leg giving way due to weakness of quadriceps muscle. The exact localization of the lesion depends upon electromyography, to detect denervation in affected muscles, and imaging may be useful to reveal a tumour or haematoma.

19.6   Mononeuritis multiplex

This name refers to multiple involvement of a number of different nerves, for example a radial in one arm, and a common peroneal in one leg.

The most frequent cause world-wide is leprosy (Section 17.6). In the lepromatous form, invasion of nerves by bacilli occurs at an early stage, although the patient usually presents with dermal lesions before a classical neuropathy becomes apparent. In the tuberculoid form, granulomas form within peripheral nerves, resulting in local palsies. Some affected nerves may be readily palpable under the skin.

Nerve infiltrates may also occur with leukaemia and lymphoma. Local destruction by carcinoma often occurs, but metastases within nerves are very rare. Sarcoidosis may cause a mononeuritis multiplex, with involvement often of cranial as well as peripheral nerves. Finally, mononeuritis multiplex may result from microvascular infarctions in diabetes mellitus, polyarteritis nodosa, the Churg–Strauss syndrome, rheumatoid arthritis, and poorly differentiated connective tissue diseases such as Wegener's granulomatosis and Sjögren's syndrome.

19.7   Autonomic neuropathy

Table 19.8 classifies the causes of autonomic insuf-

Table 19.8   Classification of autonomic insufficiency

Failure of afferent drive to autonomic nervous system
   Diabetes mellitus
   Acute infective polyneuropathy
   Anderson–Fabry disease—α-galactosidase deficiency
Failure of efferent output
   Primary neuronal degeneration of intermediolateral
      cell column (multi-system atrophy)
   Spinal cord lesions
   Acute dysautonomia
      cholinergic
      adrenergic
   Familial dysautonomic neuropathy—the Riley–Day
      syndrome
   Pharmacological blockade, e.g. atropine, ganglion-
      blocking agents
Localized autonomic failure
   Syndromes affecting the pupil
      Isolated pupillotonia, or with hyporeflexia (Adie's
         syndrome)
      Pupillotonia and segmental sudomotor failure
         (Ross's syndrome)
   Achalasia of the cardia
   Hirschsprung's disease
   Trypanosomiasis

---

ficiency, only some of which are neuropathies. Nevertheless, it is convenient to consider the symptoms, signs, and investigation of autonomic failure here.

19.7.1 Clinical features

Orthostatic hypotension, diarrhoea or constipation, bladder dysfunction, erectile impotence, and abnormalities of sweating are all symptoms of autonomic failure.

19.7.2 Investigations

19.7.2.1 Vascular reflexes

The maintenance of normal arterial pressure on standing depends on baroreceptor reflexes. A prominent symptom of autonomic insufficiency is a feeling of unease or faintness on standing, due to orthostatic hypotension, which may lead to syncope. The integrity of the baroreceptor reflexes can be assessed by observing if the pressure measured supine is maintained or slightly increased, as is normal, on standing. In cases of autonomic failure, it may take several minutes before the pressure falls.

The integrity of the efferent limb of the reflex arc can be measured by noting if there is a pressor response when the subject is asked to perform mental arithmetic while being harassed to perform more quickly. The afferent limb can be tested by firm massage of the carotid sinus. The system as a whole can be assessed by the Valsalva manoeuvre. In normal subjects, forced expiration against resistance causes a decrease in effective cardiac filling pressure. Cardiac output falls. There is a peripheral vasoconstriction. On release of the forced expiration, the heart fills and expels blood into the vasoconstricted circulation. There is thus a transient overshoot in blood pressure with, in turn, a baroreceptor response which slows the heart. In patients with autonomic neuropathy there is a failure of peripheral vasoconstriction, no overshoot of pressure, and no baroreceptor-mediated cardiac slowing. This test can be performed at the bedside by noting changes in the RR interval on electrocardiography. The ratio between the RR interval in the straining phase, when there is tachycardia, and the bradycardia following release of

forced expiration should be at least 1.2. Ratios of 1.1 or less suggest impaired baroreceptor reflexes.

In patients with cardiovascular problems due to autonomic failure, the adrenergic receptors in vessel walls are supersensitive to infused noradrenaline, so a brisk pressor response will be obtained in response to an intravenous infusion at 5 ng/min, which will do little in a subject with an intact autonomic nervous system.

19.7.2.2 Impotence

Many patients with autonomic failure complain of erectile impotence (Section 6.12). This can be investigated by strain gauge measurements of penile tumescence during rapid eye movement sleep.

19.7.2.3 Sweating

Sweating is often impaired in autonomic failure. This may be tested by cautious elevation of the body core temperature, using a heat cradle, and observing the areas of sweating, having dusted the skin with a mixture of starch and iodine. Less messy methods involve quantitative tests with the local iontophoresis of pilocarpine.

19.7.2.4 Ocular changes

Lesions of autonomic cholinergic fibres serving the eye may affect lacrimation, and lesions of the adrenergic fibres may affect the sympathetically innervated portion of levator palpebrae muscle. The most obvious changes, however, are in the pupil. A localized cervical sympathetic palsy is known as a Horner's syndrome, in which there is a slight drooping of the upper eyelid and a slightly smaller pupil, which does not dilate in response to shade.

Adie's syndrome is the name given to partial failure of cholinergic innervation of the iris. The pupils appear initially not to respond to light, but eventually a slow tonic contraction occurs. It is believed that this is due to acetylcholine, liberated normally from a few surviving nerve endings, diffusing through the muscle and depolarising supersensitive denervated receptors. The tendon reflexes are often suppressed as well, presumably because the neuropathy, which is usually symptomless, has affected afferent nerve fibres of large diameters from spindles. The interest in the syndrome is related to its possible confusion with the Argyll Robertson pupil of tabes dorsalis (Section 17.4.1.3).

The normal pupil will not dilate in response to eye drops containing 1 per cent adrenaline. However, if there is sympathetic denervation, the supersensitive smooth muscle fibres will respond to a solution of this strength, and dilate. Similarly, if there is parasympathetic denervation of the pupil, a 2.5 per cent solution of methacholine will cause a marked constriction, this being ineffective on a normal pupil.

None of the syndromes listed in Table 19.8 is common, with the exception of diabetes mellitus, in which postural hypotension and impotence often occur. In acute infective polyneuropathy, paroxysmal skin flushing and paroxysmal hypertension may be seen, as well as hypotension and impaired urinary control. Orthostatic hypotension is a prominent feature of some of the multisystem atrophies (Section 13.2). Acute dysautonomic syndromes are rare, but pure cholinergic and pure adrenergic failure have both been described, probably due to immunologically mediated damage to unmyelinated nerve fibres. Such fibres are also reduced in number in the Riley–Day syndrome, but in this case impairment of pain perception is prominent as unmyelinated afferents are also involved.

Failures of localized groups of autonomic neurons are at the root of Hirschsprung's disease, Chagas' disease, and achalasia of the cardia, in which normal peristaltic movements of the bowel are interrupted by absence or loss of neurons in the myenteric plexus.

19.8   Further reading

Diabetic neuropathy

Coppack, S. W. and Watkins, P. J. (1991). The natural history of diabetic femoral neuropathy. *Quarterly Journal of Medicine New Series* **79**, 307–13.

Dyck, P. J. (1992). New understanding and treatment of diabetic neuropathy. *New England Journal of Medicine* **326**, 1287–8.

Dyck, P. J., Zimmerman, B. R., Vilen, T. H., *et al.* (1988). Nerve glucose, fructose, sorbitol, myoinositol and fibre degeneration and regeneration in diabetic neuropathy. *New England Journal of Medicine* **319**, 542–8.

Editorial (1991). Understanding diabetic neuropathy. *Lancet* **331**, 1496–7.

Watkins, P. J. (1990). Natural history of the diabetic neuropathies. *Quarterly Journal of Medicine, New Series* **77**, 1209–18.

Amyloidosis

Pepys, M. B. (1988). Amyloidosis: some recent developments. *Quarterly Journal of Medicine, New Series* **67**, 283–98.

Acute infective polyneuropathy

Hughes, R. A. C. (1990). *Guillain–Barré syndrome*. Springer, London.

Oakley, C. M. (1984). The heart in the Guillain–Barré syndrome. *British Medical Journal* **288**, 94.

The Guillain–Barré syndrome study group (1985). Plasmapharesis and acute Guillain–Barré syndrome. *Neurology* **35**, 1086–104.

Winer, J. B. (1992). Guillain–Barré syndrome revisited. *British Medical Journal* **304**, 65–6.

Winer, J. B., Hughes, R. A. C., and Osmond C. (1988). A prospective study of acute idiopathic neuropathy. I. Clinical features and their prognostic value. *Journal of Neurology, Neurosurgery and Psychiatry* **51**, 605–12.

Winer, J. B., Hughes, R. A. C., Anderson, M. J., *et al.* (1988). A prospective study of acute idiopathic neuropathy. II. Antecedent events. *Journal of Neurology, Neurosurgery and Psychiatry* **51**, 613–18.

Winer, J. B., Gray, I. A., Gregson, N. A., *et al.* (1988). A prospective study of acute idiopathic neuropathy. III. Immunological studies. *Journal of Neurology, Neurosurgery and Psychiatry* **51**, 619–25.

Chronic inflammatory demyelinating polyradiculopathy

Barohn R. J., Kissel, J. T., Warmholts, J. R., and Mendell, J. R. (1989). Chronic inflammatory demyelinating polyradiculopathy. *Archives of Neurology* **46**, 878–84.

Bell's palsy

Wolf, S. M., Wagner, J. R., Davidson, S. O., and Forsythe, A. (1978). Treatment of Bell's palsy with prednisone: a prospective randomized study. *Neurology* **28**, 158–61.

Entrapment neuropathies

Dawson, D. M., Hallett, M., and Millender, L. H. (1990). *Entrapment neuropathies*. Churchill Livingstone, Edinburgh.

Editorial (1987). Electrodiagnosis of ulnar neuropathies. *Lancet* **2**, 25–6.

Gilliatt, R. W. and Harrison, M. J. G. (1984). Nerve compression and entrapment in *Peripheral nerve disorders* (ed. R. W. Gilliatt and A. K. Asbury). Butterworths, London.

Heywood, P. L. (1987). Through the carpal tunnel. *British Medical Journal* **1**, 660–1.

Nerve injuries

Sunderland, S. (1990). *Nerve injuries and their repair*. Churchill Livingstone, Edinburgh.

Causalgia and reflex sympathetic dystrophy

Hannington-Kiff, J. G. (1991). Does failed natural spinal modulation in regional sympathetic ganglia cause reflex sympathetic dystrophy? *Lancet* **338**, 1125–7.

Withrington, R. H. and Wynn Parry, C. B. (1984). Management of painful peripheral nerve disorders. *Journal of Hand Surgery* **9B**, 24–8.

Injuries of the brachial plexus

Wynn Parry, C. B. (1984). Brachial plexus injuries. *British Journal of Hospital Medicine* **32**, 130–0.

Brachial plexopathy

Tsairis, P., Dyck, P. J., and Mulder, D. W. (1972). Natural history of brachial plexus neuropathy. *Archives of Neurology* **27**, 109–17.

Mononeuritis multiplex

Hawke, S. H. B., Davies, L., Pamphlett, R., Guo, Y.-P., Pollard, J. D., McLeod, J. G. (1991). Vasculitic neuropathy. A clinical and pathological study. *Brain* **114**, 2175–90.

Autonomic neuropathy

Watkins, P. J. (1990). Diabetic autonomic neuropathy. *New England Journal of Medicine* **322**, 1078–9.

20 Two types of degenerative neuronal disease—motor neuron diseases and the spinocerebellar ataxias

---

Two groups of degenerative diseases are considered in this chapter—those in which the primary changes appear to lie in the anterior horn cell (motor neuron diseases), and those degenerative disorders in which cerebellar ataxia is the most prominent clinical feature. Many other degenerative diseases are considered elsewhere in this book (e.g. Parkinson's disease in Section 13.1 and multiple system atrophy in Section 13.2). The two disorders considered in this Chapter do not fit in comfortably elsewhere. It is to be hoped that with greater understanding of neuron biology, diseases now considered 'degenerative' will soon have specific aetiologies uncovered.

20.1 Motor neuron disease (synonym: amyotrophic lateral sclerosis)

The term 'motor neuron disease' is used in the UK to define a disease that affects both upper and lower motor neurons supplying bulbar and/or limb muscles. The characteristic motor signs (Section 20.1.4) are unaccompanied by sensory involvement. This disorder is known in the USA as amyotrophic lateral sclerosis (ALS). The word 'amyotrophic' was used in the original descriptions from the French school of neurologists to indicate a failure of trophic influences on muscles, which become prominently wasted. The words 'lateral sclerosis' refer to the gliotic changes in the lateral (pyramidal tracts) found in those with prominent upper motor neuron signs in life.

Many authors now refer to motor neuron disease*s*, applying the name not only to the specific clinical picture next described, but also as a group name for some of the less common disorders listed in Table 20.1, and further described in Section 20.2.

20.1.1 *Epidemiology*

Motor neuron disease occurs throughout the world. In Western countries, with good rates of case ascertainment, the incidence is about 2.0 cases per 100 000 per year. Men are affected about twice as often as women. The peak age of onset is in the mid-fifties, although the disease can occur in the

Table 20.1   Motor neuron diseases

1. Motor neuron diseases, with upper and lower neuron lesions
    Synonym: amyotrophic lateral sclerosis
2. Variants of motor neuron diseases, with upper and lower motor neuron lesions:
    familial form
    Guamanian form
    hereditary spastic paraplegia (upper motor neuron only)
    hexosaminidase deficiency
3. Inherited spinal muscular atrophies:
    infantile onset (Werdnig–Hoffmann)
    childhood onset
        proximal (Kugelberg–Welander)
        other distributions
    neuronal type (type II) of Charcot–Marie–Tooth disease
    hexosaminidase deficiency
4. Inherited infantile bulbar palsy (Fazio–Londe)
5. Acquired motor neuron disease:
    acute viral infection, e.g. poliomyelitis, herpes zoster
    intoxications e.g. lead, possibly Guamanian form
    metabolic, e.g. hypoglycaemia
    immunological, e.g. paraproteinaemias
    trauma
    electric shock
6. Motor neuron involvement as part of a more widespread degenerative disorder:
    e.g. as part of spinocerebellar degeneration, Creutzfeldt–Jakob disease, Shy–Drager syndrome.

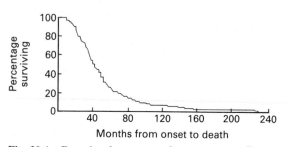

Fig. 20.1 Duration from onset of motor neuron disease (ALS) to death. (Reproduced with permission from Mulder and Howard 1976.)

twenties. The prevalence is about 5–6 per 100 000, giving an average duration of illness to death of 3–4 years (Fig. 20.1). These figures indicate that a family doctor will see a new case only about once every 25–30 years. However, motor neuron disease causes so many unusual clinical problems that every doctor should know something about it.

20.1.2 *Pathology*

Motor neurons in the brain stem and spinal cord show simple atrophy without any inflammatory response. The number of motor neurons per unit volume of tissue in the anterior horn and lower bulbar regions falls, and there is a moderate degree of astrocytic gliosis. The oculomotor nuclei and Onuf's nucleus (see p. 57) are virtually entirely spared. In those cases in which upper motor neuron signs had been prominent in life, there is loss of Betz cells and large pyramidal neurons from the fifth layer of the motor cortex. Degenerating pyramidal axons in the internal capsule and spinal cord can be demonstrated by Marchi staining. Some anterior horn cells contain eosinophilic intra-cytoplasmic inclusion bodies (Bunina bodies). Spheroidal bodies containing 10 nm neurofilaments may be found in the proximal parts of the axons. Afferent pathways in the spinal cord are generally spared, although there may be some degenerative changes in the posterior columns and in the spinocerebellar pathways in the rare familial cases (Section 20.1.3.1). Histological changes in the denervated muscle are described in Fig. 20.2.

20.1.3 *Causes of motor neuron disease*

It is not at all clear how relevant are the factors next discussed to the genesis of the specific clinical picture of motor neuron disease. The factors are of theoretical importance in indicating avenues for future research, but seem at present to be irrelevant to the vast majority of patients with motor neuron disease.

20.1.3.1 *Genetic factors*

About 90–95 per cent of patients with motor neuron disease have no family history of the disorder. Recently, intensive genetic analysis of the few families with autosomal dominantly inherited

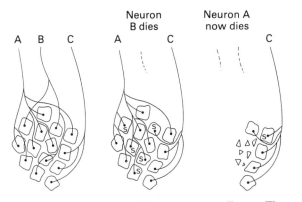

Fig. 20.2 Axon sprouting in motor neuron disease. The left hand part of the figure shows three normal neurons supplying a group of 14 muscle fibres. In the centre, neuron B has died; neuron A incorporates by sprouting (S) four of the newly denervated muscle fibres, and neuron C incorporates one. At this stage the histological appearance of the muscle fibres will be normal, but electromyography will show larger motor units than normal. As the geographical distribution of the motor unit is also larger, the duration of the motor unit potential is longer. In the right-hand part of the figure, neuron A has now died. Neuron C is now only capable of sprouting to a limited extent (S); the denervated fibres atrophy and become angulated. Grouped fibre atrophy of this type is characteristic of motor neuron disease.

adult-onset disease have shown that the gene almost certainly lies on chromosome 21q. However, linkage to four known DNA markers in this region gives evidence of considerable genetic heterogeneity. As the inherited form is very similar in its clinical nature to the sporadic form, it is likely that identification of the messenger transcript and gene product will have an enormous influence on our understanding of the basic molecular defect causing motor neuron degeneration. In sporadic cases, the presence of HLA A3 haplotype correlates with rapid progression, and of B12 with slow progression. A recessively inherited disorder similar to motor neuron disease has been identified as being associated with hexosaminidase A deficiency.

20.1.3.2 'Toxins'

Lead, manganese, selenium, and mercury have all, at various times, been allegedly found in higher concentrations in the tissues of those with motor neuron disease, but the evidence of a causal relationship is unconvincing. Other studies have shown elevated neuronal levels of calcium and aluminium. Exposure to various organic pesticides and fertilizers has also been suggested, with little sound epidemiological evidence.

Interest has focused for a number of years on the nature of the particular type of motor neuron disease found in Guam and some of the other Marianas Islands of the western Pacific. In parts of these islands the incidence of motor neuron disease has been up to 100 times the incidence in the Western world, although it has fallen as Western influences have affected the islands' cultures. The relevance of these geographical isolates of motor neuron disease has never been clear, particularly as a clinical variant includes features similar to Parkinson's disease, associated with dementia. A staple article of diet in Guam is the seeds of the false sago palm *Cycas circinalis*. Spencer and colleagues have shown that β-*N*-methylamino-L-alanine, a constituent of these seeds, produces a state like motor neuron disease when fed to primates for a few weeks.

Lathyrism is a neurological syndrome associated with excessive consumption of the seeds of *Lathyrus sativus*, characterized by some features of motor neuron disease such as spasticity and muscle atrophy. The seeds contain the excitatory amino acid β-*N*-oxalylamino-L-alanine. Excitatory amino acids open calcium channels, allowing excessive calcium entry and death of the cell. It is possible that in some forms of apparently 'spontaneous' neuronal death, as occurs in motor neuron disease, abnormalities of glutamate metabolism may mediate the neurodegenerative process. The circumstantial evidence is, first, that glutamate and its analogues are neurotoxic, possibly through excessive excitatory action, opening calcium channels. Secondly, glutamate dehydrogenase has been found to be reduced in some forms of multisystem atrophy. Finally, *N*-methyl-D-aspartate (NMDA) receptors, a subtype of the glutamate receptors, are markedly reduced in number in the affected brain regions of patients dying from other 'degenerative' disorders, such as Alzheimer's or Huntington's disease. Many interneurons are glycinergic, and one hypothesis is that free glycine in the brain stem and spinal cord increases the frequency of opening of the NMDA receptor channel, leading,

in the relative deficiency of glutamate dehydrogenase activity, to excessive neuronal activity and
ultimately neuronal death. Branched-chain amino
acids stimulate the activity of this enzyme, and
have been used in one trial.

20.1.3.3 *Immunological basis*

A number of studies suggest an immunological
basis for motor neuron disease. Serum from some
patients with neuron disease has been shown to
inhibit neonatal mouse neural cell cultures and
axonal sprouting in culture, but this work cannot
be replicated. Some studies have shown circulating
immune complexes containing Ig and C3 complement in motor neuron disease. Cases of motor
neuron disease have been reported in association
with IgG, IgM, and IgA paraproteinaemias. However, plasmapheresis and immunosuppression have
been tried, and been shown to be ineffective.
There is a suggestive association with bronchial
carcinoma, but this may be no more than coincidence. Trauma, including surgery, has been found
to figure in the histories of patients with motor
neuron disease more commonly than would be
expected by chance, again suggesting a possible
immunological basis.

20.1.3.4 *Viruses*

The selective degeneration of anterior horn cells in
both poliomyelitis and motor neuron disease, and
the reports of a motor neuron disease-like syndrome affecting some patients many years after
contracting poliomyelitis (Section 17.12.6.4), have
suggested that there is some relationship between
the disorders. However, virus-related antigen or
nucleic acid sequences have never been demonstrated in tissue from patients with motor neuron
disease, even though it is recognized that persistent
polio infection can occur in some immunodeficient
animals. Russian workers have reported transmission of motor neuron disease to primates, but
this work has not been replicated elsewhere.

There are clearly widely diverse suggestions for the
cause of motor neuron disease. A linking hypothesis is that a number of different mechanisms can
result in reduced levels of ribosomal RNA, and
decreased synthesis of essential neuronal proteins,
with subsequent degeneration. A variant of this

explanation is that motor neuron disease represents an abiotrophic exaggeration of normal
ageing, perhaps determined polygenetically. Progressive loss of neurons in cerebrum and spinal
cord does occur with age.

20.1.4 *Clinical features*

Motor neuron disease may present initially with
wasting and weakness of a hand, or a lower motor
neuron foot drop with wasting of the leg. This type
used to be called progressive muscular atrophy,
first described in 1850 by Aran. (Note that there is
a risk here of confusing an abbreviation for this
disorder (PMA) with the much more benign peroneal muscular atrophy, Section 19.3.8.) Alternatively, the weakness may affect initially the bulbar
muscles, with dysarthria and dysphagia—progressive bulbar palsy, first described by Duchenne in
1860. Charcot, in 1869, distinguished the third
variant—amyotrophic lateral sclerosis—with a
mixture of upper and lower motor neuron signs. It
was soon realized that each of these variants were
expressions of the same disease with different
degrees of emphasis. A patient who presents with
a wasted hand may go on to develop a profound
bulbar palsy.

Difficulty in coping with buttons, or with car
ignition keys, or some similar manual activity is
the most frequent presenting symptom of motor
neuron disease. By the time that such a patient
first presents to a physician there will usually
be some wasting of the interosseous or thenar
muscles, and obvious clinical weakness of the small
muscles of one or both hands. An alternative limb
presentation is with a painless foot drop, accompanied by wasting of the anterior tibial or calf
muscles.

About two-thirds of patients present with problems in a hand or foot, and most of the remainder
with dysarthria or dysphagia. A few present with
cramping pains in the limbs. Some medical students or physicians are concerned that they might
have motor neuron disease when they notice
benign fasciculations, but, although fasciculation is
prominent in motor neuron disease, fasciculation
is virtually never the only feature at presentation,
and, if there is no wasting or weakness, the worrier
can be safely reassured.

As the disease progresses, disabilities become
more and more prominent. Dysarthria may in-

itially have lower motor neuron features, such as nasal emission, hypernasality, and poor lip seal. However, even if starting in this fashion, upper motor neuron features usually become more prominent, and speech becomes slow and strained, a so-called spastic dysarthria. This is associated with other clinical evidence of upper motor neuron involvement of bulbar muscles, such as a brisk jaw jerk or pout reflex (Section 6.4.2). Many patients are unintelligible in the weeks or months preceding their death. Occasionally a severe dysarthria may exist before any other evidence of motor neuron disease.

Dysphagia also progresses during the course of the illness. A major problem associated with this is drooling of saliva. Weakness of chewing and difficulty in forming a bolus and propelling it to the back of the mouth and initiating the pharyngeal movements of swallowing all contribute. Failure of the palate to elevate may result in nasal regurgitation of fluids. Poor reflex elevation of the larynx results in failure of the seal between it and the epiglottis, and may result in partial inhalation of food and fluids, and episodes of choking.

As motor neuron disease advances in its effects upon the limbs, progressive paralysis results, and patients require more and more physical aids (see Section 26.6). The loss of muscle mass results in a marked fall in weight. The preservation of sensation and of sphincter control means that pressure sores are rare. Intellect, personality, and memory are entirely preserved, so that the patient is fully aware of his distressing symptoms.

The findings on clinical examination in the fully developed case are characteristic, with widespread wasting, fasciculation, and weakness, a spastic dysarthria, and exaggerated reflexes elicited from the tendons of wasted muscles. In spite of these pyramidal signs, the plantar responses are often flexor until the disease is far advanced. Examination of the tongue in cases of bulbar palsy may show fasciculation and wasting. Sensory signs are absent, with the exception of vibration sense which may be impaired, suggesting to some authorities that this sense travels rostrally in the lateral rather than the posterior columns, as usually accepted.

20.1.5 Diagnosis and investigation

The diagnosis rests almost entirely upon clinical grounds. It is discouraging to diagnose at a glance an illness that will almost certainly prove mortal, so it is common practice to perform a number of investigations, even though the chances of finding an alternative diagnosis are remote. In the earlier stages, however, there are important differential diagnoses to be considered.

Wasting and weakness of the muscles of one hand may be caused by ulnar or median mononeuropathies (see Sections 19.4.2.4 and 5 and Table 19.6). In these cases, the wasting lies solely in the distribution of one or other affected nerve; in an ulnar neuropathy, for example, the thenar muscles are spared. In motor neuron disease, interosseous and thenar muscles are almost always affected together, but simultaneous wasting of both groups occurs in the presence of a cervical rib, or of a syrinx or medullary glioma involving the first thoracic segment. However, in these cases, impairment of perception of painful and thermal stimuli is usually obvious.

Multiple cervical radicular lesions due to spondylosis, in association with a spondylotic myelopathy, can cause lower motor neuron signs in the arms and upper motor neuron signs in the legs, but in such circumstances sensory symptoms and signs are common. However, it may be necessary to proceed to imaging studies to exclude this possibility. Imaging will also exclude the rare case of a tumour, such as a meningioma, at the foramen magnum, which may produce wasting of the hands by its effects upon medullary venous drainage.

Purely bulbar motor neuron disease of lower motor neuron type may be mistaken for myasthenia gravis, so an edrophonium test (Section 21.12.2.4) may be required.

Electrodiagnostic studies will help distinguish cases of motor neuron disease from chronic neuropathies affecting predominantly motor function. The hallmark of the physiological findings in motor neuron disease is evidence of chronic partial denervation (Section 8.7), widespread fasciculation potentials, normal sensory nerve action potentials, and motor maximal nerve conduction velocity that is within normal limits, or slightly reduced due to a selective loss of motor nerve fibres of the largest diameter. Peripheral neuropathies, even if clinically largely motor, are usually accompanied by some reduction in amplitude of sensory nerve action potentials, and, as many of the chronic motor polyneuropathies are demyelinating (Section 19.2), maximal motor nerve conduction velocities in these cases is greatly reduced.

A single fasciculation potential in motor neuron disease cannot be distinguished on the oscilloscope from the benign fasciculation potentials that are often found in the gastrocnemius and deltoid muscles. Benign fasciculations are motor unit discharges at rates of about one a second. Fasciculations in association with chronic partial denervation are more widespread and occur at lower frequencies, perhaps once every 3–4 seconds, and often at intervals beyond this.

Examination of the spinal fluid is seldom informative, but the protein concentration may be elevated, though seldom above 1.0 g/l. In days when neurosyphilis was common, a variant known as syphilitic pachymeningitis (Section 17.4.1.1) could cause a motor neuron disease-like picture, so the VDRL test should be performed.

Blood tests are of little value, although an elevated serum phosphocreatine kinase may indicate rapidly advancing muscle necrosis. Muscle biopsy is seldom indicated but, if performed, the characteristic finding is of group fibre atrophy. The appearance, and the proposed mechanism, are illustrated in Fig. 20.2.

20.1.6 Prognosis

The median time from diagnosis to death is about 4 years, but survival may occasionally be much longer. Patients with prominent bulbar symptoms do worst, and those with muscle atrophy best. Those with prominent pyramidal signs have an intermediate prognosis.

20.1.7 Treatment

No pharmacological intervention has been shown to alter the natural history of the disease, but a number of studies have shown a very brief effect upon muscle strength of thyrotrophin releasing hormone (TRH). TRH is an excitatory transmitter of the anterior horn cell, and may also have as yet unexplained trophic effects. Pyridostigmine may transiently improve muscle strength, presumably by improving transmission at unstable sprouting or degenerating neuromuscular junctions. Other agents that have been tried over the years include antiviral agents such as amantadine, immunosuppression, chelating agents, steroids, and various

vitamins, reflecting beliefs about the illness that were current at the time. None has ever been shown to be of benefit. A multicentre study of branched-chain amino acids is currently under way.

The absence of any worthwhile pharmacological treatment is sometimes taken to mean that the neurologist has nothing to offer. It is indeed difficult to face impotently a patient who is steadily deteriorating, but patients undoubtedly value the continuing contact and support that a good general practitioner and neurologist can give.

20.1.7.1 Weakness

A weak muscle cannot be made stronger, but simple devices may considerably lessen the patient's reliance on others. Examples include a toe-raising spring for those with foot drop, a head support to prevent the head toppling forwards if the posterior neck muscles are weak, and mobile forearm supports which can be attached to a chair or wheelchair. All too often, a slow response from social services and an orthotist may prevent the supply of an aid at a stage when it can still be useful, before further deterioration has occurred.

20.1.7.2 Muscle cramps and spasticity

Cramp is often a difficult symptom to treat, but quinine or a hypnotic such as flurazepam taken on going to bed may allow better rest. Baclofen, diazepam, or dantrolene may relieve spasticity, as described in Section 18.1.4.4 but these also cause drowsiness.

20.1.7.3 Drooling of saliva

It may be possible to reduce this by altering the posture of the head with a head support. Anticholinergic agents, such as atropine 0.6 mg two or three times a day, may be useful. If dribbling continues, a discreet bag into which soaked tissues can be disposed of is useful. Bibs are demoralizing for all concerned, but a 'false' polo-neck sweater, in which the isolated front fastens round the neck with Velcro, serves the same purpose.

20.1.7.4   *Swallowing and nutrition*

Changes in the consistency of supplied food may improve swallowing for some months, the easiest to swallow being semisolid foods that can be prepared in a food blender. Attention to head position is again important. Drinking straws with valves are available which reduce the number of repeated efforts at suction of fluids.

It is not infrequent to see patients with motor neuron disease whose bulbar palsy is so severe that choking attacks and inhalation, or dehydration and starvation are threatening survival at a time when the disease is not far advanced in other areas. Many patients can therefore have their life prolonged for months, or longer, by feeding through a percutaneous endoscopic gastrostomy. Alternatively, but less satisfactorily, a nasogastric tube can be passed, or the larynx bypassed with a tracheostomy with glottal closure, although this last procedure obviously indicates that a complete loss of voice must be accepted.

20.1.7.5   *Communication*

Speech therapy probably has little influence upon the course of dysarthria, but a good therapist may prolong intelligibility by teaching strategies such as using short sentences, exaggerating expression and intonation, and adding gesture. Such patients can continue to write messages when severely dysarthric. For those more severely disabled, various electronic communication aids are now available, and are improving monthly. An example is a personal computer with a large store of messages that can be displayed by the action of a single key.

20.1.8   *The final stages*

Some hospices have extended their work with patients with terminal malignant disease to motor neuron disease, and have built up an impressive experience. Many patients, however, will die at home, cared for by their relatives, who should receive appropriate support (see Chapter 26). The judicious use of morphine in the terminal stages diminishes distress, and at this stage any possible depressant effect upon respiration is irrelevant. Most patients die as a result of a bronchopneumonia.

20.2   Other motor neuron diseases

20.2.1   *Familial form of motor neuron disease*

In any large series of patients with motor neuron disease, about 5 per cent of cases have a family history of the disease. Analysis of these shows that inheritance is through an autosomal dominant gene. The median age of onset is about 10 years younger than the sporadic cases, the modal age of onset being in the mid-forties. The duration of the illness to death is even shorter than in the sporadic form. A few families have been reported with juvenile onset. In such cases, inheritance is through an autosomal recessive gene.

20.2.2   *Inherited spinal muscular atrophy*

Corticospinal tract degeneration and pyramidal signs are not present in these conditions, which affect only anterior horn cells. Although classically referred to by the following eponymous names, both acute and chronic forms of infantile spinal muscular atrophy are associated with a mutant gene on chromosome 5q13 in most instances, but there are occasional atypical families in which this is not the case. That is to say, there is some genetic heterogeneity. Within families linked to 5q, there is also some phenotypic heterogeneity, variations in phenotypic expression, reflecting probably a number of different allelic mutations at the gene locus.

20.2.2.1   *Acute infantile onset (synonyms: type I spinal muscular atrophy, Werdnig–Hoffmann disease)*

Infants with this recessively inherited condition are born 'floppy' due to gross denervation, or develop progressive paralysis by the age of 5 months. They do not survive beyond the age of 3 years. The incidence is about 1 in 20 000–30 000 births.

20.2.2.2   *Chronic infantile spinal muscular atrophy (synonym: type II spinal muscular atrophy)*

Infants with this variant have a slightly later age of onset, and a much longer survival than those described above.

20.2.2.3 Juvenile onset spinal muscular atrophy (synonyms: type III spinal muscular atrophy Kugelberg–Welander disease)

This syndrome is characterized by proximal muscular weakness and atrophy, particularly pronounced in the legs. It is sometimes associated with pseudohypertrophy of the calves. Not surprisingly, this disorder is often initially mistaken for a muscular dystrophy (see Section 21.6). The genetic origin of this phenotype is more mixed, some cases being clearly inherited by an autosomal recessive gene (on chromosome 5q13 in some families), and some by a dominant gene.

Variations of spinal muscular atrophy of juvenile onset include topographic variations with scapuloperoneal involvement, and distal forms which are usually grouped as type 2 Charcot–Marie–Tooth disease (see Section 19.3.8).

20.2.2.4 Hexosaminidase deficiencies

This multi-subunit liposomal enzyme acts on GM2 ganglioside, and some oligosaccharides, globosides, and glycoproteins. Deficiency of the enzyme has been recognized in a number of rare neurological conditions, many of which are characterized by anterior horn cell destruction and muscular wasting. Patients with disorders clinically identical to motor neuron disease (ALS) and to juvenile onset chronic spinal muscular atrophy have been described.

20.2.3 Inherited infantile bulbar palsy (synonym: Fazio–Londe disease)

Although the tongue may be seen to fasciculate in some cases of infantile-onset spinal muscular atrophy (Section 20.2.1.1), in this variant the denervation affects predominantly bulbar muscles with prominent dysphagia and inspiratory stridor. Spinal anterior horn cells may be affected later. The disorder is inherited through an autosomal recessive gene.

20.2.4 Acquired motor neuron diseases

20.2.4.1 Acute viral diseases

Poliomyelitis is the most frequent acute disorder

of anterior horn cells and bulbar motor neurons. It is considered in Section 17.12.6. Spinal and bulbar motor neurons may also be affected by herpes zoster (Section 17.12.7.4) and by infection with enterovirus 70, which causes an acute haemorrhagic conjunctivitis in addition to paralysis.

A disorder superficially resembling acute infective polyneuropathy (Section 19.3) but with electrophysiological evidence of terminal motor neuron or anterior horn cell dysfunction has recently been reported from north China. The cause of the syndrome, quite common in rural areas, is so far unclear.

20.2.4.2 Toxins

The recent interest in the possibility that consumption of a toxic plant might be responsible for Guamanian motor neuron disease has already been discussed in Section 20.1.3.2.

Lead poisoning in children usually causes an encephalopathy or peripheral neuropathy. Adults may develop a wrist drop. Neurophysiological studies suggest that the lesion probably lies in the anterior horn cells, but there has never been an adequate pathological description.

20.2.4.3 Metabolic causes

A syndrome similar to spinal muscular atrophy has been described following repeated severe hypoglycaemic episodes, and in association with disorders of calcium and phosphate metabolism.

20.2.4.4 Immunological causes

Cases of motor neuron disease have been reported in association with IgG, IgM, and IgA paraproteinaemias.

The incidence of cancer does not appear to be greater in patients presenting with motor neuron disease. Occasional cases have been described in which an acute inflammatory necrosis of anterior horn cells is associated with a cancer. This may represent the effects of an opportunistic viral infection; the histology is quite different from classical motor neuron disease.

20.2.4.5 Trauma

Patients with motor neuron disease give a history

of previous trauma more often than do age-matched controls.

20.2.4.6 *Electric shock*

A number of patients have been reported who developed a disorder indistinguishable from motor neuron disease after a severe electric shock. A significant current passes through the spinal cord whether the contacts are hand to hand or hand through foot to ground.

20.2.5 *Motor neuron involvement as part of a more widespread degenerative disorder*

Amyotrophy (muscle wasting) may be prominent as part of a spinocerebellar degeneration (Section 20.3.2), Creutzfeldt–Jakob disease (Section 17.15.1), Shy–Drager syndrome (Section 13.2.1), and other degenerative disorders.

20.2.5.1 *Familial spastic paraplegia (Strümpell's paraplegia)*

This is a relatively benign disease, inherited by an autosomal dominant gene, in which there is a slowly progressive spastic weakness of the legs. Pathological examination shows degeneration most evident in the caudal end of the corticospinal tracts. Anterior horn cells are not affected in this disorder.

20.3 The hereditary ataxias and related disorders

Nowhere in neurology have there been so many eponymous syndromes and so much confusion. Fortunately, the taxonomy of these inherited disorders is easing as new studies in genetics allow understanding of the potential variability of large genes. A comparison may be made with sex-linked muscular dystrophy, the clinical features of which vary between the mild Becker type and the more common, severe, Duchenne type in relation to the amount of dystrophin produced. This in turn is related to the extent of the deletion or base changes in the p21 region of the X chromosome (Section 21.6.1.2). In the case of cerebellar ataxias,

within large kinships there may be such variation in the expression of the abnormal gene that a clinician could reasonably classify the clinical manifestations as a number of different disorders. None the less, there are a number of defined syndromes which are still worthy of eponymous titles. The nomenclature is, however, likely to change within the next few years to classification by the abnormal gene or gene product.

20.3.1 *Recessively inherited ataxias*

20.3.1.1 *Friedreich's ataxia*

This is the best-known of the hereditary ataxias, and the first to be described, by Friedreich in 1863. The disorder is of autosomal recessive inheritance, with age of onset around puberty, and virtually always before the age of 20 years. The prevalence of the disorder is about 1:50 000.

Clinical features

Although motor development is not delayed, unsteadiness of gait begins in later childhood, and is soon accompanied by dysarthria. Impaired sense of passive movement and vibration sense in the lower limbs follow, as do lower limb areflexia and muscle weakness. These signs are invariable in the fully developed case. The majority have extensor plantar responses, pes cavus, and, less commonly, nystagmus, optic atrophy, and sensorineural deafness.

Other organ systems are involved. Most of the patients develop a kyphoscoliosis as they grow, and this may be sufficiently marked to interfere with respiratory function. Electrocardiographic abnormalities are frequent, occurring in between 30 and 90 per cent of patients in different series. The most common abnormality is the presence of inversion of T waves in left ventricular leads. There is also electrocardiographic evidence of left ventricular hypertrophy. Paroxysmal atrial tachycardia or established atrial fibrillation are common. Diabetes occurs in about 20 per cent of patients, possibly due to islet cell atrophy, possibly due to increased peripheral insulin resistance.

Genetic and biochemical aspects

The disorder is inherited as an autosomal recessive. The gene lies in the centromeric region of chromosome 9. Cases with cardiomyopathy and diabetes tend to cluster within the same sibships. The abnormal gene product may give rise to disorders of lipoprotein metabolism, but the exact metabolic deficit remains uncertain.

Pathology

There is degeneration of the dorsal root ganglion cells and 'dying back' of their peripheral axons, leading to loss of large myelinated fibres in peripheral nerves. The central processes in the posterior columns also die back, and similar morphological changes of degeneration are seen in the lateral columns and spinocerebellar pathways. In the cerebellum there is a patchy loss of Purkinje cells, gliosis of the dentate nucleus, and degeneration of the superior cerebellar peduncle. The morphological changes in the heart are those of a chronic interstitial fibrosis.

Investigations

The diagnosis is essentially a clinical one. Nerve conduction studies show slight slowing of motor nerve conduction and reduced or absent sensory nerve action potentials. Examination of the cerebrospinal fluid is not helpful, although the protein is sometimes a little elevated. Imaging studies shows cerebral atrophy in about one-fifth of cases and cerebellar atrophy in fewer still.

Prognosis and management

The average age at death is about 35–40, about 30 years after clinical onset. Many die in cardiac failure. Scoliosis may be, at least in part, corrected by a brace, and some benefit from more radical orthopaedic corrective procedures. However, any long period of bed rest often results in increased ataxia, and this has to be weighed against any possible benefits from surgical therapy. The diabetes often responds to oral hypoglycaemic agents. Otherwise, the management is that of education and support, as outlined in Chapter 26, as no biochemical treatment has been shown to influence the progress of the disease.

20.3.1.2   *Other types of recessively inherited ataxia*

Although Friedreich's ataxia is the commonest of the early onset autosomal recessive hereditary ataxias, another type is characterized by retained or exaggerated tendon reflexes. The disease advances more slowly, and cardiomyopathy and diabetes are not features. Hypogonadism is found in some patients.

20.3.2   *Dominantly inherited ataxias*

Dominantly inherited cerebellar ataxias include a series of clinical phenotypes characterized by ataxia, dysarthia, and intention tremor, resulting from the involvement of the cerebellum and its afferent and efferent pathways. Frequently, however, other pathological changes are found in the anterior horn cells and white matter of the spinal cord, basal ganglia, and peripheral nerves. The clinical classification, therefore, is extraordinarily difficult, and, as noted above, within a single family there may be considerable variations in phenotypic expression. Those syndromes, separated in the older literature under such names as olivopontocerebellar atrophy and Joseph's disease, include cases associated with ophthalmoplegia, optic atrophy, extrapyramidal features, and sometimes deafness and dementia. Phenotypic variation could either be due to variation in the extent of allelic mutation or gene deletion, as in Duchenne dystrophy, or modification of expression of the gene by other host genes. Until there is better molecular correlation, current classifications of dominantly inherited ataxias are based upon phenotypic expression, and are no more than descriptions of constellations of clinical syndromes. Variations in phenotypic expression of probably closely similar or identical mutations are also seen in the inherited neuropathies (Section 19.3.8) and in the infantile muscular atrophies (Section 20.2.3). Alternatively, closely similar phenotypes may be due to widely different genetic mutations.

Many of these cerebellar syndromes are characterized by marked loss of neurons in the olive, and often marked atrophy of the dentate nucleus in the cerebellum. Studies have linked some families with olivopontocerebellar-type atrophy to the human leucocyte antigen (HLA) locus on the short arm of chromosome 6. However, other families, with very similar clinical disorders, have undergone analysis without finding any linkage to the HLA antigen system.

As discussed in Section 23.1.3, recessively inherited disorders are commonly associated with the accumulation of a metabolite related to a metabolic pathway which is already understood, or the deficiency of a known primary protein. In dominantly inherited disorders such as the inherited cerebellar degenerations, neither type of marker is, as yet, available. Earlier work suggested a deficiency in glutamate dehydrogenase activity in fibroblasts and leucocytes in some patients with olivopontocerebellar atrophy. There was considerable enthusiasm for the concept that a deficiency of this enzyme would allow accumulation of glutamate, a cerebellar granule cell neurotransmitter, which could produce excitotoxic degeneration of cerebellar neurons. However, further studies failed to show similar changes in the brain. Enzyme reductions in non-nervous tissue may not parallel levels in the brain, and may be something of a genetic epiphenomenon.

20.3.3   Other types of cerebellar ataxias

In contrast to the causes of uncertain nature discussed above, some patients with ataxia as one feature of their illness have a clearly recognized metabolic defect, such as hypothyroidism, abetaliproteinaemia, adrenoleucomyeloneuropathy (Section 23.1.3.3), and hexosaminidase A deficiency.

Other inherited ataxias may occur in association with mitochondrial myopathy (Section 21.8.2). Some of these are associated with myoclonus (the Ramsay Hunt syndrome) and some with myoclonus and seizures (Baltic myoclonus).

20.3.4   Treatment of cerebellar ataxias

Thyroxin benefits ataxia associated with hypothyroidism and vitamin E supplements significantly slow the course of ataxia associated with abetaliproteinaemia, but, apart from this instance, no metabolic treatment has been shown to be of value. Patients require advice and support along the lines suggested in Chapter 26. Wise genetic counselling is particularly difficult in these disorders.

20.4   Further reading

General

Rowland, L. P. (ed.) (1991). *Amyotrophic lateral scler-*

osis and other motor neuron diseases. Raven Press, New York.
Smith, R. A. (ed.). (1992). *Handbook of amyotrophic lateral sclerosis.* Marcel Dekker, New York.

Motor neuron disease

Epidemiology

Buckley, J. P., Warlow, C., Smith, P., *et al.* (1983). Motor neurone disease in England and Wales 1959–1979. *Journal of Neurology, Neurosurgery and Psychiatry* **46**, 197–205.

Genetics of chronic spinal muscular atrophies,

Munsat, T. L., Skerry, L., Korf, B., *et al.* (1990). Phenotypic heterogeneity of spinal muscular atrophy mapping to chromosome 5q 11.2–13.3 (SMA 5q). *Neurology* **40**, 1831–6.

Causation

Editorial (1987) A poison tree. *Lancet* **2**, 947–8.
Kennedy, P. G. E. (1990). On the possible role of viruses in the aetiology of motor neurone disease: a review. *Journal of the Royal Society of Medicine* **83**, 784–7.
Martyn, C. N., Barker, D. J. P., and Osmond, C. (1988). Motoneuron disease post poliomyelitis in England and Wales. *Lancet* **1**, 1319–21.
Mitsumoto, H., Hanson, M. R., and Chad, D. A. (1988). Amyotrophic lateral sclerosis: recent advances in pathogenesis and clinical trials. *Archives of Neurology* **45**, 189–203.
Plaitakis, A. (1990). Glutamate dysfunction and selective motor neurone degeneration in amyotrophic lateral sclerosis: a hypothesis *Annals of Neurology* **28**, 3–8.
Siddique, T., Figlewicz, D. A., Pericak-Vance, M. A., *et al.* (1991). Linkage of a gene causing familial amyotrophic lateral sclerosis to chromosome 21 and evidence of genetic-locus heterogeneity. *New England Journal of Medicine* **324**, 1381–4.
Tandan, R. and Bradley, W. G. (1985). Amyotrophic lateral sclerosis: part 2—Etiopathogenesis. *Annals of Neurology* **18**, 419–31.

Care

Carey, J. S. (1986). Motor neurone disease–a challenge to medical ethics. *Journal of the Royal Society of Medicine* **79**, 216–20.

Cochrane, G. M. (ed.) (1987). *The management of motor neuron disease*. Churchill Livingstone, Edinburgh.

Norris, F. H., Smith, R. A., and Denys, E. H. (1985). Motor neuron disease: towards better care. *British Medical Journal* **291**, 259–62.

O'Brien, T., Kelly, M., and Saunders, C. (1992). Motor neurone disease, a hospice perspective. *British Medical Journal* **304**, 471–3.

Pollard, D. (1984). Personal view. *British Medical Journal* **288**, 481.

Report of a Working Group (1990). Standards of care for patients with neurological disease: a consensus. *Journal of the Royal College of Physicians of London* **24**, 91–7.

Prognosis

Mulder, D. W. and Howard, F. M. (1976). Patient resistance and prognosis in amyotrophic lateral sclerosis. *Mayo Clinic Proceedings* **51**, 537–41.

Hereditary ataxias

Harding, A. E. (1984). *The hereditary ataxias and related disorders*. Churchill Livingstone, Edinburgh.

Rosenberg, R. N. (1990). Autosomal dominant cerebellar phenotypes: the genotype will settle the issue. *Neurology* **40**, 1329–31.

21 Diseases of muscles and of the neuromuscular junction

The activity of muscles is one of the most obvious means whereby activity of the nervous system is expressed to the external world. Patients with many disorders of muscle function therefore have traditionally come under the clinical care of neurologists, although rheumatologists and orthopaedic surgeons are often also involved. More recently, geneticists and biochemists have made considerable strides in our understanding of some muscle diseases, and immunologists in disorders of the neuromuscular junction.

21.1 Definitions

Myopathy is an all-embracing word indicating some primary structural or biochemical abnormality of muscle fibres. The term excludes, however, changes that are obviously secondary to pathological changes in other systems, for example following a fracture or secondary to denervation, as in the chronic spinal muscular atrophies (Sections 20.1 and 20.2). An inflammatory myopathy is referred to as a myositis, although, as many muscles are usually affected, the term polymyositis is more often seen. Muscular dystrophy refers to a group of myopathies that are genetically determined, characterized by progressive degenerative changes in muscle fibres. However, some sporadic cases without any obvious family history but with related clinical and pathological features are often also termed dystrophic. Substantial inroads of understanding into this poorly defined group have been made in recent years, and the biochemical lesion in some instances defined. Such examples are then known as metabolic myopathies. Drug-induced, toxic, and endocrine myopathies also occur. Myotonia refers to a continuing contraction of muscle fibres after termination of the initiating stimulus—a voluntary act, or an electrical or mechanical stimulus. Cramps are strong contractions of muscle, often occurring after use, which cannot be inhibited by the will. The electrophysiological distinction between different types of involuntary contractions is referred to in Section 8.7. Contracture refers to irreversible shortening of muscles and tendons that follow on disuse. They may complicate traumatic paraplegia, for example (Sections 18.1.4.4), but contractures also occur secondary to the degenerative changes in muscular dystrophy.

21.2 General clinical features of muscle diseases

A cardinal feature of a myopathy is muscle weakness. Other phenomena, such as wasting, hypertrophy, pseudo-hypertrophy, or myotonia, may also occur. These changes are virtually invariably symmetrical. Some myopathies affect the cranial musculature, for example wasting of the sternomastoids is prominent in myotonic dystrophy. In other dystrophies, the brachioradialis muscles are affected at an early stage. However, it is usually the proximal limb girdle muscles that are most prominently affected. It has been suggested that the cause for the predominant affection of proximal muscles is, at least in part, mechanical. The disadvantageous lever ratios against which the proximal muscles work mean that small forces applied at the end of the limbs result in large forces tending to stretch and damage proximal muscle fibres. This is probably not the sole explanation, however. The different patterns of muscle involvement probably reflect different biochemical systems in muscles specialized in different ways.

Proximal weakness is often first manifest in adults by difficulty in getting out of a low chair or in climbing stairs—movements that employ glutei and quadriceps. Weakness of the shoulder muscles is often first noted when brushing or washing the hair, or putting an object up on to a high kitchen shelf.

Most myopathies are painless, but pain may be present in the inflammatory myopathies (Section 21.3) or in some of the metabolic myopathies (Section 21.8). The tendon reflexes are often depressed at an early stage. There are, of course, no sensory signs, and this, and the proximal distribution, distinguishes a myopathy from a neuropathy. Occasionally both nerves and muscles are affected by toxins or drugs, resulting in a 'neuromyopathy' (Section 21.10.7).

21.3 Inflammatory myopathies

This type of acquired myopathy is characterized by inflammatory infiltrates in skeletal muscle, usually in association with destruction of muscle fibres. A summary of these myopathies is given in Table 21.1.

Table 21.1 Inflammatory myopathies

Inflammatory myopathies due to identified infective
agent
  Bacterial myositis
    tropical myositis, usually staphylococcal
    clostridial myositis
  Parasitic myositis
    trichinosis
    cysticercosis
    toxoplasmosis
    echinococcosis
    trypanosomiasis
  Viral myositis
Idiopathic inflammatory myopathies
  Isolated polymyositis
  Polymyositis with skin involvement =
  dermatomyositis
    juvenile or adult onset
      associated with malignancy
      associated with connective tissue disorders
      induced by drugs
  Inclusion-body polymyositis
  Polymyalgia rheumatica
Inflammatory myopathies due to drugs
  Hydralazine, procainamide, sulphacetamide,
  zidovudine

21.3.1 *Bacterial myositis*

Bacterial myositis is rare outside tropical countries, but in Uganda and Papua New Guinea the incidence can reach 1 per 1000 per year. For these reasons the disease is sometimes called tropical myositis. However, Europids in these countries are seldom, if ever, affected. Large muscles of the buttock, thigh, and shoulder are affected by acute abscesses, which usually contain *Staphylococcus aureus*. Sometimes signs of acute inflammation may be absent, and the muscle may be infiltrated with diffuse inflammatory tissue, so that it feels hard and woody. There is some evidence that staphylococcal infection is secondary to another focal type of myositis, possibly viral in origin. The treatment involves surgical drainage, accompanied by penicillin or other appropriate antibiotic therapy in high dosage.

One specific form of bacterial myositis is that due to *Clostridium welchii*, the gas gangrene organ-

ism. Extensive local necrosis may occur in the neighbourhood of contaminated wounds.

21.3.2 *Parasitic myositis*

Muscle pain, tenderness, and mild weakness may be caused by infection with *Trichinella spiralis*. Trichinosis is usually acquired by eating inadequately cooked pork or horse meat. Oral steroids may be used if muscle pain is severe. Thiobendazole, 25–50 mg/kg day for 5 days, may be used to reduce the population of larvae encysted in muscle.

Parasitic infections of muscles also commonly result from cysticercosis, echinococcosis, and toxoplasmosis. Treatment of these infections is reviewed in Section 17.10.

21.3.3 *Viral myositis*

The entity 'Bornholm disease' refers to severe muscle pain in the upper part of the trunk occurring in association with coxsackie B infection. Diffuse muscle aches and pains are common in influenzal infections. Occasionally an acute myositis can follow about 1 week after the initial symptoms of influenza. The status of continuing muscular aching and weakness after a viral infection (chronic fatigue syndrome) remains uncertain (Section 25.2.4).

21.3.4 *Idiopathic polymyositis and dermatomyositis*

21.3.4.1 *Epidemiology*

Polymyositis and dermatomyositis are unusual disorders. The annual incidence is about 1 in 100 000, with a prevalence of about 5 per 100 000. The peak incidence in adults is between the ages of 45 and 65, and in children between 5 and 14. At all ages males are affected twice as frequently as females.

21.3.4.2 *Clinical features*

Occasionally the onset of the disorder is acute, with fever, muscle pain, and oedema and tenderness of the limbs. The process of muscle destruction may be so acute that myoglobinuria results, and the serum level of phosphocreatine kinase may be strikingly raised. Muscle weakness may be so profound that artificial ventilation is required.

More frequently, the symptoms of polymyositis develop over several weeks or months. Patients notice increasing proximal weakness, often with little or no pain. The weakness may be greater than the degree of atrophy would suggest. The muscles of the neck are commonly involved, but rarely those of the face. The tendon reflexes may be preserved, even in muscles that are very weak. There are no sensory signs.

Cutaneous changes accompany the myositis in about one-third of patients. The most typical rash is a dusky discolouration of the skin in a 'butterfly' distribution over the face, with lilac discolouration and some oedema of the eyelids. A pinker, scaling eruption may also be seen on the front and back of the chest, and the backs of the hands, where the skin becomes swollen and tight. Subcutaneous calcification may occur in chronic cases, particularly in children. There are dilated capillary loops at the base of the nails, which may be ridged and cracked.

Other tissues may also be involved in the inflammatory process. There may be dysphagia, Raynaud's phenomenon, and a non-erosive arthritis, even in patients who do not have an associated connective tissue disorder. Myocarditis and interstitial pulmonary fibrosis rarely occur.

21.3.4.3 Aetiology

About 20 per cent of those aged over 50 with dermatomyositis will have an occult or overt malignancy. The most frequent associations are with carcinoma of the bronchus and gastrointestinal tract in men, and of the breast, ovary, and gastrointestinal tract in women. Another 20 per cent of patients with polymyositis and dermatomyositis have an associated connective tissue disorder, such as systemic lupus erythematosus, mixed connective tissue disease with antibodies to ribonucleoprotein, and, less often, systemic sclerosis, rheumatoid arthritis, or Sjögren's syndrome. Polymyositis may also be associated with monoclonal gammopathies. Patients with polyarteritis nodosa may have focal ischaemic muscular lesions secondary to vasculitis, but do not show the overall clinical picture of patients with polymyositis.

An inflammatory myopathy may occur during treatment of rheumatoid arthritis with D-penicillamine. Hydralazine, procainamide, and sulph-acetamide have also been reported to cause a myopathy.

The primary cause of idiopathic polymyositis or dermatomyositis is not known, but there is good evidence that immunological factors are involved. Analysis of the types of lymphocytes at different tissue sites on muscle biopsy implies sensitization of cytotoxic T-cells to an antigen associated with muscle fibres. Studies of T-cell subsets have shown in dermatomyositis a higher ratio of CD4+ (helper) cells to CD8+ (suppressor-cytotoxic) cells in the inflammatory infiltrates, with OKT8+ cells invading muscle fibres; there are also smaller numbers of killer and antibody-secreting B-cells. Genetic factors are also important in polymyositis, as some studies have shown an increase in HLA types DR3 and DRw5s.

There is considerable evidence that an immune-complex-mediated vasculopathy is an important mechanism of muscle injury. Using immunohisto-chemical techniques, it is possible to demonstrate neoantigens of the terminal C5b-9 complement membrane attack complex in the intramuscular microvasculature in the childhood form of polymyositis, and dermatomyositis. In polymyositis and inclusion body myositis, there is evidence not of a vasculopathy as just described but of an antigen-directed cytotoxicity mediated by cytotoxic T-cells and directed against muscle fibres.

In the vast majority of patients, no obvious trigger to these abnormal immunological mechanisms can be identified. Various viruses have, from time to time, been incriminated on two grounds: first, that virus-like particles can be seen in the muscle fibres of some patients on electron microscopy, though very rarely can virus be recovered from biopsy specimens; secondly, that raised antibody titres have been found against a variety of viral or rickettsial agents. A significant proportion of patients also have evidence of previous infection with *Toxoplasma*. The very variety of these findings suggests that infective agents may be involved only in initiating a self-perpetuating auto-immune process, either by interfering with regulatory mechanisms, or because immune responses directed against the agent cross-react with some muscle antigen. One hypothesis is related to the occurrence of antibodies to the enzyme histidyl-transfer RNA synthetase, known as anti-Jo-1. Antibodies to Jo-1 are found only in patients with myositis. The enzyme is capable of interacting with the genomic RNA of some picornaviruses, the structure of which presumably resembles that of transfer RNA. Autoantibodies directed against this enzyme may arise as a result of the enzyme–virus interaction.

Infection with the human immunodeficiency virus (HIV) may result in a polymyositis, probably by triggering at T-cell-mediated cytotoxic process rather than by direct infection. The situation is complicated by the fact that zidovudine, a treatment for HIV, may also produce a myopathy.

21.3.4.4 *Investigation*

The clinical diagnosis of poly- or dermatomyositis is supported by elevated serum levels of phosphocreatine kinase, electromyography, and muscle biopsy. There are two traps for the unwary, which may lead falsely to a diagnosis of polymyositis. First, the tissue damage caused by the insertion of a concentric needle electrode for electromyography may cause a transient elevation of phosphocreatine kinase levels. Secondly, biopsy, by ill-chance, of a site of needle insertion will result in histological findings of necrotic muscle fibres surrounded by inflammatory cells. It is important, therefore, that electromyographer and surgeon liaise about the sites of their respective investigations. Polymyositis is characterized electromyographically by short-duration myopathic potentials on volition, and by spontaneous positive sharp waves and fibrillation potentials (Section 8.7). This spontaneous activity is presumably due to inflammatory damage to end-plate regions and subterminal nerve endings. Some patients also show repetitive high-frequency pseudomyotonic discharges on movement of the needle.

21.3.4.5 *Pathology*

Muscle biopsy shows necrosis of muscle fibres, and interstitial and perivascular infiltrates of lymphocytes and macrophages. In dermatomyositis the inflammatory infiltrates are predominantly perivascular and around, rather than within the fascicles. In polymyositis and inclusion body myositis (Section 21.3.5) the infiltrates are mostly in the fascicles surrounding individual muscle fibres. Patients with juvenile dermatomyositis may show a vasculitis characterized by swelling of capillary endothelial cells with resulting capillary infiltration and

microinfarcts. Electron-microscopic observations suggest that the vascular endothelium is an early site of immunologically mediated damage. These changes are particularly marked at the periphery of fascicles, where there may be atrophy of muscle fibres. Other patterns seen include muscle necrosis without much in the way of an inflammatory response. This is particularly common in poly- or dermatomyositis associated with malignant disease (Section 21.3.4.3).

In all types of myositis, regenerating fibres may be seen, characterized by central rows of nuclei in basophilic fibres.

21.3.4.6 *Treatment and prognosis*

The mainstay of treatment is corticosteroid therapy, usually with a dose of 60–80 mg of prednisone daily for about 6 weeks, with gradual reduction as muscle strength improves and serum levels of phosphocreatine kinase fall. One problem is that of the patient who develops a steroid myopathy (Section 21.10.5) as a complication of therapy. The distinction between this and a recrudescence of the myopathy may require further biopsy or juggling with the daily dosage of steroids. A high serum level of phosphocreatine kinase implies an active myositis rather than a steroid myopathy. Some steroid-resistant cases may benefit from immunosuppression. Benefit has been claimed for treatment with azathioprine, methotrexate, and cyclophosphamide. Plasmapheresis or whole-body irradiation have occasionally been used in life-threatening acute polymyositis.

Figures for prognosis vary greatly, according to the numbers of children and of those with malignancies or severe connective tissue disorders in the published series. It is believed that early treatment with corticosteroids influences the prognosis. Broadly speaking, the prognosis of those with malignancy is the prognosis of that malignancy. Of the remainder, about 10–20 per cent will die from their disease, about 50 per cent will enter a prolonged remission within a few months, and the remaining 30–40 per cent will suffer a relapsing and remitting course for many years.

21.3.5 *Inclusion-body myositis*

This is a distinct variety of inflammatory myopathy not associated with malignant disease or connective tissue disease. It affects particularly older men, with slowly progressive but painless weakness of both proximal and distal muscle groups.

The characteristic pathological feature, which gives the disease its name, is the presence of granular inclusions within muscle fibres. These inclusions are often formed around the edge of slit-like vacuoles. They stain blue with haematoxylin, but their nature remains unknown. Corticosteroids are not as effective in inclusion-body myositis. Immunosuppression with azathioprine may improve the prognosis.

21.3.6   *Other types of myositis*

Granulomatous changes are often found in the muscles of patients with sarcoidosis. However, these seldom result in a clinically evident myopathy. Focal or nodular areas of myositis are often found in muscle biopsies from patients with a variety of connective tissue disorders, but these again seldom result in symptoms.

An eosinophilic polymyositis may occur in association with peripheral eosinophilia, anaemia, and cardiac and pulmonary involvement by eosinophilic infiltrates.

21.4   Polymyalgia rheumatica

This is a relatively common disorder of the elderly, affecting at least 100 per 100 000 per year of those over the age of 50. The cause is unknown, but there is a relationship to cranial arteritis (Sections 9.7 and 10.2.5.1), as some patients develop overt cranial arteritis during the course of their illness. Although arteritis is not apparent on routine muscle biopsy, autopsy studies often show arteritis in the aorta and its branches. Probably many of the symptoms arise from an associated inflammatory arthropathy affecting the shoulder and sternoclavicular joints. The knee and finger joints may also be affected.

Characteristic clinical features are pain and stiffness in the shoulder girdle muscles that is worse on first waking. The upper arm muscles may be tender on squeezing. Systemic features, such as loss of weight and depression, are common.

Another characteristic feature is an elevated sedimentation rate, although it must be remembered that the normal sedimentation rate in the healthy elderly is higher than in younger adults. Sedimentation rates under 40 mm in the first hour are not likely to be significant. There may also be a mild anaemia. Other investigations, such as electrodiagnostic studies, seldom show any abnormality.

Patients with polymyalgia rheumatica respond very rapidly to treatment with corticosteroids. Muscle stiffness and pain is usually relieved within a few days if the diagnosis is correct. A dose of 10–20 mg of prednisone per day is often sufficient. A small dose (5–10 mg/day) may be required for some years to suppress symptoms.

21.5   Inflammatory myopathy induced by drugs

Hydralazine, procainamide, and suphacetamide may all precipitate a syndrome similar to lupus erythematosus, accompanied by a polymyositis.

Other drug-induced myopathies are described in Section 21.10.

21.6   Recessively inherited muscular dystrophies

A simplified classification of these genetically determined myopathies is shown in Table 21.2. As already mentioned, some sporadic cases of myopathy with similar clinical features are grouped with the dystrophies, but biochemical advances are defining these syndromes more clearly.

21.6.1   *Duchenne muscular dystrophy (synonym: pseudohypertrophic muscular dystrophy)*

Duchenne muscular dystrophy is an allelic X-linked disorder affecting about 1 in 3000 of all live male births. The location of the gene on the X-chromosome and the gene product are now known.

21.6.1.1   *Clinical features*

The development of an affected child is often slow, the average age at walking being delayed by about 6 months. Many never learn to hop or skip or jump. Acquisition of speech is often a little

Table 21.2   Classification of muscular dystrophies

X-linked
  Duchenne–Becker
  Emery–Dreifuss
Autosomal recessive
  scapulohumeral
  childhood forms
  late-onset proximal
Autosomal dominant
  facioscapulohumeral
  scapuloperoneal
  late-onset proximal
  oculopharyngeal
  myotonic
Metabolic myopathies
  disorders of glycogen metabolism
  acid maltase deficiency
  myophosphorylase deficiency
  phosphofructokinase deficiency
  mitochondrial myopathies

delayed, reflecting an associated mild intellectual retardation. When the boy is aged about 4 years old the family notices that he has difficulty in getting up from playing on the floor. He adopts a technique of rolling on to his face, pushing up on to all fours, and then climbing his hands up his legs and thighs. This manoeuvre, necessary because of proximal muscle weakness, was first described by Gowers, and the observation bears his name— Gowers' sign. Clinical examination shows some hypotonia at the shoulders, best appreciated by attempting to pick the boy up by his armpits, proximal muscle weakness, and pseudohypertrophy of the calf muscles, which are weak in spite of their bulk.

21.6.1.2   *Inheritance*

There have been enormous advances in our understanding of the inheritance of Duchenne dystrophy. Research efforts in the years 1965–85 (approximately) were largely directed to detection of maternal carriers, and attention was paid to slightly elevated levels of maternal phosphocreatine kinase and minimal maternal electrodiagnostic abnormalities. These findings were believed to represent activity of the abnormal gene incompletely suppressed by the normal allele. It had also been hoped that detection of an elevated level of fetal phosphocreatine kinase would allow selective therapeutic abortion, but there were at least 30 per cent false negative results. However, direct evidence about the gene is now available. Information has come from more than one route. Very occasionally, Duchenne muscular dystrophy affects girls. In each case it has been shown that there had been translocation of an X-chromosome in the central area of the short-arm band p21. Secondly, the discovery of DNA restriction fragment length polymorphisms (RFLP) linked to the gene also placed the gene firmly in the X p21 region. The use of different markers has disclosed that the gene is a very large one, about 2000–4000 kilobase pairs in length. It also seems to be on a particularly unstable part of the chromosome, as crossover events, which result in an exchange of DNA between two X-chromosomes, are frequent. (See also Section 23.1.3)

Cases of Duchenne dystrophy result from a deletion of a part of this large gene, which can be detected by a number of gene probes. As the availability of these increases, most cases of Duchenne dystrophy will probably prove to be due to deletions. The severity of the illness may reflect the extent of the gene deletion (Section 21.6.2).

The gene product has been now identified—a protein that has been named dystrophin. This is absent from the muscles of affected children. It is normally present on the sarcolemmal membrane. Interestingly enough, it is also present in cells other than muscles. Intense research activity is now directed towards its function. It is of great interest that an X-linked myopathy of mice (mdx mouse myopathy) is also associated with an absence of dystrophin, so an important animal model is at hand.

The instability of the Duchenne gene results in at least one-third of the affected boys being the result of a new mutation. However, the mother of an apparent new mutation should be regarded as a carrier for all practical purposes, as she may be a gonadal mosaic for normal and deleted X-chromosomes, the deletion occurring during mitosis in primordial gonadal development. Occasionally carriers may themselves have mild symptoms, and recent studies have shown that dystrophin may be missing from a proportion of their muscle fibres.

Alternative sophisticated explanations involving translocation to autosomal chromosomes are also possible.

21.6.1.3 Diagnosis

The clinical features of Duchenne muscular dystrophy are such that there are few possibilities of confusion. Children with chronic spinal muscular atrophy may have similar weakness and occasional pseudohypertrophy (Section 20.2.2.3). Electrodiagnostic studies will readily distinguish the two conditions (see Section 8.7). The level of phosphocreatine kinase enzyme is greatly elevated in affected children and may reach 2000 IU/l or more, this abnormality becoming measurable at or soon after birth. Muscle biopsy shows widespread variation in muscle size, with rounding of the cells in transverse section. Some fibres are hyalinized with loss of normal striations on longitudinal sections. Split fibres, degenerating, and regenerating fibres may all be seen. There is very little inflammatory response to the degenerating fibres.

The diagnosis of the disease and the identification of carriers is likely now to depend increasingly upon amplification of mRNA from peripheral blood lymphocytes.

21.6.1.4 Treatment

Although identification of the gene product opens up theoretical avenues of treatment, there is at present no pharmacological method of arresting the progress of the disease. Current interest lies in myoblast transfer. In mdx mice, raw DNA transferred to muscle cells results in the expression of dystrophin. However, we do not yet know how myoblasts might be dispersed. The skills of the neurologist and paediatrician lie initially in supporting families through the initial period of shock and bewilderment, as is necessary for the families of children with cerebral palsy. In the case of muscular dystrophy, however, problems mount with increasing physical disability. Many boys with muscular dystrophy become obese, through a combination of low energy expenditure and overeating, sometimes with the mistaken idea that muscle bulk will thereby be improved. Control of body weight is therefore a worthy therapeutic target in so far as mobility is likely to be prolonged. The provision of physical aids may do much to alleviate the child's

limitations by disability (see Chapter 26). Physiotherapy and the provision of splints may limit the development of contractures, and prolong walking, but in spite of valiant efforts, contractures are common, particularly of the gastrocnemius and soleus, so that the child walks on his toes. Orthopaedic procedures undertaken to relieve these contractures are often disappointing, as they may have biomechanical disadvantages which limit compensatory choices. Surgery for scoliosis may maintain adequate ventilation for a worthwhile time. For those uncomfortable on account of night-time hypoventilation, intermittent positive pressure ventilation using a nasal mask may be very useful. For some, daytime assisted ventilation is also appropriate.

21.6.1.5 Prognosis

Unfortunately, weakness progresses. Gluteal weakness leads to a forward tilt of the pelvis on walking, and a compensatory lordosis of the spine. Shortening of the calf muscles results in an equinus contracture so that the boy walks on his toes. The ability to walk is usually lost by the age of 10–12 years. As the disease progresses, kyphoscoliosis and involvement of respiratory and cardiac muscles occur. Death usually occurs by the age of 18.

21.6.2 Becker muscular dystrophy

This is a milder variant of Duchenne dystrophy, affecting about 1 per 10 000 of all male births. Onset of weakness is at about the age of 10, and most patients are able to walk until their midtwenties. The gene responsible for this disorder lies also in the p21 segment of the X-chromosome. Allelic heterogeneity occurs at the Duchenne gene locus, giving rise to myopathies of degrees of severity varying between classical severe Duchenne, mild Becker dystrophy, and quadriceps myopathy (Section 23.1.1). There does not yet seem to be a close correlation between the region of the gene deletion and the severity of the clinical phenotype. However, those with milder phenotypes do show low amounts of dystrophin, or variants of dystrophin of low molecular weight.

21.6.3 Emery–Dreifuss dystrophy

Although syndromes of muscular weakness and

wasting are much more commonly neurogenic than myogenic (see Sections 20.1 and 20.2), a number of families have been described in which there is early myopathic involvement of proximal muscles in the arms, usually with onset at about age 5 years. Contractures around the elbow joint are an early feature, and soon foot drop or contractures at the ankle joint follow. Cardiac involvement is common. The gene lies close to the tip of chromosome Xq.

21.6.4 *Autosomal recessive muscular dystrophy*

In any one family, autosomal recessive inheritance is difficult to distinguish from sporadic cases of muscular dystrophy. However, studies of some large kindreds with weakness and wasting in the scapulohumeral, scapuloperoneal, or proximal limb girdle muscles with onset in childhood or in middle age suggest that it is probable that any apparently sporadic cases probably do have a genetic basis. Many such patients used to be labelled just 'limb-girdle dystrophy', which is clinically reasonable enough, and in at least some instances the disorder is associated with a gene localized to 15p. The differential clinical diagnosis of a 'limb-girdle dystrophy' lies betwen an autosomal recessive dystrophy and a neurogenic atrophy (Section 20.1.1). Also if male, a late-onset Becker dystrophy, and, if female, a symptomatic Duchenne carrier state must be considered. Dystrophin studies do now allow the accurate classification of these cases.

A condition known as Fukuyama dystrophy occurs in Japan, where it is about half as common as Duchenne dystrophy. Associated with dystrophy are areas of cortical dysplasia, which may be sufficiently severe to result in microcephaly.

21.7 Dominantly inherited muscular dystrophies

Facioscapulohumeral dystrophy (Landouzy–Déjérine) affects, in early childhood, the muscles indicated by its name. Contractures and cardiac involvement seldom occur, and the disease is compatible with a normal expectancy of life. The prevalence is about 1 per 20 000. The disorder is inherited through an autosomal dominant gene localized to chromosome 4q. Some affected family members are without symptoms, even though clinical examination may reveal thinning and mild weakness of biceps and triceps. Both this type of myopathy and the scapuloperoneal form may only be clinically distinguishable from neurogenic atrophies by biopsy. The serum phosphocreatine kinase is usually only slightly raised.

Ocular myopathies are usually associated with abnormalities of mitochondrial metabolism (Section 21.8.2), but a few cases of non-neurogenic external ophthalmoplegia do not have a mitochondrial defect, and some of these cases are associated with dysphagia (oculopharyngeal dystrophy).

21.7.1 *Myotonic muscular dystrophy*

This type of dystrophy is inherited through an autosomal dominant gene. The prevalence is about 5 per 100 000.

21.7.1.1 *Clinical features*

Muscles are not the only tissue affected by this disorder, which involves also the ocular lens, gonads, heart, and hair. Myotonia (Section 8.7.1.4) or weakness are usually the first symptoms of the disorder. Myotonia becomes much more pronounced in cold weather. One patient, for example, was a keen dinghy sailor who found that he had increasing difficulty in letting go of the sheets as his hands became cold during a race. Dystrophic weakness is also prominent in forearm and anterior tibial muscles, so patients may notice weakness of grip and difficulty in walking due to foot drop. The first symptoms usually occur between the ages of 15 and 30. Dystrophic wasting and weakness subsequently affect the cranial muscles so that ptosis and wasting of temporalis muscles may be prominent. The sternomastoids are also usually prominently affected. Other clinical features include premature baldness in a male distribution, premature cataracts, testicular atrophy, diabetes mellitus, and electrocardiographic abnormalities with evidence of conduction defects or cardiomyopathy. The central and peripheral nervous systems are also affected, with some degree of mental retardation being common. The tendon reflexes are depressed or absent, and nerve conduction studies show minor slowing of velocity.

21.7.1.2 *Inheritance*

The relatives of probands with myotonic dystrophy may only show evidence that they carry the gene by demonstrating premature cataracts, for example, without obvious myotonia or dystrophy. The gene lies on chromosome band 19q 13.3. A normal restriction fragment in this region is replaced in affected individuals by a larger fragment which varies in length both between unrelated affected individuals and within families. The unstable nature of this region may explain variation in age of onset and severity of disease. Linkage dysequilibrium studies suggest that most cases are descended from one original mutation.

21.7.1.3 *Diagnosis, prognosis, and treatment*

The diagnosis depends upon the characteristic myotonic discharge on electromyography (Section 8.7.1.4) in association with the appropriate dystrophic clinical features that distinguish myotonic dystrophy from other myotonic syndromes. Slit-lamp examination will show bright dust-like particles in the lenses of most patients after the age of 40. The level of phosphocreatine kinase may only be slightly elevated. Muscle biopsy shows nuclei lying in the centre of muscle fibres and splitting of muscle fibres. Type I fibres tend to be atrophied, and type II hypertrophied.

Severe disability usually results within 15 years in those family members presenting with muscle weakness. There is no useful treatment for the dystrophic features. Myotonia is not usually a sufficiently troublesome feature to warrant treatment, but phenytoin may occasionally be useful.

21.7.1.4 *Congenital myotonic dystrophy*

Occasionally a child carrying the gene will be affected from birth, being profoundly hypotonic, and with grossly delayed motor and intellectual development.

21.7.2 *Central core disease*

Central core disease is a mild, usually non-progressive myopathy, presenting in infancy or early childhood with hypotonia and proximal muscle weakness. The 'cores' are central zones seen in type I muscle fibres; histochemical stains show a deficiency of mitochondrial oxidative enzymes and glycogen. The disorder is inherited as an autosomal dominant, localized to chromosome 19q. Children with central core disease or their relatives may be liable to malignant hyperthermia (Section 21.10.4).

21.7.3 *Nemaline (rod) myopathy*

This is a slowly progressive myopathy presenting in middle life. The characteristic finding is of rods in the centre of muscle fibres, without evidence of inflammation. Rods originate in the Z disc; their main constituent is actin and α-actin. Nemaline myopathy has been reported in HIV infection, and it may be that viral or immune factors play some part in the disruption of these muscle proteins.

21.8 Metabolic myopathies

There are a number of metabolic disorders of muscle. Classification now is more appropriately based upon the identified biochemical lesion rather than on the clinical presentation.

21.8.1 *Disorders of glycogen metabolism*

21.8.1.1 *McArdle's disease*

In McArdle's disease there is a deficiency in myophosphorylase, readily revealed by histochemical techniques. Patients with myophosphorylase deficiency develop generalized muscular 'cramps' (which are electrically silent) and stiffness after exercise. Blood lactate and pyruvate fail to increase as they should on exercise, as the enzyme deficiency prevents the breakdown of muscle glycogen. Vigorous exercise may be accompanied by myoglobinuria. The disorder is further discussed in Section 23.1.4.1.

21.8.1.2 *Acid maltase deficiency*

Acid maltase (α-1,4- and 1,6-glucosidase) deficiency usually presents in infancy with hypotonia, cardiomegaly, hepatomegaly, and enlargement of the tongue due to excess glycogen storage (Pompe's disease). Inheritance is through an autosomal recessive gene. However, less severe levels of enzyme deficiency may present in childhood with clinical features reminiscent of Duchenne dystrophy, and in adult life with features of a limb-girdle dystrophy. Muscle biopsy shows distortion of the normal muscular architecture by large intracellular vacuoles packed with glycogen. These reveal their lysosomal origin by staining with acid phosphatase.

21.8.1.3 Glycogen de-branching enzyme deficiency

Deficiency of the debranching enzyme amylo-1,6-glucosidase is again characterized by hypotonia and hepatomegaly if presenting in infancy, but in adult life the disorder presents with muscular fatiguability and distal muscular wasting. Deficiency of the debranching enzyme allows the enzymatic breakdown only of the outer chains of the glycogen molecule. Muscle biopsy again shows glycogen stored in vacuoles, but these do not contain acid phosphatase.

21.8.2 Disorders of mitochondrial metabolism

Mitochondria have their own DNA, which codes for the enzymes responsible for the respiratory (electron-transport) chain, and for the oxidative phosphorylation system. Other mitochondrial systems are concerned with substrate transport and substrate utilization. Disorders associated with abnormalities of mitochondrial metabolism are characterized by a variable lactic acidaemia and mitochondrial proliferation in peripheral muscle. Severely affected patients usually present in early life with an encephalopathy, mitochondrial encephalopathy with lactic acidosis and stroke-like episodes (the MELAS syndrome), or with profound muscle weakness resulting in hypotonia, or myoclonic epilepsy with ragged red muscle fibres (the MERFF syndrome). There is considerable phenotypic diversity among these syndromes, but recent studies show point mutations of mitochondrial DNA in association with MERFF and MELAS (at different points), and these mutations can be detected in blood cells as well as muscle fibres, an advance which will allow increased understanding of these disorders.

Less severely affected patients may present in middle life with a myopathy, often affecting the external ocular muscles as well as distal muscles (Section 21.8.2.2). However, there is often other evidence of metabolic derangements, such as retinitis, peripheral neuropathy, ataxia, dementia, and seizures. Muscle biopsy shows accumulations of abnormal mitochondria in the subsarcolemmic space. Muscle fibres are seen to have a ragged, red appearance when stained with the Gomori trichome stain.

21.8.2.1 Defects of substrate transport and utilization

Carnitine   (L-β-hydroxy-N-trimethylaminobutyric acid) is a necessary carrier for the entry of fatty acids into mitochondria. Free fatty acids are an important source of energy during prolonged exercise when muscle stores of glycogen have become depleted. Deficiencies of carnitine synthesis may occur in the liver and muscle, or in muscle alone, both types being inherited through an autosomal recessive gene. Carnitine deficiency presents as a slowly progressive myopathy, in which muscles of the face, neck, and jaw are prominently involved. Muscle biopsy shows accumulation of neutral lipids, particularly in type I fibres. Electron microscopy shows an excess of mitochondria, many of which have abnormal shapes.

Patients with carnitine deficiency may improve if given oral supplements of carnitine and medium-chain triglycerides. Oral steroids may also be useful.

Carnitine depletion can occur secondarily to other metabolic defects, such as deficiency of one of the fatty acid acyl CoA dehydrogenases. As a result of the metabolic block, acylcarnitines are transported out of the mitochondria and excreted in the urine, draining carnitine stores. The build-up of acyl CoA compounds in the mitochondrial matrix inhibits a number of mitochondrial enzymes, leading to ATP depletion. This may present as an encephalopathy. Some patients may improve on riboflavin.

Apart from deficiency of carnitine itself, there may be deficiency of carnitine palmityl transferase, the enzyme that controls the entry of long-chain fatty acids into mitochondria. Deficiency of the enzyme is inherited through a recessive gene. Muscle activity is followed by painful cramps and muscle necrosis, leading to myoglobinuria.

21.8.2.2 Defects of respiratory chain enzymes

Other defects of mitochondrial metabolism involve deficiencies of the multimeric enzymes of the respiratory chain and oxidative phosphorylation system embedded in the mitochondrial inner membrane. The most frequently affected enzyme complexes are NADH-CoQ reductase, CoQ-cytochrome c reductase and cytochrome c oxidase. Clinical presentations of these deficiencies depend upon the extent of and tissue distribution of the deficiency. The spectrum includes infantile hypotonia with myopathy, often associated with encephalopathy, a later-onset myopathy, or a late-onset encephalopathy. In the context of this chapter, special reference is made to a limb girdle dystrophy characterized by ragged red fibres, with large numbers of abnormal mitochondria, some of which contain paracrystalline inclusions. Other mitochondrial myopathies include a syndrome of what has been termed 'ophthalmoplegia plus'— external ophthalmoplegia associated with retinal pigmentation, cerebellar optic atrophy, ataxia, and cardiac conduction defects. This is known as the Kearns–Sayre syndrome, and appears to be due to a defect in mitochondrial protein translation, associated with either large gene deletions or duplications in mitochondrial DNA.

21.8.2.3 Defects of energy production

Luft's syndrome is characterized by hypermetabolism of non-thyroid origin, with fever, sweating, diffuse muscular weakness, and excessive numbers of mitochondria of abnormal structure on microscopical examination. There are defects in oxidative phosphorylation.

21.8.3 Disorders of potassium flux—the syndromes of periodic paralysis

Weakness in otherwise healthy subjects may result from hypokalaemia induced by drugs (Section 21.10.6). The thiazide diuretics are most frequently incriminated. There are, however, three inherited syndromes in which profound weakness is associated with spontaneous fluctuations in the distribution of potassium.

21.8.3.1 Hypokalaemic periodic paralysis

Hypokalaemic periodic paralysis usually begins in adolescence, affecting males more often than females, although inheritance is through a dominant gene. Episodes of paralysis occur on waking, after a heavy carbohydrate meal, and after exercise. The leg muscles are predominantly affected, but arm and cranial muscles are also sometimes affected. Fortunately, bulbar and respiratory muscles are spared. Paralysis usually lasts for several hours. During an attack the serum potassium falls to 2.5 mmol/l or less. Attacks may be precipitated under laboratory control by large doses of glucose or by the injection of insulin, which induces potassium entry into muscle cells. Muscle biopsy during an attack shows vacuolation, and evidence of dilatation of the sarcoplasmic reticulum. Severe attacks may be shortened by the use of oral potassium salts. Attacks may be largely prevented, or reduced in severity, by the use of thiazide diuretics, in spite of their potassium-losing properties. The mechanism of their action in this syndrome is not clear.

The diagnosis of hypokalaemic periodic paralysis is not difficult once the disorder has been suspected, as the affected muscles are electrically inexcitable, and the serum potassium is low. However, the profound weakness of sudden onset, with preserved consciousness and function of bulbar muscles may lead the unwary to suspect hysteria.

Episodes of paralysis become less frequent in middle age. However, a fixed proximal weakness may occur after many episodes of paralysis.

21.8.3.2 Hyperkalaemic periodic paralysis

Hyperkalaemic periodic paralysis is also known as adynamia episodica hereditaria. This is inherited through an autosomal recessive gene, now mapped to chromosome 17q. Paralytic episodes tend to occur earlier in life than in the hypokalaemic form, and are of shorter duration—usually less than 1 hour. The serum level of potassium rises during the period of paralysis as potassium leaks from muscle fibres into the circulation. Myotonia may be seen in the periocular muscles during an attack. Electromyography shows fibrillation potentials and myotonic discharges between attacks and, as in the hypokalaemic form, the muscle is inexcitable or only partly excitable by electric stimulation during an attack.

21.8.3.3   *Normokalaemic periodic paralysis*

Normokalaemic periodic paralysis is a poorly understood disorder in which paralytic attacks may last for days at a time. There may be some improvement after infusion of sodium chloride. Acetazolamide may prevent some attacks in this variety.

21.9   Endocrine myopathies

21.9.1   *Thyrotoxic myopathy*

Weakness and wasting of muscles around the shoulder girdle are common in acute thyrotoxicosis, and may occasionally be the presenting symptoms. Bulbar and external ocular muscles are also sometimes involved, but this may represent the coexistence of another immune disorder—myasthenia gravis. Muscle biopsy shows fibres containing central nuclei and fibre atrophy. There may be focal collections of lymphocytes. The myopathy improves as the thyrotoxicosis is brought under control.

In thyrotoxic oriental men, episodes of hypokalaemic periodic paralysis are frequent. This appears to be associated with a genetically determined overactivity of the sodium pump.

21.9.2   *Hypothyroid myopathy*

Hypothyroid myopathy is characterized by muscle pain, stiffness, and cramps. Muscles characteristically show pseudomyotonia—a prolonged contraction after percussion without continuing electrical discharge. This is due to a change in proportions of type I and type II fibres, and changes in myosin light-chain patterns, both resulting in slower relaxation than normal. This is clinically manifest by unusually slowly relaxing ankle tendon reflexes, which may alert the neurologist to a previously overlooked diagnosis of myxoedema.

Occasionally hypothyroidism is accompanied by an inflammatory myopathy, both presumably immunologically mediated.

21.10   Drug-induced myopathies

21.10.1   *Focal myositis*

Repeated intramuscular injections of antibiotics in acute illness or of drugs of abuse may lead to local fibrosis and contraction, presumably due to the effects of repeated needle tracks and haemorrhage.

21.10.2   *Acute generalized drug-induced myopathies*

A number of drugs cause diffuse muscle aching and mild weakness without progression to a severe myopathy. Danazol, salbutamol, cytotoxic agents, cimetidine, zidovudine, and lithium are examples.

A more severe necrotizing myopathy has been reported after ε-aminocaproic acid, emetine, and clofibrate. Emetine is widely used in the treatment of amoebiasis, and may be abused in the form of ipecac by those with bulimia. The myopathy caused by ε-aminocaproic acid may come on some weeks after beginning treatment (usually for subarachnoid haemorrhage, although the benefits of the drug are uncertain, Section 10.6.4). Sometimes the intensity of muscle necrosis caused by drugs can be so great that rhabdomyolysis, myoglobinuria, and renal failure may result. A similar picture may result from abuse of heroin and alcohol.

21.10.3   *Acute drug-induced inflammatory myopathies*

D-Penicillamine, hydralazine, and procainamide may result in a lupus-like picture in which polymyositis is a prominent feature.

21.10.4   *Acute myopathy after anaesthesia (synonym: malignant hyperpyrexia, malignant hyperthermia)*

This condition is inherited, usually through an autosomal dominant gene localized to chromosome 19q, although recessive inheritance has also been described. Tightly linked flanking markers have been identified. Affected family members may or may not have a mild myopathy, as judged clinically or by the finding of elevated serum levels of phosphocreatine kinase. What is unique about this condition, however, is that general anaesthesia results in a potentially lethal syndrome. Within 30 minutes or so of induction of anaesthesia, patients develop hyperpyrexia, metabolic acidosis, muscular rigidity, and sometimes myoglobinuria. The anaesthetic agents most often incriminated include halothane, methoxyflurane, enflurane, trichloroethylene, cyclopropane, ether, chloroform, and ketamine. It appears that these agents trigger entry of calcium ions into the sarcoplasmic reticulum that leads to muscle rigidity, hypermetabolism, with pyrexia and sarcolemmal disruption. This results in hyperkalaemia and myoglobinaemia. The primary defect lies in the calcium induced calcium release channel known as the ryanodine receptor for which the gene codes.

An episode of muscle rigidity may be aborted by dantrolene sodium intravenously. A similar disorder affects one strain of Landrace pigs, which provide a good experimental model of this intriguing disorder.

21.10.5   *Chronic proximal myopathy due to drugs*

A chronic, painless proximal myopathy is the commonest type of drug-induced myopathy. Fluorinated steroids, such as triamcinolone, dexamethasone, and betamethasone are most often responsible. The myopathy is to some extent related to the dose of steroids used, but individual susceptibility is also important. The quadriceps muscles are often particularly involved, and wasting is prominent. Electrodiagnostic studies show typical myopathic changes (Section 8.7), but the serum level of phosphocreatine kinase is usually normal. Biopsy shows a selective atrophy of type II fibres.

Difficulties sometimes arise in treating inflammatory myopathies (Section 21.3.4.6) with steroids. It may be difficult to decide if proximal weakness is due to continuing disease or to its treatment. Estimation of the serum level of phosphocreatine kinase or further biopsy may help the decision.

21.10.6   *Drug-induced hypokalaemic myopathy*

Prolonged use of diuretics, purgatives, liquorice derivatives such as carbenoxolone, and amphotericin B may all induce transient hypokalaemic muscular weakness, but if the plasma potassium is chronically maintained at a low level there may be persistent changes on biopsy, similar to those found in hypokalaemic periodic paralysis (Section 21.8.3.1).

21.10.7   *'Neuromyopathy'*

Some drugs, such as colchicine, amiodarone, vincristine, and chloroquine, produce a syndrome in which a myopathy is associated with a distal axonal neuropathy. Electrodiagnostic studies show findings reminiscent of polymyositis, with evidence of denervation in the form of fibrillation potentials, as well as myopathic motor unit potentials. In both colchicine myopathy and chloroquine myopathy there are autophagic vacuoles.

21.11   Toxic myopathy

21.11.1   *Alcoholic myopathy*

After a prolonged bout of drinking, alcoholics may develop swollen and tender muscles, with severe proximal weakness. Necrosis of muscle fibres may be so rapid that myoglobinuria and renal failure result, as in cases of heroin abuse. The prognosis is reasonable if the patient is treated by dialysis and eschews alcohol thereafter.

Other patients develop a chronic proximal myopathy with type IIb fibre atrophy. Not surprisingly, a neuropathy is usually also present (Section 23.4.2.7).

21.12   Disorders of neuromuscular transmission

Our understanding of the disorders of neuromuscular transmission has increased enormously in the past 20 years. Before discussing the clinical features of myasthenia gravis and the various myasthenic syndromes, the physiology of the normal neuromuscular junction is outlined.

21.12.1   *Physiology of the normal neuromuscular junction*

Motor nerve terminals synthesize acetylcholine, which is stored in membrane-bound vesicles. Even at rest there is a continuous random spontaneous release of acetylcholine into the synaptic cleft, by exocytosis of vesicles. Each vesicle stores 5000–10 000 molecules of acetylcholine, released together as a packet or 'quantum'. The spontaneous release of acetylcholine can be detected by a microelectrode inserted into the muscle fibre near the end-plate, as the release of each vesicle results in a miniature end-plate potential (mepp). The amplitude of the mepp is proportional to the number of acetylcholine molecules in the vesicle.

On arrival of a nerve impulse as a result of some reflex action or act of volition, depolarization of the terminal axon results in a sudden surge of Ca^{2+} ions into the terminal. This results in an almost synchronous release of perhaps 50–60 vesicles. The acetylcholine released binds to receptors on the folded surface of the end-plate region of the muscle fibre. There are about 5000 receptor sites/ μm^2 of receptor, concentrated on the terminal expansions of the junctional folds. The receptor protein has a considerable amount of homology across many genera. As the acetylcholine molecule binds to the receptor, ion channels are briefly opened, allowing Na^{2+} ions to enter, causing a depolarization of the end-plate region. This end-plate potential (epp) usually exceeds the threshold membrane potential for depolarization of the muscle fibre, so that an action potential is propagated along the muscle fibre surface. This in turn results in the release of Ca^{2+} ions from the sarcoplasmic reticulum, and the myofibrils contract.

This complex system could fail because of

(1) an inability to create actylcholine;

(2) an inability to form acetylcholine into vesicles;

(3) a failure of preterminal neural conduction, so that Ca^{2+} ions do not enter the terminal;

(4) a failure to exocytose the vesicles into the synaptic cleft;

(5) an accelerated catabolism of acetylcholine before binding with a receptor can occur;

(6) receptor blockade;

(7) degradation of, or insufficient, receptors;

(8) a failure of propagation of the muscle action potential; or, finally,

(9) a failure of Ca^{2+} release from the sarcoplasmic reticulum.

A number of these potential faults are reflected in clinical syndromes, of which the best known is myasthenia gravis.

21.12.2 *Myasthenia gravis*

Myasthenia gravis is an illness characterized by weakness of periocular, facial, bulbar, and girdle muscles. It is associated with the presence of antibodies to acetylcholine receptor protein. A patient with what was probably myasthenia was described by Willis in 1672, and the clinical picture was well recognized by the end of the nineteenth century. Landmarks include the recognition of the benefits of cholinesterase inhibitors by Walker in 1934, and of the role of receptor antibodies by Patrick and Lindstrom in 1973.

21.12.2.1 *Epidemiology*

The prevalence of myasthenia gravis is about 5 per 100 000. Females are affected twice as often as males. The modal age of onset is at age about 20, but younger and much older patients may be affected, the older patients tending to present with weakness of bulbar muscles. The initiating factor of the illness is not known, but sometimes the onset is abrupt after a febrile illness, or during pregnancy, both factors being known to alter immunological balance.

As would be expected from the immunological nature of the disease (see Section 21.12.2.2), evidence of a genetic factor is present. White patients can be divided into four main subgroups by age and thymic histology. Those presenting before age 40 are predominantly female, have high titres of acetyl choline receptor antibody, and a strong association with HLA-B8 and -DRw3. After the age of 40, there is a slight predominance of men, antibody titres are lower, and there is a weak association with B7 and DRw2. The genes predisposing to myasthenia gravis are probably located within the variable region of the Ig heavy chain loci. However, these haplotypes are not obligatory, and indeed myasthenia gravis in each of twins is rare. However, subclinical disease, as reflected in increased jitter (Section 8.8.1), may occur in close relatives. The thymus gland shows lymphoid hyperplasia, with T-lymphocytes in the cortex and medulla. Although the myoid cells found in the thymus express acetylcholine receptor on their surface, they are not obviously a focus of immune destruction. About 10 per cent of patients with myasthenia gravis, almost invariably those with a later age of onset, have a thymona, which is usually cystic and calcified, but which may spread by local invasion, and by nodal spread to lymph glands in the thorax and neck. No HLA bias is apparent in this group, nor in the fourth group with signs confined to the ocular muscles for at least 2 years.

Although anti-acetylcholine receptor antibody can be shown to be released from the thymus, the major role of the thymus appears to be in sensitizing lymphocytes to the receptor; these lymphocytes are then exported from the thymus.

21.12.2.2 *Pathophysiology*

Antibodies to the acetylcholine receptor will be found in about 85 per cent of patients with undoubted clinical and electrophysiological evidence of myasthenia, and in about 70 per cent of those whose myasthenia is limited to the ocular muscles. It is not thought that the antibodies directly block the receptor, but rather that there is complement-mediated lysis of the receptors on the post-synaptic membrane, and also that accelerated modulation of receptors and internal degradation by lysosomes are responsible for the reduced number of binding sites. The numbers of these can be demonstrated by radiolabelled α-bungarotoxin. The reduction of the number of binding sites results in small miniature end-plate potentials and end-plate potentials, both of which can be demonstrated by microelectrode studies of affected human intercostal muscles. In normal subjects, sustained voluntary activity or repetitive nerve stimulation results in progressive reduction of transmitter release. In myasthenic subjects, this normal decline is unmasked by the reduced safety factor for neuromuscular transmission, due to the reduced number of binding sites for acetylcholine.

The titre of antibodies is lowest in patients with purely ocular myasthenia, intermediate in those with thymic hyperplasia, and highest in those with a thymoma. There is a loose correlation between the height of the antibody titre and the clinical severity of the disease, and the titre falls during immunosuppressive treatment (Section 21.12.2.5). Occasional patients are found, with otherwise clinically typical myasthenia gravis, whose serum does not contain acetylcholine receptor antibodies. In spite of this, some respond to plasmapheresis or immunosuppression. It is probable that such patients have a pathogenetic immunoglobulin antibody that binds to determinants at the neuromuscular junction that are not acetylcholine receptors. Thymic hyperplasia may be absent at thymectomy, suggesting that this may be inappropriate treatment for such patients.

21.12.2.3 *Clinical features*

The external ocular muscles are commonly first involved, causing ptosis and diplopia. The shoulder girdle muscles are also frequently involved, so that a young woman may complain of difficulty in raising her arms above her head to brush her hair or to put an object on a high shelf. Other early features may include difficulty in chewing meat, a nasal voice, and difficulty in swallowing due to involvement of bulbar muscles. Pelvic girdle and distal limb muscles are affected later in the illness.

Although external ophthalmoplegia is a common presenting symptom, the disease only remains limited to these muscles in 10–15 per cent of patients. Generalization to other muscles usually begins within 2 years of onset.

Although fatiguability is an important diagnostic point on examination, many patients do not stress this in the history, although when specifically asked they may report that chewing, for example, tends to be more difficult towards the end of a meal.

Examination of a patient early in the course of the illness may show no more than a slight ptosis, and external ocular muscle weakness resulting in a diplopia that is difficult to 'sort out', as variable failure of neuromuscular transmission constantly alters the pattern of oculomotor weakness. A clinically doubtful weakness of the shoulder girdle muscles may become quite clear-cut after 20 repetitive abductions of the shoulders, confirming both the weakness and its fatiguability. During the course of taking the history, progressive nasality of speech may be noted.

Later in the illness muscle wasting may become prominent. The facial muscles may become flattened, and the jaw sags. The tongue may waste in a typical way, three furrows appearing on its surface.

21.12.2.4   *Investigation*

The short-acting anticholinesterase, edrophonium, can be injected intravenously in the clinic, and will reverse, for 1–5 minutes, many of the clinical features of early myasthenia. It is essential to have a marker muscle which is undoubtedly weak. Care must be taken to avoid a positive placebo response in a patient with non-myasthenic 'fatigue' (Section 25.2.4), and for this reason an initial control injection of saline may be useful.

One minute after an initial test dose of 2 mg, a further 8 mg of edrophonium chloride is given by bolus injection. The patient should be warned that he may experience uncomfortable intestinal peristalsis, fasciculation, and lacrimation. Bradycardia is not usually a problem, but some authorities recommend the previous intravenous injection of 0.6 mg atropine.

Clinical neurophysiological tests are also helpful. Fatigue on repetitive stimulation of the ulnar nerve at the wrist at 3 Hz results in diminution of the amplitude of the compound muscle action potential evoked from abductor digiti minimi for the reasons explained in Section 21.12.2.2. A positive result is illustrated in Fig. 8.7. Section 8.8.1 describes the jitter phenomenon, a more sensitive test of failure of neuromuscular transmission.

Clinical examination and investigation should also be directed at the possibility of associated immunological diseases, such as hypothyroidism, failure of vitamin B_{12} absorption, vitiligo, and systemic lupus erythematosus.

Other necessary tests include the imaging procedures, chest X-ray and CT scan, to show the anatomy of the thymus gland. Hyperplasia is usually obvious in patients with myasthenia gravis under the age of 40; sometimes a cystic or calcified thymoma may be seen.

21.12.2.5   *Treatment and prognosis*

For many years the primary treatment of myasthenia gravis was with anticholinesterase compounds. Neostigmine, in an oral dose of 15 mg, has an action that is no longer than about 2 hours. Smoother control may be given with the longer-acting pyridostigmine, the action of which lasts for about 4–6 hours. With these drugs, there is a danger of passing without remark from a myasthenic block, and weakness sensitive to anticholin-

esterases, to a depolarization block caused by excessive acetylcholine at the end-plate, accumulated there by an excess dose of the cholinesterase inhibitor. In a sick patient, increasing weakness may incorrectly be thought to be due to an exacerbation of myasthenia, as can occur during intercurrent infections. If the increased weakness is really due to depolarization block, then a further dose of anticholinesterase may have disastrous effects, resulting in respiratory paralysis.

Long-term follow-up studies show that spontaneous remissions can occur in up to 20 per cent of all patients treated with anticholinesterases alone. However, it is now usual practice to attempt to modify the course of myasthenia gravis by treatment directed at the immune system: immunosuppression, plasmapheresis, and thymectomy.

Immunosuppression is usually commenced with corticosteroids. Alternate-day treatment with prednisolone up to 100 mg a day is effective in inducing a remission, and is associated with a decline in circulating concentrations of anti-acetylcholine receptor antibody. However, there may be a temporary exacerbation of the illness before any remission is induced. This may be so severe that artificial ventilation is required briefly. Exacerbations are believed to be due to the direct effects of corticosteroids on ion flux across the muscle membrane. Once improvement has been achieved, the dose can be reduced, but gradual reduction (e.g. 5 mg/day at monthly intervals) is wise in order to avoid the precipitation of a relapse.

Immunosuppression can also be accomplished with azathioprine (2–5 mg/kg/day) or with cyclosporin (6 mg/kg/day). The latter drug has a rather faster effect, some improvement occurring within 2–3 weeks. However, nephrotoxicity limits the use of this drug to patients otherwise unresponsive to treatment.

Plasmapheresis undoubtedly induces a clinical remission in many patients, but probably does no better than immunosuppression alone in reducing circulating levels of anti-acetylcholine receptor antibody and in inducing clinical improvement. However, plasmapheresis has a place in helping to cope with a myasthenic crisis, or in getting a patient fit enough for thymectomy.

Thymectomy is undoubtedly effective, inducing a complete remission in about a fifth of patients, and improvement in about a further 40 per cent. The benefits appear to be greatest if the patient is young, if the length of history before thymectomy is short, and in those with bulbar symptoms. The benefits are not proven in those aged more than 40. Although thymomas should be removed because of their propensity for local invasion, the chances of improvement of myasthenia in these cases are unfortunately slim.

After a thymectomy, there may be considerably less requirement for anticholinesterase inhibitors, so that most physicians stop these drugs a few hours before the operation, and electively ventilate the patient thereafter, with monitoring of ventilatory volumes. Cholinesterase inhibitors at about two-thirds of the pre-operative daily dose should then be reintroduced at about 48 hours after operation. The full benefits of thymectomy may not be apparent for 1–2 years.

21.12.2.6   Neonatal myasthenia

About 10–15 per cent of pregnant myasthenic mothers will give birth to infants who suck poorly, cry poorly, and are at risk from respiratory insufficiency due to neonatal myasthenia. The phenomenon disappears after 10–20 days, suggesting the passive transfer of acetylcholine receptor antibody from the mother. An alternative hypothesis is that the infant makes its own antibody in response to transplacental transfer of a cell clone from the mother.

21.12.3   Myasthenic syndromes

This name is given to a group of disorders of neuromuscular transmission in which the physiology of the defect is different from that found in myasthenia gravis.

21.12.3.1   The Lambert–Eaton myasthenic syndrome

This disorder was first recognized clinically in the 1950s in association with lung cancer, although it is now recognized that no cancer is found in about half the patients with typical clinical features.

Clinical features
The presenting symptom is usually gradual onset of weakness of the legs, the arms being less often affected. The muscles may ache on exercise. The usual age of onset is 50–60. Males are more often affected. Although patients often complain of fatiguing weakness on exercise, it is characteristic of this condition that there is a brief augmentation of strength for the first few seconds of a voluntary effort, the physiological explanation of which is discussed below. Other clinical features include autonomic symptoms such as a dry mouth, impotence, and constipation. Limb reflexes are usually depressed or absent. About half the cases have a ptosis but, in contrast to myasthenia gravis, there is no other evidence of an external ophthalmoplegia.

The neurological features of those with or without cancer are identical. Cancers are usually small-cell carcinomas of the lung, but occasional adenocarcinomas or extrathoracic carcinomas have been reported (e.g. breast). The symptoms of the myasthenic syndrome usually precede the diagnosis of the cancer. The median interval is 10 months (range, simultaneous diagnosis to nearly 4 years). If no carcinoma has emerged by then, it is unlikely to do so in the future.

Pathophysiology
The disease appears to be caused by circulating antibodies to voltage-gated calcium channels. Blockage or loss of these channels results in a reduction of Ca^{2+} entry during nerve terminal depolarization, and thus a decrease in transmitter release. Freeze-fracture electron-microscopic study has shown a paucity of 'active zones' known to be related to acetylcholine release. The immunological basis for the disorder is supported by the association of the Lambert–Eaton syndrome with other auto-immune disorders, and the presence of a range of organ-specific antibodies in about half the patients. Furthermore, plasma exchange produces a short-lived improvement in patients with the Lambert–Eaton syndrome, and the physiological abnormality can be transmitted to mice by the intra-peritoneal injection of plasma from patients with the syndrome. The transmitted antibodies reduce the number of functional voltage-gated Ca^{2+} channels.

Physiological studies on nerve–muscle preparations, obtained by intercostal muscle biopsy of affected patients, show that there is a decrease in the number of packets (quanta) of acetylcholine released by each nerve impulse. Conversely, the spontaneous release of individual quanta by exocytosis, resulting in miniature end-plate potentials, is not affected. The end-plate potential, in response to the liberation of the smaller than usual number of quanta of acetylcholine as the nerve action potential invades the terminal, increases in size as a result of repetitive stimulation at rates of higher than 10 Hz, accounting for the initial augmentation of strength during a voluntary contraction. On electromyography, an initial small compound muscle action potential is increased in size many-fold after repetitive stimulation. As the number of quanta released in response to a nerve impulse is continually varying, jitter is seen, as it is in myasthenia gravis.

Small-cell lung carcinomas may be of neural crest origin, contain neurosecretory granules, and secrete neurohormones such as antidiuretic hormone and adrenocorticotrophic hormone. The cells of these tumours can be shown to have voltage-gated Ca^{2+} channels. The initial auto-antibody response in the Lambert–Eaton syndrome in those cases associated with cancer may therefore be to block the voltage-gated Ca^{2+} channels on tumour cells, with a secondary blockade of normal nerve terminals.

Treatment

Treatment of the primary tumour may result in a partial remission of the myasthenic syndrome. Immunosuppression may produce a useful long-term response, and the weakness may be helped by 3,4-diaminopyridine, which enhances the release of acetylcholine from the nerve terminals. A suitable dose is 25 mg four times a day. Tingling of the extremities, headache, and fatigue are unwanted effects of the drug.

21.12.3.2 *Drug-induced myasthenic syndromes*

Some drugs may induce pre-synaptic inhibition of nerve action potentials by inhibition of calcium flux. Others produce a curare-like post-synaptic receptor blockade, or inhibit ionic conductance across the muscle membrane. Drugs particularly incriminated include antibiotics of the aminoglycoside and polymyxin group, β-adrenoreceptor-blocking drugs, and phenytoin.

Penicillamine used in the treatment of rheumatoid arthritis may induce true myasthenia gravis, with the presence of circulating acetylcholine receptor antibodies. Patients usually recover over several months after the drug is withdrawn.

21.12.3.3 *Congenital myasthenia*

A number of rare syndromes have been characterized. Familial infantile myasthenia is an autosomal recessively inherited disease in which there appears to be a pre-synaptic abnormality in acetylcholine synthesis or transport into synaptic vesicles, and a defect in acetylcholine resynthesis by choline acetyltransferase. In another sex-linked or autosomally recessive condition, there is an inherited deficiency of acetyl cholinesterase. A further variant is the 'slow-channel' syndrome in which the acetylcholine receptor ion-channel closes slowly, prolonging the duration of the end-plate potential, and allowing the accumulation of calcium in the post-synaptic region. There is also a syndrome of congenital acetylcholine receptor deficiency, with unusually simplified end-plate anatomy.

21.12.4 *The stiff-man syndrome*

This rare disorder begins subacutely in adult life, with worsening over weeks or months. The cardinal features are generalized aches and stiffness, giving way to spasms precipitated by movement, emotion, or by sensory stimulation. Trismus does not occur, in contrast to tetanus. Attempted passive movements of the muscles by the examiner reveal generalized stiffness. Electromyography shows continuous motor-unit activity in the rigid muscles that, on the oscilloscope screen, looks like ordinary voluntary activity. A few patients have increased production of IgG in the cerebrospinal fluid. In one patient antibodies against glutamic acid decarboxylase have been demonstrated. This is the enzyme that synthesizes the inhibitory neurotransmitter γ-aminobutyric acid (GABA). It appears, therefore, that the stiff-man syndrome may be due to an auto-immune disorder directed against suprasegmental or spinal inhibitory GABA-ergic neurons. Drugs that enhance GABA-mediated central inhibition, such as diazepam and baclofen, may help to relieve the stiffness partially.

21.13 Cramps

Cramp may be defined as a powerful involuntary painful muscle contraction, usually lasting for less than 1 minute. What may reasonably be termed 'ordinary' cramps occur in the calves when settling for sleep at night, after exercise, or sometimes after a voluntary movement of plantarflexion. Nocturnal 'ordinary' cramps often disturb the sleep of older people. The pain and cramp may be relieved by forced passive extension of the muscle.

The physiology of 'ordinary' cramps is not known, but the contraction appears to be of peripheral rather than central origin. Nocturnal cramps may be inhibited, or at least partly relieved, by quinine sulphate (200 mg at night) if necessary.

Although 'ordinary' cramps are common enough, cramps indistinguishable from these may be symptoms of Parkinson's disease, motor neuron disease, peripheral neuropathy, muscular dystrophy, and some of the metabolic myopathies such as myophosphorylase deficiency. Cramp is also seen in association with dehydration and salt depletion, and with some drugs, such as terbutaline, salbutamole, cimetidine, and nifedipine.

21.14   Further reading

Tropical myositis

Shepherd, J. J. (1983). Tropical myositis: is it an entity and what is its cause? *Lancet* **2**, 1240–2.

Polymyositis and dermatomyositis

Lotz, B. P., Engel, A. G., Nishino, H. *et al.* (1989). Inclusion body myositis; observations in 40 patients. *Brain* **112**, 727–47.

Plotz, M. D., Dalakos, M., Leh, R.L., *et al.* (1989). Current concepts in the idiopathic inflammatory myopathies: polymyositis, dermatomyositis, and related disorders. *Annals of Internal Medicine* **111**, 143–7.

Dalakos, M. C. (1991). Polymyositis, dermatomyositis and inclusion body myositis. *New England Journal of Medicine* **325**, 1487–98.

Polymyalgia rheumatica

Sewell, J. R. (1986). Polymyalgia rheumatica. *British Journal of Hospital Medicine* **35**, 299–301.

Muscular dystrophies

Brooke, M. H., Fenichel, G. M., Griggs, R. C., *et al.* (1989). Duchenne muscular dystrophy: patterns of clinical progression and effects of supportive therapy. *Neurology* **39**, 475–81.

Editorial (1988). Central core disease. *Lancet* **1**, 866.

Harley, H. G., Rundle, S. A., Reardon, W. *et al.* (1992). Unstable DNA sequence in myotonic dystrophy. *Lancet* **339**, 1125–8.

Roberts, R. G., Bentley, D. R., Barby, T. F. M., *et al.* (1990). Direct diagnosis of carriers of Duchenne and Becker muscular dystrophy by amplificiation of lymphocyte RNA. *Lancet* **336**, 1523–6.

Rowland, L. P. (1988). Clinical concepts of Duchenne muscular dystrophy. The impact of molecular genetics. *Brain*, **111**, 479–95.

Metabolic myopathies

Case records of the Massachusetts General Hospital (1986). (Acid maltase deficiency.) *New England Journal of Medicine*, **315**, 694–701.

Editorial (1989). Mitochondrial DNA and genetic disease. *Lancet* 1989 **1**, 250–1.

Editorial (1990). Carnitine deficiency. *Lancet* **335**, 631–2.

Goto, Y., Horai, S., Matsuoka, T. *et al.* (1992). Mitochondrial myopathy, encephalopathy, lactic acidosis, and stroke-like episodes (MELAS): a correlative study of the clinical features and mitochondrial DNA mutation. *Neurology* **42**, 545–50.

Hammans, S. R., Sweeney, M. G., Brockington, M., Morgan-Hughes, J. A., and Harding, A. (1991). Mitochondrial encephalopathies: molecular genetic analysis from blood samples. *Lancet* **337**, 1311–13.

Layzer, R. B. (1991). How muscles use fuel. *New England Journal of Medicine* **324**, 411–12.

Drug-induced myopathies

Blain, P. G. (1984). Adverse effects of drugs on skeletal muscle. *Adverse Drug Reaction Bulletin* **104**, 384–7.

Editorial (1987). Colchicine myoneuropathy. *Lancet* **2**, 668.

Toxic myopathies

Hodgson, P. (1984). Alcoholic myopathy. *British Medical Journal* **288**, 584–5.

Palmer, E. P. and Guay, A. T. (1985). Reversible myopathy secondary to abuse of ipecac in patients with major eating disorders. *New England Journal of Medicine* **313**, 1457–9.

Myasthenia gravis

Durelli, L., Maggi, G., Casadio, C., Ferri, R., Rendine,

S., and Bergamimi, L. (1991). Actuarial analysis of the occurrence of remissions following thymectomy for myasthenia gravis in 400 patients. *Journal of Neurology, Neurosurgery and Psychiatry* **54**, 406–11.

Fonseca, V. and Havard, C. W. H. (1990). The natural course of myasthenia gravis. *British Medical Journal* **300**, 1409–10.

Ousterhuis, H. J. G. H. (1989). The natural course of myasthenia gravis: a long term follow up. *Journal of Neurology, Neurosurgery and Psychiatry* **52**, 1121–7.

Myasthenic syndrome

McEvoy, K. M., Windebank, A. J. Daube, J. R. and Low, P. A. (1989). 3, 4-diaminopyridine in the treatment of Lambert–Eaton myasthenic syndrome. *New England Journal of Medicine* **321**, 1567–71.

O'Neill, J. H., Murray, N. M. F., and Newsom-Davis, J. (1988). The Lambert–Eaton myasthenic syndrome. A review of 50 cases. *Brain* **111**, 577–96.

Congenital myasthenic syndromes

Engel, A. G. (1988). Congenital myasthenic syndromes. *Journal of Child Neurology* **3**, 233–46.

The stiff-man syndrome

Solimena, M., Folli, F., Aparasi, R., Pozza, G., and de Camilli, P., (1990). Autoantibodies to GABAergic neurons and pancreatic β-cells in stiff-man syndrome. *New England Journal of Medicine* **322**, 1555–60.

Cramps

Henry, J. (1985). Quinine for night cramps. *British Medical Journal* **291**, 5.

Joekes, A. M. (1982). Cramp: a review. *Journal of the Royal Society of Medicine* **75**, 546–9.

22 Congenital defects of the nervous system, spina bifida, and hydrocephalus; cerebral palsy

The maturation of the developing nervous system, from first formation of the neural plate at about 18 days after conception to full myelinization many months after birth, depends upon the interaction of genetic and environmental factors. Some defects of neural development clearly originate from the effects of a maternal environmental agent acting during pregnancy. An example is hydrocephalus or microcephaly resulting from maternal rubella. Other defects are entirely dependent, as far as we are aware, on chromosomal abnormalities (e.g. Down syndrome) or genetic abnormalities (e.g. tuberous sclerosis). More often, there is a complex interaction between maternal environmental and genetic causes. For example, maternal rubella, or the use of sodium valproate for epilepsy during early pregnancy, clearly increase the risk of neural tube defects. However, genetic factors also play a part, as subsequent children of the same mother, unexposed on this occasion to sodium valproate, do have a risk of a neural defect that is substantially higher than the general population.

Pre-natal structural damage of the developing brain, or damage acquired during birth, or in the neonatal period, for example a parenchymal haemorrhage, may result in abnormalities of later motor development, known as congenital cerebral palsy (Section 22.4). Acquired cerebral palsy refers to similar syndromes resulting from insults such as infarcts or infections in later infancy.

In this book, a traditional division will be followed. Genetic disorders such as von Recklinghausen's neurofibromatosis and tuberous sclerosis are considered in other chapters (see Index). In this chapter, abnormalities of development of the neural tube, such as spina bifida, are first considered, followed by hydrocephalus and then by other disorders of neural development. Cerebral palsy is then considered in Section 22.4.

22.1 Spina bifida and other neural tube defects

22.1.1 *Epidemiology*

There are wide geographical differences in the incidence of neural tube defects, the rate being several times higher in the UK than in Asia. Even within the UK there are wide local variations in incidence. Furthermore, for uncertain reasons, the overall incidence is changing rapidly. The incidence of meningomyelocele and anencephaly, both at about 2 per 10 000 live births, is about one-third to one-half of what it was in 1972. Some of the difference can be accounted for by the selective abortion of affected fetuses discovered by pre-natal ultrasound scanning, but, even allowing for this, neural defects are less common than they were.

22.1.2 *Types of neural tube defect*

The neural plate begins to be infolded from the ectodermal plate at 18 days after conception. The infolding is rapidly pinched off dorsally so that a separate neural tube is formed between 22 and 26 days. Closure of the tube begins in the mid-dorsal region and proceeds rostrally and caudally, as does closure of the subsequently developing bony ele-ments, the vertebrae. Defects of closure, there-fore, are seen near the two ends of the neuraxis and spinal column. At the caudal end, the defect may be no more than a failure of fusion of verteb-ral spines at around L5 or S1. This so-called spina bifida occulta is seen on radiography of about 5 per cent of symptomless subjects, or of patients who are having lumbar X-rays for chronic low back pain, although there is no reason to suppose that the defect causes pain. A more prominent defect is an overlying dimple or plaque of unusually formed and often hairy skin in the lumbosacral region. A lipoma or dermal sinus may be associ-ated with such a lesion. More extensive defects result in a sac of meninges extending to the surface, a meningocele. If nerve roots or malformed dys-plastic cord tissue are incorporated into the sac the defect is known as a meningomyelocele. At the cephalic end of the neural tube, defects in devel-opment on closure may result in anencephaly—virtually no development of forebrain structures—hydrocephalus, or defects such as a meningocele or Arnold–Chiari malformation (Section 22.1.4) at the cranio-cervical junction.

22.1.3 *Causes of neural tube defects*

As already mentioned, both environmental and genetic factors seem to be important in the genesis of neural tube defects. However, the environ-mental factors have not been clearly identified. One example chosen above to illustrate this point, the use of sodium valproate for epilepsy in preg-nancy, is relevant in only a tiny proportion of those affected. Other environmental agents once con-sidered to be relevant, such as excessive maternal consumption of tea, or eating potatoes affected by blight, are not now thought to be relevant. Interest centres on the possible effect of relative vitamin deficiency during pregnancy, largely on the basis that vitamin supplementation around the time of conception appears to reduce the incidence of neural tube defects, although not all trials have shown such protective action.

That genetic factors are important is suggested (but not proved) by the fact that pregnancies subsequent to the birth of a child with a neural tube defect are more likely to result in a further child with a neural tube defect than would be expected by chance. Subsequent siblings carry a risk that is increased approximately tenfold com-pared to the risk for the population as a whole.

One feature that is unexplained on the basis of either a genetic or maternal environmental factor is the fact that if one monozygotic twin is affected, the other usually is not.

22.1.4 *Clinical features and management*

A meningocele may present as no more than a soft fluctuant subcutaneous mass, with no neurological involvement. More often the cyst, covered only with meninges, protrudes through the associated bony defect, increasing rapidly in size in the early days after delivery. Neural elements can be seen following a distorted course through the walls of the cyst. Sometimes the covering meninges are themselves deficient, and the dysplastic neural tissue is seen as a flattish plaque on the lumbar spine and sacrum.

If the meninges are deficient, or if the thin meningeal covering is damaged, bacterial menin-gitis rapidly supervenes. For this reason, many paediatricians formerly advocated surgical closure within the first 24 hours of life for all patients. However, the realization that many infants were being salvaged only to lead lives of very consider-able physical and cognitive disability has now led to a more selective approach. Paediatricians usu-ally do not now refer for immediate surgery infants with sacral meningomyeloceles with obvious high levels of paralysis, skeletal deformity, or hydro-cephalus. If the defect is not closed surgically, it usually does, in any event, become covered with epithelium if the child survives the early weeks.

Of considerable recent epidemiological interest is the observation that if the fetus is delivered by Caesarian section after pre-natal diagnosis by ultrasound scan, then the degree of motor paralysis is substantially less than in those infants delivered after a normal labour. It appears that the avoidance of labour-induced trauma to nerve roots should seriously be considered when planning delivery.

As the infant grows, varying degrees of neurological deficit will become apparent, dependent upon the level at which neural elements are involved. Almost always there is urinary and faecal incontinence, even if leg muscles are normally innervated. Higher lesions are accompanied by weakness of the feet and buttocks, and even higher lumbar lesions by a complete lumbar paraplegia. Sensation is affected also, so that, as the child grows, it becomes clear that there is little or no bladder or rectal sensation, and varying degrees of sensory loss on the lower limbs are found. The absence of normal neural input to the developing muscles of the lower limbs results in varying degrees of deformity, of which 'club feet'—talipes and calcaneus deformities—are best known, but there may also be hyperextension of the knees, and fixed flexion at the hips. Many of the lesser deformities can be partly corrected by orthopaedic procedures, including transplanting the tendon of a normal muscle to take over the function of an affected muscle. Supportive calipers may also be necessary. Complex axial skeletal deformities (kyphoscoliosis) may also require orthopaedic management.

Hydrocephalus is associated with meningomyelocele in at least 50 per cent of children, and many of those who survive the early weeks will subsequently require the insertion of a shunt (Section 22.2.2). Cranial ultrasound and, after closure of the sutures, CT or MRI will often show ventricular dilatation, even if the head itself is not enlarged. Ventricular hydrocephalus and meningomyelocele may be associated with the Arnold–Chiari malformation. In this complex malformation the brain stem is displaced downwards, carrying the cerebellum with it, so that the cerebellar tonsils become impacted in the upper cervical canal. Imaging shows dilated third and lateral ventricles, and a fourth ventricle that is lying unusually low in the posterior fossa, which itself is often malformed. Lower cranial nerve palsies may result as the nerves are stretched downwards.

A further complication is the occurrence of large volume of residual urine. Hydronephrosis due to detrusor–sphincter dyssynergia and repeated urinary infections may lead to renal failure.

Children with lesser degrees of spinal dysraphism also require careful and continuing assessment. Even if the spina bifida is occult, there may be an associated diastematomyelia (a divided spinal cord which may override a bony spur), or a spinal cord that is tethered by a tight filum terminale, or other fibrous band connecting the cord with a lipoma or other maldeveloped mass of tissue. As the child grows, the tight tethering and consequent stretching of the cord and nerve roots result in progressive neurological symptoms. These include asymmetrical development of muscle bulk of the legs, weakness, incontinence, and trophic ulceration of the feet.

A child with a tethered cord may develop any of these abnormalities as he or she grows, but it does not seem that their occurrence is necessarily related to linear growth, as neurological deterioration can occur at times other than those of rapid axial growth. A child with a cutaneous abnormality over the lower back, and with spina bifida should be observed carefully during development for the onset of neurological troubles, particularly the insidious onset of neurogenic bladder. Some surgeons believe that a tethered cord demonstrated by MRI should be released before the onset of neurological disability. Children with a lumbosacral lipoma and tethered cord appear to do best if operated on in infancy.

22.1.4.1   Other neural tube defects

In anencephaly there is no development of the forebrain. The skull vault is usually absent, and the anterior pituitary gland may also be absent or hypoplastic. The survival of such children is limited, but brain-stem responses allow sucking and feeding, crying, and facial grimacing. In other infants a meningoencephalocele is present, usually in the occipital region.

22.1.5   Prenatal diagnosis and prevention

Ultrasound scanning will readily detect anencephaly and some cases with a meningocele or a meningomyelocele. However, these sacs are often of comparatively small volume at birth, expanding only as the child is born free of its flotation system within the amniotic cavity in which pressures are uniform. Fortunately, however, infants with open spina bifida and anencephaly can be detected by the presence of elevated levels of α-fetoprotein in the maternal serum and amniotic fluid. Screening in this way is essential for women who have been delivered of a previously affected infant, as the risks of a second affected infant are considerable (Section 22.1.3).

22.1.6 *Prognosis*

The prognosis for survival and quality of life depends upon the extent, site, and type of the lesion. Approximately one-third of children whose meningomyelocele was not operated upon in the early days (on account of factors considered to be unfavourable) will survive to enter school 5 years later. About one-third of all survivors will be wheelchair-bound, or have their mobility severely limited. About 85 per cent will be incontinent of urine, and by the age of 16, the upper renal tracts of about 40 per cent will already be compromised. Multiple admissions to hospital for urinary infections and stones, and for pressure sores, are common.

22.2 Hydrocephalus

Some of the siblings of children with meningo-myelocele will have hydrocephalus without spina bifida, suggesting that genetic factors operate in some cases of hydrocephalus. In some, the Arnold–Chiari malformation is present. Other cases of hydrocephalus are due to atresia of the exit foramina of Luschka and Magendie, through which drains the cerebrospinal fluid from the fourth ventricle into the subarachnoid space. In this condition, known as the Dandy–Walker syndrome, the fourth ventricle and third and lateral ventricles are dilated, and the cerebellum hypoplastic. In aqueduct stenosis, the obstruction lies in the aqueduct between the third and fourth ventricles, and only the third and lateral ventricles are dilated. Aqueduct stenosis may be induced by intrauterine infection with cytomegalovirus and other viruses.

Hydrocephalus may also be due to postnatal influences. An example of the obstructive or non-communicating type is aqueduct stenosis due to post-meningitic ependymitis. Other causes include posterior fossa tumours, such as a medulloblastoma. Meningitic infiltrates, especially tuberculous infiltrates, may prevent the free circulation of CSF to the arachnoid villi. This is known as a communicating hydrocephalus.

22.2.1 *Clinical features*

Pre-natal hydrocephalus in developed countries is often now diagnosed by pre-natal ultrasound scanning, but in other cases hydrocephalus may prevent or cause difficulties in vaginal delivery. After birth, obvious degrees of hydrocephalus are noted both by parents and physicians, but lesser degrees are overlooked unless proper recourse is made to a centile chart of cranial circumference. Older signs, such as transillumination and an unusual note on percussing the head, have been replaced by modern imaging techniques, which reveal the anatomy very well.

There may well be other clinical features associated with the hydrocephalus, depending upon its cause and severity. There may be a general failure to thrive and a failure of social and motor development.

22.2.2 *Treatment*

Clinical observations and serial imaging will sometimes suggest that the hydrocephalus has 'arrested'. That is to say, a balance has been struck between production and absorption of cerebrospinal fluid. In other cases, a progressive enlargement of the ventricles and/or head requires the insertion of a shunt between ventricles and atrium or peritoneum. Shunt revision as the child grows may be necessary. Other drawbacks include shunt blockage by choroid plexus, or the colonization of the shunt by bacteria such as *Staphylococcus epidermidis* (see Section 17.3). In some cases chronic infection leads to a so-called shunt nephritis, due to the deposition of antibody complexes in the glomeruli.

The overall prognosis for children with hydrocephalus is poor, even in the absence of spina bifida. By the age of 10, one-third will be dead, and only one-third will be able to attend a normal school, the remaining third having some degree of intellectual retardation.

22.3   Other congenital anomalies

Hydranencephaly is the absence of the greater part of the cerebral hemispheres, although, in contrast to anencephaly, a normal skull vault is found. Encephaloceles are similar in embryogenesis to spina bifida. Megalencephaly is the word used to describe a large brain inside a large head. Sometimes no specific cause emerges; other cases have tuberous sclerosis or a lipidosis. Disorders of neural development and migration may result in agenesis of the corpus callosum, or abnormalities of development of the cortical mantle, leading to a diminution or distortion of the gyri (lissencephaly).

Microcephaly indicates a small brain and head, due either to developmental hypoplasia or as part of a complex associated malformation, or as the result of pre-natal damage. Porencephaly is the name given to a localized cyst in a developing brain, usually the result of an infarction in the perinatal period. Such cysts are often associated with seizures but, as the rest of the brain is normal, development is usually satisfactory. Arachnoid cysts are benign cysts of uncertain origin, filled with cerebrospinal fluid. They often arise in the middle cranial fossa, and may be associated with epilepsy.

Arteriovenous malformations (Section 10.6.6) are congenital malformations that usually present later in life with haemorrhage or epilepsy, but a malformation of the great vein of Galen may cause a shunt of such flow-rate that the infant has cardiac failure. This malformation may also cause an obstructive hydrocephalus.

The Sturge–Weber syndrome is the association of a 'port-wine' cutaneous naevus in the upper part of the trigeminal distribution with meningeal angiomatosis on the surface of the posterior part of the ipsilateral hemisphere, this malformation often causing epilepsy. The cutaneous naevus may be associated with ipsilateral glaucoma.

Congenital malformations may also affect the skull, and secondarily produce neurological deficits. Premature closure of the sutures (craniosynostosis) is usually associated with retardation, especially if sutures other than the sagittal are affected. Early operation, before 6 weeks, may prevent retardation. Artificial 'sutures' are made, and prevented from early fusion by stripping back the pericranium.

Anomalies of development may also affect the base of the skull. The posterior fossa may be unduly small (platybasia), or the odontoid peg and rim of the foramen magnum may invaginate into the posterior fossa. Such anomalies may be associated with an Arnold–Chiari malformation (Section 22.1.4), hydrocephalus (Section 22.2), or syringomyelia (Section 18.5.4.1).

22.4   Cerebral palsy

Cerebral palsy is an inclusive term that describes a group of non-progressive disorders occurring in young children in which disease of the brain affects motor function. The disorder of motor function may be impaired control of dexterous movements (a pyramidal lesion), incoordination, or dystonia. Progressive neurological disease due, for example, to inherited abnormalities of lipid metabolism are excluded by convention, as are those rare disabilities due to perinatal spinal cord injury. Even though progressive disorders are excluded, however, the effects of a static lesion are manifest by different clinical pictures at different ages, due to the interaction of the static lesion with other maturing areas of the young brain. For example, a child who has a flaccid hemiplegia at birth may later develop spasticity and dystonic movements in the affected limbs.

Although the motor effects of a brain lesion are often the most prominent clinically, it is clear that a brain lesion will seldom be so discrete as to affect motor pathways exclusively. Defects of motor function are therefore often associated with mental retardation, epilepsy, visual disturbances, and squints. Such associations by no means affect all cases, however, and preserved intelligence may be trapped in a body grossly handicapped by cerebral palsy.

22.4.1   *Epidemiology*

There are some confusions about the terms 'incidence' and 'prevalence rates' in enumerating cases of cerebral palsy. For example, if a survey is made at age 6 months, and expressed as cases per 1000 live births, many neurological lesions that will

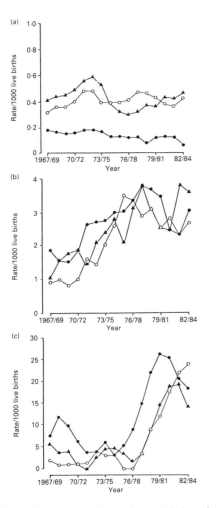

Fig. 22.1 The relationship between birth weight and the incidence of cerebral palsy: (a) birth weight >2500 g; (b) birth weight 1501–2500 g; (c) birth weight ≤1500 g. In all cases a three-year moving average was used, (▲) Quadriplegia; (●) diplegia; (○) hemiplegia. (Reproduced by permission from Pharoah *et al.* 1990.)

become apparent only as the child develops will be missed. Surveys done at the age of 5 years will fail to include those who have died earlier of their lesions. A generally accepted prevalence is that there will be two children with handicapping cerebral palsy alive at school age resulting from every 1000 live births. This is a figure that is remarkably constant among industrialized nations, and there is no evidence of any decline in the past 50 years.

The male to female ratio is about 1.5:1, suggesting a gender difference in susceptibility to pre-natal causes of cerebral palsy (see below).

22.4.2 *Causes of cerebral palsy*

Little, a London orthopaedic surgeon, first described spastic diplegia, the most common form of cerebral palsy, in 1862. He held that defects in obstetric care were largely responsible for cases of cerebral palsy. This belief has continued amongst many until today, and presumably accounts for the large malpractice premiums demanded of obstetricians in the United States. One of the many contributions of Sigmund Freud, in his first career as a neurologist, was, in 1897, to draw attention to the importance of pre-natal factors. He proposed that abnormalities of labour and delivery were often markers of pre-natal fetal abnormality, rather than themselves the cause of cerebral palsy. Whatever the causes, there is a strong association with low birth weight (Fig. 22.1). The bottom part of Fig. 22.1 gives cause for concern that the salvaging of very low birth weight infants by modern techniques of neonatal care may add to the burden of cerebral palsy in the community. There is also a strong association with social class, mothers of lower socio-economic class being more likely to bear children with cerebral palsy, particularly children with diplegia and hemiplegia. This association is only partly accounted for by the greater tendency of lower socio-economic classes to have higher pre-term birth rates.

The development of neonatal ultrasound scanning has led to the recognition of cerebral abnormalities that are likely to be associated with the later development of cerebral palsy. The initial orientation of the circulation of the developing fetus is to the central structures of brain stem and basal ganglia, and only later in development is cortical perfusion enhanced. Any failure of fetal oxygenation, for example due to placental insufficiency associated with toxaemia, may affect areas of marginal perfusion. Hypoxia–ischaemia in these areas is recognized on the ultrasound scan as periventricular zones of low density, known as periventricular leucomalacia. These zones show areas of gliosis and microscopic calcification on histological examination. These appearances are associated with a high incidence of pre-term delivery, and with the later development of spastic

Table 22.1   Types of cerebral palsy

	Percentage of cases	Associations	Neonatal ultrasound
Spastic diplegia	30	Often pre-term birth, usually weight appropriate for gestational age	Periventricular leucomalacia
Spastic diplegia with ataxia	15	Often pre-term birth, usually weight appropriate for gestational age	Periventricular leucomalacia
Tetraplegia	5	Very low birth weight, often small for gestational age, if term, may be due to post-natal infection	Periventricular leucomalacia
Hemiplegia	25	Often term births; sometimes adverse late intrapartum factors	If pre-term, may have periventricular haemorrhage due to venous infarction
Dyskinetic syndrome	10	Often term births; perinatal factors such as asphyxia and kernicterus are important	
Ataxia	5	Often genetic factors	
Unclassifiable	10		

diplegia, the most frequent type of cerebral palsy (Table 22.1). Diplegia with ataxia seems to be a very similar syndrome, and the rare cases of tetraplegia probably only a more pronounced version of spastic diplegia. Factors that affect the rate of fetal development may be implicated in the aetiology of spastic diplegia at all gestations. Hemiplegia, on the other hand, is associated with adverse late intrapartum factors, and the neonatal scan often shows asymmetrical areas of parenchymal haemorrhage due to venous infarction. Haemorrhage in the lateral ventricles, or confined to the germinal matrix, does not significantly increase the probability of later cerebral palsy. If the neonatal ultrasound scan shows ventricular dilatation, hydrocephalus, or cerebral atrophy, then there is a high rate of subsequent disabling neurological impairment, as these observations presumably reflect the degree of damage to neurons and their processes.

It must be recognized that, even though ultrasound scanning has led to a better understanding of the pathology of cerebral palsy, it adds little to our understanding of the cause. Pre-natal associations include genetic factors, social class, mater-

nal infections, pre-eclampsia, relative infertility, previous history of pre-term delivery, antepartum haemorrhage, multiple pregnancy, and even a very long maternal pre-conceptional menstrual cycle. However, there are so many interactions between these factors that the contribution of each is difficult to assign. Perinatal factors, such as breech delivery, birth asphyxia (low Agpar score and acidosis), and respiratory distress syndrome associated with cerebral haemorrhage, have often been blamed for cerebral palsy, but more recent studies show that their contribution to the total number of cases is small. Particularly convincing evidence of the role of pre-natal factors is the association of cerebral palsy with congenital malformations outside the nervous system. The relative risk of congenital malformations in a child with cerebral palsy compared to a normal child is 4:1.

It is unlikely that further improvements in obstetric management will reduce the incidence of cerebral palsy much below its present level. Continuous intrapartum monitoring, for example, has recently been shown to be of no value in reducing the incidence of cerebral palsy, although encouraging a greater rate of operative intervention. The situation is best summarized as follows: birth asphyxia has a low predictive value for cerebral palsy; most cases of cerebral palsy have no evidence of birth asphyxia.

Recent studies using magnetic resonance spectroscopy show considerable promise in predicting outcome. If the ratio between phosphocreatine and inorganic phosphate is low, then there is a high probability of death or multiple impairments.

About 10 per cent of cases of cerebral palsy arise from post-natal causes. Infections such as pertussis, and injury, including non-accidental injury, are important causes. Profound dehydration associated with gastrointestinal infections in developing countries may result in cerebral infarction.

22.4.3   Treatment

It is natural for mothers of handicapped babies to assume that appropriate intervention by therapists will improve neurological development, a belief supported by many of the therapists themselves. A number of controlled trials suggest that no benefit accrues from physical therapy, but some benefit results from what is termed 'infant stimulation'. This may be no more than 'a better or broader understanding by the parents of their infant's development and capacities, which may improve their ability to cope with and interact with their infant'. This quotation comes from the Baltimore study by Palmer and colleagues. The authors also remark that the 'motor and mental capacities at the time of enrollment were the most powerful determinants of . . . outcome, strongly outweighing any effects of treatment'. That is to say, the children with relatively minor disabilities do well, and those with severe disabilities do badly, whatever the treatment.

Children with abnormalities of posture can often be improved by appropriate orthopaedic procedures. A commonly performed operation lengthens the Achilles tendon and allows the heels of a child with an equinus deformity, due to spastic diplegia, to reach the ground, allowing the child to walk more normally. The long-term benefits of this are, however, uncertain. There are, of course, other aspects to 'treatment', including appropriate parental counselling, advising about education, and aids to mobility and to daily living (see Chapter 26).

22.5   Further reading

Neural tube defects

Ethical working group (1985). The prognosis for babies with meningomyelocele and high lumbar paraplegia at birth. *Lancet* **2**, 996–7.

Hobbins, J. C. (1992). Diagnosis and management of neural tube defects today. *New England Journal of Medicine* **324**, 690–1.

Luthy, D. A., Wardinsky, T., Shurtleft, D. B., Hollenbach, K. A., Hickok, D., Nyberg, D. A. and Benedetti, T. J. (1991). Caesarian section before the onset of labor and subsequent motor function in infants with meningomyelocele diagnosed antenatally. *New England Journal of Medicine* **324**, 662–6.

MRC Vitamin Study Group (1991). Prevention of neural tube defects: results of the MRC vitamin study. *Lancet* **338**, 131–7.

Menzies, R. G., Parkin, J. M., and Hey, E. N. (1985). Prognosis for babies with meningomyelocoele and high lumbar paraplegia at birth. *Lancet* **2**, 993–7.

Mills, J. L., Rhoads, G. G., Simpson, J. L., *et al.* (1989). The absence of a relation between the periconceptional use of vitamins and neural tube deficits. *New England Journal of Medicine* **321**, 430–5.

Rickwood, A. M. K., Hodgson, J., Lonton, A. P., and Thomas, D. G. (1984). Medical and surgical complications in adolescent and young adult patients with spina bifida. *Health Trends* **16**, 91–6.

Seller, M. J. (1987). Unanswered questions on neural tube defects. *British Medical Journal* **294**, 1–2.

Cerebral palsy

Dowding, V. M. and Barry, C. (1990). Cerebral palsy: social class differences in prevalence in relation to birthweight and severity of disability. *Journal of Epidemiology and Community Health* **44**, 191–3.

Editorial (1988). What causes cerebral palsy. *Lancet* **1**, 142–3.

Graham, M. Trounce, J. Q. Levene, M. I., and Rutter, N. (1987). Prediction of cerebral palsy in very low birth weight infants: prospective ultrasound study. *Lancet* **2**, 593–6.

Pharoah, P. O. D., Cooke, T., Cooke, R. W. I., and Rosenbloom, L. (1990). Birthweight specific trends in cerebral palsy. *Archives of Diseases of Childhood* **65**, 602–6.

Stanley, F. and Alberman, E. (ed.) (1984). *The epidemiology of the cerebral palsies*, Spastic International Medical Publications, Clinics in Developmental Medicine No. 87. Blackwell, Oxford.

Stanley, F. J. and Watson, L. (1992). Trends in perinatal mortality and cerebral palsy in Western Australia. *British Medical Journal* **304**, 1658–63.

Veen, S., Ens-Dokkum, M. H., Schreuder, A. M., Verloove-vanhorick, S. P., Brand, R., and Ruys, J. H. (1991). Impairments, disabilities and handicaps of very preterm and very-low-birthweight infants at five years of age. *Lancet* **338**, 33–6.

Volpe, J. J. (1989). Intraventricular haemorrhage in the premature infant. Current Concepts Parts I and II. *Annals of Neurology* **25**, 3–11, 109–16.

Treatment

Editorial (1988). Physical therapy in spastic diplegia. *Lancet* **2**, 201–2.

Palmer, F. B., Shapiro, B. K., Wachtel, R. C., *et al*. (1988). The effects of physical therapy on cerebral palsy. A controlled trial in infants with spastic diplegia. *New England Journal of Medicine* **318**, 802–8.

Park, T. S. and Owen, J. H. (1992). Current concepts: surgical management of spastic diplegia in cerebral palsy. *New England Journal of Medicine* **326**, 745–9.

23 Some disorders caused by genetic, metabolic, toxic, or immunologically mediated damage to the nervous system

Although all clinical disorders presumably have a metabolic basis, this chapter describes those in which the genetic or metabolic component is reasonably well understood.

23.1 Inherited metabolic diseases

Virtually all inherited metabolic disorders are rare, and many can be described as exceptionally rare. The classic text '*The metabolic basis of inherited disease*' runs to more than 3000 pages. The end pages of that book show a map of the morbid anatomy of the human genome dated 10 July 1989, which is already much out of date, such is the 'avalanche of new material'. A detailed discussion is therefore out of place in a book this size, and only general principles will be given, and brief notes about some of the better-known genetic disorders affecting the nervous system.

All biochemical processes are resolvable into a series of stepwise reactions; each biochemical reaction is under the ultimate control of a single gene; mutation of a single gene results in an alteration of the ability of the cell to carry out a single biochemical reaction; the aggregate of our genes determines our biochemical individuality; our individuality determines our biological outcomes.

In some disorders, the effect of a single mutant gene is so powerful that biological outcome is almost entirely dependent upon that gene alone. Duchenne dystrophy could be considered a good example of that type of disorder. Short of a boy, affected by Duchenne dystrophy, being knocked down at the age of 7 by a car and killed (an environmental factor), his biological career is doomed to progressive weakness and a premature death in his late 'teens. In other disorders, genes at other loci may influence the outcome considerably. An example is hypercholesterolaemia, associated with early mortality from coronary artery disease, which may in turn be influenced by a number of genes leading to hypertension, an associated risk factor also leading to a premature death from arterial disease. Yet other genes may be modified by the environment. An example here is the risk of small-cell cancer, the gene for which is carried on chromosome 3, but the risk is modified by cigarette smoking. It follows that in a book of this type, it is an entirely arbitrary decision as to where to place any of the disorders described in the preceding chapters—it is entirely a matter related to ease of use (I hope) that Duchenne dystrophy is placed in the chapter on muscle disorders rather than here.

Genetic disorders are usually considered as falling into one of three categories. *Chromosomal disorders* involve the deficiency or excess in number of chromosomes, or abnormal arrangement of one or more chromosomes. Many genes are therefore affected by these genetically massive faults. Down syndrome (trisomy-21) is an example of such a disorder.

Mendelian disorders are determined by a single mutant gene carried on the autosomes or sex chromosome. The disorder is dominantly transmitted if a clinical phenotype is manifest when an individual has a single copy of the allele (i.e. is heterozygous). The disorder is recessively inherited if the clinical phenotype occurs only when both alleles on autosomes are defective (i.e. homozygous).

The heterozygote phenotype may be clinically entirely normal in the case of some gene disorders, and yet have subtle biological differences from those homozygous for the normal allele. In Duchenne dystrophy, to continue our example, it has been known for years that heterozygotes have slightly higher serum phosphocreatine kinase levels than the norm, and occasional degenerate muscle fibres on biopsy. Occasionally, the number of affected fibres is such that the female heterozygote is mildly weak. In this sex-linked disorder, 'occult' phenotypic expression in the heterozygote carrier is due to the random inactivation of one X-chromosome (the Lyon hypothesis). Clones of cells containing the Duchenne gene deletion will be present, and, depending upon the proportion, the heterozygote carrier will show some dystrophin deficiency, with the 'occult' effects noted.

At a molecular level, both alleles in heterozygotes may be active. For example, in sickle-cell disease, electrophoretic separation of haemoglobins from heterozygotes will show that both HbS and HbA are produced.

It is theoretically possible for an individual to have two copies of a mutant dominant allele, i.e. to be homozygous for a dominant disorder. In this case, the disorder is usually exceptionally severe. In the case of Huntington's disease, however, the homozygote appears to have the same phenotype and natural history as the heterozygote. This suggests that in the (much more) usual case of heterozygous Huntington's disease, the mutant allele is truly dominant at a cellular level, the other allele making no contribution to cellular metabolism.

The third category is that of *germ cell disorders*. While there is a 50 per cent risk that the offspring of an individual with an autosomal dominant disorder will inherit the disease, it is not necessarily true that all affected individuals must have an affected parent. Leaving aside the well-known dictum that *pater non certus est* (non-paternity), mutations may arise in the germ cells of a parent who is otherwise homozygous for the healthy allele. New mutations in some disorders are rather more likely in the germ cells of older fathers. Mutations of recessive genes presumably also occur, but they are usually unidentified, because they result in an asymptomatic heterozygote.

23.1.1   *Variation in clinical expression (expressivity)*

With regard to autosomal dominant disorders, a classical phenotype may arise from apparently unaffected parents for reasons other than non-paternity or germ cell mutation—one parent may indeed carry the faulty gene but have no phenotypic expression of the gene. Or a sophisticated paraclinical examination may be necessary to determine a hint of expression. An example is myotonic dystrophy, in which, in some individuals, subcortical lenticular opacities may be the only phenotypic evidence of the abnormal allele (Section 21.7.1).

Such variation in clinical expression (expressivity) may be due to the effects of other genes, which modify the expression of the mutant allele, or, in the case of other disorders, environmental factors, as noted above. As identical twins with genetic disorders may also show some variation in expressivity, stochastic factors presumably also play a part.

It is also now realized that variations in mutations at a single locus, or a variation in length of deletion at a single locus, will result in considerable variations in clinical expression (allelic heterogeneity). 'Milder' mutations do not totally eliminate the production and/or function of the gene product. Only when the gene product is below levels to maintain intracellular metabolism do clinical symptoms and overt phenotypes occur. The mild Becker and more severe Duchenne dystrophies are examples of allelic heterogeneity, both being due to deletions of varying length on the X-chromosome. Conversely, phenotypes can appear initially clinically similar, even with different non-allelic mutations. Examples are the major clinical types of Charcot–Marie–Tooth disease (Section 19.3.8). Simple investigation such as electrodiagnostic studies and nerve biopsy, however, will show that some have quite different physiological and histological characteristics. Genetic investigation of a population of patients clinically diagnosed as having Charcot–Marie–Tooth disease will show autosomal dominant, autosomal recessive, and X-linked forms. That is to say, clinically similar phenotypes may result from mutations at widely separated chromosomal sites (non-allelic heterogeneity).

23.1.2   Chromosomal abnormalities

23.1.2.1   Down syndrome

Down syndrome is the most common cause of mental retardation due to genetic causes. The incidence in live-born children is about 1 per 650. Physical characteristics include oblique, upslanting palpebral fissures, a short (brachycephalic) head, with a flat bridge to the nose and a narrow palate, hyperflexibility and loose skin on the nape of the neck, short, broad hands with a transverse palmar crease and with a short fifth finger, which is often incurved, and a gap between the first and second toes. There is marked hypotonia and developmental delay. Other congenital lesions affecting the heart and gastrointestinal tract are frequent. Older children may have atlanto-axial instability.

Down syndrome is the phenotypic expression of an extra copy of chromosome 21 in the genome, whether the extra copy is free or fused to another. In most cases the extra copy is derived from the mother. There is a strong association with maternal age.

The pathological changes of Alzheimer's disease are virtually universal in the brains of all people with Down syndrome surviving to age 35. This is of great theoretical interest in relation to the aetiology of Alzheimer's disease in the general population. Acute leukaemia is also very common in children with Down syndrome, the risk being about 20 times that of the general population. The mechanism whereby the excess genetic material in chromosome 21 results in the phenotypic changes, and in the 'complications' such as Alzheimer's disease and leukaemia is uncertain.

Trisomy 13 (Patau syndrome) and trisomy 18 (Edwards syndrome) also occur. The associated congenital anomalies are more severe than Down syndrome, and the infants do not long survive.

23.1.2.2   Fragile-X syndrome

This is the second most common cause of mental retardation, and to a large extent accounts for the excess of males over females in institutions for the care of mentally retarded people. The term fragile-X is used because cytogenetic studies under certain conditions demonstrate a constriction towards the end of the long arm of the sex chromosome, which gives the appearance that it might break off. The gene locus is at Xq27.3. Affected boys have a rather long face, big ears, and big testes. Recent studies suggest that an unstable region of DNA at this site can expand in successive generations. This explains why about one-fifth of certain male carriers are phenotypically and cytogenetically normal, having a small 'pre-mutational' DNA abnormality and why about one-third of heterozygote women are somewhat mentally retarded, having a large 'dose' of abnormal DNA on one of their X chromosomes.

23.1.3   Chromosomal microdeletions

The microscopically visible chromosomal disorders, of which the fragile-X syndrome is one, shade into microdeletions of part of a chromosome that are not visible by light microscopy, but are expressed by the deletion of several contiguous genes over a length of chromosome. The Prader–Willi syndrome is one such microdeletion. The length deleted is so small that the inheritance is, for all practical purposes, Mendelian. Another example is a patient who had a complex phenotype which combined four known X-linked diseases (Duchenne dystrophy, chronic granulomatous disease, McLeod syndrome, and retinitis pigmentosum). It could be seen with high-resolution cytogenetic analysis that there was a very small deletion of the short arm of the X-chromosome. This gave the clue to the locus of the Duchenne gene. Deletion of the Duchenne gene by itself is not yet visible by cytogenetic analysis.

23.1.3.1 *Ataxia-telangiectasia*

Ataxia-telangiectasia is a genetic multisystem disorder inherited in an autosomal recessive manner. The disorder is genetically heterogeneous, with evidence suggesting chromosomal breaks sometimes on 14q and sometimes on 7q. DNA in fibroblasts from both homozygotes, and to a lesser extent from heterozygotes, is excessively sensitive to radiation damage and delayed repair.

The disease is characterized by the association of telangiectasia, involving principally the conjunctivae, and cerebellar ataxia, choreoathetosis, ocular motor apraxia, immunodeficiency (usually of immunoglobulins A and E), and a high incidence of neoplasia. The serum levels of α-fetoprotein and carcinoembryonic antigen are increased.

Progressive cerebellar ataxia is usually noted towards the end of the second year of life. Telangiectasia appear usually first on the bulbar conjunctiva and flexor aspects of the forearms a few years later.

Patients with ataxia-telangiectasia have a high incidence of lymphomas and T-cell leukaemia, and primary carcinomas of the breast, oral cavity and salivary glands and stomach occur. Heterozygotes also have an increased risk of neoplasia, particularly of breast cancer. Here there is a further example of the interaction of environmental and genetic factors. Breast cancer is distinctly more common in heterozygotes who have had thoracic radiation than those who have not.

23.1.4 *Mendelian disorders*

A greater degree of molecular understanding comes from those disorders that are recessively rather than dominantly inherited. Recessive disorders causing neurological diseases are often associated with the accumulation of a metabolite related to an already understood metabolic pathway. Examples are the mucopolysaccharidoses, the leucodystrophies, the aminoacidopathies, and the gangliosidoses. For dominant disorders, such as neurofibromatosis, myotonic dystrophy, tuberous sclerosis, and Huntington's disease, there is no storage product that helps identify the biochemical pathway involved. It is true that abnormal products such as 'amyloid' may accumulate, but it is not certain that these are not simply secondary cellular degradation products.

The chromosomal sites of some dominantly inherited genes have been identified by linkage analysis. Examples are myotonic dystrophy on 19q (Section 21.7.1.2), Huntington's disease on 4p (Section 13.6.2.4), neurofibromatosis 1 on 17p (Section 16.8.1.1) and 2 on 22q (Section 16.8.1.2), idiopathic torsion dystonia on 9 (Section 13.5), and tuberous sclerosis on 9q (Section 16.8.2). Because the mechanism of gene action has not been identified, these disorders are considered elsewhere in the book in the Sections indicated. A brief description of the metabolic abnormalities associated with some of the recessively inherited disorders follows.

23.1.4.1 *Muscle disorders*

The gene determining myophosphorylase deficiency (McArdle's disease; type V glycogenosis) is on chromosome 11q. Myophosphorylase cleaves the 1–4 bond of glycogen. Its absence results in accumulation of glycogen in the muscle. Histochemistry readily demonstrates the absence of the enzyme, and excess muscle glycogen. The patients characteristically present with muscle pain and weakness on exercise. Serum lactate falls or fails to rise during exercise, especially during ischaemic work. Phosphorus nuclear magnetic resonance shows an excessive reduction in phosphocreatine on exercise.

Phosphofructokinase deficiency (type VII glycogenosis) is a similar syndrome. Red cells are also affected by this deficiency, resulting in a mild haemolytic anaemia. Muscle phosphofructokinase deficiency (Tarui's syndrome) results in a complete block in muscle glycolysis and glycogenolysis, leading to muscular fatigue and cramping on exercise.

23.1.4.2 *Disorders of amino-acid metabolism*

The best known of these is phenylketonuria,

caused by a deficiency of phenylalanine hydroxylase. Detection of urinary ketone bodies at birth is now part of all child health screening programmes in developed countries. If undetected, high levels of phenylalanine, tyrosine, and phenylketoacids result in severe mental retardation, often accompanied by microcephaly and epilepsy. More severely affected children develop spastic paraparesis. Histopathologically, there is hypomyelination and vacuolation within the brain. Since the mid-1950s it has been known that feeding a diet deficient in phenylalanine can prevent the adverse effects of hyperphenylalanaemia, phenylketonaemia, and hypotyrosinaemia. There is very good epidemiological evidence that it is essential to continue a low phenylalanine diet well into adolescence.

Severe hyperammonaemia will result from deficiencies of any of the enzymes responsible for processing carbamoyl phosphate through citrulline, arginosuccinic acid, arginine, and ornithine, with the exception of arginase deficiency. Hyperammonaemia usually results in a severe encephalopathy in the new-born. Some children with partial enzyme activity present later in childhood with recurrent confusion and irritability, especially after high-protein meals. Arginase deficiency results in progressive mental retardation, spasticity, and occasionally choreoathetosis.

23.1.4.3 Disorders of branched-chain amino-acid metabolism

The characteristic odour of branched-chain ketoacids in the urine due to a deficiency of branched-chain α-ketoacid dehydrogenase has led to phenotypes being said to have 'maple syrup urine' disease. Patients are usually normal at birth, but lethargy, hypotonia, and convulsions soon occur, due to excessive tissue concentrations of the ketoacid derivates of leucine, isoleucine, and valine. As in phenylketonuria, dietary restriction of these branched-chain acids is beneficial to development. Early diagnosis is essential to prevent retardation. Infection or fasting commonly results in metabolic decompensation with increased serum levels of branched-chain acids, associated with metabolic acidosis and a potentially fatal encephalopathy. Dialysis or maintenance of nutrition by an intravenous solution deficient in these acids may resolve the crisis.

23.1.4.4 Disorders of peroxisome structure and biochemistry

Peroxisomes are tiny intracellular organelles concerned with sterol metabolism, peroxide metabolism, and fatty acid metabolism.

Zellweger syndrome
A complete absence of peroxisomes results in disturbed neuronal migration during development, and is one cause of microgyria and pachygyria—the Zellweger syndrome.

Adrenoleucodystrophy
This is a disorder of very long chain fatty acid metabolism, an X-linked disorder. Very long chain fatty acids accumulate in the cholesterol ester and ganglioside fractions of the white matter and in the adrenal cortex. The brain is also infiltrated by lymphocytes, but the significance of this is uncertain. It is possible to normalize plasma very long chain fatty acids by restricting the dietary intakes of these, and by dietary supplementation with oleic acid, but there is, as yet, no indication that the clinical course of progressive mental and psychological decline is affected. Adrenal infiltration results in Addison's disease. Characteristic changes are seen on MRI, with areas of high signal around the occipital horns of the lateral ventricles.

A milder form of the disorder, known as adrenomyeloneuropathy, also sex linked, usually presents in adolescents as Addison's disease. Yet another form is transmitted as an autosomal recessive.

Refsum disease
Patients with Refsum disease have an isolated deficiency of phytanic acid dehydroxylase. Phytanic acid is exclusively dietary in origin. Phytanic acid levels can be controlled by dietary measures, avoiding dairy products and the fats of ruminants.

The clinical features of Refsum disease include retinitis pigmentosa, peripheral neuropathy, ataxia, nerve deafness, and thickening of the skin.

23.1.4.5 Sterol storage disease

A deficiency of hepatic mitochondrial 26-hydroxylase allows the accumulation of cholestanol and cholesterol in brain, bile, and in the skin as xanthomas. The disorder is sometimes known as cerebrotendinous xanthomatosis. Sterol deposits replace much of the white matter. The disease results in dementia and spastic quadriparesis. The storage of further cholesterol and cholestanol can be inhibited by chenodeoxycholic acid.

23.1.4.6   Lysosomal disorders

Lesions of lysosomal enzymes allow undegraded or incompletely degraded macromolecules to accumulate in the lysosomes, distorting the anatomy and function of the cell. All are rare—together arising in perhaps 50 per 100 000 births—but they are of considerable theoretical interest.

Sphingolipidoses

Anderson–Fabry disease is the name given to an X-linked deficiency of α-galactosidase A, which results in the progressive lysosomal deposition of neutral glycosphingolipids. Deposition of sphingolipids in vascular endothelium results in premature stroke, or progressive renal failure. Unexplained but severe pain and paraesthesiae in the extremities are common. This may respond to carbamazepine. Characteristic vascular lesions ('angiokeratoma corpora diffusum') are found over the lower part of the trunk, clustered in a 'bathing trunk' distribution. Corneal opacities, myocardial involvement and hypo-hidrosis are other clinical features.

Deficiency of arylsulphatase A results in *metachromatic leucodystrophy*, in which cerebroside sulphate accumulates in the lysosomes. This results in progressive demyelination of central white matter, and of peripheral nerves. Progressive intellectual deterioration, weakness, progressive ataxia, paraparesis, and optic atrophy all occur. The age of onset is very variable, reflecting genetic heterogeneity.

Gaucher's disease is caused by a deficiency of lysosomal glucocerebrosidase. In type I, there is marked hepatosplenomegaly and bone marrow involvement, with no neural involvement. In type II disease, both viscera and nervous system are involved, and early death results. Type III disease presents with neurological involvement in later childhood.

Tay–Sachs disease is caused by a deficiency in β-N-acetylhexosaminidase A, resulting in accumulation of GM2 gangliosides. Progressive early infantile neurological deterioration is accompanied by a 'cherry-red spot' at the macula. The gene is largely confined to those of Ashkenazi Jewish stock.

Other sphingolipidoses are due to accumulation of galactocerebroside (Krabbe's disease), sphingomyelin (Niemann–Pick disease), ceramide (Farber's disease), and mucosulphatides. α-N-acetylgalactosaminidase deficiency is one cause of infantile neuroaxonal dystrophy.

Mucopolysaccharidoses

Mucopolysaccharides accumulate due to failure to degrade the glycosaminoglycans such as hyaluronic acid, chondroitin, and heparan. Those affecting the nervous system particularly are the Hurler, Hunter, and Sanfilippo types, all with mental retardation and other major somatic abnormalities.

There are a number of therapeutic strategies that have been tried for the lysosomal storage disorders, including orthotopic liver, spleen, or bone marrow transplantation and direct injection of enzyme, none of which has proved to be successful. The enzyme produced outside the brain cannot enter through the blood–brain barrier.

A strategy that has already proved successful for X-linked disorders is the biopsy of oocytes at the eight-cell stage, and the reimplantation only of those embryos that contain no Y-specific genetic material, as detected by amplification by the polymerase chain reaction.

23.1.4.7   Wilson's disease (synonym: hepatolenticular degeneration)

Wilson's disease is a rare autosomal recessive disorder, the gene lying on chromosome 13. The metabolic defect results in the accumulation of copper in the liver, brain, kidney, cornea, and bone. The clinical and biochemical manifestations are described in Section 13.5.5.

23.1.4.8   The porphyrias

Porphyrins are constructed of four pyrrole rings linked by methylenes. Haem is a porphyrin, which, besides its role in oxygen carriage, is concerned in the cytochrome P_{450} oxidase system. Partial deficiencies in the enzymes involved in the biosynthesis of haem result in a number of different syndromes.

Acute intermittent porphyria

δ-Aminolevulinic acid (ALA) synthetase is the

enzyme that mediates the condensation of glycine and succinyl coenzyme A to form ALA. This hepatic enzyme is inducible by drugs, in a fashion similar to the induction of hepatic hydroxylating enzymes by phenytoin (Section 12.8).

The next step in the porphyrin pathway is the conversion of ALA to porphobilinogen. This monopyrrole in turn is metabolized by porphobilinogen deaminase (also called uroporphyrinogen I synthetase) to form the tetrapyrrole, uroporphyrinogen.

Patients with acute intermittent porphyria have a dominantly inherited partial deficiency in porphobilinogen deaminase due to a faulty allele on chromosome 11. The deficiency rarely causes any problem until the flow through the porphyrin pathway is increased. The porphobilinogen deaminase cannot then cope with the increased production of porphobilinogen and this and ALA increase markedly. These biochemical changes result in abdominal pain, vomiting, constipation, hypertension, confusion, seizures, and peripheral neuropathy, which may be severe enough to require ventilation. The mental changes may mimic an acute psychosis, or behavioural changes suggestive of hysteria rather than confusion. Death may occur in an acute porphyric crisis. The diagnosis may be made by estimating the urinary excretion of porphobilinogen (normally <8 μmol/day). If present in great excess, the urine colours purple on standing.

Not all people with deficiencies of porphobilinogen deaminase necessarily express this clinically, for reasons which are not yet clear.

The most frequent inducers of ALA synthetase, increasing flow through the porphyrin pathway, are drugs, notably barbiturates, sulphonamides, griseofulvin, phenytoin, chlordiazepoxide, and ergot preparations. All these should be avoided in patients known to have porphyria, and the pharmacy consulted before *any* drug is prescribed.

Treatment of acute intermittent porphyria consists of controlling hypertension and tachycardia with propranolol. Seizures must not be treated with barbiturates, phenytoin, or carbamazepine, and recourse to bromides or paraldehyde is necessary. Glucose suppresses the activity of ALA synthetase, so a high-carbohydrate diet should be given. More specific suppression of ALA synthetase can be obtained by haematin infusions.

Variegate porphyria

This is most common in South Africa. Protoporphyrinogen oxidase is present in reduced amounts. The disorder presents with chronic skin eruptions and acute neuropsychiatric crises.

Hereditary coproporphyria

This is the least common of the porphyrias, and is due to a partial deficiency of coproporphyrin oxidase. The clinical features are similar to variegate porphyria, except that the skin lesions only occur in the acute attacks.

23.1.5 Disorders inherited through mitochondria

Mitochondria are cytoplasmic organelles containing a small quantity of DNA—the only site outside the nucleus in animals. The mitochondria play a central role in oxidative phosphorylation.

An individual's mitochondrial DNA is inherited from his or her mother, the sperm contributing none. This results in interesting patterns of inheritance for the disorders due to mutations in mitochondrial DNA—Leber's optic atrophy (see below) and the mitochondrial myopathies (Section 21.8.2).

23.1.5.1 Leber's optic atrophy

This is characterized by the acute or subacute loss of vision in young men, due to an optic neuropathy. The first change in vision is enlargement of the blind spot, the scotoma gradually extending towards fixation—a pattern of visual impairment different to multiple sclerosis, in which a paracentral scotoma first appears. Inspection of the optic fundus of an affected person shows a swollen hyperaemic optic disc, tortuous arterioles, and telangiectatic (dilated) vessels in the retina near the disc. Virtually all those who are affected are men, but as their sperm do not carry mitochondria, their children will not be affected. However, the male children of their sisters may be affected. Not all are, suggesting a possible interaction between nuclear and mitochondrial DNA.

Males in families with Leber's disease are more likely to be smokers than not. Metabolic studies suggest a failure to convert cyanide, present in tobacco smoke, to thiocyanate. Leber's subjects have been shown to be deficient in the enzyme thiosulphate sulphur-transferase (rhodanase), an intramitochondrial enzyme. Cobalamin may help reverse or prevent the visual loss associated with the abnormal gene.

23.2   Other metabolic events affecting the nervous system

23.2.1   *Hepatic encephalopathy*

In fulminant acute liver failure due to viral hepatitis, or in chronic hepatic failure secondary to cirrhosis, the patient may develop an encephalopathy characterized by clouding of consciousness (progressing to coma), incoordination, and a flapping tremor.

23.2.1.1   *Pathophysiology*

Ammonia is generated in the gut by colonic bacteria and mucosal enzymes acting on dietary protein. In a healthy liver, the ammonia reaching the liver through the portal system is detoxified to urea. In a failing liver, hyperammonaemia exists. This has a direct sedative effect, and also stimulates glucagon secretion, which leads to increased hepatic gluconeogenesis from amino acids, and further production of ammonia. When ammonia reaches the brain, it reacts with glutamic acid to form glutamine. The extent of the encephalopathy correlates reasonably well with CSF glutamine levels, but other malfunctions are probably also important, such as high serum levels of methionine, tryptophan, short-chain fatty acids, and octopamine, a 'false neurotransmitter' synthesized either by bowel bacteria or by the brain from excessive free amino acids. Ammonia detoxification in the brain is also inhibited in those with chronic hepatic encephalopathy, as levels of glutamine synthetase, the enzyme primarily responsible, are reduced.

The EEG in hepatic encephalopathy shows characteristic triphasic waves in paroxysmal bursts, and runs of delta waves.

The treatment of hepatic encephalopathy is by lactulose, a synthetic disaccharide which is metabolized by bacteria in the lower bowel, resulting in a reduction in pH. Ammonia is then trapped as ammonium ion, and excreted in the stool. Lactulose treatment can result in a substantial loss of free water, through osmotic diarrhoea, resulting in hypernatraemia. Another approach is to restrict protein intake and prevent bacterial decomposition of protein to ammonia by the use of oral neomycin or ciprofloxacin. The fact that a benzodiazepine antagonist can briefly reverse the depressed conscious level in hepatic encephalopathy suggests that inhibitory neurotransmitters such as GABA have an important role in its pathophysiology.

23.2.2   *Hyponatraemia*

Patients with hyponatraemia may present with, or develop, stupor, seizures and coma with serum sodium concentrations of less than 110–115 mmol/l. This situation may arise in patients with inappropriate secretion of antidiuretic hormone in association with, for example, bronchial carcinoma, or as part of a generalized metabolic disturbance secondary to severe hepatic disease, alcoholism, or major burns. Some patients with severe hyponatraemia develop central pontine demyelinating lesions (central pontine myelinolysis (CPM)). There has been some discussion as to whether CPM may be precipitated by too rapid a correction of serum sodium. A prospective MRI study indicated that an initially very low sodium, and a fast rate of correction, were both likely to be associated with CPM. It seems safest to keep the increase in serum sodium to less than 25 mmol/l in the first 48 hours of therapy, and to less than 2.5 mmol/l/hour at any time. CPM probably depends upon an osmotic shift rather than upon any specific property of the sodium ion.

23.2.3   *Hypoglycaemia*

The central nervous system uses oxidative metabolism as its only source of energy. If the blood sugar falls as a result of an insulin injection, or due to secretion from an insulinoma, there will be a marked adrenergic response with anxiety, palpitations, and sweating. Irritability and confusion follow. The symptoms are rapidly aborted by the ingestion of glucose. Sometimes markedly asymmetrical signs can occur, for example transient cranial nerve palsies or a hemiplegia. The reasons for such asymmetry in the context of a global metabolic disturbance are not clear.

Repeated episodes of hypoglycaemia will damage neurons in the middle layers of the cerebral cortex and hippocampus. Anterior horn cells are also selectively involved, resulting in distal wasting and weakness. Profound and long-lasting hypoglycaemia may result in a continuing coma with only partial recovery.

Although the blood sugar falls on starvation of healthy people, particularly some time after a heavy meal (reactive hypoglycaemia), there is little evidence that the light-headedness and dizziness and other vague symptoms reported are due to hypoglycaemia as such.

Recently, there has been a report of two infants with a defect in the protein that transports glucose across brain endothelial cells, resulting in a brain deficient in glucose in the presence of a normal blood sugar.

23.2.4   *Vitamin deficiencies*

23.2.4.1   *Deficiency of thiamine*

Deficiency of thiamine (vitamin B_1) and other B vitamins result in a peripheral neuropathy (Section 19.3.4) and of thiamine alone in Wernicke–Korsakoff encephalopathy (Section 23.4.2.4).

23.2.4.2   *Deficiency of pyridoxine*

Deficiency of pyridoxine (vitamin B_6) results in a confusional state. Pyridoxine deficiency may be induced by the therapeutic use of isoniazid, which increases the rate of pyridoxine excretion. Excessive xanthenuric acid will be found in the urine as a marker of pyridoxine deficiency.

23.2.4.3   *Deficiency of vitamin E*

Deficiency of vitamin E (α-tocopherol) can occur in patients with a lipid malabsorption syndrome, in cystic fibrosis, and in patients with abetalipoproteinaemia. Deficiency results in a peripheral neuropathy and ataxia due to dying back of the long fibres in the posterior columns of the spinal cord. Supplementation of the diet with large doses of vitamin E will prevent or partly reverse these abnormalities.

23.2.4.4   *Deficiency of vitamin B_{12}*

Deficiency of vitamin B_{12} (cobalamin) leads to two major syndromes. The first is attributable to impaired DNA synthesis, and is therefore most clearly expressed in rapidly dividing cells: in the bone marrow, where a deficiency results in a megaloblastic anaemia, on the surface of the tongue (a glossitis), and in the testes (hypospermia). The second or neurological syndrome, although classically associated with a megaloblastic (pernicious) anaemia, is not necessarily so, and can arise without any hint of anaemia. Cobalamin deficiency may affect the peripheral nervous system, resulting in distal tingling and numbness, and depression of the ankle reflexes. In more advanced cases, the lateral and posterior columns of the spinal cord degenerate—so-called subacute combined degeneration of the cord. As long as the diagnosis is made early, the symptoms and signs are reversed by cobalamin, which, if due to intrinsic factor deficiency, must be given by intramuscular injection.

It has been suggested that smoking may play a role in deciding whom of those deficient in cobalamin develops neurological symptoms. The suggestion is that cyanide in tobacco smoke converts cobalamin coenzymes to cyanocobalamin, which is metabolically inert. Certainly, one type of toxic amblyopia is attributable to heavy smoking, and responds, at least in part, to abstention and cobalamin supplements.

There are two cobalamin-dependent enzymes. One is concerned in a methyl transferase reaction, the regeneration of methionine from homocysteine, that indirectly affects DNA synthesis. The second, methylmalonyl CoA mutase, is concerned in the catabolism of fatty acids. It is not clear which enzyme is primarily concerned in the genesis of the neurological syndrome, but the second seems more likely as an accumulation of methylmalonyl CoA causes the incorporation of branched-chain fatty acids into myelin.

Cobalamin deficiency may also be one cause of the neuropsychiatric problems of old age. Certainly, a very low serum cobalamin can cause a dementing illness, and there has been increasing interest in the concept that 'low-normal' values, between 75 and 150 μg/ml may be associated with neuropsychiatric disease. Measurement of serum methylmalonic acid and serum total homocysteine levels has been suggested as confirmatory evidence that the low serum cobalamin is of biological importance in this older age-group. There are reports of improvement in cognitive function when cobalamin is given.

23.3 Neurological disorders due to external toxins

Many neurological syndromes are iatrogenic, induced by drugs. Examples include the ataxia and nystagmus associated with phenytoin toxicity, seizures secondary to isoniazid or the use of water-soluble contrast media, and neuropathies secondary to vincristine or amiodarone.

Other neurological syndromes are secondary to exposure to industrial agents. Examples include neuropathy secondary to exposure to *n*-hexane, acrylamide, or lead, premature vascular disease after prolonged exposure to cadmium sulphide, and an encephalopathy after exposure to lead or mercury. Debate continues on the extent to which environmental exposure to lead influences cognitive development, but there is renewed concern about this in the USA. Although there are good histopathological and electron-microscopic descriptions of these toxic effects, how the toxin works at a cellular level is often poorly understood.

Carbon monoxide may cause death by intoxication, but survivors may be demented and have prominent extrapyramidal signs. Urgent hyperbaric oxygenation is recommended.

Toxins present in food may cause profound neurological illness. Botulinum toxin (Section 17.7.2) causes irreversible neuromuscular blockade. Consumption of puffer fish, *Ciguatera* (turban shellfish), and bivalve and gastropod molluscs can all cause paralysis, including respiratory paralysis. Toxins within the flesh, roe, and liver block sodium channels in nerves. Shellfish are particularly likely to contain high levels of toxin when they have consumed certain dinoflagellate phytoplankton, which multiply in the sea as 'red tides' when thermal and other conditions are right. The puffer fish (*Fugu*) tetrodotoxin has been of great biological use in studying the physiology of neuromuscular transmission.

Another syndrome induced by the consumption of contaminated mussels has been shown to be due to domoic acid, produced by the marine vegetation *Nitzschia pungens*. Ingestion of contaminated mussels results in headache, seizures, agitation, and bizarre alternating hemiplegias. On recovery, those affected may have significant defects in memory and recall of visual material. Domoic acid is related to kainic acid, an agent that can act as a hyperexcitatory transmitter in experimental an-

imals, resulting in hippocampal neuronal damage. In those patients who died in the Canadian domoic acid event, severe neuronal loss was found in the hippocampus.

Finally, mention should be made of the organophosphorous compounds, used as insecticides. They produce an acute cholinergic crisis, due to the inhibition of acetylcholinesterase, followed by a delayed dying-back neuropathy. There is also evidence of permanent impairment of neuropsychological performance after acute exposure. Other organophosphorous compounds are stored as nerve gases in the event of war. It has been shown that pyridostigmine given *before* exposure protects a proportion of the total quantity of cholinesterase against subsequent attack by the nerve gas. When the nerve agent is metabolized, a proportion of pyridostigmine-bound cholinesterase dissociates from the pyridostigmine, so that a supply of uninhibited enzyme becomes biologically available. Initial treatment after exposure to nerve gases is atropine 2 mg, pralidoxime 500 mg, and diazepam 5 mg, self-administered by intramuscular injection.

23.4 Syndromes associated with excessive consumption of alcohol

Alcohol consumption is best measured in units—one unit is a single measure of spirits, a glass of sherry, a glass of wine, or a half pint of beer. Each of these contains about 8 g of alcohol. Epidemiological evidence suggests that weekly consumption of over 14 units a week by women and 21 units a week by men leads to a significantly increased mortality from accidents and cirrhosis.

Most developed countries now have defined blood alcohol limits above which an offence is committed if the subject drives. In the UK it is 80 mg per 100 ml. This level is likely to be exceeded if more than three units are drunk in an evening, and, in people of small build, may be exceeded by an even smaller consumption. There is good epidemiological evidence that motor vehicle accident rates are linked to the blood alcohol level, and there is no threshold blood level below which the accident rate is the same as that of those who have not consumed alcohol. It is likely that the threshold beyond which prosecution results will be reduced in future years. It is already lower in some countries.

23.4.1 *Acute intoxication*

Social drinking is enjoyable partly because of the mild release of some learned inhibitions that prevent enjoyable social discourse. It is, however, a narrow line between such pleasurable personal feelings and unwanted disinhibition that is a bore to one's friends.

The rapid consumption of large quantities of alcohol produces the well-recognized syndrome of drunkenness—slurring of speech, unsteadiness, poor motor coordination, nystagmus, and either maudlin depression or the release of previously inhibited personality defects of aggression and violence. Naïve young drinkers particularly are at risk from the further toxic effects of stupor and cardiorespiratory arrest, sometimes precipitated by the inhalation of vomit.

Those who drink excessively every day develop some tolerance to alcohol, by which they may show no clinical evidence of intoxication at blood levels that would severely incapacitate a naïve drinker. Tolerance probably involves adaptive changes in membrane lipids and neurotransmitter receptors. There is cross-tolerance between alcohol, benzodiazepines, and barbiturates, and the clinical symptoms of intoxication with each have much in common. This, and experimental evidence, suggest that one likely site for alcohol's intoxicating effect is a complex of membrane proteins containing a receptor for the inhibitory neurotransmitter γ-aminobutyric acid (GABA) and an associated chloride ion channel. A benzodiazepine inhibitor, R0 15-4513, binds to the benzodiazepine receptor and has been shown to reverse transiently the clinical manifestations of alcohol intoxication in spite of a continuing high blood alcohol level.

Subjects may be amnesic for all or part of a heavy drinking bout, even though their behaviour seemed normal (for them) in the course of the evening. Such episodes are reminiscent of transient global amnesia. The mechanism may be due to a transient disorder of serotoninergic transmission or of other neurotransmitters, such as glutamic acid.

Table 23.1 Neurological syndromes associated with alcohol

Acute intoxication
Withdrawal syndromes
   irritability, tremulous, anxiety—'the shakes'
   delirium tremens
   seizures
Syndromes associated with malnutrition
   the Wernicke–Korsakoff syndrome
   alcoholic neuropathy
Alcoholic dementia
Alcoholic cerebellar degeneration
Central pontine myelinolysis
The Marchiafava–Bignami syndrome
Alcoholic myopathy

23.4.2 *Chronic alcoholism*

Table 23.1 lists the neurological syndromes associated with chronic alcoholism.

23.4.2.1 *Withdrawal states*

Those who drink heavily refer to the 'morning shakes'—tremulousness, irritability, and a feeling of anxiety that is rapidly relieved by another drink ('a hair of the dog that bit me'). If the temptation to drink is resisted, the irritability and tremor decline slowly over the next 12 hours or so.

At a more advanced stage of chronic alcohol poisoning, the subject may, on withdrawal from alcohol, experience delirium tremens ('DTs'). After 2–3 days of increasing tremulousness, irritability, restlessness, and agitation, the subject develops vivid auditory and visual hallucinations. Consciousness may be clouded and the sleep–wakefulness cycle disturbed. Tonic–clonic seizures may occur. There is usually marked tachycardia, fever, sweating, and other autonomic phenomena. Many medical students and young doctors meet the syndrome for the first time when a patient who has drunk heavily for many years is admitted to hospital for a routine procedure, and is thereby deprived of alcohol. The syndrome of delirium tremens then supervenes unexpectedly on about the third hospital day.

The patient with delirium tremens should be nursed in a well-lit room, as one source of agitation is misinterpretation of objects or shadows in the room (illusions) as threats. The agitation may be so profound that the patient is a danger to himself or to his nurses. Sedation with diazepam, 40–50 mg/day orally, or chlormethiazole, 4 g/day orally, may be successful. If, as sometimes happens, the patients cannot be persuaded to take oral medication, then an intramuscular injection of haloperidol, 2–5 mg, can be given initially, in order to allow the establishment of an intravenous infusion of chlormethiazole. Chlormethiazole's beneficial effect may be due to blockade of alcohol receptors, a suggestion supported by the observation that some alcoholics are also addicted to chlormethiazole if they can obtain it.

Atenolol is also useful in reducing tachycardia and anxiety in delirium tremens. Thiamine supplementation should also be given, as many patients are likely to be vitamin deficient.

Patients with delirium tremens are at risk from intercurrent infection, and sometimes an intercurrent infection appears to precipitate an episode of delirium tremens. This will require its own specific treatment.

With vigorous treatment along the lines suggested here, an episode of delirium tremens usually settles with 3–7 days.

23.4.2.2 Alcohol and seizures

Seizures commonly occur in alcoholics, either as a direct effect of alcohol or, more commonly, on withdrawal, although there has been some recent evidence that the influence of withdrawal from alcohol in causing seizures is exaggerated. Long-term prophylactic medication is not usually effective in preventing seizures associated with alcoholism.

23.4.2.3 Syndromes caused by malnutrition

The high calorie content of alcohol, and the social disruption caused by chronic alcoholism result in many alcoholic patients failing to eat a proper diet. Thiamine deficiency plays a major part in the Wernicke–Korsakoff syndrome, and probably plays at least some part in the other syndromes next described.

23.4.2.4 The Wernicke–Korsakoff syndrome

Wernicke described, in 1881, two alcoholics who

developed a syndrome characterized by confusion, ataxia, and ophthalmoplegia. He also described a young woman with the same syndrome who had vomited repeatedly after poisoning by sulphuric acid—a hint already of the nutritional cause of Wernicke's encephalopathy. Six years later Korsakoff described a profound amnesic syndrome, with characteristic confabulation (the subject's invention of events in a conscious or unconscious attempt to conceal the gaps in the recollection of his life's events). More recently it has been realized that those who recover from an episode of Wernicke's encephalopathy may show a severe amnesic syndrome of the type described by Korsakoff. It is now clear that both have a common aetiological and pathological basis.

The initial symptoms are a mild confusion, dullness and apathy, and amnesia, particularly for recent events. A sudden ophthalmoplegia then occurs, with a complex mixture of disrupted eye movements and nystagmus. There is also marked ataxia of gait. Sometimes the focal brain-stem signs precede the onset of the organic mental state. If untreated, the disorder proceeds to coma and death. Histological examination shows varying degrees of vacuolation and disruption of myelinated fibres, with a proliferation of capillary endothelium and punctate haemorrhages. These are symmetrically placed around the inferior parts of the third ventricle, particularly in the region of the medial dorsal and anterior medial nuclei and mamillary bodies, and in the floor of the fourth ventricle, particularly in the region of the dorsal nucleus of the vagus and the vestibular nuclei. The anterior part of the cerebellum is also affected.

Immediate treatment with intravenous thiamine, 20–100 mg, reverses the drowsiness and ophthalmoplegia over a few hours, if the encephalopathy has not advanced too far. The nystagmus, ataxia, and amnesia take longer to recover, and some patients may be left with a permanent amnesic syndrome—the Korsakoff syndrome.

Thiamine is a cofactor for transketolase, α-ketoglutarate dehydrogenase, pyruvate dehydrogenase, and branched-chain α-ketoacid dehydrogenase. How thiamine deficiency is related to the metabolic and structural lesions of Wernicke's encephalopathy is not clear. Experimental drugs that block ion currents activated by N-methyl-D-aspartate glutamic acid receptors protect the rat against Wernicke-like pathological changes induced by experimental thiamine deficiency, suggesting that excitotoxicity may contribute to neuronal death in Wernicke's encephalopathy. As only some alcoholic patients develop the syndrome, it has been suggested that another factor is necessary—possibly an inherited variation in transketolase, which reduces its affinity for thiamine.

The characteristic features of the Korsakoff syndrome (also known as the alcohol amnesic syndrome) include a loss of past memories and an inability to form new memories, with loss of insight and initiative. Confabulation, as described above, is not an invariable feature, and tends to become less as the years go by. This permanent state is not responsive to thiamine.

Korsakoff's syndrome is comparatively infrequent in non-alcoholic patients who have had an acute Wernicke's syndrome (e.g. in association with hyperemesis), which suggests that the amnesic syndrome is most fully developed in those who have alcoholic damage to other parts of the brain, particularly the frontal lobes.

23.4.2.5   *Alcoholic dementia*

Those who drink heavily throughout life show significant impairment of cognitive function on intellectual testing when sober, a factor which must lead to impaired performance at work, quite apart from the behavioural disturbance which is usually the precipitating factor that terminates employment. Frontal lobe atrophy, as mentioned above, is often prominent on CT scanning or MRI. Cognitive deterioration may be exacerbated by the effects of repeated head injuries due to falls or brawls.

23.4.2.6   *Alcoholic cerebellar degeneration*

Chronic alcoholics develop persistent ataxia of gait and dysarthria which is no longer related to acute intoxication. This is probably due to a direct neurotoxic effect upon Purkinje cells, but may also be due to repeated subclinical episodes of Wernicke's encephalopathy.

23.4.2.7   *Alcoholic neuropathy*

A distal sensorimotor neuropathy, with painful burning feet and tender calves, is common in chronic alcoholics. It is not certain whether this is due to nutritional deficiencies of thiamine and other vitamins, or to a direct toxic effect of alcohol. Probably both factors are important.

23.4.2.8   *Central pontine myelinolysis*

This syndrome, associated with hyponatraemia and/or its correction by intravenous electrolyte therapy, is described in Section 23.2.2. It is particularly likely to occur in alcoholic patients.

23.4.2.9   *The Marchiafava–Bignami syndrome*

The aetiology of this rare disorder of alcoholic patients is not known. It is characterized by necrosis of the corpus callosum and adjacent subcortical white matter, clinically manifest by dementia, dysarthria, and a spastic ataxic gait.

23.4.2.10   *Myopathy*

An acute form of alcoholic myopathy occurs, sometimes after a binge, characterized by weakness, pain, tenderness, and swelling of proximal muscles. The serum phosphocreatine kinase is elevated, and biopsy shows intense muscle fibre necrosis, which may be sufficiently severe to cause myoglobinuria and renal failure.

Chronic alcoholics may also develop an insidious proximal myopathy with preferential involvement, on biopsy, of type II fibres. Many chronic alcoholics show a pseudo-Cushing's syndrome with truncal obesity and wasted limbs, the latter being due in part to an alcoholic myopathy.

Other syndromes associated with excessive consumption of alcohol include stroke (Section 10.1.4.3), recurrent cranial trauma, and hepatic encephalopathy (Section 23.2.1). A number of studies suggest that alcohol-related problems account for about 10 per cent of all acute hospital admissions.

23.4.2.11   *The treatment of chronic alcoholism*

Alcoholism is a chronic disease, of multifactorial origin. There is certainly a genetic component, as witnessed by the high incidence of alcoholism in the children of alcoholic parents, even if reared in non-alcoholic families. Environmental and cultural factors are also important, as is psychiatric co-morbidity, particularly affective and panic disorders.

Current standard treatment is based upon the principle of total abstinence; it is believed that few, if any, alcoholics can return to controlled social drinking. Typical treatment includes a period of in-patient hospitalization for detoxification, adequate nutrition, and, most importantly, separation from the previous environment. This is followed by a period of individual and group psychotherapy, usually involving the family, and possibly involving lay support groups such as Alcoholics Anonymous.

23.5 Some disorders due to immunologically mediated damage to the nervous system

An immune basis clearly underlies myasthenia gravis (Section 21.12.2), and plays a large role in acute infective polyneuropathy (Section 19.3.9), chronic relapsing polyneuropathy (Section 19.3.6.1) and multiple sclerosis (Section 14.2), and other diseases described in this book. This section describes some other immunologically mediated disorders.

23.5.1 Paraneoplastic syndromes

Secondary deposits of carcinomas of the breast, bronchus, and other primary tumours occur frequently in the brain, as described in Chapter 16. Some tumours, however, produce immunological or biochemical effects on the nervous system at sites remote from the occurrence of tumour cells.

23.5.1.1 Immunologically mediated paraneoplastic syndromes

These are believed to result in part from the immunological response of the patient to his or her tumour, with the production of antibodies that react with tumour antigens, and which may play some part in limiting its growth. However, if the tumour antigen is identical or closely similar to a neuronal antigen, neuronal function may be compromised by the same antibodies directed against these neuronal components.

The paraneoplastic cerebellar syndrome

This is a rare complication of bronchial, breast, and ovarian cancer, manifest by the acute or subacute onset of ataxia of the limbs and trunk, nystagmus, and dysarthria, sometimes preceding clinical evidence of the tumour. Histologically, there is a severe loss of cerebellar Purkinje cells and often submeningeal lymphocytic infiltration. It is believed that the tumour antigen corresponds to a specific cerebellar neural protein, so that the tumour-generated immune response is misdirected against Purkinje cells. Tumours from patients with paraneoplastic cerebellar degeneration express a specific Purkinje-cell protein (CDR 62) that is not detected in the breast or ovarian tumours of those without cerebellar degeneration. The antibody generated by this antigen is known as the anti-Yo antibody.

The paraneoplastic visual syndrome

A few patients with bronchial carcinoma suffer acute loss of vision occurring over a few days. Histological examination of the retinae of such patients shows a loss of retinal ganglion cells and immunologlobulin deposition in the ganglion cell layer. There is cross-reactivity with similar or identical antigens in cloned retinal ganglion cells and cloned tumour cells.

Paraneoplastic sensory neuropathy

This syndrome, complicating or preceding clinical evidence of small-cell lung carcinoma, is characterized by the subacute onset of a severe sensory neuropathy, which may cause a prominent ataxia due to sensory deafferentation. Histological examination shows marked loss of neurons in the dorsal root and trigeminal sensory ganglia. The serum of such patients contains an antibody known as anti-Hu directed against both neurons and tumour.

More common than a pure sensory neuropathy is a mixed motor and sensory neuropathy associated with a wider variety of tumours, the immunological basis of which is less clear.

Opsoclonus

This is the name given to intermittent bursts of very rapid conjugate eye movements occurring in the vertical, horizontal, and oblique planes. This is believed to be due to loss of inhibitory control over the system in the pretectal region that produces ocular saccades—brief, high-velocity movements

necessary for fixing a target on the fovea. Opsoclonus may occur in multiple sclerosis, but it is also
seen as a paraneoplastic syndrome in patients with
neuroblastoma, or carcinomas of the breast or
lung. Some patients with opsoclonus and tumours
also have loss of Purkinje cells. The mechanism of
neuronal damage in the pretectum in opsoclonus is
assumed to be similar to that seen in paraneoplastic
cerebellar degeneration.

The Lambert–Eaton myasthenic syndrome
This is described in Section 21.12.3.1. In a few
patients with tumours, particularly bronchial carcinoma, there are circulating auto-antibodies
against the voltage-gated Ca^{2+} channel at the neuromuscular junction. This produces a myasthenic-
like weakness affecting particularly the proximal
muscles.

23.5.1.2   *Limbic encephalitis*

This is another paraneoplastic syndrome, seen
particularly in association with small-cell lung
cancer, presenting with brain-stem symptoms and
signs, and disordered personality and behaviour.
Histologically, there are zones of perivascular lymphocytic infiltrates and microglial nodules in the
amygdala, the hippocampal formation, the cingulate and orbital gyri, and the hypothalamus, which
together make up the limbic system, and in the
brain stem. It is not yet clear whether this is an
immunologically mediated disorder, or due to an
opportunistic virus infection similar to that causing
progressive multifocal leucoencephalopathy (Section 17.14.3.2).

23.5.1.3   *Other paraneoplastic syndromes*

These include dermatomyositis (Section 21.3.4),
opportunistic viral infections (Section 17.12.12.4),
and inappropriate secretion of antidiuretic hormone by small-cell lung carcinomas, resulting in
hyponatraemia and confusion (Section 23.2.2).

23.6   Further reading

General

Baraitser, M. (1990). *The genetics of neurological disorders*. Oxford University Press, Oxford.

Baraitser, M. and Winter, R. M. (1991). *The London
neurogenetics database*. Oxford Medical Databases,
Oxford.
Kingston, H. M. (1989). Treatment of genetic disorders.
British Medical Journal **298**, 1499–1501.
Scriver, C. R., Beaudet, A. L., Sly, W. S., and Valle,
D. (ed.) (1989). *The metabolic basis of inherited dis-
ease*. McGraw-Hill, New York.

Ataxia telangiectasia

Woods, C. G. and Taylor, A. M. R. (1992) Ataxia
telangiectasia in the British Isles: The clinical and
laboratory features of 70 affected individuals. *Quarterly Journal of Medicine*, New Series, **82**, 169–79.

Phenylketonuria

Thompson, A. J., Smith, I., Brenton, D., *et al.* (1990).
Neurological deterioration in young adults with phenylketonuria. *Lancet* **336**, 602–5.

Maple syrup urine disease

Berry, G. T., Heidenreich, R., Kaplan, P., *et al.* (1991).
Branched-chain amino-acid free parenteral nutrition
in the treatment of acute metabolic decompensation in
patients with maple-syrup urine disease. *New England
Journal of Medicine* **324**, 175–9.

Adrenoleucodystrophy

Aubourg, P., Blanche, S., Jambque, I., *et al.* (1990).
Reversal of early neurologic and neuroradiologic manifestations of X-linked adrenoleukodystrophy by bone
marrow transplantation. *New England Journal of Medicine* **322**, 1860–6.

Lysosomal disorders

Editorial (1990). Anderson–Fabry disease. *Lancet* **336**,
24–5.
Menkes, J. H. (1990). The leukodystrophies. *New England Journal of Medicine* **322**, 54–5.
Polten, A., Fluharty,A. L., Fluharty, C. B., *et al.* (1991).
Molecular basis of different forms of metachromatic
leukodystrophy. *New England Journal of Medicine*
324, 18–22.
Watts, R. W. E. and Gibbs, D. A. (1986). *Lyosomal
storage diseases: biochemical and clinical aspects*.
Taylor and Francis, London.

The porphyrias

Kushner, J. P. (1991). Laboratory diagnosis of the porphyrias. *New England Journal of Medicine* **324**, 1432–3.

Sack, G. H. (1990). Acute intermittent porphyria. *Journal of the American Medical Association* **264**, 1290–3.

Mitochondrial disorders

Poole, C. J. M. and Kind, P. R. N. (1986). Deficiency of thiosulphate sulphurtransferase (rhodanase) in Leber's hereditary optic atrophy. *British Medical Journal* **292**, 1229–30.

Hepatic encephalopathy

Fraser, C. L. and Arieff, A. J. (1985). Hepatic encephalopathy. *New England Journal of Medicine* **313**, 865–73.

Hypoglycaemia

Boyle, P. J., Schwartz, N. S., Shah, S. S., *et al.* (1988). Plasma glucose concentrations at the onset of hypoglycemic symptoms in patients with poorly controlled diabetes mellitus. *New England Journal of Medicine* **318**, 1487–92.

Fishman, R. A. (1991). The glucose-transporter protein and glucopenic brain injury. *New England Journal of Medicine* **325**, 731–2.

Hyponatraemia

Berl, T. (1990). Treating hyponatraemia: what is all the controversy about? *Annals of Internal Medicine* **113**, 417–18.

Brunner, J. E., Redmond, J. M., and Hagger, A. M. (1990). Central pontine myelinolysis and pontine lesions after rapid correction of hyponatraemia: a prospective magnetic resonance imaging study. *Annals of Neurology* **27**, 61–6.

Vitamin E deficiency

Traber, M. G., Sokol, R. J., Ringel, S. P., *et al.* (1987). Lack of tocopherol in peripheral nerves of vitamin E-deficient patients with peripheral neuropathy. *New England Journal of Medicine* **317**, 262–5.

Cobalamin deficiency

Beck, W. S. (1990). Cobalamin and the nervous system. *New England Journal of Medicine* **318**, 1752–4.

Neurotoxicology

Meredith, T. and Vale, A. (1988). Carbon monoxide poisoning. *British Medical Journal* **296**, 77–9.

Schaumburg, H. H. and Spencer, P. S. (1987). Recognising neurotoxic disease. *Neurology* **37**, 276–8.

Senanayake, N. and Karalliedde, L. (1987). Neurotoxic effects of organophosphorus intoxication. *New England Journal of Medicine* **316**, 761–83.

Teitelbaum, J. S., Zatorre, R. J., and Carpenter, S. (1990). Neurologic sequelae of domoic acid intoxication due to the ingestion of contaminated mussels. *New England Journal of Medicine* **322**, 1781–7.

The neurological effects of alcohol and chronic alcoholism

Brennan, F. N. and Lyttle, J. A. (1987). Alcohol and seizures: a review. *Journal of the Royal Society of Medicine* **80**, 571–3.

Charness, M. E., Simon, R. P., and Greenberg, D. A. (1989). Ethanol and the nervous system. *New England Journal of Medicine* **321**, 442–54.

Editorial (1990). Korsakoff's syndrome. *Lancet.* **336**, 912–3.

Harper, C., Kril, J., and Daly, J. (1987). Are we drinking our neurones away? *British Medical Journal* **294**, 534–6.

Klerman, G. L. (1989). Treatment of alcoholism. *New England Journal of Medicine* **320**, 394–5.

Lerner, W. D. and Fallon, H. J. (1985). The alcohol withdrawal syndrome. *New England Journal of Medicine* **313**, 951–2.

Simon, R. P. (1988). Alcohol and seizures. *New England Journal of Medicine* **319**, 715–6.

Paraneoplastic syndromes

Furneaux, H. M., Rosenblum, M. K., Dalmau, J., *et al.* (1990). Selective expression of Purkinje-cell antigens in tumour tissue from patients with paraneoplastic cerebellar degeneration. *New England Journal of Medicine* **322**, 1844–51.

Kornguth, S. E. (1989). Neuronal proteins and paraneoplastic syndromes. *New England Journal of Medicine* **321**, 1607–8.

Limbic encephalitis

Case records of the Massachusetts General Hospital (1988). *New England Journal of Medicine* **319**, 849–60.

Opsoclonus

Case records of the Massachussetts General Hospital (1988). *New England Journal of Medicine* **318**, 563–70.

24 Sleep and its disorders

Sleep is a recurring state of inactivity, accompanied by a loss of awareness of and a decrease in responsiveness to the environment. Regular cycles of sleep are determined by intrinsic pacemakers or biochemical clocks. These require resetting when crossing several time zones, as external factors such as the alternation of night and day also play a part in determining sleep, as do, of course, simple factors such as social engagements and previous heavy exercise.

24.1   The nature of sleep

The past 25 years have seen a considerable body of research into the nature of sleep and its disorders. Principal among the methodologies used in research into sleep has been the electroencephalogram. At the onset of sleep, the alpha rhythm at 9–12 c/s recorded over the occipital regions of the scalp spreads further forwards, and becomes rather slower in frequency, then tends to wax and wane in amplitude, before giving way to a low-voltage irregular pattern with generalized slower rhythms at 4–7 c/s. This is stage I of non-rapid eye movement sleep (NREM sleep). If stimulated at this stage, subjects usually describe being drowsy rather than fully asleep. In stage II of NREM sleep, brief bursts of 12–15 c/s activity are recorded, each lasting about 1–2 seconds. As the amplitude in the middle part of this burst is larger

than at onset and at termination, the discharge on the electroencephalogram has a spindle shape, so that these bursts are known as sleep spindles. Also found in stage II NREM sleep are K complexes, occurring 2–3 times a minute. Each K complex is triphasic, with an initial negative wave followed by a positive wave occurring simultaneously over all regions in the head. Small-amplitude vertex sharp waves may also be seen at this stage. In stage III of NREM sleep, the dominant voltage becomes even slower, usually down to 2 c/s, and of higher amplitude, usually more than 75 μV. As stage III passes into stage IV, slower waves become more and more abundant.

The time taken to reach stages III and IV is about 30–45 minutes in healthy people, and then there is a gradual lightening to stage II before the first burst of REM sleep—rapid eye movement sleep. REM sleep is characterized by the occurrence of conjugate rapid eye movements in all planes of gaze, and is accompanied by muscle twitching. In between the twitching, muscles are characteristically electrically silent, and deep tendon reflexes are very depressed or abolished. During REM sleep, blood pressure and respiration rate both increase, and, in men, erections or penile tumescence occur.

In a typical night, there are usually about five NREM–REM cycles, the duration and intensity of REM increasing with each cycle; in the NREM phases of the later cycles, stages III and IV are not usually reached. The last part of the night is therefore spent largely in REM sleep alternating with stage II NREM sleep.

24.1.1 *Attention during sleep*

Whatever the depth of sleep, the brain seems able to maintain some attention. For example, a mother with a young child is readily awoken from sleep by her baby crying. It is also a commonplace experience to awake a few minutes before an alarm is set off, if the alarm is set for an important engagement, such as catching an aeroplane. Automatic motor behaviour can continue during sleep. Many animals and birds sleep while standing up, and soldiers may apparently sleep during long marches.

24.1.2 *Duration of sleep and deprivation of sleep*

The duration of sleep 'required' by an individual is very variable. Some reported subjects manage to get by with only 1–2 hours' sleep each night for many years. Others feel exhausted and deprived if they do not have 8 or 9 hours' sleep. Long sleepers tend to have more REM sleep than short sleepers. Long sleepers appear no more or less energetic than short sleepers, but short sleepers may, if they get up, be able to accomplish more during the working day by dint of having more time awake for focused activity.

The amount of a 24-hour day spent in sleep alters markedly during life. New-born babies spend 18 hours or more a day asleep, much of it in REM sleep. The amount of sleep taken each day declines rapidly, so that by the age of 1 year children are spending about 13 of each 24 hours asleep, 30 per cent of which is in REM sleep, and, by adolescence, adult levels are reached. Many late-teenagers, however, seem to go into a second phase of days in which much time is spent asleep, or at least in bed, before a fully adult pattern is reached. With increasing age, time taken to onset of sleep increases, with 'lighter' sleep, which is more readily disturbed. The amount of REM sleep, however, remains more-or-less constant from the age of 5 years to very old age.

Deprivation of sleep, for example, by being on duty as a medical resident or registrar, results in diminished performance in psychological tests the following day, the disturbance being greater in the afternoon and evening rather than in the morning immediately after deprivation. With longer periods of sleep deprivation, impaired performance is accompanied by subjective feelings of depression and an increasing desire to sleep, and by aggression. Longer periods of deprivation of sleep are associated with 'micro-sleeps'—short bursts of stage I or stage II NREM sleep, as seen on the electroencephalogram, with brief lapses of awareness. Prolonged sleep deprivation of 100 hours or so is accompanied by very frequent micro-sleeps, and, if carried to extremes, confusion and depersonalization. It is presumably for these reasons that deprivation of sleep is used by the agents of totalitarian regimes when interrogating their opponents. With electroencephalographic monitoring, it is possible to wake subjects at the onset of REM sleep, and such experiments show that after a period of REM sleep deprivation there is, on subsequent nights, a considerable increase in the proportion of REM sleep, and a reduction in latency to onset of REM sleep.

24.1.3 *The nature of dreams*

Throughout history, humans have considered the nature of dreams, and their possible meaning in relation to the individual's daily life. Sigmund Freud proposed in his book *The interpretation of dreams* that an analysis of the content of dreams allowed access to the unconscious mind, and an analysis of dream content might reveal the reasons for his patients' underlying neuroses. Subjects woken in NREM or REM sleep may both report being awakened from dreams, but most dreams reported on waking from REM sleep are vivid and personal, whereas awakening from NREM sleep is less frequently accompanied by dreams. If these are present they are more in the way of ill-formed and poorly described thoughts.

Mammals show REM cycles similar to those of humans, and these observations have allowed the exploration of neural activity by means of depth electrodes in experimental animals. Neural control of REM sleep is centred in the brain stem. During REM sleep, large spikes can be recorded projected from the pontine region to the geniculate bodies and thence to the occipital cortex. It has been suggested that dreaming consists of imagery elicited from the neocortex in response to random brain-stem signals such as these pontine–

geniculate–occipital (PGO) spikes. In this model, dreams are the best 'fit' that the neocortex can provide to this input from the brain stem. The plot of dream stories, and their inner significance to the individual, reflect only the different probabilities of the cortex responding to this brain-stem input. Although an attractive hypothesis, this is in a sense an unscientific one, as are all hypotheses so far about human dreaming, as they are untestable. Other hypotheses suggest that other cerebral activities, such as the sinusoidal 6 c/s rhythm found in the hippocampus during REM sleep, are important in consolidating psychologically and sociologically important memories received during the day.

Aspects of sleep such as circadian rhythms and their effects upon sleep when disturbed by shift-work or transmeridianal jet flights, variations in hormone secretion with sleep, sleep and depression, and insomnia, although of great theoretical interest, are not covered in this book as these phenomena do not usually fall within the domain of clinical neurologists. Readers are referred to the book by Parkes (1985).

24.2   The parasomnias

The parasomnias (events occurring in relation to sleep) do clearly fall within the neurological domain. In general, they are episodic but non-epileptic abnormalities of neural behaviour reflected in abnormalities of movement (for example, nocturnal myoclonic jerks), thought content, and nightmares.

24.2.1   *The motor parasomnias*

24.2.1.1   *Hypnic jerks*

Hypnic jerks are small-amplitude, single or multiple jerks occurring at the onset of sleep, usually in stage I or stage II of NREM sleep. Sometimes these jerks are associated with a sensation of falling. They are entirely normal.

24.2.1.2   *Sleep myoclonus*

Sleep myoclonus (sometimes called periodic movements in sleep) is confined to NREM sleep, but during this may occur at intervals of about 40

seconds throughout the night. The movements are not really myoclonic in so far as they are not as brief as myoclonic jerks seen with neurological disorders. The 'jerks' are muscular contractions, often affecting the extensors of the foot, and may last up to 5 seconds.

About one-third of those with periodic movements in sleep also suffer the phenomenon known as restless legs, a perception occurring before sleep so that the sufferer feels that he must move his legs to relieve an unbearable but difficult to describe discomfort in the legs, particularly in the calves. In order to relieve this discomfort, the person with restless legs may kick his legs around the bed, or rub them vigorously in order to gain some relief.

Occasionally, restless legs are associated with organic neurological disease such as motor neuron disease or a mild diabetic neuropathy. However, most patients with restless legs are entirely healthy, although the sensation may be so unpleasant that they dread going to bed. Both clonazepam and carbamazepine have been used with some effect, but, in general, treatment is not very beneficial.

24.2.1.3   *Bruxism*

This is the name given to grinding of the teeth during sleep that may be sufficiently loud to wake a sleeping partner. Bruxism occurs in the early stages of NREM sleep. Sometimes it seems more prominent at times of personal stress.

24.2.1.4   *Headbanging*

This occurs in stage I or stage II NREM sleep. A variant of overall body rocking, it is more common in boys than girls, and may affect children without any apparent family stress or unhappiness. Usually the stage of headbanging is comparatively short-lived, and no specific treatment is necessary, but a small dose of a benzodiazepine may be useful.

24.2.1.5   *Sleep-walking*

More complex motor behaviour may occur during sleep, in which young children aged between about 4 and 12 years get out of their bed. They may perhaps sit on the end of their bed or wander round their bedroom, making purposeless repetitive movements, such as opening and closing a drawer. A child will not respond if spoken to, but if awakened, he or she may be disorientated and confused for a few minutes. Sleep-walking occurs in the deeper stages of NREM sleep. Sleep-walking is commonly associated with night terrors.

24.2.2 Night terrors and nightmares

24.2.2.1 Night terrors

It is alarming to be the parent of a child with night terrors, although they have no sinister significance. In stage III or IV NREM sleep, the young child cries out with a piercing scream, and, when the parents rush to the bedroom, the child appears terrified, with dilated pupils, and other signs of extreme adrenergic activity such as tachycardia.

Although usually self-limiting, the distress caused to the family is such that it is usually worth trying some treatment. Probably the best method is to wake the child about 1 hour before the terror is due, and as they typically occur within about 90 minutes of sleep onset this is not too hard to arrange. This often seems to abort a series of night terrors.

24.2.2.2 Nightmares

In contrast to night terrors, nightmares occur in stage III or REM sleep, and presumably reflect no more than dreams with an unpleasant psychic content. Nightmares can be induced by drug treatment, notably by reserpine and by L-dopa.

24.2.3 Sleep paralysis

Sleep paralysis—a complete flaccid paralysis with atonia and areflexia—may occur at sleep onset or on first waking. The subject is aware that he or she is unable to move, and may therefore, understandably, be terrified. Some individuals can abort the paralytic attack by moving the eyes, or perhaps by being able to move one digit, this then making possible the activation of other digits and limbs. Another sensory input, such as a light touch from another person, will abort the paralytic attack. Sometimes the paralysis is accompanied by vivid hallucinations.

Isolated episodes of sleep paralysis are quite common in the general population, occurring perhaps in as many as a third of the entire population on at least one occasion. Repeated attacks of sleep

paralysis may occur as a familial disorder, and are commonly associated with narcolepsy (see below).

Repetitive sleep paralysis may be prevented by clomipramine (25 mg) on going to bed at night.

24.2.4 The narcolepsy–cataplexy syndrome

More is understood about the narcolepsy–cataplexy syndrome than about most of the other parasomnic disorders.

24.2.4.1 Narcolepsy

Narcolepsy is the intense desire to go to sleep. As with normal sleepiness, narcoleptic sleepiness is most apparent in rather boring sedentary situations, but it may occur during active conversation, for example. The association with cataplexy and other parasomnias indicates that narcolepsy is quite distinct from other causes of excessive daytime somnolence, considered below.

About one-third of all patients with narcolepsy have a family history of the disorder. In the past decade it has been recognized that there is a strong association with certain histocompatibility antigens. About 95 per cent of White people with narcolepsy are positive for the DRw15 subtype of DR2, while the normal population frequency of DR2, although varying geographically, is only of the order of 20–35 per cent. In black Americans, the association with a narcolepsy is with the DQw6 subtype of DQwl. However, there are a few well-documented cases of classic narcoleptics who do not have these antigens, suggesting that the gene responsible for narcolepsy may be just outside the DQ and DR subregions on the short arm of chromosome 6.

In spite of the apparent close relationship of the gene for narcolepsy to the HLA system, there is no evidence of narcolepsy being associated with auto-immune diseases. Although there is an apparent relationship between narcolepsy and multiple sclerosis, a disease which certainly has some relationship to the body's immune system (see Chapter 14), it may be that narcoleptic patients with multiple sclerosis do have a plaque causing a narcoleptic-like syndrome, rather than the two disorders sharing a common origin.

The occurrence of REM sleep at the onset of sleep or shortly after sleep onset is the most characteristic physiological abnormality observed in narcolepsy. This is the basis of the multiple sleep latency test. In this investigation, the patient with suspected narcolepsy is asked to try to get to sleep at intervals of 2 hours throughout the day. The length of time to the onset of sleep and the types of sleep that occur are monitored with the electro-encephalogram. More than 80 per cent of patients with narcolepsy have a mean latency to sleep of less than 5 minutes, and at least two REM periods at the onset of sleep during this procedure. It is of great theoretical interest that many normal subjects without narcolepsy who are DR2 positive have a shorter latency to REM sleep than those who are DR2 negative.

24.2.4.2   *Cataplexy*

About 5 per cent of patients with narcolepsy initially have cataplexy, and within 10 years the number with associated cataplectic attacks increases to about 25 per cent overall. Occasionally cataplexy is the first symptom, narcolepsy following. Cataplexy is an episode of muscular atonia, often precipitated by excitement or strong emotions, such as a gale of laughter or anger. It is interesting that when schoolgirls 'laugh themselves sick' they may stagger around as if their legs are weak. True cataplectic attacks are very dramatic. For example, a patient of mine was playing on a beach and was trying very hard to catch a ball thrown by his young son. The excitement of doing so caused his legs to buckle under him, and he was unable to get up for 20 seconds or so. A few patients have been examined by neurologists during cataplectic attacks, and the absence of all tendon reflexes and extensor plantar responses has been observed.

24.2.4.3   *Hypnagogic hallucinations*

Rather less common than cataplexy, but also associated with the narcolepsy–cataplexy syndrome are episodes of sleep paralysis, as described above, and hallucinations occurring at onset of sleep (hypnagogic hallucinations). These are not dreams, but half-awake sensory errors with fragments of waking imagery incorporated into near dreams that can be summoned, and sometimes dispensed with, at will. Similar waking hallucinations can occur in a small proportion of patients with narcolepsy.

Other symptoms associated with narcolepsy include periods of automatic behaviour for which the patient is amnesic, and disturbed night-time sleep with frequent awakenings, periodic bodily movements, and apnoeic episodes.

24.2.4.4   *Treatment*

The effects of narcolepsy upon a patient's life are often substantial. Many fall asleep at work, and many while driving. It is highly probable that many unexplained single-vehicle accidents are associated with unrecognized narcoleptic attacks. The embarrassment of falling asleep in social gatherings is also substantial, and patients understandably want effective treatment. The mainstay of treatment is dexamphetamine, and this may be taken in doses of between 5 and 25 mg/day. Although substance abuse may occur, the vast majority of patients manage to control the dose of dexamphetamine within reasonable limits. Methylphenidate is no longer available to new patients in the UK, but is available in the USA. Other stimulant drugs that have been employed include mazindol and fencamfamin. Tyrosine, a precursor of tyramine, was at one time thought to be beneficial, but further trials have shown no benefit. γ-Hydroxy butyrate is under active study in the USA, and is proving to be a promising drug.

Clomipramine, a tricyclic antidepressant, is moderately effective in the treatment of cataplexy. Tricyclic antidepressants act principally by inhibiting the re-uptake of noradrenaline and serotonin. However, cataplexy is seldom as troublesome to the patient as is narcolepsy, and clomipramine seems relatively ineffective in the treatment of daytime somnolence.

If patients with narcolepsy can find times during the day in which they can allow themselves to sleep, they may be able to abort narcoleptic attacks at unwanted times, and reduce their requirement for dexamphetamine.

24.2.5   *Other causes of excessive daytime drowsiness*

There can be few readers of this book who have not experienced drowsiness at, say, 3 o'clock in the afternoon after lunch and faced with a boring lecture. Such daytime drowsiness is commonplace, and is minimized by the avoidance of alcohol, taking a light lunch, and following an interesting life. There is, presumably, a distribution of normality for alertness and somnolence at different times of the day, and some are more gifted than others at staying awake in boring circumstances, such as after dinner with guests who have outstayed their welcome. However, in the past few years there has been an increasing interest in excessive daytime somnolence in association with disrupted nocturnal sleep secondary to sleep apnoea, and this is considered next.

24.2.6   *The sleep apnoeas*

Central apnoea is said to occur when there is no detectable air flow at the nose or mouth, and when there are no respiratory movements. The failure of respiratory movements must be due to disturbances of primary neural control, often an apparent insensitivity to hypoxia and hypercapnia even when the subject is awake. Sometimes one meets an intelligent child who asks how one continues to remember to breathe while one is asleep. Rarely, disorders of breathing during sleep do occur, named by some Ondine's curse. Ondine was a mythical water nymph whose lover was cursed to lose automatic functions while asleep, so he had always to stay awake. Central apnoea may play some role in some cot deaths.

Much more frequent is obstructive apnoea, in which the airflow through the nose or mouth is reduced, even though ventilatory efforts continue. Usually this is caused by obstruction of the pharynx and other upper airways during REM sleep. Many patients with obstructive apnoea are considerably overweight, and have a rather small lower jaw and large tongue, all of which tend to reduce the diameter of the available airway. Snoring, if not due to otherwise trivial nasal obstruction, is due to vibration of the lax pharyngeal walls during inspiration. Inspiratory snores often increase gradually in volume with increasing depth of REM sleep and increasing pharyngeal obstruction. There is then a sudden choking inspiratory gasp and bodily movement as the occlusion is overcome, and the subject briefly aroused. The repeated arousals effectively deprive the subject of REM sleep, secondarily resulting in excessive daytime somnolence.

Epidemiological surveys have shown that there is an association between snoring and hypertension, angina, consumption of alcohol, and stroke. The interaction of these variables is such that the risk ratio of cerebral infarction between those who snore and do not snore is as high as 10 (confidence limits 3–30). Hypothyroidism is another predisposing factor.

The most effective treatment for snoring and sleep apnoea, and for the daytime somnolence arising from repeated arousal at night, is continuous positive airway pressure applied through the nose (nasal CPAP). This may be accomplished simply by fitting a well-sealed mask to the nose, through which is delivered air from a compressor. A positive pressure of 5–10 cmH$_2$O is maintained throughout the breathing cycle, adjusted by altering the outlet resistance. This keeps the pharynx inflated, abolishes snoring, and markedly improves alertness during the day. Before considering such manoeuvres, abstinence from alcohol and hypnotics, and loss of weight in those who are extremely overweight, should be the first lines of treatment. Occasionally very large adenoidal lymph nodes may obstruct the airway in adults, to a degree sufficient to warrant surgical removal.

24.2.7   *Disorders of sleep due to organic brain disease*

The normal sleep cycle may be disturbed by a severe cranial injury. There is then often restlessness and agitated behaviour at night, with excessive somnolence during the day. Excessive somnolence may also follow an episode of encephalitis, or be associated with tumours in the pineal region, the floor of the third ventricle, or hypothalamus. Those with hypertension and secondary cerebrovascular disease (multiple lacunar infarctions), may also have excessive daytime somnolence. A syndrome of periodic hypersomnolence associated with grossly increased appetite and sometimes hypersexuality, with normal alertness, behaviour, and sleep cycles between episodes, is known as the Kleine–Levin syndrome. No cause has been identified. Finally, familial fatal insomnia has recently been described, characterized also by dysautonomia and motor signs. This is associated with a prion protein gene variant (see Section 17.15).

24.3   Other phenomena associated with sleep

Epileptic seizures may occur only at night, or, in

the case of primary generalized epilepsy, in the first few minutes after waking. Sleep may precipitate episodes of bronchial asthma, and the horizontal position assumed during sleep may precipitate episodes of cardiac asthma. Nocturnal enuresis is not related to any particular stage of the sleep cycle, but may reflect, in part, an inadequate arousal response to a full bladder. Treatment with imipramine may be successful. This may not necessarily depend upon any central action of the drug, as it has been shown that contractile activity is reduced by instillation of imipramine into the bladder.

24.4   Further reading

Aldrich, M. S. (1990). Narcolepsy. *New England Journal of Medicine* **323**, 389–94.

Douglas, N. J., Thomas, S., and Jan, M. A. (1992). Clinical value of polysomnography. *Lancet* **339**, 347–50.

Medori, R., Tritschler, H-J., LeBlanc, A. *et al.* (1992). Fatal familial insomnia, a priori disease with a mutation at codon 178 of the prion protein gene. *New England Journal of Medicine* **326**, 444–9.

Parkes, J. D. (1985). *Sleep and its disorders*. W. B. Saunders, London.

Prinz, P. N., Vitiello, M. V., Raskind, M. A., and Thorpy, M. J. (1990). Current concepts in geriatrics: sleep disorders and aging. *New England Journal of Medicine* **323**, 520–6.

van Cauter, E., and Turek F. W. (1990). Strategies for resetting the human circadian clock. *New England Journal of Medicine* **322**, 1306–8.

25 The borders of neurology

In this chapter I consider some of the problems that are not, by most definitions, due to diseases of the nervous system, but which beset the neurologist in outpatient practice.

25.1 Psychological symptoms

The division and interactions between mind and brain have been the subject of philosophical discussion since the time of Aristotle. Mental perceptions arise through the structure and function of the brain. A thought must have a neurophysiological basis. Some aspects of this can now be demonstrated directly: cerebral blood flow can be shown to be increased in different parts of the cortex depending upon whether the subject is mentally solving a mathematical problem, or thinking using verbal constructs; thinking about a planned action results in a 'readiness potential' that can be recorded by scalp electrodes.

Some psychological symptoms, such as anxiety, probably are based in an extension of normal neurophysiology. Others, such as those that arise in bipolar affective illness or schizophrenia, may well in time prove to be due to disorders of neurotransmission, some of which may have a genetic basis. The division between 'mental' (psychological) and neurological symptoms is therefore largely an artificial one, and yet still useful in clinical practice.

25.1.1 Symptoms not due to obvious structural disease

About one-quarter of all neurological consultations are for symptoms that are not clearly due to structural disease (see Section 3.2). Headache is the prime example. Whatever the various hypotheses about the genesis of common headache (see Section 9.3), the fact has to be faced that clinical examination and investigations fail to define a cause in the vast majority of patients. Although it is usual to explore aspects of the patient's life for 'stress', most patients have not had unfavourable life events preceding the onset of the headache, and many patients deny that they are any more stressed at this time of their life, at which they have headaches, than at other times when they have been free from headaches.

Most patients with headache are psychologically entirely normal (see Section 9.3) and they are no more neurotic than their friends and relatives without headache. Many such patients have fears about organic illness, such as an impending stroke, or a brain tumour. After giving the patient the opportunity to ventilate the problem, and after a negative clinical examination, reassurance is usually remarkably effective (see Section 9.11). Investigations undertaken solely to reassure the patient are inappropriate and unnecessary.

Another common symptom presented to neurologists in outpatient practice is paraesthesiae. Of course, many patients with paraesthesiae do have an organic basis for them; for example, the median nerve may be compressed in the carpal tunnel. Other patients complain of peculiar feelings running down the spine, or 'tingling all over'. A negative clinical examination and an early resolution suggest that these symptoms never had an organic basis. Some patients, often women, fear a diagnosis of multiple sclerosis in these circumstances, and again reassurance specifically about this often helps resolve symptoms and the associated specific anxiety.

25.1.2 *Hypochondriasis*

The preceding paragraphs have stressed the normal psychology of many patients who have anxieties about organic illness. It is usually comparatively easy to reassure such patients. Occasionally, however, a neurologist meets a patient who has had many earlier consultations, of which he is vocally critical, and who has failed to be reassured about the absence of physical illness. In neurological practice, most such patients fear that they have a brain tumour or multiple sclerosis.

The descriptive basis of hypochondriasis is a patient convinced that he or she has a disease, fearing the disease, and being preoccupied by the disease. Hypochondriasis often arises without a basis of affective illness, although a few patients do respond to appropriate antidepressant therapy.

The most inappropriate way to manage such a patient is to be seen to be perfunctory in taking the history or giving reassurance. There is some evidence that detailed reassurance, especially if directed also through the family, is beneficial.

25.1.3 *Alexithymia*

Although the subject of a major review article, I must confess that this word has not 'caught on' in clinical practice, yet it usefully describes patients who present repeatedly with vague, ill-described physical symptoms. The principal clinical features are a limited ability to describe emotions verbally; a description, albeit a poor one, of physical symp-

toms rather than emotions; a difficulty in recognizing and acting on inner affect; a limited inner fantasy life; conversation that is mundane, concrete, and closely tied to external events. All of these attributes prevent a physician 'getting to grips' with what the patient is attempting to describe. Faced with a history such as 'my head feels bad . . . I can't tell you any more about it', the physician may take refuge in inappropriate numerous investigations. Limited explanatory therapy may help some patients achieve an increased feeling of being in control of their own lives, and relinquish illness as their principal mode of communication and ordering their lives.

25.1.4 *Depression*

Patients whose primary symptom is depression of mood are usually appropriately referred, if the severity of the depression justifies it, to a psychiatrist rather than a neurologist. However, some mildly depressed patients present with symptoms, such as headache, that lead to a neurological consultation. Other patients with organic illnesses, such as stroke or Parkinson's disease, may be depressed for biological reasons—there is some evidence that specific neuronal damage in these disorders precipitates depression (see Sections 10.1.9 and 13.1.6.6). Yet other patients recently labelled with an unfavourable neurological diagnosis, such as multiple sclerosis, become depressed for a time, as do others with advancing disabilities.

Faced in his everyday practice with all these types of, and reasons for, depression of mood, the neurologist has to be a bit of a 'do-it-yourself' psychiatrist. Indeed, in many European and Arab countries, neurology and psychiatry are practised as a conjoint speciality, but they are separate specialities in the UK and the USA.

Experienced neurologists may recognize depression of mood as they take their patients' histories. However, a study by Bridges and Goldberg showed that the extent of psychiatric illness in neurological inpatients was considerably underestimated by neurologists. The questions listed in Table 25.1 have been shown to be particularly helpful in detecting depression in general medical settings. Rather surprisingly, in the study just quoted, about half the patients remarked that they did not wish to discuss their mood with their neurologists. A lack of appropriate modes of inter-

Table 25.1 Scales for detecting depression and anxiety in general medical settings (from Goldberg *et al*. 1988)

Depression scale (score one point for each yes)
1. Have you low energy?
2. Have you lost interests?
3. Have you lost confidence in yourself?
4. Have you felt hopeless?

If 'yes' to any question, go on to ask:
5. Have you had difficulty in concentrating?
6. Have you lost weight due to poor appetite?
7. Have you been waking early?
8. Have you felt slowed up?
9. Have you tended to feel worse in the mornings?

Anxiety scale (score one point for each 'yes')
1. Have you felt keyed up, on edge?
2. Have you been worrying a lot?
3. Have you been irritable?
4. Have you had difficulty in relaxing?

If 'yes' to any *two* questions, go on to ask:
5. Have you been sleeping poorly?
6. Have you had headaches or neckaches?
7. Have you had any of the following: trembling, tingling, dizzy spells, sweating, frequency of passing urine, diarrhoea?
8. Have you been worried about your health?
9. Have you had difficulty in falling asleep?

Interpretation: patients with depression scores of 2, or anxiety scores of 5 have a 50 per cent chance of having a clinically important disturbance. Above these scores, the probability rises sharply.

action, and facilities for private talk appeared to be inhibiting factors.

Appropriate treatment for depressed patients seen by neurologists varies from case to case. Some patients depressed about the probable effects of a new and unfavourable diagnosis upon their future life and expectations respond well to two or three consultations in which a full explanation of the nature of the illness is given, combined with firm promises of professional support if the worst happens. Other patients require treatment with antidepressants. For example, nortriptyline has been shown to be more effective than placebo in the management of depressive illnesses following stroke. Mianserin has been shown to be more

effective than placebo in the depressive illness associated with cancer. This observation may reasonably be extrapolated to the management of patients with advancing and disabling neurological illness. In depressed patients presenting with 'non-organic' symptoms, such as headache, consideration should be given to non-pharmacological treatments, such as psychotherapy or exercise.

25.1.5 *Anxiety*

Patients may come to neurologists with somatic symptoms of anxiety, often related to hyperventilation. Symptoms such as giddiness, chest pain, paraesthesiae, and nausea are frequent, and are often associated with headache. Such symptoms may be due to chronic or intermittent hyperventilation with hypocarbia. The hyperventilation is often not readily apparent, but investigation shows that the $P_{a\,CO_2}$ is low, and the ventilatory response of such patients to emotional stimuli is much greater than that of control subjects. Behavioural techniques to help retrain breathing patterns may be remarkably effective.

25.1.6 *Functional signs, hysteria, and malingering*

Words such as 'functional weakness', 'functional sensory loss', or 'functional visual disturbance' quite commonly appear in neurological reports, particularly when those reports are being prepared for the purposes of litigation after personal injury. What are meant by these terms? Let us take 'functional weakness' as an example.

A subject who is psychologically perfectly normal who has, say, a frozen shoulder (Section 25.2.2), may, if asked to abduct his shoulder against resistance, suddenly 'give way' and reduce his force, for the entirely sensible reason that the force he is applying is hurting him. A timid examiner may be unsuccessful in getting an anxious patient to exert full power in each muscle group on request, and may record a statement that a limb is 'globally weak'. He or she will then be surprised to see a more skilled and persuasive examiner obtain full muscle power from all groups. A patient who has a moderate weakness due to organic disease may, for the simple reason that he is keen that his doctor takes him seriously, exaggerate the degree of weakness that he has. All these are examples of 'functional weakness'—weakness due to inadequate cortical drive to anterior horn cells.

Few clinicians would hold that such functional weakness was consciously simulated. Yet most are happy to accept a distinction between a hysterical conversion paralysis, and malingering. As a neurological disability such as paralysis or loss of vision is gross and obvious, pretended symptoms are not infrequently seen by neurologists. If the gain for which the disability is being simulated is pecuniary, or associated with some obvious evasion of duty, then the simulation is said to be malingering. If the gain is said to be an unconscious communication of psychological distress, then the illness is said to be hysterical. The truth of the matter, of course, is that such a distinction is an act of faith by the neurologist, as there is no test to distinguish them.

The manifestations of hysteria correspond to an idea of illness in the mind of the patient. The idea may be comparatively unsophisticated. For example, hysterical sensory loss usually involves the whole of the distal part of a limb—a glove or stocking sensory loss, not conforming to the territory of dermatomes or peripheral nerves. A muscle may be totally paralysed for some movements, yet seen to function normally in others. Impairment of visual activity may not follow the laws of optics, so that a subject claims to see only the larger letters on a Snellen chart, regardless of his distance from it. Another patient may speak in a 'stage-whisper', with no neurological or laryngeal structural abnormality.

The manifestations of hysteria are also culturally determined. For example, swooning used to be, by all Victorian accounts, an acceptable way of showing even minor psychological distress. It is now rare in England, though an important differential diagnosis of apparent loss of consciousness in less sophisticated cultures. During the First World War, 'paralysis' due to shell shock was a common (organic) diagnosis. This is now recognized as an understandable psychological reaction to conflict. Due to different army medical policies in the Second World War, shell shock was not seen. Simulated illnesses conform to the medical ideas of the time. With the present 'hi-tech' approach in clinical practice, it is not surprising that patients in pretended coma may end up on ventilators.

The distinction between real and presented neurological dysfunction depends upon internal inconsistencies of the type remarked upon above.

Unconscious pretence (hysteria) may be due to a significant psychiatric illness such as an affective disorder, and it is wise to seek psychiatric advice. However, the pretence is often comparatively lightly held, and firm reassurance and encouragement by, for example, a physiotherapist may rapidly relieve a hysterical paralysis.

25.2 Musculoskeletal symptoms

25.2.1 'Non-neurological' causes of low back pain

Back pain in association with radicular syndromes (prolapsed intervertebral discs, degenerative lumbar spondylosis) is described in Section 18.3.

25.2.1.1 Regional back pain not associated with other disease

Low back pain of mechanical origin is the most frequent symptom amongst patients referred to clinics in rheumatology or physical medicine, and accounts for 5 per cent of all new hospital outpatient consultations. Low back pain accounts for about 8 per cent of all sickness absence from work. The vast majority of patients with low back pain not due to a prolapsed intervertebral disc will have poorly characterized mechanical derangements of the spine and paravertebral ligaments and muscles. An exact analysis of the cause defies conventional medicine, although other systems of medicine, such as osteopathy, seem to be more successful. Some younger patients will have clear-cut mechanical causes, such as spondylolisthesis allowing subluxation, for which fusion is required.

Most low back pain of mechanical origin settles spontaneously, or with some rest. In only 5 per cent of patients does it last longer than 4 months. One trial has shown that those who rested in bed for 2 days did as well as those who rested for 7 days. There is no good evidence that non-steroidal anti-inflammatory agents are more effective in relieving pain than simple analgesic drugs. There is no good evidence that facetal injections of corticosteroid drugs are more effective than placebo.

For those few patients whose pain lasts longer than a week or two, consideration may be given to the provision of a spinal support, manipulation, traction, short-wave diathermy, or exercise. Physical exercises may be one of three types: hyperextension exercises to strengthen the paravertebral muscles, exercises designed to increase generally the mobility of the spine in all planes, and isometric spinal flexion with secondarily increased abdominal pressure.

The very variety of treatments suggests that none has been shown by experience to be clearly superior. A number of controlled trials have also failed to give clear guidelines. Probably the best pragmatic treatment of chronic low back pain is to control pain with the sensible use of analgesia, to advise the obese patient to lose weight in order to reduce the strains on the spine, to avoid heavy lifting, and to keep the spine as supple as possible by gentle exercise each day. In periods of relative freedom of pain, the patient may usefully attempt to increase the strength of the paravertebral muscles; swimming seems helpful in this regard. It is worth recording that a controlled trial has shown that those with low back pain of mechanical origin who undertake back flexing and strengthening exercises have a greater degree of pain relief than those who do not exercise. Moreover, a trial has also shown that transcutaneous nerve stimulation is no more effective than exercise alone.

There is no doubt that the patient's perception of the extent of his disability and different illness behaviours influence the outcome.

Repeated investigation and, above all, operation in the absence of clearly defined indications of radicular compression or vertebral instability should be avoided.

25.2.1.2   Back pain associated with systemic disease

In ankylosing spondylitis, backache first occurs before the age of 30, may last many months without remission, and is characterized by the pain worsening with rest and improving with activity.

Backache at rest, particularly at night, is a common feature of vertebral metastases (characteristically from bronchus, breast, or prostate), infectious disease, including tuberculosis, and primary bone disease, including osteomalacia and Paget's disease.

Backache may also arise from intra-abdominal disease. Causes include a pancreatic carcinoma, a fixed penetrating duodenal ulcer, or a large aortic aneurysm.

25.2.2   Frozen shoulder

Some patients with pain in the shoulder and upper arm are seen by neurologists as the differential diagnosis includes a cervical radiculopathy (see Section 18.2.2). The pathological basis of a primarily frozen shoulder remains obscure. Indeed, one worker has suggested that the acronym HGAC (humero-glenoid acromioclavicular syndrome) can also stand for 'haven't got a clue!'. There is little evidence for a capsulitis of the joint, although isotope scans in the active phase may show areas of increased uptake. Clinical examination readily reveals limitation of movement of the joint, particularly on medial rotation, and tenderness over the anterior aspect of the joint.

Many patients recovering from a hemiparesis find that their progress is impaired by the onset of a painful shoulder, resulting from a capsulitis of the joint. Stretching of the capsule may occur as the patient is lifted, and every effort should be made to avoid partially subluxing the joint in this way. However, minor degrees of physical trauma are probably not the only cause, as capsulitis of the shoulder may occur in association with a number of other neurological disorders of insidious onset, such as Parkinson's disease, and become a prominent symptom.

Capsulitis also results from the use of some anticonvulsant drugs, notably phenytoin and phenobarbitone.

Apart from physiotherapy to maintain and improve the range of shoulder movement by passive movement, many patients require one or more injections of methylprednisolone acetate, 40 mg plus 1 per cent lignocaine, guided to the point of malfunction identified by the method of selective tissue tension. Other methods showing promise include pulsed electromagnetic field therapy, as has been shown to accelerate bone repair and the healing of skin ulcers.

25.2.3   The overuse syndrome (synonym: repetitive strain injury)

The overuse syndrome is a disorder characterized by pain, tenderness, and sometimes impaired function in muscle groups and ligaments subjected to repetitive action. The syndrome occurs in those engaged in repetitive movements in the course of their work, such as those using word-processing keyboards and musical instruments. Physical examination is unrewarding, but there may be co-contraction of muscle groups on examination, and various tender points in the muscles at their points of insertion. There is sometimes said to be associated dermatographia. Various minor structural variants in muscle biopsies have been reported, but the importance of these is doubtful; epidemiological evidence suggests that the disorder is particularly frequent in cultures in which it is recognized as a work injury for which compensation is paid, as is the case in Australia.

25.2.4   *The chronic fatigue syndrome*

The tension exerted by contraction of a muscle may fatigue due to disordered neuromuscular transmission (see Section 21.12), or due to a failure of central neural pathways to drive anterior horn cells. Patients after a stroke, for example, may find attempts to move the hemiplegic limbs extremely fatiguing. There are few problems in understanding this. What are far more difficult to comprehend and analyse are the vague symptoms of lack of energy and easy fatiguability that commonly follow acute viral infections, such as infectious mononucleosis. Occasionally these symptoms are so severe and so persistent that concern is expressed about a persistent Epstein–Barr (EB) or enterovirus viral infection, but such patients do not have any convincing evidence of continuing replication of EB virus, or defects in cellular immunity, nor do antiviral agents, such as acyclovir, relieve symptoms. One study, however, suggests the presence of enteroviral RNA sequences in muscle biopsy specimens.

Changes in muscle metabolism have been reported in studies using nuclear magnetic resonance spectroscopy in patients with post-viral fatigue syndrome. On exercise, intracellular acidosis may occur out of proportion to the associated rise in high energy phosphates. Malaise and fatigue are common in those given interferons in trials of treatment of multiple sclerosis, suggesting that these agents might play some part in causing fatigue after spontaneous viral infections. Other evidence of an immunological basis for the chronic fatigue syndrome comes from evidence of CD8 cell activation, associated with a reduction in numbers of CD8 cells. Treatment with intravenous immunoglobulin has failed to show convincingly any benefit.

As it is probable that the chronic fatigue syndrome will prove to have multiple somatic and psychosomatic causes, it has been suggested that in further studies the disorder is defined by simple clinical criteria. The principal criteria are the new onset of persisting or relapsing debilitating fatigue that is not resolved with bed rest, and a reduction in daily activity to less than half the patient's premorbid activity level, and which continues for 6 months. Other known causes of similar symptoms such as specific infections, neoplasms, overt psychiatric disorders (such as depression), or endocrine disease must be excluded. However, it is likely that this definition will include many patients who also fulfil criteria for major depression or other psychiatric disorders.

25.3   Other syndromes on the borders of neurology

25.3.1   *Schizophrenia*

There are three strands of evidence that suggest that schizophrenia has an organic base, whatever the social and psychological circumstances that precipitate the onset and subsequent relapse. Evidence from family and twin studies strongly suggests the importance of a genetic factor, although there is good evidence that psychological stress can influence the timing of onset and relapse. CT scanning and MRI show definite, albeit minor, abnormalities in the brains of people with schizophrenia, most consistently an increase in the size of the frontal and temporal horns of the cerebral ventricles. The first rank symptoms of schizophrenia may be substantially alleviated by neuroleptic drugs that block dopamine receptors. There is also evidence from positron emission tomography that there is relative hypometabolism in the frontal lobes of the brain, and increased glucose metabolism in the left temporal lobe. The difficulty with this last evidence, and to some extent with the evidence showing ventricular dilatation, is that it is very difficult to find patients for studies such as this who have not been exposed to neuroleptic medication for many years. It is not yet clear whether the ventricular dilatation and hypometabolism represent changes secondary to many years of psychosis and antipsychotic medication, or whether they are important primary features. Recent studies suggest a striking and specific loss of the messenger RNA that encodes a non-*N*-methyl D-aspartate receptor in the temporal lobes of schizophrenic patients, but again some of these patients had been treated for many years. It is very likely that the next decade will show an increasing understanding of the neurobiology of this serious mental illness.

25.3.2   *Autism*

This unusual syndrome of childhood was first described by Kanner in 1943. Children with autism show profound social disinterest, marked disturbances in communication, and unusual repetitive stereotyped motor behaviours. Although at one time thought to be a variant of childhood schizophrenia, the clinical features, genetics, and course of the illness appear to be different. Autism may be associated with a variety of biological insults to the nervous system, such as congenital rubella, and may occur with varying degrees of mental retardation. The organic basis for the unusual mental state of autism is supported by MRI findings of significant hypoplasia of the cerebellar vermis in some autistic children. Variants include Rett's syndrome, characterized by autistic behaviour, dementia, ataxia, and loss of purposeful hand movements in girls aged under five years, and Asperger's syndrome, characterized by autistic behaviour, clumsiness, preserved intelligence and a rather better social outlook.

25.3.3   *Dyslexia*

Developmental dyslexia (as distinguished from acquired dyslexia or alexia with lesions in adult life of the left cerebral hemisphere) is a disorder manifested by difficulty in learning to read despite conventional instruction, adequate intelligence, and adequate opportunity. Dyslexia appears to be dependent upon cognitive disabilities that are of constitutional origin. Dyslexic children often have a history of impairment of language skills other than reading. They may have been late in starting to talk, and may show deficits in spoken as well as written language, and have impaired recall for verbal material. The difficulty in reading therefore

appears to be the most prominent manifestation of a generalized language impairment. The primary defect appears to be in the process of the internal representation of speech sounds, and in maintaining and manipulating these phonological representations in memory. Learning to read probably involves the internal decomposition of complex sounds into single sounds that can then be matched to letters. Increased attention to this task is very much the basis of all remedial therapy.

There is now some evidence of a neurobiological disturbance in dyslexia. First, twin studies show some degree of concordance for difficulties with verbal processing for monozygotic twins. Larger family studies suggest sometimes a single gene locus, but more often polygenic transmission. Secondly, careful measurements of the brains of young adults who had been dyslexic in childhood, who have then died, show symmetry of the planum temporale, which contains the auditory association cortex between the two sides of the brain. In those without dyslexia, the planum temporale is distinctly larger on the left side. Furthermore, histological examination of the brains of previously dyslexic young adults shows some cortical anomalies, such as neuronal ectopias.

Interest has also centred recently upon the eye movements of dyslexic readers. It has been suggested that ocular exercises may improve reading skills, but it is more likely that the abnormal eye movements during reading are secondary to the language problem rather than primarily causing it.

There is, therefore, some biological evidence that dyslexia is an abnormality of information processing based upon structural differences in the brain, with an inherited component. However, one large epidemiological study from the USA suggests first that the diagnosis of dyslexia is unstable over time, and second that reading ability follows a normal distribution, with dyslexia at the lower end of the continuum. From this perspective, dyslexia is not an all or none phenomenon, but is like hypertension. The threshold for 'treatment' of dyslexia will depend upon societal views and resources.

25.3.4   *Hyperactivity in childhood*

Easy distractability, with a short attention span and an aimless restlessness with increased motor activity, both partly unresponsive to normal social parental correction, affects between 1 and 5 per cent of all children, depending upon the cultural threshold for diagnosis. Boys display these features much more frequently than girls. The characteristic behaviour is present early in childhood before school age. There is probably no single cause for hyperactivity, the features representing a failure of the developing brain to respond to normal social influences. About 25 per cent of children with hyperactivity do have specific learning disabilities, and others are of less than average intelligence. However, the syndrome can occur in children with normal cognitive function and memory.

For many children, the restlessness spills over as they grow older to a conduct disorder, with disobedience, fights, and lying and stealing. In about half these children the conduct disorder and hyperactivity remit as the child enters adult life, but there is good evidence that educational achievement and work status in adult life are, for some, below that which would have been expected from the family background and cognitive ability. Those who were hyperactive in childhood tend to have more car accidents, make more suicide attempts, and have a higher incidence of drug and alcohol abuse.

Hyperactivity in childhood may be treated with behavioural therapy, including simple training in social skills, and with drugs. Stimulant drugs such as methylphenidate given to a hyperactive child may have a settling effect and may greatly improve the quality of family life. Although dramatic in the short term, the long-term outcome does not seem to be influenced by methylphenidate or other stimulant treatment.

Recently it has been shown by positron emission tomography that adults who had been hyperactive since childhood had areas of reduced cerebral glucose metabolism, particularly in those areas of the brain known to be associated with a regulation of attention and of motor activity. Here, then, is another example of how a syndrome on the borders of neurology is being shown to have, at least in part, an organic base.

25.4   Further reading

The interactions between mind and brain

Searle, J. (1984). The Reith Lectures 1984. 1. A froth on reality. *The Listener* 8th November, 14–16.

Reassurance

Warwick, H. M. C. and Salkovskis, P. M. (1985). Reassurance. *British Medical Journal* **290**, 1028.
Creed, F., Mayou, R., and Hopkins, A. (ed.) (1992). *Medical symptoms not explained by organic diseases*, The Royal College of Psychiatrists and the Royal College of Physicians, London.

Psychological symptoms

Appleby, L. (1987). Hypochondriasis: an acceptable diagnosis. *British Medical Journal* **294**, 857.
Lesser, I. M. (1985). Alexithymia. *New England Journal of Medicine* **312**, 690–2.

Depression

Bridges, K. W. and Goldberg, D. P. (1984). Psychiatric illness in patients with neurological disorders: patients' views on discussion of emotional problems with neurologists. *British Medical Journal* **289**, 656–8.
Editorial (1986) Treatment of depression in medical patients. *Lancet* **1**, 949–50
Gold, P. W., Goodwin, F. K., and Chrousos, G. P. (1988). Clinical and biochemical manifestations of depression. Relation to the neurobiology of stress. *New England Journal of Medicine* **319**, 348–53 and 413–20.
Goldberg, D., Bridges, K., Duncan-Jones, P., and Grayson, D. (1988). Detecting anxiety and depression in general medical settings. *British Medical Journal* **297**, 897–9.
House, A. (1987). Depression after stroke. *British Medical Journal* **294**, 76–8.
Lum, L. C. (1987). Hyperventilation syndromes in medicine and psychiatry: a review. *Journal of the Royal Society of Medicine* **80**, 229–32.
Marsden, C. D. (1986). Hysteria—a neurologist's view. *Psychological Medicine* **16**, 277–88.
Metcalfe, R., Firth, D., Pollock, S., and Creed F. (1988). Psychiatric morbidity and illness behaviour in female neurological inpatients. *Journal of Neurology, Neurosurgery and Psychiatry* **51**, 1387–90.

Low back pain

Deyo, R. A. (1983). Conservative therapy for low back pain: distinguishing useful from useless therapy. *Journal of the American Medical Association* **250**, 1057–62.
Deyo, R. A., *et al.* (1990). A controlled trial of transcutaneous electrical nerve stimulation (TENS) and exercise for chronic low back pain. *New England Journal of Medicine* **322**, 1627–34.

Deyo, R. A. (1991). Fads in the treatment of low backpain. *New England Journal of Medicine* **325**, 1039–40.

Editorial (1989). Risk factors for back trouble. *Lancet* **1**, 1305–6.

Gilbert, J. R., Taylor, D. W., Hildebrand, A., and Evans, C. (1985). Clinical trial of common treatments for low back pain in family practice. *British Medical Journal* **291**, 791–4.

Hadler, N. M. (1986). Regional back pain. *New England Journal of Medicine* **315**, 1090–2.

Frozen shoulder

Bunker, T. D. (1985). Time for a new name for 'frozen shoulder'. *British Medical Journal* **290**, 1233–4.

Jacobs, L. G. H., Barton, M. A. J., Wallace, W. A., Ferrousis, J., Dunn, N. A., and Bossingham, D. H. (1991). Intra-articular distension and steroids in the management of capsulitis of the shoulder. *British Medical Journal* **302**, 1498–501.

Overuse syndrome

See correspondence in *Lancet* (1988) pp. 1464–6.

Chronic fatigue syndrome

Editorial (1991). Chronic fatigue syndrome—false avenues and dead ends. *Lancet* **337**, 331–2.

Gow, J. W., Behan, W. M. H., Clements G. B., Woodhall C., Riding, M., and Behan. P. O. (1991). Enteroviral RNA sequences detected by polymerase chain reaction in muscle of patients with postviral fatigue syndrome. *British Medical Journal* **302**, 692–6.

Kendell, R. E. (1991), Chronic fatigue, viruses and depression. *Lancet* **337**, 160–1.

Landay, A. L., Jessop, C., Lennette, E. T., and Levy, J. A. (1991). Chronic fatigue syndrome: clinical syndrome associated with immune activation. *Lancet* **338**, 707–12.

Swartz, M. N. (1988). The chronic fatigue syndrome, one entity or many? *New England Journal of Medicine* **319**, 1726–8.

Wessely, S. (1989). Myalgic encephalomyelitis—a warning: discussion paper. *Journal of the Royal Society of Medicine* **82**, 215–17.

White, P. (1989). Fatigue syndrome: neurasthenia revived. *British Medical Journal* **298**, 1199–200.

Schizophrenia

Harrison, P. J., McLaughlin, D., and Kerwin R. W. (1991). Decreased hippocampal expression of glutamate receptor gene in schizophrenia. *Lancet* **337**, 450–2.

Mesulam, M. N. (1990). Schizophrenia and the brain. *New England Journal of Medicine* **322**, 842–5.

Autism

Editorial (1991). The autistic dimension. *Lancet* **337**, 1192–3.

Frith, U. (ed.) (1991). *Autism and Asperger syndrome.* Cambridge University Press, Cambridge.

Dyslexia

Editorial (1989). Dyslexia. *Lancet* **2**, 719–20.

Pennington, B. F., Gilger, J. W., Pauls, D., Smith, S. A., Smith S. D., and DeFries, J. C. (1991). *Journal of the American Medical Association* **266**, 1527–34.

Shaywitz, S. E., Escobar, M. D., Shawitz, B. A. *et al.* (1992). Evidence that dyslexia may represent the lower tail of a normal distribution of reading ability. *New England Journal of Medicine* **326**, 145–50.

Hyperactivity in childhood

Weiss, G. (1990). Hyperactivity in childhood. *New England Journal of Medicine* **323**, 1413–15.

Part IV

Coping with chronic physical disability

26 Rehabilitation of physical disabilities due to neurological disease

Pharmacological therapy is available for some of the disorders considered in this book, notably for epilepsy and Parkinson's disease, and further pharmacological interventions are very effective in those with neuroendocrine disorders; for example, the use of bromocriptine in reducing the size of a prolactinoma. Other neurological disorders, such as myasthenia gravis, can be treated by a variety of effective methods: anticholinesterases to correct the primary biochemical defects of neuromuscular transmission; immunosuppressant agents, such as steroids, to suppress the abnormal cells interfering with the architecture of the myoneural junction; and surgical therapy, such as thymectomy, to remove part of the system that activates lymphocytes to abnormal behaviour. The recent discovery of the gene product (dystrophin) in Duchenne muscular dystrophy indicates that we are on the brink of further important understandings of the biochemical nature of many neurological illnesses. However, it has to be acknowledged that for other disorders, such as multiple sclerosis, pharmacological therapy plays a comparatively small part, and for yet others, such as stroke and spinal injury, virtually no part at all except in the acute phase. However, survivors of stroke and of head and spinal injuries, and those who are further advanced in the course of their multiple sclerosis or Parkinson's disease undoubtedly benefit from rehabilitative therapy.

It is traditional to distinguish rehabilitation—the attempted restoration of patients to their fullest possible physical, mental and social capability—from the support of those with chronic advancing diseases, such as motor neuron disease, and from the support of the frail elderly, many of whom have impairments of vision and hearing as well as physical frailties. The techniques of physical rehabilitation and the support structures are much the same across all groups, and the only distinction that it is necessary to make is to maintain a realistic appreciation of what is possible, so that resources are not wastefully expended upon, for example, physical therapy which is achieving no measurable outcome beyond the feeling that 'something is being done'. This chapter provides a brief overview of the principles of neurological rehabilitation, and draws attention to those areas the effectiveness of which is clearly proven.

26.1   The size of the problem

Estimates of the number of people who require some sort of rehabilitative service vary much according to the criteria used in defining disability and its severity, and in the need for treatment. Tables 26.1 and 26.2 indicate the prevalence of various disabling disorders. The tables show that the principal causes of severe physical disabilities are neurological disease and arthritis. The report from which the tables are taken states that 'in an average health district, there will be about 1810 people with a wheelchair, about 11 000 people with regular urinary incontinence, and 25 000 adults with severe deafness . . . There will be 500 people with Parkinsonism, of whom 55 will be severely or very severely disabled. There will be at least 200 patients with multiple sclerosis, and there could be up to 6000 with rheumatoid arthritis.' Tables 26.1 and 26.2 also show that in an average health district there will be about 1375 survivors of

Table 26.1   Estimated numbers of disabled people and of those who are severely or very severely disabled or handicapped in various categories in a District with a population of 250 000 people reflecting the national age distribution

| Category | Estimated number in category | | | Estimated number severely or very severely disabled or handicapped in District |
	Per 10 000 population, e.g. typical group practice	Per 250 000 population e.g. typical Health District	Per cent severely or very severely disabled or handicapped	
All physically 'disabled' people				
National Sample Survey	670 adults	16 750 adults	20	3350 adults
Local Authority Surveys	557	13 925	30	4180
Lambeth Survey	1150 adults	28 750	–	4170
Impaired hearing				
Min. 35 dB HL, at 0.5, 1, 2 and 4 kHz in better ear	1000 adults	25 000 adults	10 (66–95 dB HL)	2500 adults
Impaired vision				
Less than 6/18 with Snellen with glasses	52 adults	1300 adults	32 (6/60 or less)	408 adults
Regular urinary incontinence	440	11 000	–	–
Use of wheelchairs	72	1810	–	–

Reproduced from *Physical disability 1986 and beyond*, Royal College of Physicians, 1986, with kind permission.

Table 26.2   Estimated number of persons with major physical disabling conditions and of those who are severely or very severely disabled or handicapped thereby in a district with a population of 250 000 people reflecting the national age distribution

Disabling conditions	Estimated prevalence of disease/condition (various sources)		Estimated number of severely or very severely disabled or handicapped in District Based on Harris Survey*
	Per 10 000 population	Per 250 000 population	
Osteoarthritis	2900	72 500	860 all forms and unspecified
	1280	32 000	arthritis
Rheumatoid arthritis	250	6250	
	100	2500	
Ischaemic heart disease	c.700	17 500	60
Other heart disease	–	–	110
Respiratory conditions (excluding cancer of lung)	c.800	20 000	115
Stroke (survivors)	55	1375	340
Parkinsonism	20	500	55
Multiple sclerosis	8	200	80
Motor neuron disease	1	15	–
Muscular dystrophy	1	15	–
Epilepsy	50	1250	not known
Paraplegia	–	–	35
Colostomies	16	400	–
Injuries	About 2500 people per 'District' are treated as in-patients in hospital each year.		40 (head injuries excluded)
Head injuries	About 675 people per 'District' are treated as inpatients in hospital each year.		
Amputations	About 30 people per 'District' are referred annually for the first time to a Limb Centre.		–
Major congenital malformations	Incidence is about 2 per cent of all live births.		

* The Harris survey deals mainly with physical disability.

Reproduced from *Physical disability 1986 and beyond*, Royal College of Physicians, 1986, with kind permission.

stroke, of whom 340 will be severely or very severely disabled.

26.2   Impairment, disability, and handicap

Our concepts of physical disability have been advanced in the past decade by the increasing use of three terms: impairment, disability, and handicap. The words are used as follows. A disease or disorder may lead to an *impairment*, defined as any disturbance of the normal structure and functioning of the body, including the systems of mental function. Impairment may lead to *disability*—the loss or reduction of functional ability to perform an activity consequent upon impairment. It is characterized by deficiencies of functions customarily expected of the body or its parts. Disability represents objectification of impairments in everyday life and activities. Impairment and disability may lead to *handicap*—'the disadvantage experienced as a result of impairment or disability, characterized by a discordance between the individual's performance or status and the expectations of a particular group of which he or she is a member, including the individual's own expectations. Handicap thus represents the social and environmental consequences of impairments and disabilities.' To take an example from outside neurology, a man after a severe myocardial infarction has *impaired* cardiac function with a reduced left ventricular ejection fraction, his *disability* is breathlessness and angina on going upstairs, and his *handicap* may be his inability to go and visit his grandchildren because of his disability. To take a further example from within neurological practice, a man after a stroke has *impaired* left hemisphere function, is *disabled* by dysphasia and a right hemiplegia, and may be *handicapped* by his inability to drive to the shops because of the right hemiplegia.

Although many physicians first viewed this architecture of disability with some suspicion, the concepts contained in these definitions have proved useful in clarifying what it is reasonable to expect of rehabilitation. For example, appropriate assessment of the man with a stroke whose history has just been described may allow relief of his handicap by advice about modification to the steering control of his car (by placing a knob for one-handed use on the rim of the steering wheel) but may have no influence upon the impairment or disability.

Impairment and disability give rise to handicap by the interaction of other influences, such as the environment in which the patient lives. To go back to the other example of the patient with angina, for example, his impairment may not be manifest as a disability if he moves to a bungalow without stairs.

It becomes clear that resources are also important in the interaction between impairment and disability and handicap. For example, the move of our patient with angina from a house with stairs to a bungalow is dependent either upon his own financial resources or the resources of his family, or the assistance of a local housing authority which provides subsidized accommodation, and the willingness of that authority to set up mechanisms for appropriate housing of people with impairments and disabilities.

Resources are not only financial. An important external supporting resource for those with physical disabilities is the network of family, neighbours, and friends who may provide physical support from time to time, or social support, such as taking the disabled person out to the cinema or to visit friends, thereby reducing his handicap. A final resource is the 'resourcefulness' of the individual. All neurologists are familiar with patients who lead very successful lives in spite of severe physical disability, and who are, by their own resourcefulness, barely handicapped. At the other extreme are patients who have comparatively mild neurological impairments, and yet who become grossly handicapped by these impairments.

26.3   The politics of disability

As already noted, the handicapping effect of a disability is to some extent dependent upon resources. In a welfare state, the provision of resources by the state becomes a political issue, and it is therefore not surprising that the financial needs of disabled people have for many years been a political issue. A landmark in the UK was the Chronically Sick and Disabled Persons Act, 1970, which placed an obligation on local authorities to inform themselves of the number of disabled people and their needs, and to take steps to meet their needs. Since then, as might have been surmised, the difficulty has always been that the more vigorous an authority was in seeking out the needs of disabled people in its area of local government, then the greater the demands upon the financial resources of that authority to meet those needs. However, the Act and events leading up to it have been responsible for a considerably increased perception of the handicapping effects of society upon people with physical disabilities. All public buildings now have to have access for people with wheelchairs, and over the years an increased range of supporting monetary allowances have become available to people with physical disabilities (see Section 26.9 and Appendix A).

There is, however, another area of 'politics of disability'. Some sociologists and many disabled people feel that society locates the 'problem' of disability within the individual, whereas the 'problem' is really due to the failure of society to provide appropriate services, and to ensure that the needs of disabled people are fully taken into account in its social organization. Furthermore, the consequences of this failure do not fall randomly upon individuals, but systematically upon disabled people as a group, who experience this failure as discrimination institutionalized throughout society. Disability in this context is a social state and not a medical condition. In many instances, medical expertise is inappropriate, as the disabled person knows more about how to reduce the handicapping effects of his or her disability than anyone else.

26.3.1 'Finding able minds in disabled bodies'

This is the title of a paper in the *Lancet* in 1986. The authors cite a further paper to illustrate their point: 'the social value attached to *mens sana in corpore sano* is strongly persistent, and with it the corollary that an impaired body implies an impaired mind.' The totally irrational perspective of otherwise intelligent people that physically disabled people are also mentally suspect is a source of anguish. For example, talking across a patient with an expressive aphasia to his spouse is extremely hurtful, bitterly recognized in the title of a radio programme of a decade ago entitled *'Does he take sugar?'*. Patients with severe disorders of communication, such as aphasia or virtual anarthria, associated with cerebral palsy are particularly at risk of being thought to have no inner emotional or intellectual life. It is unfortunately too much to hope that Christy Brown's book and subsequent film *My left foot* will have laid this canard to rest once and for all.

26.3.2 Psychological responses to disability—the importance of age and of abruptness of onset

Those who are disabled from very early childhood, such as those with cerebral palsy, grow up with the disabling and handicapping effects of their impairment, and develop their own personality and mechanisms for coping with their disability, and very often lead fulfilled lives because of this. Growth and maturation within the brain may allow the performance of physical functions which to an able-bodied person appear remarkable, as witnessed by the success of many of the victims of the thalidomide disaster.

An able-bodied young man who becomes paraplegic as a result of a motor cycle accident (see Chapter 15) is in a completely different situation. He has developed expectations of his life, including his emotional life and career, which have to be abruptly adjusted as a result of the spinal injury. Those caring for people with spinal injuries recognize a number of psychological stages through which such an injured person has to pass—typically denial, then anger, which may include anger directed at the medical carers, then depression, and finally gradual acceptance and reconstruction of a new life. A number of sociological studies have been directed at this topic. Insights gained include the gradual release of information by doctors about the lack of recoverability (called 'cooling the mark' by Goffman), and the concept of the patient's need to timetable stages in his or her illness career, and of his or her determination to 'pass' as normal. These are insights which all sensitive doctors should have, but they have been formulated in an understandable and imaginative way by medical sociologists in the past 30 years.

A young man with a spinal injury has much to face, but he can at least be aware that his illness is static (although older age will bring an increasing and different range of problems). However, people with muscular dystrophy, for example, or Parkinson's disease, or multiple sclerosis characterized by frequent relapses, are all aware that their disease is progressive, and they have the additional tasks of coming to terms with the uncertainty about the rate of progression, and about whether they will be able to accomplish at least some of their personal ambitions before physical disability makes some of these impracticable. The subject's uncertainties are compounded by medical uncertainty, too, because few of us can predict in other than rather vague and general terms about the likely rate of progress of any individual's disorder.

26.3.3 Particular aspects of disability due to brain disease

As the brain is the organ of the mind, it is immediately apparent that any neurologically disabling condition due to brain disease may have some influence upon cognitive function and behaviour, as well as upon physical ability and upon ability to communicate. This is particularly apparent in those who are physically disabled by the effects of severe brain injuries, in whom lack of insight, increased irritability and disinhibition, and cognitive change all conspire to make support more difficult for their carers than for carers of those with other disabilities of locomotor function, such as rheumatoid arthritis or spinal injury. There is also some evidence that depression in association with disability is particularly likely to follow if the cause of the physical disability is intracranial. For example, a disabling depression of mood is not uncommon after stroke (see Section 10.1.9).

26.4   Functional assessment

Integral to any proper efforts at rehabilitation is some measure of how effective is that rehabilitation in restoring a disabled person towards a better level of function. In order to measure effectiveness of rehabilitation, it is therefore necessary to have some measure of functional capability before and after the intervention.

A simple, unstructured, and informative way of assessing functional capability is to ask the disabled person how he or she spends an average day. This will give some measure of his or her ability to get out of bed, to shave, wash, and dress, to prepare breakfast, perhaps to look after children and prepare them for school, perhaps to travel to work and from work, and to enjoy recreation. The main areas of disability and handicap can thereby readily be grasped. However, for the evaluation of the effectiveness of therapy, and for comparison between patients, it is helpful to use one of the more formal scales. A vast number of these are available, many being only minor variations on old favourites.

26.4.1   Physical disability

For physical disability the Barthel scale is extremely useful (Table 26.3), and correlates well with the perceptions of patients and their carers as to their overall ability. It is, however, comparatively insensitive to minor levels of disability—a so-called 'ceiling effect'.

26.4.2   Tests of cognitive function

The Abbreviated Mental Test reviewed in Chapter 11 is a reliable and valid way of screening for impaired cognitive function, but for those who have suffered cranial injuries or stroke, a more sophisticated neuropsychological assessment may uncover important defects in spatial orientation

Table 26.3   The Barthel scale

		With help	Independent
1.	Feeding (if food needs to be cut up = help)	5	10
2.	Moving from wheelchair to bed and return (includes sitting up in bed)	5–10	15
3.	Personal toilet (wash face, comb hair, shave, clean teeth)	0	5
4.	Getting on and off toilet (handling clothes, wipe, flush)	5	10
5.	Bathing self	0	5
6.	Walking on level surface (or if unable to walk, propel wheelchair) *score only if unable to walk	10 0*	15 5*
7.	Ascend and descend stairs	5	10
8.	Dressing (includes tying shoes, fastening fasteners)	5	10
9.	Controlling bowels	5	10
10.	Controlling bladder	5	10

Note: A score of zero is given where patients cannot meet the defined criterion.

(Section 6.1.2.1), communication (Section 6.1.1), or memory.

26.4.3   Sphincter control

Some neurologically disabled people, particularly those with spinal disorders, have urgency or incontinence of micturition. Some of these also have impaired control of bowel sphincters. In others, relative physical immobility is reflected in chronic constipation. More often, physical disability and poor design of lavatories handicap people with intact sphincters so that journeys and attendances at social engagements become a misery because of poor access to lavatories. A simple record of difficulties with control of bowel and bladder usually suffices.

26.4.4   *Education, work, and financial support*

An initial assessment of a disabled person before rehabilitation requires a knowledge of that person's previous educational attainments, work experience, and enjoyment of different types of work, and the financial support that he or she has available in terms of capital resources and, possibly, insurance benefits. For example, it may be inappropriate to attempt to rehabilitate a spinally injured scaffolder to work as a computer analyst if neither his educational background nor prior interests in any way indicate that he could successfully accomplish such retraining.

26.4.5   *Family and social relationships*

Details about the immediate family and social network within which the disabled person operates should also be obtained at the initial assessment. For example, experience shows that a man is far more likely to be able to return home from hospital after a stroke if he has a caring spouse at home than if he is a widower of the same age, even if the physical impairments are the same.

26.4.6   *Housing*

An initial assessment should also include a record of the disabled person's housing, and his or her perception of the difficulties that might be encountered on return to that housing.

26.4.7   *Sexual life and disablement*

An initial abrupt onset of physical disablement is nearly always associated with impaired sexual function for a time, due to the destruction of the disabled person's self-image as an attractive and well-formed person. Acceptance that one can still receive and give sexual love often, but unfortunately by no means always, returns. Apart from these psychological aspects of sexual function, there may be organic causes for impotence (see Section 6.12), or physical impairment due to spasticity or impaired control of bodily movements may interfere with the physical aspects of sex. Simple advice about changes in bodily position for intercourse may be very effective in restoring sexual life in the latter cases. Aids for erectile

impotence are described in Section 6.12.1. More important than the provision of aids is skilled counselling of the disabled person and partner about meeting their expectations of each other.

26.5   Mechanisms of recovery

Neurons that die are not replaced. How is it, therefore, that some degree of functional neurological recovery usually occurs after apparently severe initial damage to the central nervous system? The transected axon, in the case of a spinal transection, sprouts vigorously, but the sprouts reach only a few millimetres in length, and, un-directed by the architecture of Schwann cells as they are in the peripheral nervous system, form a useless tangle. Although there is a very considerable body of ongoing research about how the effectiveness of neural regeneration might be improved, current rehabilitation depends upon encouraging the development of residual function, aided by physiotherapy, speech therapy, and occupational therapy.

26.5.1   *Physiotherapy*

Before a neurological illness, few of us other than dancers or athletes are consciously aware of how our bodies move. Walking, for example, is largely a reflex activity, and can even be induced in a decerebrate cat on a treadmill under certain conditions. After a neurological catastrophe such as a stroke, a person is painfully and consciously aware of attempting to move a paralysed limb. 'Voluntary effort', whatever that is, attempts to gain access to stereotyped patterns of activity organized at a lower level in the nervous system. Physiotherapy aims to facilitate appropriate patterns of movement, such as balancing the trunk, and to inhibit inappropriate patterns, such as flexor spasms. Outside research centres, an evaluation of the effectiveness of physiotherapy continues to be bedevilled by a lack of objective assessment of results, and by the loose terminology adopted by some therapists. None the less, no neurologist doubts that physiotherapy is effective in appropriate circumstances, even though the methods are empirical, and the arguments used to justify the methods are not always soundly based upon physiological observations. A patient whose hemiplegia has been neglected will recover spontaneously to some extent, but, without physiotherapy will retain a clumsy spastic gait and distorted posture of the arm, abnormal postures which might well have been largely avoided by appropriate physiotherapy at the appropriate time.

26.5.1.1 *Spasticity*

Repeated passive movement of a joint gradually 'breaks down' spasticity through mechanisms that are uncertain. This is one of the principal ways by which a physiotherapist both prevents and subsequently treats spasticity. Abnormal postural drives may also place a spastic limb into a position in which it functions poorly, as well as looking socially less than acceptable. For example, the untreated hemiplegic arm is flexed at the elbow and the wrist is often strongly pronated and flexed. A physiotherapist may be able to improve the posture of such a limb by repeated extension of the elbow and wrist joints, encouraging the patient to undertake the same range of activities many times each day.

Spasticity in the lower limbs, as may occur after a thoracic spinal injury, may be prevented by similar passive stretching, and the abnormal postural drive, which tends to bring the hips and knees into flexion, may be prevented by a period of lying prone each day. Unfortunately, however, passive stretching is sometimes not enough. Some physiotherapists use ice-packs to reduce spasticity, although the effectiveness of this treatment is not certain. Nociceptive afferent impulses from the bladder, bowels, and the skin may all play a part in generating or exaggerating spasticity. For example, a person with a spinal injury may be much more troubled by flexor spasms at a time of a urinary tract infection. Attention to the care of bladder, bowel, and skin may do much to reduce spasticity.

If spasticity does not respond to simple measures such as passive stretching, then drugs are available, although none are dramatically effective. The first choice is baclofen, a derivative of γ-aminobutyric acid (GABA). Baclofen reduces the pre-synaptic release of excitatory neurotransmitters such as substance P, and also acts post-synaptically, reducing the firing of both α and γ motor neurons. The initial dose should be of the order of 10 mg/day in adults, and the drug increased slowly up to 70 or 80 mg/day. Unfortunately, drowsiness may prevent use of the drug even in modest dosage, but sometimes patients are well helped by this medication. An alternative is diazepam, which has much the same disadvantage of drowsiness, but sometimes useful benefit is achieved at a dosage level that would seem high by everyday standards (e.g. 40 mg/day) without producing significant drowsiness. Diazepam increases pre-synaptic inhibition, probably by facilitating GABA transmission. The third available drug is dantrolene sodium, which decreases the release of calcium ions from the sarcoplasmic reticulum, reducing the coupling between the process of electrical discharge of the muscle membrane and activation of the myofibrils. Dantrolene is therefore different from the two previous drugs, in so far as it acts peripherally rather than centrally. Unfortunately, however, there is a significant risk of hepatic failure with this drug.

A useful way of treating long-established spasticity is by disruption of the stretch reflex by injection of phenol at the motor end points previously identified by threshold electrical stimulation. Remarkable reduction in hip flexor spasms, hamstring spasm, and adductor spasm in the lower limbs may be achieved. It is often necessary to repeat the injection after an interval of a few months, presumably on account of neural regeneration. The reflex arc can also be interrupted at the level of the nerve root by the subarachnoid injection of 5 per cent phenol in glycerol. Glycerol is heavier than cerebrospinal fluid, so that if it is planned to treat spasticity in the left leg, the patient would lie on his or her left side, and the mixture allowed to sink around the left lumbar and sacral roots. It must, however, be remembered that the roots that are affected by the phenol cannot be selected with any degree of accuracy, and there is a real risk of incontinence following this procedure. For this reason, it is usually reserved for patients with severe spasticity who are already incontinent of urine and faeces. Another unwanted effect is deafferentation of the skin, as somatosensory fibres in the nerve roots are also damaged by the phenol; this leads to an increased incidence of pressure sores.

26.5.1.2 *Surgical treatment*

In patients who have had spastic deformities for

Mechanisms of recovery 457

many months, secondary structural shortening in muscles and their tendons, and contractures in the capsules of the joints often occur, so that interruption of the reflex pathways is no longer sufficient to allow the limb to be moved to a position of extension. Operations designed to lengthen the tendons, or to sever them, and to make various releasing incisions into the joint capsules may then be necessary.

Apart from the corrective operations just described, an orthopaedic surgeon may be able to reduce disability by other procedures. For example, a patient who has a traumatic tetraplegia with preservation of the sixth cervical spinal cord segment, and loss of all function below, will still be able to contract the brachioradialis muscle, and the extensors of the wrist. He or she will, however, not be able to flex the fingers, as these are supplied by the eighth cervical segment. In this situation the flexor tendons can be fixed to the front of the wrist, so that with active dorsiflexion through the C6 root innervated extensors of the wrist, the fingers are passively pulled down towards the palm. It may also be possible to transfer the tendon of brachioradialis to flexor pollicus longus so that some active thumb flexion is possible.

Orthopaedic surgery has an important role to play in improving the physical function of children with cerebral palsy. The most common procedure is to lengthen the Achilles tendon, so allowing the reduction of an equinus deformity. In developing countries, where poliomyelitis remains a problem in spite of the availability of immunization, an orthopaedic surgeon will have more complex tendon transfer operations to undertake. However, a country that is unable to afford adequate immunization programmes is unlikely to be able to afford orthopaedic surgeons with the necessary skills.

As can be seen from the foregoing list of procedures, prevention of spasticity by early attention to stretching muscles and preventing flexion deformities is much better than secondary treatment. The physiotherapist has a major role to play in preventing contractures and deformities, as has the patient in stretching his or her muscles as far as he or she can within the limits of overall disability.

26.5.1.3 *Ataxia*

Ataxia of hand movements and of gait, as may

occur, for example, in multiple sclerosis or in the cerebellar degenerations, is resistant to physiotherapy. At an early stage an unsteady gait may be made a little better by encouraging the patient to walk on a narrow base, and to concentrate on holding an erect posture. Visual feedback with mirrors has not been shown to have much effect, nor has the previously fashionable treatment of increasing the inertial mass of the limb by placing heavy weighted bracelets of lead around the wrist or ankle.

26.5.2 *Speech therapy*

The effect of what may be termed 'non-specific care and attention' has been seen in an interesting comparative trial of the effectiveness of speech therapy given by volunteers interested in the subject, but without any formal training, and speech therapists. No differences in outcome could be identified. Most neurologists remain sceptical of the value of speech therapy in disorders of language, bearing in mind that the organization of the internal dictionary remains obscure, and therapy at present has little scientific basis. Speech therapy does, however, have some part to play in improving phonation and in articulation in diseases of the extrapyramidal system and brain stem, and is of striking benefit in other fields of medicine, such as re-educating patients to talk after a laryngectomy.

For those whose possibilities of normal communication remain severely limited by aphasia or anarthria, the provision of simple aids such as picture and symbol charts through which the patient can indicate his needs and ideas are useful. Many patients with an anterior dysphasia (Section 6.1.1.1) can read, and can therefore assemble sentences by the use of cards with common prechosen words. The advent of microcomputer systems has enabled many of those with disordered communication to communicate through means of a keyboard and screen. Function keys can be programmed to bring up common complete phrases or sentences on the screen. Patients with additional severe physical disability, who cannot point or operate a keyboard, may be able to operate a switch-operated scanning method, whereby a cursor moves over a series of messages on the screen, and is halted at the appropriate one by operating a micro-switch which may be closed by very limited pressure, such as chin pressure.

More sophisticated devices allow the use of word-processing packages and printers.

Jayne Easton has some useful points for those communicating with a person using a communication system. She writes, 'Make sure the equipment is accessible to the patient. Remember that he or she may not be able to ask for it. Encourage the use of communication systems by conversing with the patient, not admiring the equipment and directing your conversation to the accompanying relative or spouse. Allow time for patients to communicate; do not frustrate them by answering your own questions, guessing ahead, and closing the conversation before they have had a chance to complete the message in answer to your first question. If you have not time to wait, ask patients to prepare any questions that they may have for you in advance. Doctors should be positive in their attitude towards the use of communication equipment. Comments relating to 'dalek-like voices', 'toys', and 'gadgets' may discourage acceptance. Remember it takes a lot of courage to use this equipment outside a cossetted clinical environment. Encourage patients to use any speech that they may have in addition to the communication aid.'

Ms Easton's publication contains a number of useful addresses for the provision of communication aids in the UK.

26.5.3 Occupational therapy

The role of occupational therapy is even harder to evaluate in a formal way. Rehabilitation ideally means the return of the neurologically disabled person to his or her previous or similar work. However, social factors such as the unwillingness of employers to take on disabled employees, and the general level of unemployment in the community, may mean that return to work is not a reasonable measure of outcome of the effectiveness of occupational therapy. Regardless of formal assessment, occupational therapists and physiotherapists provide, at a common-sense level, answers to many of the 'simple' problems that bedevil the lives of many disabled people. For example, it is difficult to visualize how one might scrub one's fingernails if one has a hemiplegia, and yet the answer is simple—have a nail brush fixed securely to the wall immediately above the hand basin, so that either the good or the impaired hand can be drawn briskly through the bristles. Occupational therapists are often instrumental in reducing the handicap of disabled women to a functional level at which they can run their own home. In association with psychologists at industrial retraining units, they can advise on making the best use of remaining manual and intellectual skills in the neurologically disabled.

Therapists of all types often make the point that if they had access to patients for intensive and early treatment, then the outcomes of their therapy would be better. Such evidence as there is does suggest that intensive therapy gets patients slightly quicker to a level of function which they would, in any event, have achieved with less intensive therapy. There is suggestive but less convincing evidence about speech therapy after stroke. However, these accelerated gains, which are, in any event, of small magnitude, have to be seen against the consumption of resources by intensive therapy. A curious anomaly of therapists' perspectives also has to be considered—that, with natural sympathy, they tend to concentrate their services upon the severely disabled, even though in terms of gains in performance they might do better to concentrate on the less severely disabled. This is particularly illustrated by repeated efforts to restore function to the hemiplegic hand, long after the time at which there is good research evidence that expected gains are at all likely.

26.6   Aids and adaptations

An aid is any item designed to help functional ability, and includes obvious items such as spectacles, dentures, and hearing aids. Adaptations are aids that are fixtures in the home. Communication aids have been considered in Section 26.5.2.

26.6.1 Aids to mobility

26.6.1.1 Sticks and frames

The simplest aid, used by many with minor locomotor disabilities, is a walking stick, which reduces anxiety about instability, and can relieve pain by giving support. Outside the realm of neurological disability, sticks are very useful for those with arthritis of the hip, as the static force of the body can be transmitted partly through the stick rather than through the painful joint. A simple stick increases the size of the area through which the patient's centre of gravity is carried to the ground, and therefore considerably aids balance and increases confidence. The area through which the body weight is transmitted can be increased by terminating the stick with a tripod or tetrapod, but these do not work very well if the ground is uneven, and they may be impractical on stairs. The stick should be chosen so that the distance from the handle to the ground is equal to the distance from the proximal wrist crease to the ground, with the elbow held flexed to 15°, and the patient wearing his normal shoes. The flexion of the elbow is necessary so that the stick can be swung ahead with the arm extended, while walking, without the tip catching on the ground. In hemiplegic patients, the stick should be held in the contralateral hand, often the only hand in which it can be held, as this encourages a better pattern of reciprocal walking.

Patients who are very unsteady, particularly if elderly, may find that a walking frame (e.g. Zimmer frame) considerably increases mobility with safety. Variations are available with wheels on the front legs, or articulating frames to allow alternating gait, but the standard fixed four-point frame is very reliable and sturdy. It has the advantage that a shopping bag may be hung on one corner. It is also reportedly often used for supporting clothes near a radiator to dry!

26.6.1.2 *Wheelchairs*

Many patients with progressive neurological disorders understandably dread the thought of becoming reliant upon a wheelchair, but a well-chosen wheelchair may considerably reduce handicap by increasing mobility in and outside the home. The provision of an appropriate wheelchair is a specialist function, and an unsuitable wheelchair may be worse than no wheelchair at all. Points that have to be considered include whether the wheelchair is for use indoors, or outdoors, or both; whether it is for occasional use; whether it should be collapsing so that it can be transported into a car; whether the patient has the ability to propel it himself or herself; whether it should be manual or electric; whether the arm rest should be removable to allow sideways transfers; and what accessories, such as a Roho cushion, are required. The braking mechan-

isms are often less effective than one would like to see, and often so inadequate as to be dangerous. It is necessary to adapt the braking mechanism for hemiplegic patients so that brakes on both wheels can be operated by the one arm. For hemiplegic patients, it is possible, by a system of dual rims on one end of the axle, to drive wheels alternately with the unaffected hand. However, many patients prefer a rather erratic propulsion with the unaffected hand and foot rather than the double-hand rim on the normal side. Until recently, electric wheelchairs have suffered from poor control mechanisms that accelerate and decelerate too abruptly.

Many medical students and doctors are ignorant about the best way to push a wheelchair and to help someone out of it. If, for example, you are helping a newly hemiplegic patient from wheelchair to bed, you must first consider whether you and the patient together are going to be strong enough to make the transfer, and what you are going to do about any attachments such as catheters. Next you must ensure that the brakes are not only 'on' but working. The foot rests must be up and folded well clear. You must then stand in front of the patient, blocking his feet from sliding forwards with your own, and, if the patient's good arm is strong enough, lock that arm behind your neck. Then liaise with the patient on an appropriate count-down to lift. In order to protect your own back, you must squat and use your own quadriceps, rather than the extensor muscles of your spine.

If you attempt to push a wheelchair forwards over a kerb, the patient will topple forwards out of it. It is essential to tilt the chair backwards so that the centre of gravity is over the rear wheels, and then go slowly over the edge of the kerb.

In the UK, wheelchairs are obtained by posting a completed appliance order form 5 (AOF5G) to the nearest artificial limb and appliance centre. These centres have now been brought much more firmly within the mainstream of the National Health Service.

26.6.1.3 *Orthoses*

Orthoses may be used to redistribute a load, to support an unstable joint, or to provide a mechanical means of compensation for weak or absent muscles. Consider the patient with a flaccid foot drop. The simplest orthosis is made from polypropylene moulded around the ankle and underneath the heel, extending forwards under the foot to just behind the metatarsal heads. It is sufficiently light to fit under the sock and shoe. A more complex orthosis may be developed using a toe-raising spring. More sophisticated still is an active orthosis, if the common peroneal nerve is intact, it may be electrically stimulated behind the head of the fibula. The stimulator is designed to be cut out by a switch in the heel when there is pressure by the foot on the ground. When the pressure is off, the stimulator is switched on, and the foot actively dorsiflexed.

More complex orthoses, supporting movement at the knee and ankle as well as at the foot, may be used for those with cauda equina lesions. A hinged knee joint allows the patient to sit down in relative comfort, the hinge being locked when the patient wishes to stand upright and move forwards. For those with higher lesions in the low thoracic cord, a hip-guidance orthosis may be used, with reciprocating interlock, so that as one hip flexes the other extends and supports the body weight. As might be expected, such orthoses are cumbersome, and it is only the occasional active and reasonably lightweight person who thinks that this complicated device is worthwhile.

Over the past few years there has been increasing interest in computer-driven functional electrical stimulation of lower limb muscles, combined with orthoses, for patients with spinal lesions. Work is advancing rapidly in this field.

26.6.1.4   *Other simple aids*

Many patients, particularly those with spinal injuries, readily learn lateral transfers, for example between bed and wheelchair. The most important point is to ensure that the two surfaces are at about the same height. A smooth board on which the bottom can slide aids such transfers. For those with graver disabilities, hoists may be required in the home. It may be better to consider the provision of an overhead track hoist rather than a clumsy mobile hoist if the disabled person's room is big enough, and if he or she is largely confined to that room.

A number of other simple domestic aids may make a considerable difference to reducing the handicap of those with neurological disability. A plate-surround clips on to a dinner plate, offering a surface against which food can be pushed, thus helping a hemiplegic patient who only has one hand for eating. Such a patient can also use a Dyna fork, one prong of which is of extra width and sharpened to be used for cutting. A Nelson knife—a knife and fork combined for one-handed eating—is preferred by some. A non-slip plate-holder and a suction egg-cup are all useful devices. For dressing, Velcro fastening rather than shoe laces may be preferred. There are also button-fasteners which can be used one handed, and a sock and shoe aid, which allows these to be put on with one hand without bending. Other useful devices include self-pasting toothbrushes for one-handed use, and a wedge that can be screwed on to the kitchen wall, allowing the lid of a jar to be trapped in the wedge so that it can be twisted open or closed.

26.6.1.5   *Aids and adaptations in the lavatory and bathroom*

Many modern lavatories are low, and a disabled or elderly patient may find it difficult to rise from them. In one recent survey, a number were found to use the lavatory door handle as the principal aid to get up! A disabled person may well require a raised lavatory seat and rails appropriately fitted. For those in wheelchairs, there must be sufficient space to allow wheelchair access, usually through a sideways transfer from chair to lavatory seat. Sophisticated lavatories are now available which will flush the perineal area with warm water after evacuation, followed by drying with a blast of warm air.

Getting in and out of the bath is often difficult for people with quite minor locomotor disabilities. The simplest aid is the provision of a non-slip mat. Also very useful is a bath stool on which the patient sits while washing himself or herself, so that it is not necessary to raise the centre of gravity from a very low position when attempting to get out. Many older and disabled people rely on holding on to the bath taps to aid getting out. This is unsatisfactory, the provision of appropriately placed rails being a safer alternative.

A recent advance is the provision of a Parker bath, a tilting bath that allows easy access. Many young people prefer a shower. A wheelchair user can use a shower in a lightweight, wheeled, shower chair.

26.6.1.6 *Other adaptations to the home*

The provision of an exterior ramp allows wheelchair access. The gradient should not exceed 1 in 20 for a disabled person propelling his or her own wheelchair. It may be necessary to widen doors for wheelchair use, a minimal acceptable clear opening being 75 cm. A kitchen usually requires extensive adaptation for wheelchair use, as the normal range of cupboards under the worktop prevents a wheelchair-user from approaching the sink or worktop. It is necessary to adjust the height of the worktop and clear the space beneath. Adaptations to taps are often necessary. Other possible adaptations in the home include the provision of a stair lift or a through-ceiling lift.

This brief outline of the aids and adaptations that may reduce the handicap of disabled people is only an introduction to the various handicapping aspects of the usual environment that must be considered. The handicap of each disabled patient must be individually assessed, and here the occupational therapist has a key role to play. Useful resources in the UK include autonomous disabled living centres and the Disabled Living Foundation.

26.6.2 *Disabled people and driving*

Mobility outside the home is understandably highly prized by all of us. Many disabled people can drive with minimal adjustments to the car. For example, patients with a right hemiparesis can often drive again if provided with a car with automatic transmission. The brake pedal and accelerator can both be operated by the left foot, although in practice it is usually safer to fit a hand throttle. The steering wheel can be turned by the functioning hand, using a knob mounted on the wheel. Restriction of the visual field may impair driving safety more significantly than restriction of physical mobility. Those who have had a non-dominant hemisphere lesion may have such spatial disorientation that it is clearly quite unsafe for them to drive. Patients with Parkinson's disease tend to go on driving rather longer than they should, until it becomes clear from a number of minor or more serious accidents that the speed of their response to other road users is insufficient. For people with epilepsy (in the UK) the occurrence of seizures prevents driving until 2 years have elapsed from the date of the last seizure. (Section 12.14.)

In the UK, the Mobility Advice and Vehicle Information Service (MAVIS) provides 'a comprehensive information assessment and vehicle familiarisation service to disabled drivers'. After a neurological event, the Medical Advisory Board at the Drivers and Vehicle Licensing Agency at Swansea may ask for a medical examination by an independent doctor before issuing a new licence.

26.7 Rehabilitation of those with specific neurological disabilities

The previous sections have laid out some general principles for all those with neurological disabilities. References to the rehabilitation of specific neurological disorders can be found in Section 26.12, and in relation to stroke in Section 10.1.9, to spinal trauma in Section 18.1.5 and to cranial injury in Section 15.7.2.

26.8 The problems of carers

Carers of people with chronic neurological disability, and particularly carers of elderly disabled people and those disabled by dementia, carry an enormous and largely unrecognized burden. Anderson points out that 'the daily grind, the repetitiveness of tasks, and the need for constant watchfulness cause declining energy and morale'. The stress on carers is related not only to the severity of the disability of the person that they care for, but also to the mood and social behaviour of the disabled person. Clinically significant depression is common amongst carers. This warrants therapy in its own right, but it has also been shown that social rehabilitation after a stroke is less successful if the carer is depressed.

Carers require an identified key person amongst the proliferation of helping agencies to whom they can turn for general support, and for help at times of crisis. They also need financial and emotional recognition of their work, and respite time.

26.9 Monetary support

How much financial support is given to those

unable to work on account of neurological disability varies between different societies. In some cultures, family ties are so strong that a family will regard it as a primary function to maintain and support their less able members—a policy which maintains the prestige of the extended family unit. In Western industrial cultures, these responsibilities appear to have weakened, and have partly been replaced by social welfare benefits. What is available does, of course, vary enormously between countries. Although benefits may be legislated for nationally, their uptake may vary between different wards of the same city, being dependent largely upon the energies of those responsible for informing potential clients of their rights. Some of the benefits available in the UK are explained briefly in Appendix A.

26.10   The role of self-help groups

Until recently, doctors have been uneasy about the role of self-help groups, possibly because, as Mary Black has written, 'doctors may . . . fear being called to account by a vociferous group at a meeting outside the safe confines of their consulting rooms or a hospital'. None the less, for those with chronic disabling conditions, which may well be lifelong, self-help groups have much to offer. Not only does a self-help group provide information about the neurological disorder, often more clearly than a doctor seems to be able to do within the pressures of a consultation, but also because members of the self-help group reinforce each other. They do so not only in sharing common goals, for example at a local level, by improving access for disabled people to a socially important local building, but also by providing a forum for collective willpower and belief, within which members of the group can look to each other for validation of their feelings and attitudes. The group may also reinforce disabled people's concepts of normality, and, through a common experience of members, provide practical help and support by those who are less disabled by a disorder to those who are more disabled by a disorder. Finally, self-help groups are instrumental in raising important amounts of finance for research into the disorder.

The addresses of some of the self-help groups in the UK for those with chronic neurological disorders are listed in Appendix B.

26.11   Co-ordination of rehabilitative services

As can be seen from the foregoing sections, the multiplicity of support agencies that a person disabled by a neurological disorder may need to contact is formidable. Fortunately, demarcation disputes about the territories of various professional groups are becoming less each year, but these may become more prominent with tighter monetary controls, and anxiety about to which budget an item of support should be charged. The practical management of a team of carers is a formidable task, not least because each member of the team, be he or she physiotherapist or occupational therapist or other type of rehabilitative or social worker, has his or her own captain—often non-playing—off the field. Such integrated management as does take place in health authorities or social service departments is far removed from the needs of patients, which are specific and individual, and often small in scale. The non-monetary help that is required is virtually always entirely practical in nature, such as help with shopping, household cleaning, physical help with bathing and getting dressed. Many of the tasks now done by highly trained staff in professions from which there is a high wastage rate could as effectively be carried out by practical helpers, who could individually carry out many of the tasks for which a co-ordinated team of professionals is now employed.

26.12   Further reading

General

Goodwill, C. J. and Chamberlain, M. A. (ed.) (1988). *Rehabilitation of the physically disabled adult*. Croom Helm, London.
Hopkins, A. (1984). Practical help. *Lancet* **139**, 1393–6.
Physical disability in 1986 and beyond. A report of the Royal College of Physicians (1986). *Journal of the Royal College of Physicians of London* **20**, 160–94.

Sociology of disability

Goffman E. (1986) *Stigma: notes on the management of spoiled identity*. Touchstone Books, New York.
Wilson, S. L. and McMillan, T. M. (1986). Finding able minds in able bodies. *Lancet* **2**, 1444–6.

Rehabilitation of the head-injured

Levin, H. S. (1990). Cognitive rehabilitation. *Archives of Neurology* **47**, 223–4.

Financial benefits for the disabled in the UK

Ennals, S. (1990). Doctors and benefits. *British Medical Journal* **301**, 1321–2, 1386–8.

Aids and appliances

Easton, J. (1988). Communication aids. *British Medical Journal* **296**, 193–5.

Mulley, G. (1990) and (1992). *Everyday aids and appliances*, and *More everyday aids and appliances*. British Medical Journal Publications, London.

Royal Association for Disability and Rehabilitation (1988). *Directory for disabled people*, (5th edn). Royal Association for Disability and Rehabilitation, London.

Appendix A: The range of benefits available in the UK

Statutory Sick Pay (SSP) is paid by the employer of those who pay Class I National Insurance (NI) contributions, including married women's reduced rate contributions. SSP is paid for up to 28 weeks in an episode of sickness. Episodes with 8 weeks or less between them count as one spell. SSP is paid only if the person is off sick for 4 days or more in a row. SSP is currently £43.50, or if average weekly earnings are more than £175, £52.50. The employer must deduct any tax and NI due from SSP. (See DS leaflet N.I. 244.)

Sickness Benefit (SB) is payable to those who cannot get Statutory Sick Pay (SSP), for example, the self-employed. It is not available to those who have paid insufficient NI contributions at the right time, unless they are claiming because of an accident at work or an industrial disease. SB is paid for up to 28 weeks. It may be allowable to undertake some work in order to improve health but earnings must be less than £39.00 per week. SB is currently £41.20 a week for a single person under pensionable age. (See DS leaflet N.I. 16.)

Invalidity Benefit (IB). If a person is unable to work after 28 weeks, when SSP or SB ends, invalidity benefit may be claimed. Invalidity Benefit is tax free, and is made up of Invalidity Pension, Invalidity Allowance, and an additional pension. Invalidity Pension is usually paid if the subject is incapable of work after 28 weeks of sickness, when SSP or SB ends. Invalidity Allowance is paid on top of Invalidity Pension if the subject's illness began before the age of 55 (women) or 60 (men). The additional pension is based upon earnings since 1978. As with SB, some work may be carried out while receiving invalidity benefit—earnings up to £35 a week are allowed. Invalidity Pension is currently £54.15 a week for a single person, free of tax. The rate of Invalidity Allowance depends upon the age at which incapacity for work started.

Extra payments are made for spouses and dependent children. (See DS leaflet N.I. 16A.)

Severe Disablement Allowance (SDA) is a benefit for those with long-term illness or disability (more than 28 weeks), as may arise in patients with neurological illness. It may be possible to get SDA even if insufficient NI contributions have been paid to obtain IB. For young people incapable of work on or before their twentieth birthday, disability need not be assessed. For those incapable of work after their twentieth birthday, disability must be assessed as at least 80 per cent. There are obvious difficulties about scoring disability in this simplistic way. SDA is not payable if a person is in receipt of an Invalidity Pension.

SDA is payable only to those aged over 16, and is payable only to women over 59 and men over 64 if they had a right to SDA before their sixtieth or sixty-fifth birthday. SDA is currently £32.55 a week with age-related supplements, and is free of tax. Extra benefit is payable for each child (£10.70 a week) and a spouse or other adult who looks after the subject's children (£16.85 a week). (See DS leaflet N.I. 252.)

Attendance Allowance This is paid to people whose disabilities start after the age of 65. It is paid for those needing personal attention a lot of the time, for example help with walking, and moving about generally, help with using the lavatory, help with eating, and with other activities of daily living. Attendance Allowance is also paid to those who require a lot of watching to prevent them hurting themselves or others. A patient with Alzheimer's disease would qualify under this last rule, for example. Normally, the subject must have needed a lot of help for at least six months before he or she qualifies for the Attendance Allowance, but an immediate allowance may be paid to those suffering a terminal illness. (Form DS 1500).

Attendance Allowance is currently £28.95 if attendance is required by day or by night, or £43.35 if attendance by both day and night is required. It is tax free and is not affected by savings or income. Further details are available in Leaflet DS 702.

Disability Living Allowance (DLA) This is a tax free benefit which has replaced and extended the help previously given by Attendance Allowance (for people disabled before the age of 65) and Mobility Allowance. It is not income related, contributory or taxable. DLA has two components to help people with the extra costs which arise from care and mobility needs. The care component is for people who need help with personal care. There are three rates depending upon the amount of care a person needs. The criteria for obtaining the higher (£43.55) and middle (£28.95) rates are the same as the criteria for obtaining Attendance Allowance, described above, and the rates are currently the same. The lower rate of £11.55 is paid to a person needing some help during some of the day, but less help than for the middle rate, or, if over age 16, to a person who needs help in preparing a cooked main meal. Again, people who are terminally ill are able to qualify for the highest rate of the care component.

The other component of DLA is the Mobility component, payable at two rates to people age 5 or over. The higher rate (currently £30.30) is payable if a person cannot walk at all, or has had both legs amputated at or above the ankle, or was born without legs or feet, or is both deaf and blind, or is severely mentally impaired with severe behavioural problems and qualifies for the highest rate of the care component. The lower rate (£11.55) is payable if a person can walk but needs someone with them to make sure that they are safe or to help them find their way around. The allowances may be used for the purchase of private transport of various types, for example, taxi rides, or towards hire-purchase on a car, often in the UK through Motability, a voluntary organization backed by the Department of Social Security.

If a person qualifies for the Mobility component of DLA before the age of 65, it is payable for life. It is not possible to claim the Mobility component for the first time after age 66.

There is a three month qualifying period for both components of DLA which is waived for people who are terminally ill. Medical assessment is not always necessary. A decision can usually be reached by information supplied on the assessment forms supplemented by other professionals such as a social worker. (See leaflet DS 704.)

Disability Working Allowance (DWA). This is a new means-tested benefit which tops up the income of those who can work, but whose illness or disability limits their earning capacity. The idea is to provide a platform from which people who wish to try some work could do so without being penalized by total loss of benefits. A person qualifies if aged over 16, is disadvantaged by illness or disability, and if working at least 16 hours a week. Savings must not exceed £16,000 for a couple. The applicant must have been in receipt of IB, SDA, DLA or various other benefits for at least 8 weeks before the claim. It is not possible to receive both IB and DWA, but if a person tries work and fails, he can again return to IB. DWA is not taxable. (See leaflet DS 703.)

Additional help is available in the form of *income support*, which is taxable, and not paid to those working more than 24 hours a week, or to those whose partner is working 24 hours a week, or those whose savings exceed £8,000. Income support is sometimes used to top-up shortfalls when it is believed that other benefits are insufficient to maintain a family. If income support is provided, then National Health Service Prescriptions and dental treatment are free, and there may be some help with the provision of spectacles. The level of income support is variable, but a couple both aged 18 or over, requiring support, is eligible for £62.25 per week. Additional support is available for dependent children and young people (up to £31.15 per young person aged 18). (See DS leaflet I.S. 20.)

In addition to the benefits detailed above, additional support may be available in terms of Housing Benefit from the local authority. If injured during the course of employment, or suffering from a recognized industrial disease, other benefits apply. (See DS leaflet N.I. 6.)

Short-term loans are sometimes made from the Social Fund, for example to help people meet their immediate short-term expenses in an emergency. Loans are repayable from future benefits. People on income support qualify for a grant of at least £500 on moving to unfurnished accommodation.

Means tested grants are sometimes made from the Independent Living Fund, a charitable Trust funded by the Government. The Trustees may make small grants to enable a disabled person to remain in a community setting rather than institutional residential care. The address of the fund is PO Box 183, Nottingham NG8 3RD. (See DS leaflet SB 16.)

Further advice about the admittedly complex benefits system in the UK can be obtained from any local social security office, or from the social services department of any local authority. A free telephone enquiry service is available on 0800–666–555.

Further Reading

Rowland, M. (1991). *The rights guide to non-means-tested benefits* (14th edn). Child Poverty Action Group.

Rowland, R., Webster, L., (ed.) (1991). *National welfare benefits handbook*. Child Poverty Action Group, London.

Benefit rules and rates will certainly change, but are recorded here as current in July 1992.

Appendix B: Self-help groups in the UK for sufferers from chronic neurological disorders

Alzheimer's Disease Society,
158/160 Balham High Road,
London SW12 9BN.

The Amnesia Association (AMNASS),
St. Charles Hospital,
Exmoor Street,
London W10 6DZ.

Chest, Heart and Stroke Association,
123–127 Whitecross Street,
London EC1Y 8JJ.

Action for Dysphasic Adults,
Canterbury House,
Royal Street,
London SE1 7LL.

Dystonia Society,
Omnibus Workspace,
39–41 North Road,
London N7 9DP.

British Epilepsy Association,
Anstey House,
40 Hanover Square,
Leeds LS3 1BE.

National Society for Epilepsy,
Chalfont Centre,
Chalfont St. Peter,
Gerrards Cross,
Bucks. SL9 0RJ.

Friedreich's Ataxia Group,
Copse Edge,
Thursley Road,
Elstead,
Godalming,
Surrey GU8 6DJ.

Guillain-Barré Syndrome Support Group,
Foxley,
Holdingham,
Sleaford,
Lincs NG34 8NR.

Headway,
National Head Injuries Association Ltd.,
200 Mansfield Road,
Nottingham NG1 3HX.

Huntington's Disease Society,
108 Battersea High Street,
London SW11 3HP.

National Meningitis Trust,
Fern House,
Bath Road,
Stroud,
Glos. GL5 3TJ.

British Migraine Association,
178A High Road,
Byfleet,
Weybridge,
Surrey KT14 7ED.

Migraine Trust,
45 Gt. Ormond Street,
London WC1N 3HD.

Motor Neurone Disease Association,
PO Box 246,
Northampton NN1 2PR.

Action for Research into Multiple Sclerosis (ARMS),
4A Chapel Hill,
Stansted,
Essex CM24 8AG.

Multiple Sclerosis Society,
    of Gt. Britain & N. Ireland,
25 Effie Road,
London SW6 1EE.

Muscular Dystrophy Group of Gt. Britain,
Nattrass House,
35 Macaulay Road,
London SW4 0QP.

British Association of Myasthenics,
Central Office,
Keynes House,
77 Nottingham Road,
Derby DE1 3QS.

Narcolepsy Association UK,
South Hall,
High Street,
Farningham,
Kent DA4 0DE.

Neurofibromatosis Association (LINK),
120 London Road,
Kingston upon Thames,
Surrey KT2 6QJ.

Parkinson's Disease Society,
22 Upper Woburn Place,
London WC1H 0RA.

British Polio Fellowship,
Bell Close,
West End Road,
Ruislip,
Middx. HA4 6LP.

The Spastics Society,
12 Park Crescent,
London W1N 4EQ.

Spinal Injuries Association,
Newpoint House,
76 St. James Lane,
London N10 3DF.

Association for Spina Bifida and Hydrocephalus,
ASBAH House,
42 Park Road,
Peterborough PE1 2UQ.

For families with members with unusual genetic disorders, advice may often be obtained from: Contact a Family, 16, Strutton Ground, London SW1P 2HP.

Index

dipyridamole in transient ischaemic attack
  patients 153
disability, physical 449–63
  age and abruptness of onset 453
  aids and adaptations 458–61
  assessment 454–5
  benefits available in UK 465–7
  carers, see carers
  definition 451, 452
  financial/monetary resources and support
    452, 455, 461–2
  increasing 7
  politics of 452–3
  recovery mechanisms 455–8
  rehabilitation, see rehabilitation
  sexual function with 61, 455
Disability Living Allowance 466
Disability Working Allowance 466
discs, intervertebral, lumbar
  prolapsed 337–8
  protrusion 338
    cervical 335–7
disorientation in space, vertigo defined as
    consciousness of 44
dissection, arterial 156
disulphiram, neuropathies and 354
diuretics in head injury 262
dizziness 44–9
doctors/physicians
  family, neurological work 11
  specialist, neurological work 11
doll's eye in unconscious patient 67
domoic acid, toxicity 424
L-dopa
  adverse effects, early 218
  in dystonia 225
  in Parkinson's disease therapy 216,
    217–22
    beginning/starting 218, 219–20
    long-term use of, management 218–19
dopa decarboxylase inhibitors in Parkinson's
    disease 218
dopamine
  agonists, in Parkinson's disease therapy
    220
  antagonists/blockers, in Gilles de la
    Tourette syndrome 231
  Parkinson's disease and 212–13
  potentiators, in Parkinson's disease
    therapy 220
dopamine β-hydroxylase deficiency 223
dopaminergic pathways/system in
    Parkinson's disease 210–11, 212–13,
    216, 217
dorsal roots in neurosyphilis 295
double vision 53–4
Down syndrome 417
doxycycline in Lyme disease 297
dreams, nature 432–3
dressing apraxia 27
driving
  disabled persons and 461
  epilepsy and 206, 461
  head injuries associated with 257–8
drop attacks 150
drowsiness, daytime, causes 434–5, 435–6
drugs
  confusional states caused by 171
  dementia caused by 181
  history 17

illicit, cerebrovascular disease associated
    with 139
interactions, involving anticonvulsants
    199
movement disorders induced by 234–7
myasthenic syndromes induced by 403
myopathy induced by 390, 397–8
  inflammatory 390, 397
neuropathies caused by 352, 353–4
seizures precipitated by 194
see also specific (types of) drugs and
    chemotherapy
Duchenne muscular dystrophy 390–2, 415
duplex sonography, see sonography
dura (mater)
  beneath, see entries under subdural
  external to, see entries under extradural
dying-back (axonal) neuropathies 348,
    349–50
dysarthria 43–4
  cortical 26
  in motor neuron disease 376–7
  spastic 43
dysdiadochokinesis 35
dysgraphia 26
dyskinesia
  in Parkinson's disease 214–15
  in Parkinson's disease therapy with
    L-dopa 218, 218–19, 219, 220
  tardive, drug-induced 235, 236
dyskinetic syndrome in cerebral palsy 412
dyslexia 26, 444–5
  acquired 26
  developmental 444–5
dysphagia (swallowing difficulties) in motor
    neuron disease 377, 379
dysphasia
  aphasia and, synonymity/near-synonymity
    25
  nominal 25
  speech therapy 457
dysphonia 43–4
dysplasia, fibromuscular 156
dysreflexia, autonomic, spinal injury patients
    333
dysrhythmias, cardiac 159–60
  seizures and, distinction 196
dystonia 224–7
  drug-induced acute 235
  focal 224
  idiopathic 224
  symptomatic 224
  syndromes with 224–7
  treatment 225
dystrophies
  of extremities, post-traumatic 360
  muscular 390–4, 415, 416
dystrophin gene 391

ECG, see electrocardiography
Echinococcus granulosus 305
echolalia 230
edrophonium test in myasthenia gravis 401
education of disabled persons 455
Edward's syndrome 417
EEG, see electroencephalography
efferent supply, somatic, bladder
    dysfunction with disorders of 57–8
ejaculation 59

retrograde 61
electric shock
  motor neuron disease following 381
  myelopathy following 344
electrocardiography (ECG)
  in epilepsy 196
  in Friedreich's ataxia 381
  in subarachnoid haemorrhage 163
electrocorticography 81
electrodes
  in electroencephalography 81
  in electromyography 83
  in nerve conduction studies 86
electroencephalography (EEG) 79–81
  in epilepsy 80, 190, 192, 193, 196, 197
  information derived from, presentation
    81
  long-term 81
  spikes in, see spikes
  in stroke 144
electromyography (EMG) 83–5
  in Bell's/facial palsy 358
  in tremor of Parkinson's disease 214
emboli
  cerebral 130–1, 159
    investigation/imaging 144
    transient ischaemic attacks associated
      with 151
  paradoxical 159
  pulmonary, in spinal injury patients 333
  see also thrombo-embolism
embryonic grafts in Parkinson's disease 221
Emery–Dreifuss dystrophy 392–3
EMG, see electromyography
encephalitis
  limbic 429
  parkinsonism following 211–12
  varicella–zoster virus-associated 314–15
  viral, acute 309–11
    in AIDS 318
  see also panencephalitis
encephalomyelitis
  acute disseminated 254
  experimental allergic 244–5
  myalgic (post-viral fatigue/chronic fatigue)
    320, 387, 443
  post-viral 314–15, 319
  varicella–zoster virus-associated 314–15
encephalopathy
  hepatic 422
  HIV-associated 316, 317
  hypertensive 156
  mitochondrial, with lactic acidosis and
    stroke-like episodes 395
  pertussis vaccine-induced 323
  spongiform 321–3
  varicella–zoster virus-associated 315
  Wernicke's 426–7
endocarditis, bacterial
  subacute 165
  subarachnoid haemorrhage in 165
  thrombo-embolism in 159
endocrine myopathies 397
end-plate, motor
  disorders affecting 348
  noise, in electromyography 84
energy production, defects 396
entrapment, peripheral nerve 362–6
environmental factors (in disease) 9
  genetic and, interactions 9

Index